Brief Second Edition

ACCESS
TO
HEALTH

Rebecca J. Donatelle, Ph.D., CHES

Oregon State University

Lorraine G. Davis, Ph.D., CHES

University of Oregon

Prentice Hall, Englewood Cliffs, New Jersey 07632

Library of Congress Cataloging-in-Publication Data

Donatelle, Rebecca J.
    Access to health / Rebecca J. Donatelle, Lorraine G. Davis,—
Brief 2nd ed.
        p.   cm.
    Includes bibliographical references and index.
    ISBN 0-13-007782-8
    1. Health.   I. Davis, Lorraine G.   II. Title.
    [DNLM: 1. Exercise—popular works.   2. Health.   3. Physical
Fitness-popular works.   QT 255 D677a]
RA776.D66   1993
613—dc20
DNLM/DLC
for Library of Congress   92-38673
                                                       CIP

Acquisitions editor: Ted Bolen

Editorial Assistant: Nichole Gray

Editorial/production supervision: Jordan Ochs

Development Editors: Thomas Moore and Marilyn Miller

Design Supervisor: Christine Gehring-Wolf

Cover design and interior design: Maureen Eide

Cover Photo: Warren Morgan/Westlight

Prepress buyer: Herb Klein

Manufacturing buyer: Robert Anderson

Photo editor: Lorinda Morris-Nantz

Photo research: Anita Dickhuth

 © 1993, 1991, 1988 by Prentice-Hall, Inc.
A Simon & Schuster Company
Englewood Cliffs, New Jersey 07632

Printed in the United States of America

10 9 8 7 6 5 4 3 2 1

0-13-007782-8

Prentice-Hall International (UK) Limited, *London*
Prentice-Hall of Australia Pty. Limited, *Sydney*
Prentice-Hall Canada Inc., *Toronto*
Prentice-Hall Hispanoamericana, S.A., *Mexico*
Prentice-Hall of India Private Limited, *New Delhi*
Prentice-Hall of Japan, Inc., *Tokyo*
Simon & Schuster Asia Pte. Ltd., *Singapore*
Editora Prentice-Hall do Brasil, Ltda., *Rio de Janeiro*

Contents

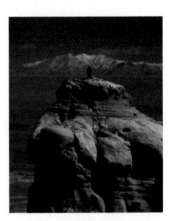

SECTION
2

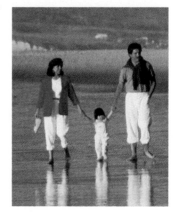

INTIMACY
AND
SEXUALITY

3 Stress: The Inevitable Reaction 37

4 Intimate Relationships and Sexuality 59

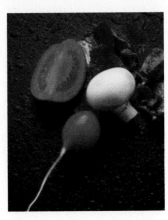

Pregnancy, Childbirth, and Birth Control   85

6 Nutrition: Eating for Optimal Health   113

7 Managing Your Weight: Consuming and Expending Energy   139

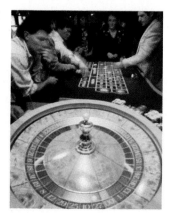

SECTION
4

ADDICTIONS
AND DRUGS

11 Alcohol and Tobacco 200

12 Prescription, Over-the-Counter, and Illegal Drugs 222

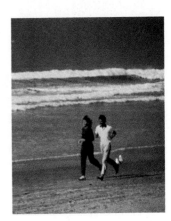

SECTION 5

AFFLICTIONS AND DISEASES

13 Cardiovascular Disease and Cancer: Understanding Your Risks 247

14 Infectious and Noninfectious Diseases 271

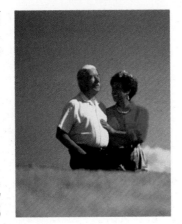
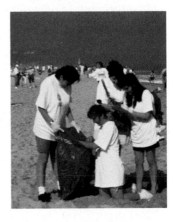

Appendix: First Aid and Emergency Care   357

Index   365

To The Instructor

The first and second editions of *Access to Health* represented our commitment to writing introductory health texts that were market leaders, rather than market followers. Having viewed the black-and-white texts of the 1970s, the colorful, insert-laden texts of the 1980s, and the early 1990s versions of texts that tried to "go where no personal health text had gone before," we found it to be a challenge to develop a text that would stand out as a superior text in a long list of competitors. Even more challenging was developing a first and second edition of a text that met the needs of an increasingly demanding, increasingly diverse group of college students.

To accomplish this, we had to incorporate our collective insights from teaching thousands of students in personal health classes, our experiences reviewing and adopting numerous health texts over the years, and the cumulative reactions and comments from professors, graduate teaching assistants, and many others teaching these courses, into a text that would best serve the needs of the largest number of potential users. We listened to your suggestions on how to improve, we analyzed the current research to determine what new information would be most vital to present to a much more sophisticated student, and we are continually trying to break new ground in the personal health market. The large number of adoptions and the favorable reviewer comments suggest that the first and second editions of *Access to Health* met the needs of many of you. The fact that many of our competitors have followed our lead and included comprehensive sections and/or chapters on such areas as interpersonal communication, addictive behaviors, and modern maladies, provides an additional indication that our "new ideas" for the personal health market were well received.

At the same time that we were listening to your comments and suggestions on how to make the second edition of *Access to Health* a market leader, we also were listening closely to those of you who were beginning to diversify in your classroom offerings. Although you liked the fact that the second edition of *Access to Health* was comprehensive, readable, interesting, understandable, and relevant to a wide range of intellectual capabilities and backgrounds, some of your course descriptions were changing to include a more "focused" approach to health, wellness, and personal fitness. You began to ask for a book that included all of the positive attributes of the more comprehensive book, but was more concentrated on the essential elements of psychological health, health behavior, stress management, nutrition, weight control, physical fitness and other vital foundations of health and wellness.

Clearly, today's health, fitness, and wellness students are among the most knowledgeable health consumers in our history. Millions of Americans are attempting to modify their lifestyles by eating less saturated fat and cholesterol, consuming more whole grains, fruits, and vegetables, striving to achieve optimal body fat levels, quitting smoking, drinking less, practicing stress management, getting into shape through aerobic exercise, toning, or strengthening body parts, demonstrating a concern for the environment, and a wide range of health promoting activities. Textbooks on wellness, fitness, eating right, living life to its fullest, having better relationships, improved sex lives, etc. have taken America by storm. Finding the most reliable, scientifically accurate written materials among this rapidly changing, highly controversial health information is often a tremendous challenge for even the most educated health consumer. Sifting through this information and trying to determine fact from fiction and right from wrong has become a daily struggle for the typical adult. Many students have had the benefit of comprehensive health education classes in public schools and come into college courses ready for new; and more extensive information. They have also been exposed to health information in the mass media and are ready for a more in-depth, thought-provoking approach to high interest health and wellness topics. This edition of *Access to Health*, although abbreviated in length and reduced in cost, is not short on content. We have carefully selected those areas that are most critical for inclusion in today's wellness-oriented health classes, and fitness courses and expanded our coverage and emphasis in these areas. We have also retained and updated those chapters deemed essential to any contemporary discussions of health and wellness, such as environmental health, HIV diseases, and other sexually transmitted diseases. We have also attempted to portray the multiple dimensions of health accurately, emphasizing personal responsibility for health behaviors, environmental and social factors that predispose people to behave in a particular manner, and positive decision-making for health and wellness. This edition has been designed not only to be read and enjoyed, but to expand student's knowledge in key health areas, while serving as a catalyst for individual change.

CONTENT INFORMATION

This text is organized into 16 chapters. Much of the content of the full version of Access Second Edition has been revised, updated, and expanded, particularly in the fundamental areas of personal health and wellness. Instructors looking for a course that is focused primarily on the core areas of physical fitness, stress, nutrition, weight control, emotional health, addictions, drugs, psychosocial elements of wellness, environmental health, and the major health topics of our times, will find this book to be especially well suited for their students. Rather than being just a superficial approach to these areas, this text provides a medium for student thinking, knowledge acquisition, and individual decision making that is based on rigorous scientific research in the core health areas. The text focuses on adult problems that have relevance to adult populations who are at critical points in their own lifestyle behaviors and offers options without preaching or talking down to the reader. The book represents our attempt to actively engage the reader in the promotion of their own health and the prevention of premature death, dysfunction, and/or disability in the physical, social, spiritual, emotional, and environmental elements of their lives.

New To The Brief Edition

Two New Chapters in the areas of Aerobic and Muscular Fitness In response to many of your requests, we have made dramatic changes in our emphasis on the physical aspects of health and wellness. This edition includes two completely new chapters on Physical Fitness (aerobic exercise) and Muscular Fitness (strength and toning) for those college and university classes where such content coverage is required. No discussion of health and wellness would be complete without providing an in-depth, comprehensive, "cutting edge" treatment of these topics. Those students who are particularly interested in improving their own physical health/wellness status, will find that these chapters provide answers to many common "getting started" and "keeping going" kinds of questions in the domain of physical health.

Revised and Expanded Nutrition and Weight Control Chapters These sections have been greatly expanded with increased emphasis on lifestyle changes that may improve overall dietary health. In addition, these chapters will include more comprehensive information on making dietary decisions with respect to fat as a percent of total calories, myths and misconceptions about fats, fibers, and other nutritional facts. Information on the new food pyramid, endorsed nationally as a guide for improved dietary practices, and the national objectives of the nation are included in this chapter.

Communication and Interpersonal Relationship Emphasis In keeping with our many positive responses about these chapters in previous editions, we have retained much of our earlier emphasis on the importance of effective communication in interpersonal relationships. Boxes, chapter sections, and interactive, thought-provoking health promotion exercises are designed to encourage each person to examine his or her own communication style and make improvements as necessary. The meaning of "love" and the role of love in relationships is also explored.

Revised Coverage of HIV disease and other STDs One of the difficulties in writing any health-related text is that by the time the text goes to press, much of the information is already "dated." Recognizing the inherent difficulties in remaining current in areas such as HIV disease (AIDS), we have incorporated the most current information into this chapter as the book nears its final production phases. We have also expanded our coverage of the sexually transmitted diseases and enhanced our emphasis on high risk "behaviors" rather than on the out-dated "high risk groups" that many health texts continue to discuss.

Infectious Diseases and the Modern Maladies As with the HIV epidemic, there are many additional disease areas that have begun to reach epidemic proportions in the United States today. We have expanded our coverage of relevant diseases such as tuberculosis, to increase national awareness of these growing threats to health.

Stress and Psychosocial Aspects of Health and Wellness No text featuring fundamentals of health and wellness would be complete without an enhanced section on the role of stress on individual well-being and the importance of selected psychosocial variables in determining overall fitness for quality living. Rather than adopting a "blame the victim" approach, we have emphasized the importance of individual responsibility while acknowledging that sometimes health is influenced by factors that may be outside of our individual control. Responsibility to self and to others within the broader environment is a key dimension of a healthy perspective on life.

SPECIAL FEATURES

A major goal of the first and second editions of *Access to Health* was to provide extensive, comprehensive, and interesting coverage of relevant health topics in an effort to help students make informed health decisions. Another major goal was to stimulate thinking, to enhance personal environmental awareness, and to promote positive personal health behaviors. In the Brief Edition of *Access to Health,* we have retained the same goals with the additional goals of providing an updated, focused approach to central health/wellness topics. In each chapter, several special features enhance our content areas, and encourage the reader to actively participate in the thinking, reasoning, and decision-making process.

Boxed Features

Promoting Your Health These boxes are designed to complement key concepts in each chapter and to translate theory into practical applications relevant to each student's lifestyle decisions. Many of these boxes are designed as self-assessments or offer advice on changing specific behaviors.

Health in Your Community In the true spirit of the health and wellness movements, these boxes are designed to encourage students to think more globally about the impact of their personal actions on the larger environment. Rather than only focusing on "self" these boxes encourage students to demonstrate concern and consider actions designed to help others or to improve the social and environmental conditions in which they live.

Highlight Boxes These general boxes are designed to highlight key topics relevant to information discussed in each chapter. Issues relevant to special populations, global health, myths and misconceptions and other topics will be the focus of these areas.

Other Features

Chapter Objectives Designed to help the reader focus on essential points highlighted in each chapter.

Chapter Outline Provides reader with a quick reference for "what's included" in each chapter and the progression of selected points.

Running Glossary Glossary of key terms for review in each chapter. Terms are defined as they appear, eliminating the need to locate information elsewhere in the text.

Appendix on First Aid and Emergency Care A brief, easy-to-read appendix that includes basic information about first aid and emergency care.

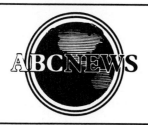

ABC News/PH Video Library for Health The media age has established video as a dominant influence in American life. Video is one of the most dynamic and effective means of communication you can use to enhance learning in the classroom. But the quality of the video material and how well it relates to your course can make all the difference.

Prentice Hall and ABC News have brought together their talents in academic publishing and global reporting and are proud to present the most comprehensive video ancillaries available in the college market today. Prominent and respected anchors, such as David Brinkley, Ted Koppel, and Peter Jennings, bring together their insights in health into your classroom. ABC and Prentice Hall offer your students a resource of these feature and documentary-style videos, which relate directly to the issues and applications in *Access to Health: Brief Second Edition*.

The ABC News/PH Video Library pulls together critically acclaimed selections from Nightline, This Week with David Brinkley, and World News Tonight. The programs are of extremely high production quality, present substantial content, and are hosted by well-versed, well-known anchors. Carefully researched selections effectively complement and enhance the material in *Access to Health*.

pening in today's society. Students who deepen their appreciation of print in the learning environment will remain devoted to the medium throughout their lives.

Instructor's Resource Manual Offers the instructor detailed outlines, discussion questions, and in and out-of-class activities for each chapter. Includes a video guide to the ABC/Prentice Hall Video Library.

Test Item File A compendium of over 2,000 multiple choice, matching, short answer, and essay questions.

Testing Software The test item file on disk, available for IBM and Macintosh computers, gives the instructor the ability to edit or delete existing questions and create and edit new questions.

Prentice Hall Health Transparencies A complete set of beautiful full-color transparancy acetates produced from a wide range of illustrations from the text and from other sources. Available free to qualified adopters.

Slide Sets for AIDS and Other Sexually Transmitted Diseases This valuable resource is available free to qualified adopters. Please ask your Prentice Hall representative for details.

Study Guide and Workbook (For Sale Item) This handy student resource offers learning objectives, self-quizzes on text material, additional self-assessment activities, and behavior change strategies.

The New York Times

The New York Times Contemporary View *The New York Times* and Prentice Hall, two leading publishers in academia and world news, are proud to cosponser **A CONTEMPORARY VIEW**, a program designed to enhance student access to current and relevant information in the world of health.

Your students will receive a 16-page dodger—a student version of *The New York Times* containing approximately 30 articles to be used in conjunction with *Access to Health: Brief Second Edition*. The stories in the dodger are actual articles that appeared in current issues of *The New York Times* and relate specifically to the world of health. The selected articles include events and new developments in personal health, health-related services and technologies, and national and international issues in health.

Knowledge of world events is invaluable. Reading a premier news publication such as *The New York Times* establishes a practice of staying abreast of the events hap-

Acknowledgments

As with any major undertaking, this book represents the combined efforts of many people. The authors wish to express their sincere appreciation to the many talented professionals who provided us with constructive reviews and criticism and helpful, thought-provoking ideas. First and foremost, we would like to extend our thanks to the editorial, production, marketing, and sales staff at Prentice Hall for their efforts in making the first and second editions of *Access to Health* a success, and to those staff members who continued the fine tradition of excellence into the Brief Edition. In particular, we would like to thank Ted Bolen for his leadership and guidance in directing this project and seeing it through to its completion; Thomas Moore and other members of the developmental editorial staff for their careful attention to detail and capable assistance with the reworking individual chapters into a cohesive, comprehensive, overview of key health/wellness components; Jordan Ochs, for his capable management of the production phases of the text; and many other key Prentice Hall staff members who provided their time, expertise, and talents to the project. Each of the above personnel exemplifies the fine tradition that the authors have been accustomed to in a quality Prentice Hall production. To all of you, thank you.

In addition to the Prentice Hall staff, the authors are grateful to many of the health professionals who contributed either directly or indirectly to the development of selected parts of this text. Dr. Tom Thomas, well known exercise physiologist from the University of Missouri, contributed two outstanding chapters in the areas of aerobic and muscular fitness. These chapters provide a "missing" element to the Brief Edition market that has not been present in other texts to date. Cheryl Graham, health educator at Oregon State University, provided an excellent revision and updating of her well-received chapter on Addiction from the second edition of *Access to Health*. Donna Champeau, health educator at Oregon State University, utilized her background in gerontology to provide editorial assistance and direction in the revision of the chapter on Successful Life Transitions. Patricia Ketcham, Director of Student Health Education at Western Oregon State College provided invaluable assistance in the overall editing and revision of several chapters in the Brief Edition. She contributed many hours of painstaking effort to enhance the chapters on Drugs, Alcohol, (written by her in the second edition), Sexuality, Nutrition, Environmental Health and she also revised the first aid appendix. Her efforts and the efforts of each of the above individuals in the completion of this text are very much appreciated.

Several people contributed to the supplementary material provided with this book. Donna Champeau and Patricia Ketcham developed a test item file for the brief edition. The Instructor's Resource Manual and the Study Guide were compiled by Emogene Fox, University of Arkansas and Vicki Krenz, California State University, Fresno, respectively.

In addition, we would like to thank the many colleagues who provided recommendations for improvement in their constructive reviews of the first and second editions of this manuscript.

REVIEWERS OF THE FIRST EDITION

Wes Alles, Pennsylvania State University
Danny Ballard, Texas A & M University
Ken Becker, University of Wisconsin, LaCrosse
Fay Biles, Kent State University

John Bonugaro, Ohio University
Robert Bowers, Tallahassee Community College
Jerry Braza, University of Utah
Andrew Brennan, Metropolitan Life Corporation
Herman Bush, Eastern Kentucky University
Jean Byrne, Kent State University
Carol Cates, Cerritos College
Carol Christensen, San Jose State University
Margaret Dosch, University of Wisconsin, LaCrosse
Judy Drolet, Southern Illinois University
Ruth Engs, Indiana University
William Faraclas, Southern Connecticut University
Jeff Forman, DeAnza College
Erika Friedman, Brooklyn College of CUNY
Bob Fries, Fresno State University
Stephen Germeroth, Catonsville Community College
Ray Goldberg, SUNY College at Cortland
Rick Guyton, University of Arkansas
Phil Huntsinger, University of Kansas
Robert McDermott, Southern Illinois University
Karen Mondrone, M.S., R.D.
Patrick Moffitt, University of Northern Iowa
Louis Munch, Ithaca College
Judith Nelson, Burlington Community College
George Niva, Bowling Green University
Larry Olsen, Pennsylvania State University
Judy Phillips, Valdosta State College
Valerie Pinhas, Nassau Community College
James Price, University of Toledo
Kerry Redican, Virginia Polytechnic
Norma Schira, Western Kentucky University
Delores Seemayer, Palm Beach Junior College
Warren Smith, University of Oregon
Sherman Sowby, California State University, Fresno
Cheryl Tucker, North East Missouri State
Martin S. Turnauer, Radford University
James Tryniechi, Southern Louisiana University
Rita Ward, Central Michigan University
Parris R. Watts, University of Missouri, Columbia
Janice Clark Young, Iowa State University
Verne Zellner, American River College

REVIEWERS OF THE SECOND EDITION

Judy B. Baker, East Carolina University
Rick Barnes, East Carolina University
W. Henry Baughman, Western Kentucky University

Gerald Benn, Northeastern State University
Donald L. Calitri, Eastern Kentucky University
Vivien Carver, University of Southern Mississippi
Bethann Cinelli, West Chester University
Joseph S. Darden, Jr., Kean College
Steve M. Dorman, University of Florida
William C. Gross, Western Michigan University
Dickie Hill, Abilene Christian University
Marsha Hoagland, Modesto Junior College
Jack A. Jordon, University of Wisconsin, LaCrosse
John Leary, SUNY College at Cortland
Michael Lee, Joliet Junior College
Richard T. Mackey, Miami University of Ohio
Richard E. Madson, Palm Beach Community College
Judith Nelson, Burlington Community College
Ian Newman, University of Nebraska, Lincoln
Gaye Osborne, Morehead State University
Kim Roberts, Eastern Kentucky University
Stephen Roberts, University of Toledo
Sherman Sowby, California State University, Fresno
Donald B. Stone, University of Illinois
Merita Lee Thompson, Eastern Kentucky University
Parris R. Watts, University of Missouri, Columbia

REVIEWERS OF THIS EDITION

Charlene Agne-Traub, Howard University
Judy B. Baker, East Carolina University
Bud Belnap, Weber State University
Gerald Benn, Northeastern State University
Vivian Carver, University of Southern Mississippi
Carol Christensen, San Jose State University
Bethann Cinelli, West Chester University
Raymond Goldberg, SUNY College at Cortland
Jack E. Hansma, Baylor University
Jack A. Jordon, University of Wisconsin, LaCrosse
John E. Leary, SUNY College at Cortland
Sherman Sowby, California State University, Fresno
Donald B. Stone, University of Illinois-Champaign
Parris R. Watts, Missouri University
Richard W. Wilson, Western Kentucky University

ACCESS TO HEALTH

1

Personal Health Promotion

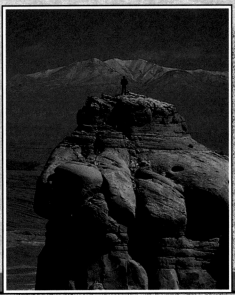

■ Objectives

- Explain why it is difficult to formulate a definition of health and then define health for yourself specifically.

- Describe the difference between quality and quantity of life and discuss why quality of life is a significant measure of health.

- Discuss some of the benefits of achieving optimal health.

- List basic behaviors associated with good health.

- Discuss the factors that influence health behavior change, drawing differences between predisposing, enabling, and reinforcing factors, and describe how you can change your health behavior.

- Explain why being well informed about health issues helps you achieve your health potential.

The old cliché "If you have your health, you have everything" has taken on special significance for today's health-conscious Americans. A quick flip through the TV channels on any given day will find program after program focusing on physical fitness, diet, weight control, stress management, environmental issues, and health care, as well as a myriad of commercials for products designed to help you become a "better you." Health clubs, weight-loss clinics, group-therapy sessions, nutrition centers, and other enterprises have capitalized on this new consumer interest to become multi-million-dollar businesses.

With such mass exposure to potential "health enhancers," each of us must certainly find it easier to achieve that firm, fit body, that large cadre of close friends and wonderful relationships, that zest for life, that illness-free existence, and that relaxed, easy approach to conflicts in our lives. Right? If you found yourself cringing a bit from that question, fear not. You are *not* alone.

Attaining health is no easy task. We are all unique products of our genetic history, our family interactions, our experiences with friends and significant others, the environment we walk through and live in, our culture, sex, socioeconomic status, and a host of subtle and not-so-subtle influences. Some of us may find few obstacles in the quest for optimum health and wellness. Others may find significant barriers, many of which may be difficult to overcome. It is important to remember that there is no one "recipe" for attaining health. We must all find our own best way to achieve our health goals within our own environment.

This text is designed to provide a framework for decision making and responses to life that will best fit your individual needs and to help you find answers to these questions: What does it mean for me to be healthy? How much change would I have to make to get there? What's in it for me? How much of this change is within my control? Where can I go for help? How will I know if the advice I get is sound? How will I know when I have succeeded?

DEFINING HEALTH AND WELLNESS

There are no simple ways to describe what it means to achieve health or wellness. One broad-based definition of health is the ability to maintain a balanced lifestyle in which one is reasonably free of pain, discomfort, disability, or unusual limitations.

Historically, the medical concept of health has focused on physical symptoms of disease and health has been defined as the absence of disease. Over the years, health experts have become increasingly aware of the inadequacy of this approach. Excluding social, emo-

tional, and spiritual health created an extremely narrow perspective on health potential.

In the 1940s, the World Health Organization (WHO) provided one of the first comprehensive definitions of health. It defined health as the "state of complete physical, emotional, and social well-being, not merely the absence of disease of infirmity." For many years, this definition of health was the reference for evaluating our health status. In the late 1970s, however, health experts began to reconsider this definition. Critics argued that based on this ideal conception of health, none of us would be considered healthy. For example, arguing that a person had to be completely healthy in the physical dimension implied that a handicapped person could never be healthy. Similar arguments were leveled against the other components of the definition.

Modern Definitions of Health and Wellness

The current definition of **health** proposes a positive view that focuses on our individual attempts to achieve optimum well-being within a realistic framework of our individual potential. In Figure 1.1, we see that health can be described as a continuum from illness to optimum well-being. Where we are on this continuum may vary from day to day as we are buffeted by life's ups and downs. However, if we are persistent in our attempts to change behaviors and reduce risk, the likelihood of remaining on the positive end of the continuum will be greatly improved.

Health relates to who we are as individuals, how we relate to others and the environment, what we value and perceive as important in our lives, and the way we respond to the daily challenges of life. Health is an ever-changing dimension of our lives, in which we strive to be the best possible physical, emotional, social, spiritual, and environmentally sensitive beings we can. The current definition of health acknowledges that each of us must attempt to achieve this optimum level of being in a "sometimes hostile environment." Each of us must come to terms with the adversity and obstacles obstructing the way to optimum health in his or her own unique way, focusing on our positive attributes whenever possible, changing those things about ourselves that we can change, and learning to recognize and deal with those that we cannot change.

"Wellness" is a term that has become popularized in the last decade. Like the modern definition of health, the term **wellness** refers to an ever-changing movement toward optimal well-being. The two terms are not mutually exclusive. In fact, most health professionals agree

---

Health A combination of the physical, emotional, social, and spiritual components of life that can be balanced to produce satisfaction and happiness.
Wellness Activities, behaviors, and attitudes that improve the quality of life and expand on that potential.

that the term *health* no longer implies the mere absence of disease but is instead a dynamic, life-long process in which physical, psychological, social, environmental, and spiritual elements are considered essential.

The *physical components* of health and wellness include such characteristics as body size and shape, sensory acuity, susceptibility to disease and disorders, body functioning, recuperative ability, and ability to perform certain tasks. *Psychological components* of health and wellness include intellectual and emotional practices and responses, and our overall outlook on life. Included here are our values and belief systems, attitudes, levels of self-esteem and self-confidence, and coping mechanisms. The *social components* of health and wellness refer to our interactions with others, our ability to adapt to various social situations, and our daily behaviors. The components of health that have often been neglected are the *spiritual components*. Although spiritual components may involve a belief in a higher form of being or a specified way of living that is prescribed by a particular religion, spiritual health goes beyond this definition. It extends to the sense of being a part of some larger form of existence—a sense of unity with the larger environment, for example. It includes a feeling of oneness with others, with nature, and with the larger environment. Anyone who has ever watched a beautiful sunset, listened to the first sounds of morning on a bright summer day, or smelled the first crisp scents of autumn can identify with the feeling of appreciation for spiritual health. Optimal spiritual health may be described as the ability to develop our spiritual nature to its fullest potential. This might include our ability to understand and express our own basic purpose in life, to feel that we are a part of a greater spectrum of existence, to experience love, joy, pain, sorrow, peace, contentment, and wonder over life's experiences, and to care about and respect all living things.

Figure 1.1 indicates that health is a dynamic process that requires our active involvement, rather than something that happens to us. Conscious efforts to make decisions to improve the health side of the continuum and battle against the illness side must be made on a daily basis.

It is important to point out that the disability component of this continuum does not imply that a physically handicapped person cannot achieve wellness. In fact, it is quite possible for a handicapped person to be very "healthy" in terms of relationships with others, level of self-confidence, environmental sensitivity, and overall attitude toward life. In contrast, a person who spends countless hours in front of a mirror lifting weights to perfect the size and shape of each muscle may be "unhealthy" in interactions with others, level of self-esteem, and attitude toward life. Although we often place a premium on physical attractiveness and external trappings, appearance is not an accurate indicator of a person's overall health status. A person who has not learned to cope with life's challenges or who participates in self-destructive activities and is abusive toward others is not healthy.

Essentially, the disability portion of the continuum indicates that as health deteriorates, the ability to function declines to the point of permanent detriment to the self. Health is multifaceted. Combining seemingly minor negative behaviors can have a *synergistic* effect, meaning that the total effect is greater than the sum of the effects of each behavior. Similarly, the more positive behaviors that can be incorporated into a person's lifestyle (even though each may seem insignificant by itself), the greater the potential for achieving a higher level of wellness.

In discussions of health and wellness, terms such as *health promotion* are often used. **Health promotion** can be defined as any combination of educational, organizational, economic, and environmental supports for behaviors that are conductive to health. More recently, health promotion has also been defined as the science and art of helping people change their lifestyles to move toward a state of optimal health. Regardless of how it is defined, health promotion identifies healthy people who are at a certain risk for disease and attempts to motivate them to improve their health status. It also encourages those whose health and wellness behaviors are already sound to maintain and improve them. Health promotion goes one step further by attempting to modify behaviors, attitudes, and values and introduce health-enhancing activities. Wellness involves a person's entire lifestyle and is directed toward individual self-fulfillment.

Whether we use the term health or wellness, it is commonly understood that we are talking about a person's overall reactions or responses to the nuances of living. Occasional dips into the ice-cream bucket and other dietary slips, failure to exercise every day, flare-ups of anger, and other deviations from optimal behavior should not be viewed as major failures. In fact, our ability to recognize that we are imperfect beings, attempting to adapt to an imperfect world, is considered an indicator of individual well-being.

We must also remember to be tolerant of others who are attempting to improve their health. Rather than being overly critical "warriors against pleasure" in our zeal to reform or transform the health behavior of others, we should try to be supportive, understanding, nonjudgmental, and positive in our interactions. **Health bashing**—intolerance or negative feelings, words, or actions toward people who fail to meet our own expectations of health—may be an indication of our own defi-

---

Health promotion   Application of any combination of educational, organizational, economic, and environmental supports for behaviors that are conducive to health.

Incidence   The numer of new cases of a given disease within a stated population

Prevalence   The numer of existing cases of a given disease at a particular time.

Health bashing   Intolerance or negative feelings, words, or actions directed toward people who don't meet our expectations of health.

Figure 1.1 The continuum from illness to wellness.

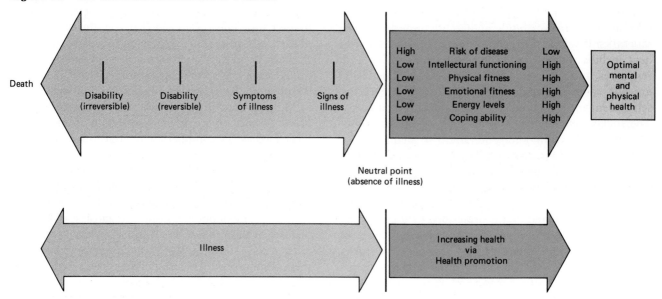

Neutral point
(absence of illness)

SELECTED CHARACTERISTICS OF ILLNESS AND WELLNESS

ILLNESS
Physically out of shape, low energy
Socially withdrawn, few friends, little interaction with others
Poor communication skills
Excessive defensiveness
Black-and-white view of issues
Minimal attention to body signals
Few social supports/networks
Dangerous risk taking
External locus of control
Limited or poor coping skills
Little capacity to recognize choices and options in problem solving
Stress-producing behaviors
Negative, critical opinion of others

Anger, depression, hopelessness

Poor attention to self-care and sound health practices
Lack of responsibility toward the environment

Negative self-image, low self-esteem
Low sensitivity, low compassion, little regard for others' feelings
Little capacity to change behaviors
Poor consumer health skills
Difficulties in maintaining satisfying relationships

Unhealthy dietary and sleep patterns
Abuse of tobacco, alcohol, or recreational drugs

Lack of sense of purpose, belonging, spirituality

WELLNESS
Physically active, energy levels medium to high
Open and receptive to others, many friends
Good communication skills
Receptivity to criticism
Integrated approach to issues and problems
Sensitivity to body signals
Many strong social ties
Risk-conscious health behaviors
Internal locus of control
Capacity to learn new coping skills
Capacity to exercise choices and options in problem solving

Stress-reducing behaviors
Acknowledgment of others' weaknesses, but understanding and flexible
Frustration and anxiety dealt with positively and usually short-lived
Keen attention to self-care and sound health practices
Environmentally responsible, capable of individual action to reduce pollution
Positive self-image, high self-esteem
High sensitivity, high compassion, high regard for others' feelings
Willingness to enhance personal, social, and other skills
Solid consumer health skills
Willingness to work toward optimally satisfying relationships
Healthy dietary and sleep patterns
Responsible use or nonuse of tobacco, alcohol, and recreational drugs
Spiritually healthy

ciencies in the psychological and social dimensions of the health continuum.

HEALTH-STATUS INDICATORS

Determining How Healthy We Are

The health status of a group of people, a community, a state, a nation, or the world is often reduced to statistical data for descriptive and comparative purposes. In 1979, the Surgeon General of the United States observed that "the health of the people has never been better." In his assessment, he looked at statistical data on death rates from disease (particularly the childhood diseases), injuries, life expectancy, and other criteria. This information helped lay the foundation for *Healthy People 2000: The National Health Promotion and Disease Prevention Objectives for the United States.* (See Table 1.1.)

Although this and other documents provide an important source of information for health planners, they typically do not offer a complete assessment of our current health status. Data used in developing documents such as these typically do not assess levels of human suffering, emotional health, spiritual health, and other *quality-of-life* measures. Instead they often focus on *quantity-of life* variables. Consider the following:*

Life Expectancy: By 1991, the average life expectancy (number of years a person is expected to live) had increased to over 78.9 years for white females, 72.6 for white males, 75.4 for black females, and 67.6 for black males. Life expectancy for a white

* The information in the following list is taken from *Statistical Abstract of the United States, 1991* (Washington, D.C.: U.S. Government Printing Office, 1991), and *Healthy People 2000: The National Health Promotion and Disease Prevention Objectives for the United States* (Boston: Jones and Bartlett, 1992).

Table 1.1 Healthy People 2000: Selected Objectives of the Nation for Children and Young Adults

1. Reduce overweight to a prevalence of no more than 20 percent among people aged 20 and older.
2. Reduce dietary-fat intake to an average of 30 percent of calories or less and average saturated-fat intake to less than 10 percent of calories. (Now nearly 40 percent for both.)
3. Increase complex carbohydrate and fiber-containing foods in the diets of adults to 5 or more daily servings for vegetables (including legumes) and fruits, and to 6 or more daily servings for grain products. (Now slightly over 2 1/2 servings of vegetables and fruits and 3 of grains.)
4. Reduce alcohol consumption by people aged 14 and older to an annual average of no more than 2 gallons of ethanol per person. (Was 2.50 gallons in 1989.)
5. Reduce to no more than 30 percent the proportion of all pregnancies that are unintended. (During past 5 years, 56 percent of pregnancies were unintended, unwanted, or earlier than desired.)
6. Reduce coronary heart disease deaths to no more than 100 per 100,000. (Now over 135 per 100,000.)
7. Reduce the prevalence of mental disorders (exclusive of substance abuse) among adults to less than 10.7 percent. (Now over 12 percent.)
8. Reduce homicides to no more than 7.2 per 100,000. (Now over 8.5 per 100,000.)
9. Reduce deaths from work-related injuries to no more than 4 per 100,000. (Now more than 6 per 100,000.)
10. Reduce destructive periodontal disease to a prevalence of no more than 15 percent among people aged 35–44. (Now 24 percent or more.)
11. Reverse the rise in cancer deaths to achieve a rate of no more than 130 per 100,000. (Now over 133 per 100,000.)
12. Reduce rape and attempted rape of women aged 12–34 to no more than 225 per 100,000. (Now in excess of 400 per 100,000.)
13. Increase to at least 30 percent the proportion of people aged 6 and older who engage regularly, preferably daily, in light-to-moderate physical activity for at least 30 minutes per day. (Only 22 percent of people aged 18 and older are active 30 minutes or more 5 times per week; only 12 percent are active 7 days per week.)
14. Increase to at least 20 percent the proportion of people aged 18 and older who engage in vigorous physical activity that promotes the development and maintenance of cardiorespiratory fitness. (Now only about 12 percent.)
15. Reduce the proportion of college students engaging in recent occasions of heavy drinking of alcoholic beverages to no more than 32 percent. (Now over 42 percent.)
16. Increase to at least 50 percent the proportion of people with high blood pressure whose blood pressure is under control. (Now an estimated 26 percent for persons 18 and older.)
17. Reduce the mean serum cholesterol among adults to no more than 200 mg/dL. (Now over 215 mg/dL.)
18. Increase to at least 20 percent the proportion of people aged 18 and older who seek professional help in coping with personal and emotional problems. (Now slightly over 13 percent.)
19. Increase to at least 60 percent the proportion of sexually active, unmarried women aged 15–19 whose partners used a condom at last sexual intercourse. (Now approximately 30 percent.)

SOURCE: *Healthy People 2000: The National Health Promotion and Disease Prevention Objectives for the United States* (Boston: Jones and Bartlett, 1992).

female born in 1990 exceeds 83.4 years, and a white male born in 1990 can expect to live to over 76 years.

Chronic Disease: During the 1980s, there were major declines in death rates for three of the leading causes of death among Americans: heart disease, stroke, and unintentional injuries. Infant mortality also decreased, and some childhood infectious diseases were nearly eliminated. Gains in these areas provides hope that the 1990s will see progress against other diseases. Heart disease continues to kill more people than all other diseases combined. Lung-cancer deaths have increased steadily since the 1960s, and breast-cancer deaths remain stubbornly high.

Risk Factors: Since the 1970s, we have made dramatic improvements in blood-pressure detection and control, experienced major declines in cigarette consumption, increased our awareness of cholesterol and dietary fats as risk factors, and reduced alcohol consumption and use of alcohol when driving.

The Environment: During the last decade, there has been increasing concern about toxic substances, solid waste, acid rain, the ozone level, dying oceans, global warming, polluted water supplies, food supplies, and many other life-threatening conditions.

Violence and Abusive Behaviors: Child abuse, spouse abuse, and other forms of intrafamilial violence threaten millions of Americans each year. The United States ranks first among industrialized nations in violent deaths, deaths caused by violent and "unintentional" misuse of firearms. Taken together, suicides and homicides constitute the fourth leading cause of potential years of life lost. Suicide is the third leading cause of death among people aged 15–24, and homicide is the leading cause of death for blacks aged 15–34.

Mental Health: Depression has been described as the common cold of mental illness and affects at least 5 percent of the population at any given time.

-Between 10 and 12 percent of children and adolescents suffer from mental disorders, including autism, attention-deficit disorder, hyperactivity, and depression.

-Over 23 million adults are severely incapacitated from mental disorders, not including substance abuse, and more than twice that number have experienced at least one diagnosable problem.

Access to Health Care: Nearly 25 percent of the American public is uninsured or underinsured, and these numbers are increasing daily. Millions of Americans are in need of medical care or will need care in the near future and will be shut out of the system.

What Does This Mean to You?

Clearly, the figures in Table 1.1 show that as individuals and as a nation, we have a long way to go when it comes to health and wellness. While the *quantity* of our lives has increased, as indicated by increases in life expectancy, the *quality* of our lives, as measured by emotional, psychological, social, environmental, and spiritual health indicators, appears to be in serious trouble.

In increasing numbers, Americans are finding themselves shut out of our health-care system. The number of homeless, undernourished, and mentally ill persons continues to grow in direct proportion to economic and social-service problems. Some critics argue that we are moving toward a society of haves and have-nots when it comes to health and well-being. While one group focuses on whether to join a health club, another group wonders if they will be safe sleeping under the bushes in the park. While one group fastidiously reads labels on food products to ensure that they don't consume too much saturated fat, another group wonders where their next bite of food may come from. The strange dichotomy between a middle-class perspective on health and the "survival" health status of many Americans and people throughout the world is reason for growing concern.

By definition, a truly healthy person possesses a sense of both individual and social responsibility. Rather than merely focusing on one's personal health, a genuinely healthy person is concerned about others and the greater environment. This concern translates into taking actions designed to help you live a high-quantity and -quality life, as well as to help others who are less fortunate. For examples of how this philosophy may become more meaningful to you, consider the box entitled "Taking Personal and Community Action (p. 9)."

BENEFITS OF OBTAINING OPTIMAL HEALTH

A quick glance at Table 1.2 provides an overview of the leading causes of death in the United States today. Risks for each of these leading killers have been shown to be reduced significantly by practicing specific lifestyle patterns. For example, consuming a diet low in saturated fat and cholesterol, exercising regularly, reducing sodium, managing stress, and other practices have been associated with decreased risk for heart disease. It is a well-established fact that nonsmokers have a greatly reduced risk for lung cancer. Lifestyle and individual behavior are believed to account for over 58 percent of your health (see Figure 1.2). Heredity, access to health care, and your greater environment are other major factors that influence your health status. While you can't change your genetic history, and changing your environment and the health-care system is difficult, you can influence your future health status by the behaviors you choose today.

Reduction in risk for major disease is just one of

the benefits that you can hope to achieve. Among the others are:

- Improved quality of life, in addition to an increased longevity
- Greater zest for living
- Greater energy levels, improved productivity, more interest in having fun
- Improved self-image
- Improved immunological functioning with enhanced ability to fight off infections
- Enhanced relationships with others due to better communication and improved "quality" time spent with others
- Improved ability to control and manage stress
- Enhanced levels of self-efficacy, more personal control in your life
- Reduced reliance on the health-care system, lower health-care costs
- Adding life to years, as well as adding years to life
- Improved cardiovascular functioning
- Increased muscle tone, strength, flexibility, and endurance, resulting in improved physical appearance, performance, and self-esteem
- More positive outlook on life, fewer negative thoughts, ability to view life as challenging and negative events as a potential for growth
- Improved self-confidence and ability to understand and reach out to others
- Improved environmental sensitivity, responsibility, and behaviors

Table 1.2 Leading Causes of Death in the United States by Age

AGES 1–15	AGES 15–24	AGES 25–64
1. Injuries	Injuries	Heart disease
2. Cancer	Homicide	Cancer
3. Congenital anomalies	Suicide	Injuries
4. Homicides	Cancer	Stroke
5. Heart disease	Heart disease	Suicide
6. Pneumonia/ Influenza	Congenital anomalies	Liver disease
7. Suicide	HIV infection	Chronic lung disease
8. Meningitis	Pneumonia/ Influenza	Homicide
9. Chronic lung disease	Stroke	HIV infection
10. HIV infection	Chronic lung disease	Diabetes

SOURCE: Center for Health Statistics (CDC), 1990. Monthly Vital Statistics Report. 1989. Health: United States, 1989.

- Enhanced levels of spiritual health, awareness, and feelings of oneness with self, others, and the greater environment

HEALTH BEHAVIORS

Although mounting evidence indicates that there are significant benefits to being healthy, many people find it difficult to become and stay healthy. Rather than realistically assessing their lifestyles, they tend to make excuses for their behavior. Taking time out for relaxation becomes impossible; exercise becomes something they must do rather than want to do; and changing dietary patterns becomes too difficult.

Typically, sleeping 7 to 8 hours a day, eating a nutritious breakfast, not eating between meals, maintaining proper weight, not smoking cigarettes, limiting intake of alcohol, and exercising regularly are recognized as essential components of a long and healthy life. These common-sense recommendations have withstood the test of time, remaining unsurpassed as sound health advice. How close do we come to meeting these goals? Table 1.3 provides an overview of how well we are doing in several of these key areas. This information clearly indicates that there are many areas in which people can make changes to improve the quality of their lives.

Change is not easy. In our culture, it is normal to eat when we're not hungry, to be overweight, to take the elevator instead of the stairs, and to drive around the parking lot for 5 minutes to avoid a 1-minute walk. We don't relax because we don't know how. We eat high-fat foods because they were a part of our upbringing. We don't exercise because exercise is often equated with work. Health behaviors are learned behaviors that are encouraged by both peers and family. Decisions to change old, negative thinking patterns or behaviors take conscious effort, planning, and an awareness of individual barriers to success.

BEHAVIOR CHANGE

Finding a successful recipe for making positive lifestyle modifications is no easy task. Determining why one person is able to lose 50 pounds and keep it off while another person cannot seem to lose an ounce, or why one person sticks to a daily exercise regimen while others quit after their first workout session, is difficult. Scientists are now concentrating on the role of behavioral factors that contribute to both illness and death. Of particular importance are lifestyle habits such as smoking, lack of exercise, poor diet, and alcohol abuse. Clearly, these behaviors contribute to a person's susceptibility to disease. Analyzing which factors influence behaviors and serve as "triggers" toward positive change is an important first step.

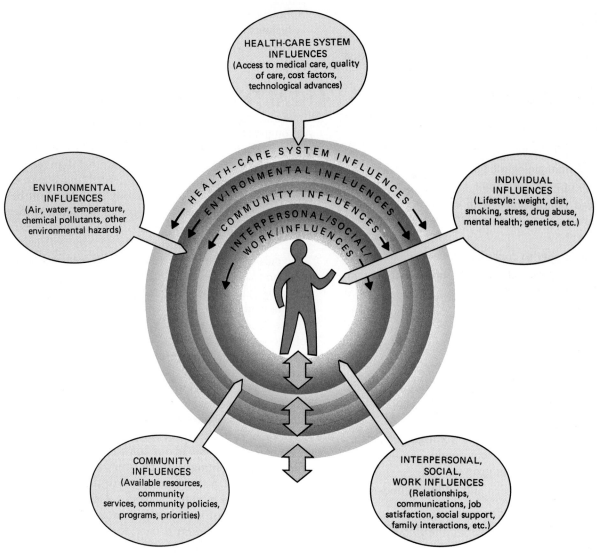

Note: each of the above influences is related to all of the others.
There is also much overlap between selected influences.

Figure 1.2 Factors that influence our health status.

Table 1.3   Overview of Selected Personal Health Behaviors in the United States, 1991 (by percentage)

Health Behavior	Sleeps 6 Hours or Less	Never Eats Breakfast	Snacks Every Day	Less Physically Active Than Contemporaries	Had 5 or More Alcoholic Drinks on Any Given Day	Current Smoker	30% or More above Ideal Weight
All persons	22.0	24.4	39.0	16.2	36.5	24.2	13.9
Age							
18–29 years old	19.8	30.4	42.2	17.1	54.4	31.9	7.5
30–44 years old	24.3	30.1	41.1	18.3	39.0	34.5	13.6
45–64 years old	22.7	21.4	37.9	15.3	24.6	31.6	18.1
65+ years old	20.4	7.5	30.7	13.5	12.2	16.0	13.2
Gender							
Male	22.7	25.2	40.7	16.5	49.3	32.6	12.1
Female	21.4	23.6	37.5	16.3	23.3	27.8	13.7
Race							
White	21.3	24.5	39.4	16.7	38.3	29.6	12.4
Black	27.8	23.6	37.2	13.9	29.3	34.9	18.7
Other	21.4	21.5	32.6	16.5	33.3	24.8	6.7

SOURCE: *Statistical Abstract of the United States 1991* (Washington, D.C.: U.S. Government Printing Office, 1991).

Health in Your Community

Taking Personal and Community Action

Although Americans are more concerned about health issues than at any time in our nation's history, many of us often feel that there is little that we can do to reduce our own risk. We find it even more difficult to bring about change at the community level. The following are but a few of the suggestions that may ultimately improve your own health status and that of those around you. The "Others?" category is provided for you to write your *own* thoughts on what individuals can do to improve individual and community health.

ACTIONS TO IMPROVE PERSONAL HEALTH

Complete a personal health history, including individual risks from your genetics, inheritance, lifestyle, environment, and health-care system. Prioritize those that *your behavior* can have an impact on, either short- or long-term

Develop a short-term plan of action to reduce your immediate risks, and begin to control your long-term risks. Improve your diet, increase your fitness levels, avoid harmful substances, improve your social skills, help others, consider spiritual issues more often, take time to control stress, get adequate amounts of sleep, practice self-care activities, use the health-care system wisely, practice responsible sexual behaviors, etc.

Act responsibly to preserve the environment. Consume fewer resources, use fewer prepackaged products, *reuse, recycle, and reduce consumption* whenever possible. Water, air, natural resources, and animals are important legacies and each of us can play a significant role in protecting them.

Others? _____
_____
_____
_____

_____
_____
_____

ACTIONS TO IMPROVE COMMUNITY HEALTH

Analyze what is going on in your school, your community, your state, and the nation. *Read, discuss, and develop opinions* about the critical health issues likely to have an impact on you, your parents, your friends, and society in general.

Listen to the opinions of your school administrators, your state elected officials, and your national elected representatives. If an important health issue is being considered, *write or call* these officials and let them know how you feel about the issues. *Become involved* in city government and in social services, particularly when the health of others is likely to be affected.

Vote for elected officials whose policies, rhetoric, and past histories have indicated that they support improvements in health care, environmental issues, education, minority health, and other critical issues facing the nation.

Purchase products and services from companies who have proven records of protecting the environment, providing safe foods and products, and who support the health and well-being of others through their organizational practices.

Others? _____
_____
_____
_____
_____
_____
_____

Factors Influencing Behavior Change

Mark Twain once said that "habit is habit, and not to be flung out the window by anyone, but coaxed downstairs a step at a time." Changing negative behavior patterns into healthy ones is often a time-consuming and difficult process. The chances of success are better when people make gradual changes that give them time to unlearn negative patterns and substitute positive ones. We have not yet developed a foolproof method for effectively changing people's behavior, but we do know that certain behaviors can benefit both individuals and society as a whole. To understand how the process of behavior change works, we must first identify specific behavior patterns and attempt to understand the reasons for our behavior.

Unfortunately, the development or maintenance of health behaviors is not necessarily a linear model in which we can assume that if we have knowledge, our attitudes and behaviors will automatically change. Were this the case, knowledgeable people would not behave in ways detrimental to their health. The reasons people behave in unhealthy ways, in spite of known risks, are complex and not easily understood. Health researchers have studied health behaviors for decades and continue to analyze the reasons that one person chooses to act in a responsible manner while another ignores obvious health risks. Figure 1.3 identifies the major factors that influence behavior and behavior-change decisions. These factors can be divided into three general categories: predisposing, enabling, and reinforcing factors. *Predisposing factors* are those things we bring to the situation, such as our life experiences, our knowledge, our cultural and ethnic inheritance, and our current beliefs and values. *Enabling factors* are those factors that make our health decisions more convenient or more difficult. For example, if you like to swim for exercise but the only available pool is inaccessible, you might be less likely to go swimming than you would if the pool were located

nearby. Although it is easy to use negative enabling factors as excuses for not behaving in a positive manner, it is often possible to devise strategies for dealing with difficult circumstances. *Reinforcing factors* relate to the presence or absence of support, encouragement, or discouragement that significant people in your life bring to a situation. For example, if you decide to stop smoking and members of your family continually smoke in your presence, you might be tempted to start smoking again. Similarly, the manner in which you reward or punish yourself for your own successes and failures may affect your chances of adopting healthy behaviors. Learning to accept small failures and to concentrate on your successes may foster further successes. Berating yourself because you binged on ice cream, allowed yourself to get into an argument with a friend, or didn't jog because it was raining might create an environment in which failure becomes almost inevitable.

Although a variety of factors influence our decisions, each of us makes either a conscious or an unconscious decision to behave in a particular manner. Our decision-making process is often motivated by a complex interaction between our values, beliefs, and selected factors in our social environment, as discussed earlier.

When we make decisions about our health, our underlying beliefs play a role. Proponents of the *health-belief model* note that people are more likely to change a given behavior if

Figure 1.3 Influences on your health decisions and behaviors.

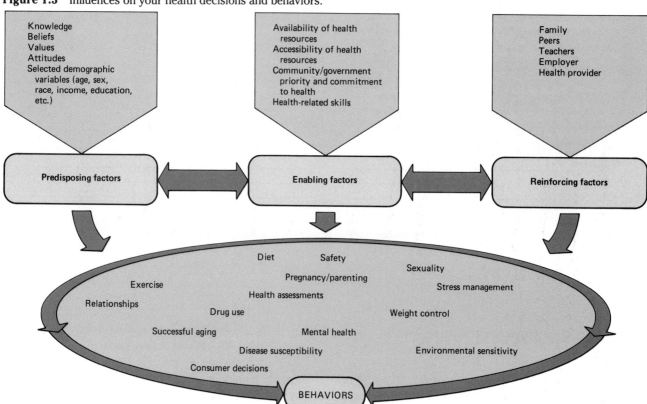

1. They believe that they may be susceptible to a given disease or health risk as a result of their behavior.
2. They believe that the consequences of their actions could be severe if they do not change.
3. They believe that they will benefit from changing their behavior.

An example of the health-belief model would be a college student who is extremely overweight but, although he has suffered several episodes of chest pain, does not believe that he is old enough to be at risk. After a brief jog he passes out, only to wake up in the emergency room. The doctor tells him that he has had a mild heart attack and that some blockage has been detected in his coronary arteries. He is warned that unless he loses 80 pounds, lowers his intake of saturated fat, and begins to exercise regularly, he faces major coronary bypass surgery or death in the months ahead. The student begins a medically supervised diet, loses weight, and begins an aerobic-exercise program. Clearly, this student responded to the risk, realized the consequences, and saw the benefits of changing his behavior.

Values are also important factors in determining behavior change. People may be more likely to engage in a weight-training or fitness program if they believe that these activities will improve other aspects of their social lives or interpersonal relationships. Selected *cues to action* may provide those underlying stimuli that motivate some people to take aggressive, firm action to change a given behavior. Finding out that your total cholesterol level is over 300 may be a "cue" that influences you to reduce your saturated-fat intake. However, everyone responds to different types of cues.

Changing Health Behaviors

Various behavioral theories have been studied as they relate to health. Ideas and concepts such as self-efficacy, locus of control, and health locus of control are becoming more widely understood. **Self-efficacy** refers to a person's appraisal of his or her own ability to change or to accomplish a particular task or behavior. **Locus of control** refers to a person's perceptions of forces or factors that control his or her destiny. **Health locus of control** focuses specifically on those factors that influence health. These constructs influence how we view ourselves and also how we behave or seek to change behaviors.

If people believe health to be a result of factors beyond their control, they will not take personal responsibility for their health. A certain sense of internal control over your health coupled with a high degree of confidence in your ability is the ideal situation for positive health-behavior change. If you believe that you can change negative health behavior (self-efficacy) and that your actions will make a difference in your health (health locus of control), positive change becomes much more likely.

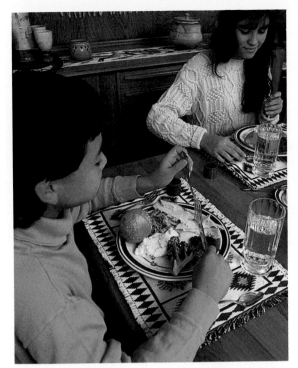

Eating a balanced diet is essential to achieving and maintaining health.

Readiness is the actual state of being that precedes the behavioral change. People who are ready to change possess the attitudes, skills, and resources that make it possible to incorporate a new positive behavior into their lifestyle. To change your behavior, you must

1. *Know what to do* (knowledge and information)
2. *Believe you can do it* (self-efficacy)
3. *Know how to do it* (skills and ability)
4. *Want to do it* (desire and motivation)

If you think you can do something, and you want to do it, you probably will do it. Figure 1.4 illustrates in detail the typical progression that a person who becomes ready for change demonstrates.

Making the Commitment to Change

Because behaviors are learned responses that often become subconscious rituals or procedures, they usually become a significant part of a person's identity. As we have noted, changing these behaviors is difficult. In general, the younger the person, the less likely that these behavior patterns will have become deeply ingrained and

Self-efficacy A person's appraisal of his or her ability to accomplish a particular task or behavior.
Locus of control A person's perception of forces or factors that control his or her destiny.
Health locus of control A person's perception of forces or factors that control his or her health status.

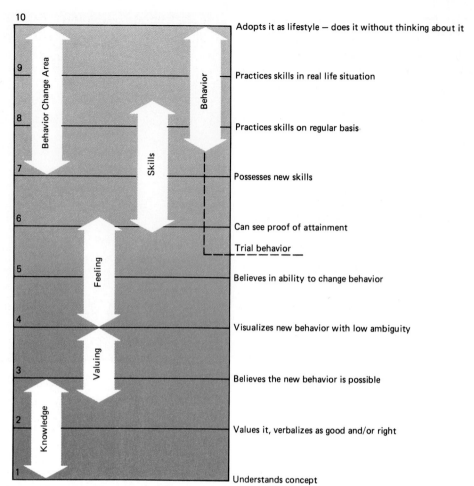

Figure 1.4 The steps and stages in becoming ready for behavioral change. This readiness scale includes five stages: knowledge, valuing, feeling, skills, and behavior.

the better the chances for change may be. The following is one set of steps for planning a positive behavior change:

1. *Decide what specifically you want to change.* Discussions with close friends may lead to some revealing information about your behaviors. A self-assessment exercise, such as the one in this chapter titled "Martin's Index of Health Behavior," may provide you with useful information and insights.

2. *Decide how things will improve or be different in your life as a result of the change.* What will really be different if you succeed? How much will the ultimate change matter to your relationships? Your health? Your self-concept? How important are these things to you?

3. *Listen to the things that you are telling yourself (self-talk) that are affecting your emotional response to change.* Are your past experiences, values, and attitudes causing you to make unrealistic excuses or to defend your past behaviors? Are you making this change because you really want to, or are you being pressured by others?

4. *Assess your resources.* What things will help you

achieve your goals? Will friends, community support groups, or other networks help you in your efforts to change?

5. *Determine what things have previously stood in the way of reaching your goals.* What are the barriers or blocking agents? Which of these can you avoid?

6. *Establish priorities for change.* Determine what things are most important for you to change now. Which is *the* most important factor? The *next* most important?

7. *Develop a plan of action.* Break the parts of your action into small components or objectives. Tackle each component one at a time, being careful not to try too many changes at a time.

8. *Determine how you will know when you have satisfactorily met your goal.* How will you evaluate success? Will you evaluate success by a series of small objectives to be met or only in terms of the ultimate goal? For example, people who begin an exercise program often find it helpful to start with a graduated program that will enable them to reach their goal after a specified period of time (say, 1 month). This is often easier than saying "By this time next year, I will be running the Boston Marathon."

9. *Determine what things will keep you going.* What will help you maintain the behavior change? The most difficult part of any behavior change strategy is to be able to continue for prolonged periods of time.

10. *Are you really ready to do whatever it takes to change?* Assess your readiness by analyzing where you are in terms of a readiness scale.

If you have already tried several of the items on this list and failed, don't be discouraged. The problems you have encountered may be due to influences you've never really thought about, or to a lack of support or encouragement. Sometimes people will even help you fail—by sabotaging your diet, for example, or encouraging you to take another drink. Positive reinforcement is essential.

 Promoting Your Health

Martin's Index of Health Behavior

Instructions: For the following questions put a check in the blank by the choice that best describes your health behavior. There are no right or wrong answers. The best answer is the one that honestly describes you.

1. How many days per week do you eat breakfast?
   _____ a. 6–7   _____ c. 2–3
   _____ b. 4–5   _____ d. 0–1

2. Which choice most closely describes your daily eating pattern?
   _____ a. eating snack foods (potato chips, soda pop, etc.) whenever I feel hungry
   _____ b. eating one balanced meal per day and eating snack foods at other times during the day
   _____ c. eating two balanced meals a day and eating snack foods at other times of the day
   _____ d. eating three balanced meals a day and eating snack foods at other times of the day
   _____ e. eating three balanced meals per day and not snacking

3. How many days per week do you eat a balanced diet that includes the minimum number of servings from the four food groups as listed below?
   2 servings of meat or protein substitutes
   2 servings of dairy products
   4 servings of breads and cereals
   4 servings of fruits and vegetables
   _____ a. 6–7   _____ c. 2–3
   _____ b. 4–5   _____ d. 0–1

4. How many servings per day of concentrated sources of sugar (soda pop, candy, cookies, etc.) do you eat?
   _____ a. 0 or less than 1   _____ c. 3–4
   _____ b. 1–2   _____ d. 5 or more

5. Considering your height and body build, how far are you from your ideal weight?
   _____ a. within 10 pounds
   _____ b. within 20 pounds
   _____ c. within 30 pounds
   _____ d. more than 30 pounds from ideal

6. Which choice most closely describes your dieting behavior?
   _____ a. never being overweight, so never dieting
   _____ b. being more than 10 pounds overweight, but not dieting
   _____ c. when overweight, going on a fad diet to lose weight quickly
   _____ d. when overweight attempting to lose weight gradually (1–2 pounds per week) by increasing exercise *or* decreasing food intake
   _____ e. when overweight, attempting to lose weight gradually (1–2 pounds per week) by increasing exercise *and* decreasing food intake.

7. What is the average number of hours per night that you sleep?
   _____ a. more than 10   _____ d. 5–6
   _____ b. 9–10   _____ e. 0–4
   _____ c. 7–8

8. How often do you use seatbelts while driving or riding in a car?
   _____ a. always
   _____ b. never in town and always on the highway
   _____ c. sometimes in town and sometimes on the highway
   _____ d. never

9. How often do you drive or ride with someone under the influence of alcohol or drugs?
   _____ a. more than once per week
   _____ b. once per week
   _____ c. a few times per year
   _____ d. never

10. Which choice best describes your consumption of alcoholic beverages?
   _____ a. not drinking
   _____ b. drinking one drink or less per day
   _____ c. drinking two drinks or less per day
   _____ d. drinking two drinks or less on weekdays, more than two drinks per day on weekends
   _____ e. drinking more than two drinks per day on most days

11. Which choice best describes your drug-use pattern (over-the-counter, prescription, and recreational drugs)?
   _____ a. using the drugs I want whenever I want
   _____ b. using the drugs I feel I need while following common sense
   _____ c. using only medically required drugs exactly as directed
   _____ d. rarely using drugs of any kind

12. How many cups of caffeinated beverges (coffee, tea, cola, etc.) do you drink per day?
   _____ a. none or less than 1   _____ c. 4–6
   _____ b. 1–3   _____ d. 7 or more

13. Which choice best describes your cigarette-smoking behavior?
   _____ a. not smoking
   _____ b. smoking less than one pack per day
   _____ c. smoking 1–2 packs per day
   _____ d. smoking more than 2 packs per day

14. How many times per week do you exercise aerobically (biking, jogging, swimming, aerobics, etc.)?
   _____ a. less than 1   _____ d. 3–4
   _____ b. 1   _____ e. 5 or more
   _____ c. 2

15. How many times per week do you do other types of exercise (weight lifting, tennis, calisthenics, racquetball, basketball, etc.) besides aerobic activities?
   _____ a. less than 1   _____ d. 3–4
   _____ b. 1   _____ e. 5 or more
   _____ c. 2

16. How often do you brush your teeth?
   _____ a. after every meal
   _____ b. twice per day
   _____ c. once per day
   _____ d. less than once per day

17. How often do you have a dental checkup?
   _____ a. never or only when something is wrong
   _____ b. every 2–3 years
   _____ c. every year
   _____ d. every six months

18. How often do you have a medical checkup?
   _____ a. never or only when something is wrong
   _____ b. only for Pap tests or other checks
   _____ c. every 3–5 years
   _____ d. at least every 2 years

19. How often do you read the labels on foods and over-the-counter drugs before purchasing them?
   _____ a. always   _____ c. sometimes
   _____ b. usually   _____ d. rarely

20. How many times per week do you make a conscientious effort to manage your stress by utilizing progressive relaxation, exercise, religion, music, or other stress-reduction techniques?
   _____ a. 6–7   _____ c. 2–3
   _____ b. 4–5   _____ d. 0–1

21. Which choice most correctly describes your closest interpersonal relationship?
   _____ a. not having a friend
   _____ b. having a friend, but I am not able to share my real feelings with the person
   _____ c. having a friendship where I can sometimes share my real feelings, but sometimes can't
   _____ d. having a friendship where I can always share my real feelings

22. How many servings per day of foods high in saturated fats or cholesterol (whole milk, eggs, sausage, bacon, red meat, etc.) do you eat?
   _____ a. 0   _____ c. 3–4
   _____ b. 1–2   _____ d. 5 or more

23. How often do you limit your consumption of salt by doing things like not salting your foods at the table, using salt sparingly when preparing foods, and limiting your intake of salty foods?
   _____ a. always   _____ c. sometimes
   _____ b. usually   _____ d. rarely

24. How often do you practice breast self-examination (female) or testicular self-examination (male)?
   _____ a. every month
   _____ b. every 2–6 months
   _____ c. less frequently than every 6 months
   _____ d. never

25. Which choice best describes your contraceptive use?
   _____ a. not sexually active, so don't use contraceptives
   _____ b. attempting to get pregnant or am pregnant, so don't use contraceptives
   _____ c. sexually active and always use contraceptives
   _____ d. sexually active and usually use contraceptives
   _____ e. sexually active and usually use contraceptives
   _____ f. sexually active and rarely use contraceptives

Scoring for Martin's Index of Health Behavior

For Items 1, 3, 4, 5, 8, 12, 13, 16, 19, 20, 22, 23, 24: a = 3, b = 2, c = 1, d = 0.

Rewards, social support, and other incentives to change may all be helpful. Although societal factors play a role, behavior change is largely an individual issue. Getting others to behave as we believe they should may be difficult, as well as inappropriate. When others behave in an unhealthy manner, it is often best to view their actions with understanding rather than contempt and to try to be supportive rather than critical.

ACCESS TO HEALTH

Health is not black-and-white, or right-or-wrong, or static and unchanging. Consensus about what constitutes health may never be reached. However, once we understand the various components of health and illness, the likelihood of positive change may be greatly enhanced. Each of us needs to be aware of current information, to evaluate our priorities, and to choose viable options. We all make decisions regarding health every day. Each day we eat, sleep, and interact with others in our environment. Basic human needs must be met, and many of these needs are health-related. *Access to Health* provides you with the opportunity to realize your health potential in an informed manner. Good health does not just happen. By being informed, you place yourself in the best position to make choices that will ensure the best future for you. What you do today may have a significant impact on what you are able to do tomorrow.

SUMMARY

- There are no simple definitions of what it means to be healthy.

- Health can be defined as the ability of an organism to achieve optimal well-being within a realistic framework of individual potential and in a sometimes hostile environment.

- Total health or wellness involves psychological, spiritual, and social components in addition to the absence of physical infirmity.

- Overemphasizing one component of the wellness continuum and ignoring other components can lead to serious health deficiencies.

- Health promotion can be defined as any combination of educational, organizational, economic, and environmental supports for behaviors conducive to health.

- The benefits of good health include improved self-image, life satisfaction, enhanced creativity, increased energy levels, and reduced medical costs.

- Lifestyle, environment, biology and heredity, health care, and other factors are major influences in individual health and longevity.

- Health status can be measured by analysis of such factors as incidence, prevalence, morbidity, mortality, and infant mortality rates. However, many nonstatistical factors must be considered as well.

- Behavior change is a complex task, and a deliberate plan is required. Logical steps include identifying a behavior change, listening to yourself, determining why it's important that you change, developing a plan of action, evaluating your progress, and maintaining the behavior change.

- Predisposing, enabling, and reinforcing factors affect our ability to change our behaviors.

- Our beliefs, values, and readiness for change may significantly affect our ability to change.

- We must each accept personal responsibility for keeping current, evaluating priorities, and choosing viable options regarding health.

2

The Foundations of Emotional Well-Being

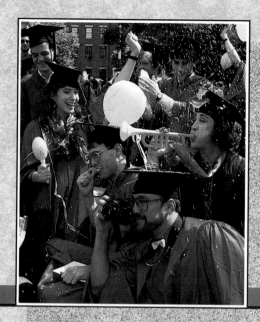

■ After Reading This Chapter, You Should Be Able to

- Explain what we mean by mental and emotional health, and list the 8 characteristics that Shapiro claims are shared by emotionally healthy people.

- Define what we mean by personality, and list the components of a healthy personality.

- Discuss various means of achieving emotional health, including maintaining self-esteem, decision making, and communication.

- Discuss various types of mental illness and their treatment, focusing on both the emotional and biological bases of these conditions.

- Explain when and how a person should seek professional help for an emotional problem.

The pursuit of a strong, physically fit body has been an important part of our American health recipe in recent decades. Prompted by a medium that glorifies the human form and personal appearance, we have responded with a seemingly endless preoccupation with what we can do to make our bodies firmer, stronger, more efficient, and more ready to respond to the nuances of life. We proudly recite statistics on our blood pressure, body fat levels, resting heart rate, strength, flexibility, and other endurance measures, and exercise, exercise, exercise to achieve these physical-fitness goals. However, when asked to assess our mental health, we give superficial responses such as, "I'm okay," "I'm great," or "Super." What we often mean is that we really don't know our mental and emotional health status, and we certainly don't know how we stack up against all of the other people in our lives in these areas. This apparent ignorance is not surprising, as very few reliable and readily available measurements of emotional and mental well-being exist.

We all know or think we can tell when someone is emotionally unstable or mentally ill. We all experience times of great turmoil in our own lives when the stress we are experiencing makes us think that we are "going crazy" ourselves. From time to time, we all wonder if we are "normal" and look at others for comparison. If they seem happy and positive, we wonder if there is something wrong with us. How do we really know if we are "normal" or if we are on the verge of some serious emotional or mental disorder?

THE FOUNDATIONS OF EMOTIONAL WELL-BEING

Mental and emotional health are generally culturally and socially determined. American standards of normalcy do not necessarily apply to other cultural groups. The Siriono people of Bolivia believe that it is healthy for children to express rage at their parents. When they feel frustrated or neglected, young Siriono children are encouraged to strike their parents with sticks or spindles. Such behavior is believed to produce valiant, brave adults. In our society, of course, such behavior would be considered abnormal and would not be tolerated.

A behavior is *normal* when it conforms to the accepted standards and patterns of a large group of people. Within each large group there are subgroups. Behaviors of subgroup members may be accepted by the subgroup but not by the large group.

Each of us may belong to a particular cultural subgroup, but we learn what types of behaviors are acceptable to the larger society in which we live. Emotional and mental health must be examined in the context of both the individual and society. Behavior that impairs the individual eventually impairs the society.

In American society today, many people have in-creased freedom to explore and develop their potentials. With that freedom comes a responsibility to pursue our own emotional well-being and mental health. During our lifetimes, we will all be faced with choices that will lead us either to growth or to stagnation. Our emotional growth and mental health depend on our ability to take an active role in the growth process.

David Heath, a psychological researcher who has examined the dynamics of emotional health, has concluded that emotional health is a *continuous process* rather than a static state of existence. He defines emotional health as the "ability of an individual to adapt constructively and positively through time to the many demands presented by living."[**] A newer, more contemporary definition of mental and emotional health is provided by psychiatrist M. Scott Peck, who defines emotional health as the "ongoing process of dedication to objective reality at all costs."[†]

Peck's definition is based on years of experience with clients, and Heath's is derived from the results of empirical and theoretical research. Together, they define emotionally healthy people as those who deliberately and purposefully devote themselves to facing and adapting to the realities of life in constructive ways.

Although this definition is broad, it does imply a set of characteristics shared by emotionally healthy people. These characteristics were outlined by psychologist Deane Shapiro in an analysis of major studies of emotional wellness.[‡] Shapiro recognized 8 common characteristics shared by emotionally healthy people:

1. Determination and effort to be healthy
2. Flexibility and adaptability to a variety of circumstances.
3. Development of a sense of meaning and affirmation of life
4. Understanding that the self is not the center of the universe
5. Compassion for others
6. The ability to be unselfish in serving or relating to others
7. Depth and satisfaction in intimate relationships
8. A sense of control over the mind and body that enables the person to make health-enhancing choices and decisions.

The concept of mental health as a process helps us understand that these 8 mental and emotional health components exist on a continuum much like the wellness continuum. Developing and integrating these com-

---

** David Heath, "The Maturing Person," in Roger Walsh and Deane H. Shapiro, eds., *Beyond Health and Normality* (New York: Van Nostrand Reinhold, 1983), p. 159.
† M. Scott Peck, *The Road Less Traveled* (New York: Simon & Schuster, 1988).
‡ Walsh and Shapiro, *Beyond Health and Normality*, p. 273.

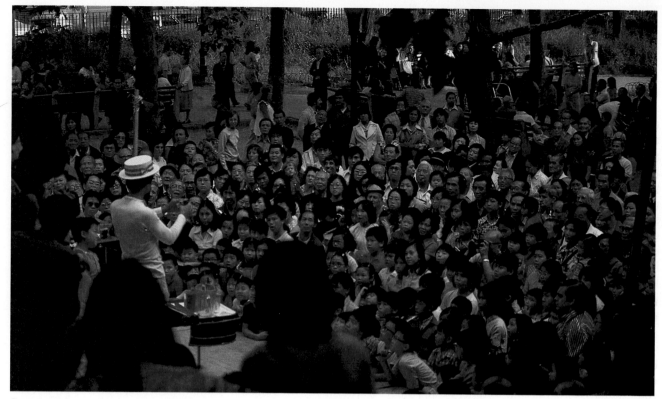

Despite differences in culture, religion, and nationality, certain behaviors are common to people everywhere.

ponents into our lives are the basis of achieving mental health.

PERSONAL EVOLUTION

Very few of us develop the 8 characteristics of mental health all at once. For most of us, learning to balance and maintain the components of mental and emotional health takes years. Americans appear to follow similar paths on their routes to mental and emotional health. The patterns and events in our lives seem to have a common basis. A study of those terms can help in the understanding of personal development.

Personality

Our **personality** is the unique mix of characteristics that distinguish us from others. Hereditary, environmental, cultural, and experiential factors influence how we develop. For each of us, the amount of influence exerted by any of these factors is different.

Our personality determines how we react to the challenges of life. It also determines how we interpret the feelings we experience in conjunction with the challenges. Our personality further determines how we resolve the conflicts we feel when we are denied the things we need or want.

Psychology is the study of the mind. Part of the task of psychologists is to explore the personality as well. As a science, psychology is relatively new. Although the importance of the workings of the human mind has been recognized for thousands of years, the actual scientific study of the mind did not begin until the early twentieth century.

The effort to understand the development of the human personality began with the teachings of Sigmund Freud, an Austrian physician who believed that the human mind had two levels: conscious and unconscious. Freud believed that observation of conscious behavior would provide clues to the workings of the hidden unconscious.

To Freud, the human personality had three components. The first, the **id**, was thought to represent our unconscious desires to enjoy the pleasures in life. The second, the **ego**, acted as a mediator and regulator for the demands made by the id. The final component, the

---

Personality A person's unique social, emotional, and behavioral characteristics.

Psychology The science of the mind, including mental processes, feelings, desires, and behaviors.

Id A Freudian term describing the part of the mind that is impulsive and directed toward satisfying desires.

Ego A Freudian term describing the part of the mind that experiences reality and, in part, controls the id's pleasure-related impulses.

superego, served as a conscience of sorts by interpreting id and ego desires as good or bad. Freud believed that the conflicts among the id, ego, and superego were manifested in behavior. He considered guilt and fear, particularly when related to sexual desires, to be the most common problems people experienced.

Other theories about the human mind began to flourish following the Freudian era. One of the earliest branches of psychology was developed by scientist B.F. Skinner. As part of the precepts of **behavioral psychology,** Skinner stated that all behavior was learned through a system of rewards and punishment. "Right" behaviors could be encouraged through rewards, and "wrong" behaviors could be eliminated through punishment. Personality was also learned, based upon the type of reinforcements a child was given.

Some followers of Skinner believed that at birth a baby's mind was a blank slate. Through directed **conditioning,** that baby could be trained to be a murderer or a priest with heredity, cultural factors, and environment playing no part in the creation of the desired behavior.

A third branch of psychology was **developmental psychology.** Those who contributed to this school of thought included Erik Erikson, Carl Jung, and others who taught that personality and emotional health were dependent on the successful completion of a series of **developmental tasks** at various stages of the life cycle.

Erikson identified and recognized eight stages of psychosocial development (see Table 2.1). He believed that at each stage we must face and resolve particular crises in order to continue growth. Successful resolution of each crisis gives us a new building block in the development of self-fulfillment and emotional health. Erikson identified these building blocks as hope, will, purpose, competence, fidelity, love, care, and wisdom.

Table 2.1 The Major Stages in Psychosocial Development as Defined by Erikson

Completion of each stage is dependent on successful completion of developmental crises at preceding stages.

Age Group	Stage	Building Blocks of Development of Emotional Health
Infancy	Trust versus mistrust	Hope
Early childhood	Autonomy versus shame and doubt	Will
Preschool age	Initiative versus guilt	Purpose
School age	Industry versus inferiority	Competence
Adolescence	Identity versus identity confusion	Fidelity
Young adulthood	Intimacy versus isolation	Love
Maturity	Creativity versus stagnation	Care
Old age	Integrity versus despair	Wisdom

In the 1950s, a group of renowned psychologists began meeting in Big Sur, California, to discuss new theories that could better describe the work they were actually doing with patients. Out of these and many other discussions emerged the theory of **humanistic psychology.** Characteristic of this movement was the belief that each of us has intrinsic value; we are "good" and "worthy" just by virtue of having been born.

One of the leaders of the movement was Abraham H. Maslow. Maslow developed the theory that people achieve emotional well-being by meeting a hierarchy of needs (see Figure 2.1). Maslow and his followers believed that there are five basic human needs: physiological (oxygen, food, water, sleep, sexual release, etc.); security (a physically and emotionally safe and consistent environment); love and belonging (to a family or other support group); self-esteem; and self-actualization (the achievement of self-fulfillment). Before achieving higher

Figure 2.1 Maslow's hierarchy of needs.

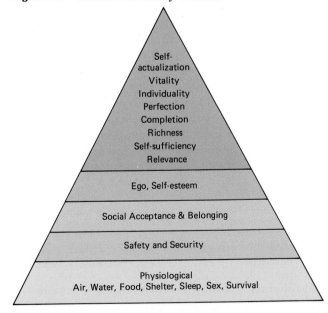

Superego A Freudian term describing the part of the mind that controls both id and ego; the conscience.
Behavioral psychology A branch of psychology that teaches that all human behavior can be learned and controlled through a process of reward and punishment.
Conditioning System of reward and punishment used in behavioral psychology to obtain desired responses to specific stimuli.
Developmental psychology A branch of psychology that holds that human development is based on the successful completion of tasks at each stage of the life span.
Developmental tasks Challenges associated with each stage of the life span from birth to death.
Humanistic psychology A branch of psychology that focuses on the intrinsic value of the individual.

levels, we must fulfill the previous levels. We therefore cannot achieve self-actualization until the more basic needs have been fulfilled.

Another well-known contributor to humanistic psychology was Carl Rogers. Rogers, a teacher and therapist, gave his students and clients what he called "unconditional positive regard." He designed a nondirective form of therapy in which the client's beliefs and interpretations of behavior were considered to be more important than the therapist's. The intrinsic worth of the individual was of primary importance.

Most of the later schools of psychological theory promote the idea that we have the power not only to understand our behavior but also to actively change our behavior and beliefs. We have the power to mold our own personalities.

Personality development probably involves some combination of all the personality theories. We feel conflicts and guilt over our desires and social rules, as Freud believed, and we have the capacity to learn behaviorally as well. For example, people who have been continually rejected in intimate relationships may give up after a time, feeling that there is no use. They have learned not to form intimate relationships because of the fear of punishment in the form of failure. We all have basic needs, as Maslow suggested, and the search for the fulfillment of those needs can certainly enrich our lives and give us life satisfaction. Most of us strive to achieve self-acceptance and self-confidence. Finally, many of us are interested in developing the ability to change and direct our own growth as the existential humanists urge us to do.

Components of a Healthy Personality

Psychologist Carol Tavris has identified four components of a healthy personality: emotionality, sociability, level of activity, and impulsiveness.** Once we recognize these components within ourselves, we can work to foster their healthy development.

Emotionality is the intensity of our emotional reactions. Some people seem to be passive in their emotional responses. Others seem cool and in control of every situation. Another group of people are described as "strong-tempered." These people display their emotions dramatically and may exhibit wide variations in mood.

Some of our emotional responses are thought to be controlled by heredity. Although we learn emotional responses through the examples set for us by our families and other associates, some experts believe that we have an inherited "reaction range" for our emotional responses. Included within this reaction range are *arousability,* or how much time elapses before we respond to emotional stimuli; *excitability,* or how much energy can

be summoned in response to emotional stimuli; and *tempo,* the speed of emotional response.

The second component of personality is **sociability.** Sociability is our tendency to want to be with others or to prefer being alone. *Introverted* people tend to direct their energies and emotions toward themselves; these people may be called "loners" or "hermits." *Extroverted* personalities are directed toward others. Tendencies toward introversion or extroversion are learned. However, they may also be genetically influenced.

Level of activity encompasses the amount and nature of the energy we expend in our responses to emotional stimuli. We may be passive, exerting little energy, or aggressive, exerting a great deal of forceful energy. Depending on the stimuli, we may also respond at some activity level between passivity and aggressiveness. Common vernacular may classify passive people as "mellow" and aggressive people as "hyper."

The final component of personality is **impulsiveness,** the tendency to respond to events without thinking. Impulsive people generally follow their emotions or "gut feelings" rather than analyzing situations. A nonimpulsive person generally thinks before responding.

None of these personality and temperament characteristics is inherently "good" or "bad." Only when practiced in the extreme do they have the potential to limit personal growth. Emotionally healthy people are able to balance their emotionality, sociability, activity levels, and impulsiveness.

Development of Personality Traits

Mental-health specialists often debate the relative influences of environment and heredity on the development of personality. This argument is referred to as *nature versus nurture.* Most professionals believe that human behavior usually results from some combination of these two factors. In the case of depression, for example, there are arguments for both environmental and genetic causes. Children can inherit certain tendencies toward depression from their parents. Suppose a person with such tendencies grows up in a positive emotional environment. As an adult, will that person show fewer symptoms of depression because of that environment? Proponents of the nature argument would say no, the person could still suffer from depression. Those in favor of the nurture argument, on the other hand, would say yes, the person would be less likely to suffer depression,

---

Emotionality Characteristics of our emotional responses to various circumstances; includes arousability, excitability, and tempo.

Sociability The methods by which we relate to others.

Level of activity The amount of energy expended on emotional responses.

Impulsiveness The degree to which we respond to problems without thinking.

** Carol Tavris, *Anger,* rev. ed. (New York: Simon & Schuster, 1989), p. 67.

or the depression would be less severe because of the positive environment.

This dispute has been difficult to resolve. However, recent studies of twins conducted at the University of Minnesota indicate that personality traits are influenced to different degrees by the environment and by heredity. The study identified common personality traits and noted the degree to which each of these traits could be inherited.* The investigators concluded that no single gene is responsible for any one trait. Rather, a great number of genes in a combination create the inheritance pattern, making it complex and indirect.

The findings of the study indicate that the trait of *social potency,* or leadership potential, has the strongest hereditary component, whereas *social closeness,* or the ability to form close emotional ties, has the weakest connection to heredity. The researchers who conducted this study stress that environment can shape the development of a child's personality. For example, a child who has not inherited a strong sense of caution or fear (*harm avoidance*) can be taught to avoid taking excessive or unnecessary risks.

The Life Span and Maturity

Although the exact determinants of personality are impossible to define, researchers do know that our personalities are dynamic entities that change as we move through the stage of our lives. In most cases, we learn to control our emotionality as we advance toward adulthood.

The work done by developmental psychologists illustrates the common stages in human development. As previously mentioned, developmental psychologists believe that emotional and spiritual growth depend on the successful completion of developmental tasks at each stage of the life cycle. Failure to meet the demands at each life stage inhibits emotional growth and can result in maladaptive behaviors.

The college years mark a critical transition period for young adults and their parents. During this time, many young adults move away from their families and establish themselves as independent adults. For most students, this step toward maturity entails changing the nature of their relationship with their parents. This transition to independence will be easier for everyone if earlier developmental tasks have been successfully accomplished. These tasks include development of the ability to solve problems, to make and evaluate decisions, to define and adhere to personal values, and to establish both casual and intimate relationships. Management of personal finances, career-management strategies, interpersonal communication skills, and parenting skills (for those who choose to become parents) are also necessary for this stage of life. Parents must accept their children's

greater independence and, in some cases, adjust to being alone after years of family interaction. Older students often have to balance the responsibilities of family, career, and school.

ACHIEVING EMOTIONAL HEALTH

As discussed earlier, emotional health can be defined by our level of self-fulfillment, or self-actualization. Attaining self-fulfillment is a life-long, conscious process that involves building self-esteem, understanding and controlling emotions, and learning to solve problems and make decisions.

Developing and Maintaining Self-Esteem

Self-esteem refers to our sense of self-worth or self-confidence. It can be defined as how much we like ourselves. If we value ourselves, then we feel good about ourselves, and achieving happiness is easier. People with low self-esteem do not like themselves, constantly demean themselves, and doubt their ability to succeed.

The roots of self-esteem are in the relationships we had with our parents when we were children. If we feel loved as children, our emotional growth proceeds smoothly. But is we are denied parental love, we grow to believe we are unworthy of love. The love and support given us by our families can be called upon to help us adjust to problems encountered at all the stages of our lives.

Boosting "I am worthy" feelings takes a little effort for all of us. Our college years present many obstacles to our feelings of worthiness. The new college student may be away from home for the first time, facing anonymity, and finding that "A's" are no longer easy to earn. Study skills developed for high school may not be sufficient for college. The ideas and opinions expressed in college classes may contradict those previously learned. At the same time, we experience pressure to loosen the ties that bind us to our families. We feel we must sever these ties in order to grow up, but we realize that those ties have been an important source of security for our entire lives.

The most important way in which we can maintain our self-esteem is through a support group. At all stages of our lives, we need peers who share our values and can offer us the nurturing that our family can no longer provide. The prime prerequisite for a support group is that it makes us feel good about ourselves.

Another way to boost self-esteem is to prepare for successful completion of required tasks. Success cannot be guaranteed in our course of study if we leave term

---

* Dan Goleman, "The Roots of Personality," *Social Issues Resource Series,* vol. 3, article 60 (1988).

Self-esteem Feeling good and comfortable about oneself; positive self-acceptance.

papers until the last minute, fail to keep up with reading, or hesitate to ask for clarification of points made in a lecture. Most college campuses provide study groups for various content areas. Such groups offer tips for managing time, understanding assignments, dealing with professors, and preparing for test-taking. Poor grades, or grades that do not meet a student's expectations, are major contributors to diminished self-esteem among college students.

Having realistic expectations of yourself is another method of boosting self-esteem. College is a time to explore your potential. The first year is also a time to learn to feel familial love from a distance. The problems inherent in college life are different from those of our earlier years. The additional stress presented by college may make our expectations for success difficult to meet. To expect perfect grades, a steady stream of Saturday-night dates, a good job, and an office in a popular club may be setting yourself up for failure.

Taking time to enjoy yourself is another way to boost self-esteem. For some, participating in a sport improves self-esteem by creating a sense of achievement. For others, meeting a new challenge, such as successfully auditioning for a university play, may improve their self-image.

Maintaining physical health also contributes to self-esteem. Regular exercise fosters a sense of well-being. Nourishing meals can help avoid the weight gain experienced by many college students.

Examining problems and seeking help when needed also boost self-esteem. Meeting and solving problems can be one of life's most satisfying experiences. We do not necessarily have to meet our problems alone. Help can come in the form of a friend, a group, or a mental-health professional.

Understanding and Expressing Emotions

The ability to express and take responsibility for emotions is an important part of achieving and maintaining emotional health. Learning to express our emotions effectively is not easy. Many of us did not learn to express our feelings in healthy ways as we were growing up. In many families, certain emotions are not even discussed. For example, many parents deny the existence of anger. Often, children growing up in such a household never learn to express their anger in healthy ways. Once we learn to understand different emotions, we can develop healthy ways to express them and thereby improve our emotional health.

Researchers have identified four basic categories of emotions: sadness, fear, anger, and joy. The first three of these are related to unmet needs—the needs for love, security, and respect. When we were children, our parents or other adults were responsible for meeting these needs, and we could express our needs easily by crying, screaming, pouting, and hitting others. As adults, however, we are responsible for arranging our lives to meet our own needs. We must learn to understand our

Participating in sports or other group activities is a good way to improve self esteem.

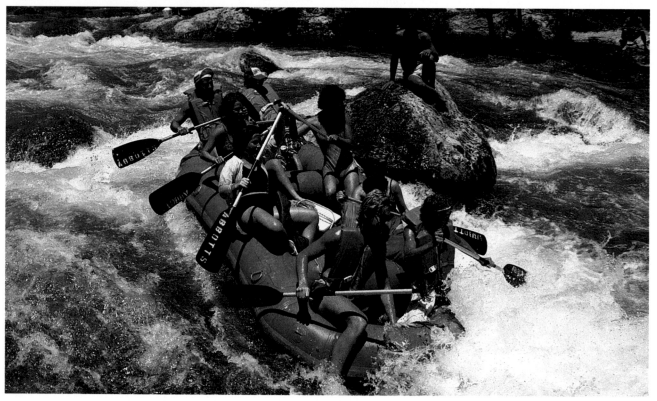

Feeling Better about Yourself

Eight Ways to Boost Your Self-Image

We all get down on ourselves from time to time. It's relatively easy to boost your own self-esteem if you are willing to relax and take the time to do it. Here are some suggestions for boosting your self-esteem.

1. Avoid putting yourself down. Accept compliments with a "thank you" and a smile.

2. Find something you do well. Whether it is writing poetry, sewing, hiking, drawing, singing, or any other activity, work to improve your skills.

3. Give yourself small rewards when you accomplish a task or finish a difficult or boring project.

4. Accept that you cannot be perfect. No one is perfect, and no one goes through life without making some mistakes.

5. Write a list of ten good things about yourself. Keep it in a place where you will see it and be reminded that you have good qualities. Avoid wasting time thinking about your negatives.

6. Look at yourself in the mirror each day. Give yourself a verbal compliment.

7. Keep yourself well-groomed. Maintain a positive attitude. Develop a sense of humor to help make the best of the trying situations we all experience.

8. Participate in activities that involve other people. Service organizations always need volunteers. Colleges usually have informal sports or other activity programs. Find something you like, or start your own group and get involved.

---

emotions in order to recognize needs that are not being met. We must also express our emotions and needs so that they can be understood and respected by others.

Sadness *Sadness* is caused by the loss of something important. Sometimes a loss is obvious; the death of a loved one and the end of a relationship are examples of obvious losses. In other cases, losses are not so obvious—for example, graduation or retirement removes us from a familiar environment and alter roles to which we have become accustomed. In response to sadness, many of us withdraw from the world. When we are sad, we are in need of comfort. Being able to express our feelings of loss can encourage others to provide this comfort.

Fear Feelings of *fear* are signals of danger, and our basic physical response to fear is usually that of "fight or flight." Fear can result in both postive and negative behaviors. It can motivate acts of heroism, such as rescuing an endangered child, as well as acts of prejudice, such as discrimination against AIDS victims. In order to deal with fear, we must reduce the sense of threat or danger. We can cope with many of our fears through education and experience.

Anger *Anger*, which has been called "the misunderstood emotion," is often associated with violence.

When anger is not recognized or is not expressed appropriately, it can result in violence. However, anger can be controlled and used constructively. Anger can be a response to an unmet need for respect. One way to deal with anger is to make your needs clear to others. When you have a need that is not being satisfied, you should express yourself using "I" statements—for example, "I felt angry because I was tired and hungry, and I had to wait an hour to eat dinner."

Joy *Joy*, or happiness, results from our meeting the needs for love, security, and respect. Our degree of happiness can range from a feeling of contentment to a feeling of ecstasy. The capacity to feel joy is as natural as the capacity to feel any of the other emotions. Yet, just as some people have difficulty recognizing their own anger or sadness, others have not learned to recognize or achieve happiness. Children raised in dysfunctional families may not have experienced love, security, and respect. When they reach adulthood, these people may find happiness difficult to achieve.

Problem Solving and Decision Making

We bring our temperaments, our experiences, our memories, and our personalities to problem-solving situations. We also bring a few other characteristics that can either help or hinder us in our pursuit of personal growth. We may practice **intuitive problem solving,** based on feelings or hunches; **creative problem solving,** based on unusual or unique solutions; or **practical problem solving,** based on the black-and-white facts of the particular challenge.

Regardless of our approach, a model for decision making exists. This model follows specific steps but allows for individuality in problem solving or decision making. The model is illustrated in the box entitled "Decision Making: How to Evaluate Your Decisions."

Some of us follow decision-making steps for all our problems. We may not even be aware that we are doing so. For others, the urge to be impulsive is strong. Impulsiveness is not harmful unless it becomes the only problem-solving method followed. At times, an impulsive decision can promote growth, especially if it helps us to have new and enjoyable experiences. However, we need to curb our impulsiveness when it becomes habitual and when our decisions repeatedly turn out to have disappointing results.

As we mature, we learn that very few of our decisions are irrevocable. Unless the decision is life- or health-threatening, we usually can select an alternative if we want to.

Mistakes do happen. We make "wrong" decisions from time to time. The growth that comes with time helps to take the edge off our mistakes. Time and experience teach us not to be devastated by those decisions that do not work out. Part of maturity is learning to pick yourself up, dust yourself off, and continue with your life.

Communication: A Key Element of Emotional Health

As we discussed in Chapter 1, health is a dynamic process of changing and adapting that involves a complex interaction of physical, psychological, spiritual, and social components. Because we do not live in a vacuum and because our daily interactions with others are critical factors in our total health, effective communication is vital to achieving wellness. Whether verbal or nonverbal, written or symbolic, public or private, communication determines the shape and substance of our social lives. It is through the process of communication that we can express our experience of living and gain access to how others feel and function. People who have developed a high degree of communication skill are more effective in their academic or professional pursuits and have the potential for deeper bonds in their personal relationships than noncommunicators.

Perhaps the arena for greatest communication satisfaction is in our close relationships. The messages being sent from us to friends, lovers, partners, and family members are often those that distinguish us as unique individuals. Relaying such information makes us vulnerable to the other person's reception of, and reaction to, information about ourselves. Intimacy develops when two people (1) like the information they hear coming from each other, and (2) can exchange messages easily and effectively. The feeling of "hitting it off" with someone comes from relating well to both the content and process of communication.

Whether we develop effective communication skills that facilitate healthy social interactions depends largely on how we learn to communicate. Parents are perhaps the greatest source of our initial learning patterns in the area of communication. Interaction between parents and their children is often critical in determining whether a child is shy and withdrawn, or outgoing and unafraid of interaction. Parents who teach good communication skills do so by encouraging all family members to express their feelings about situations and circumstances they encounter. They encourage "I" messages rather than "you" messages and reward their children for using these words with comments such as, "I'm glad you told me that. Now let's talk more about it." Nurturing parents listen to their children and allow them to talk about their fears and unhappiness. Children raised in households that foster communication find it easier to talk to others about their disappointments, fears, frustrations, and other emotions later in life. Such individuals often find that they have larger networks of social support and, ultimately, better social and emotional health.

As children grow and mature, their circle of friends, their teachers, and other significant people in their lives foster or inhibit their continued development as skilled communicators. Such interactions contribute to the nature and extent of subsequent communication with significant others in sexual and nonsexual intimate relationships. People who can't talk about their concerns, share their thoughts, or express their feelings about others often find that they are troubled by many interpersonal interactions in their lives. Can you learn to communicate effectively if you have been raised in a family setting where communication was stifled or expressing feelings was frowned upon? Fortunately, the answer is yes. Although it may take time and effort, each of us has the ability to develop new skills, improve old skills, and become socially adept in communicating with others.

UNSOUND ADAPTATIONS TO PROBLEMS

We achieve emotional growth and maturity by actively and successfully confronting and resolving our problems. Because problem solving can cause pain, we may try to avoid facing our problems from time to time.

Intuitive problem solving A method of problem solving that relies on feelings and hunches.
Creative problem solving A method of problem solving that involves uncommonly used responses to problems.
Practical problem solving A problem-solving method that uses only facts.

Decision Making

How to Evaluate Your Decisions

Educated decision making involves using a process based on some type of model for making decisions. The following model is one that might help you evaluate your own decisions. The model will work well for major decisions (where to go to college, whether to return to work full-time, whether to make a major purchase, whether to use a particular drug, whether to commit to a marriage or other type of relationship). Smaller decisions (what to serve for supper, what to wear to work, whom to invite to a party) can be made by using some modification of the model. *Note:* Some people have great difficulty in making *any* kind of decision. They feel inadequate to make the decision or overwhelmed by decision making. These people need to seek appropriate help for their problem.

Step 1: Identify the problem. This may be done orally, in writing, or by just thinking about it.

Step 2: Identify possible solutions to the problem. Again, these may be written, spoken, or thought about. If the decision is a *major* one, writing out the alternative solutions is an excellent way to make them visible. Consider alternative solutions in light of your own value system. (If you do not know your values in a particular area, you need to define those before you begin.)

Step 3: Identify the possible positive and negative outcomes for *each* alternative solution. Again, how do these outcomes relate to your value system?

Step 4: Select the alternative that best meets your needs and values.

Step 5: Evaluate your decision after it has been made. How would you change your decision if you could? What have you learned from this particular decision? How has it contributed to your own mental, emotional, physical, or spiritual growth?

Temporarily avoiding our problems can be healthful in some cases. For example, in facing major decisions, we may need additional time in which to gather facts. In some cases, temporary and deliberate avoidance of an issue can give both the time and breathing space necessary before making crucial decisions. In other cases, putting off dealing with a problem may help us to take care of more pressing business. For example, a student in the last stages of preparing a term paper may be told of a relative's death. That student may deliberately choose to put off grieving for the lost relative until the stress of the paper is removed.

In most cases, though, problem avoidance is not directed or controlled. We may choose to procrastinate indefinitely, hoping our problem will magically disappear. We may also put off facing a difficulty in hopes that someone else will step in and resolve it for us.

Defense Mechanisms

All people use **defense mechanisms** at some point in their lives. Defense mechanisms are behaviors or thought processes that we use to suppress problems so that we do not have to deal with them immediately. People do not usually choose these behaviors consciously. Among the most common are compensation, daydreaming, idealiza-

tion projection, identification, and rationalization. Although we should ideally address problems realistically as soon as they arise, in fact we sometimes need to suppress them until we are better able to confront them. When used in this manner, defense mechanisms can be considered reasonable coping mechanisms. Extensive reliance on these behaviors, however, prevents us from assessing our problems realistically and therefore works against personal growth. For a more detailed description of defense mechanisms, see Table 2.2.

Drug Abuse

When common psychological defense mechanisms fail or seem inadequate, many people turn to external defenses against the pain caused by the various problems in life. The use of alcohol and other drugs to alleviate pain is widespread, as evidenced by the numbers of alcohol- and drug-dependent people in the United States. Although these substances may seem to offer temporary relief from emotional pain, they can lead to long-term drug dependency. Drug and alcohol users may also blame their prob-

---

Defense mechanisms   Behavior used to avoid confronting problems.

Communication

How to Handle Conflicts Constructively

A good way to learn to resolve conflict is to watch your parents fight fair, write Dr. George Bach and Peter Wyden in *The Intimate Enemy: How to Fight Fair in Love and Marriage* (Avon Books). For this reason Dr. Bach encourages parents to argue in front of their children.

That sounds great, but what if your parents *don't* fight fair and aren't a good example? Fortunately our experts' tips can help:

1. "When you feel you're getting ready to blow up, imagine a big red STOP sign in front of your eyes," says Dr. Roger Bach, psychotherapist at the Bach Institute for Group Psychotherapy in Los Angeles. The first step, he says, is to halt your growing rage. This may mean taking a deep breath, or walking away for a few minutes.

2. "Identify your feelings to yourself," says Dr. Robert Hendren. Ask yourself some very important questions: What am I really angry about? Do I have a good reason to be angry with the other person, or have I been looking for an excuse to hurt him or her? Am I picking a fight because I'm in a bad mood? Or am I really mad at someone else but afraid to let that person know?

3. "If you feel you're right to be angry and you need to argue, make sure you choose your time and place carefully," says Dr. Sally Lloyd. Don't try to resolve arguments when you've got five minutes between classes or you're about to eat dinner. You might say, for example, "We're both mad. Let's talk after dinner [or on the phone at nine tonight, if the ongoing argument is outside of the family]."

   Supposing the other person says, "No way! Let's have it out here and now." You might answer, "Look this is too important for both of us to spend only a few minutes on. I think we both need time to talk and listen. And even if you don't feel you need the time, I do."

4. "The single most important thing is to talk—and feel," says Dr. Hendren. You don't have to recite your feelings like a shopping list to get them across. Put some emotion in your voice, says Dr. Hendren. Be firm when you say, for example, "I really need to tell you how I'm feeling about our relationship." The point is, to *express* your feelings without losing control of them.

5. "Once you're talking, stick to one issue at a time. It's too easy to dump on the other person and say everything that's wrong with him or her." For example, if you've been stood up by a friend, tell the person you're mad. But don't use the argument to attack your friend's "big mouth," her lousy choice of clothes, or the time she stole your boyfriend. Those are separate issues, says Dr. Lloyd.

6. "Don't blame or accuse the other person. Use 'I' [put the emphasis on yourself] to get your point across," says the Kentucky Prevention of Family Violence Series curriculum. For example, instead of saying, "You never listen to me," you might say, "I feel I'm not being listened to when I talk."

   By expressing *your* point of view, you make it easier for the other person to express his or hers without feeling threatened.

7. "You may have to repeat your point to get it across," says Dr. George Bach. Fair arguing calls for good communication skills. You may have to say more than once, for example, "I feel like you expect too much from me," or "I hate it when you're late."

8. The secret of fair fighting is arguing not to win but to seek resolutions that work for both of you. You don't have to win—and see the other person lose—to get results. Both parties win if they can keep their self-esteem in a fight and learn something from it, says Dr. Lloyd. For example, you don't have to call your friend names to let him know that it hurts to be stood up. Letting your friend know how you feel can help him change.

9. "Listen carefully to everything the other person has to say. Be prepared to change things about yourself, too," Dr. Roger Bach says. If your friend tells you she is late because she always comes by your house to get you, it may be time to meet halfway between her house and yours.

10. "Once the argument is over you must forgive," says Dr. Hendren. Forgiving is letting go of the anger that sparked the fight. A good last question to ask yourself and the other person is, "Have we gotten everything off our chests?" Then a handshake, or hug, is a good way to end an argument.

Source: *Scholastic Choices* (November 1986), pp. 6–7.

Table 2.2 Defense Mechanisms

This table illustrates various defense mechanisms, along with possible consequences and risks if the behaviors are maintained chronically.

Defense:	**Compensation**—trying to make up for weaknesses in one area by playing up strengths in another area.
Example:	*You and your roommates are planning a party. Everyone is supposed to pitch in and cook. You're a terrible cook, so you volunteer to clean up everything.*
Risk:	You may spend too much time doing only the things you can do. You might not work to overcome your weaknesses or find strength in other areas.
Defense:	**Daydreaming**—a simple imaginary escape from frustrating, boring, or otherwise unpleasant situations.
Example:	You are sitting in your sociology class. The professor is lecturing on her favorite topic. You've heard it all six times before. You tune out and fantasize about going camping.
Risk:	Daydreaming is only a temporary escape. Suppose the professor tests you on this lecture?
Defense:	**Idealization**—admiring someone else to the point that that person becomes perfect and godlike in your eyes despite the person's obvious imperfections.
Example:	Your high-school English teacher was your mentor for three years. You really admire her and have decided to major in English because of her. Your mother sends you a hometown newspaper with headlines declaring your former English teacher to be a child molester. You hotly deny it in phone calls to your parents and friends.
Risk:	When you idealize anyone, you risk being let down when you realize the person is not perfect. Continuous disappointments can lead you to mistrust others.
Defense:	**Identification**—taking on the qualities of someone you admire.
Example:	You meet an older student in the snack bar. He tells you he is studying Zen Buddhism. You like almost everything about him. You start taking courses in Zen, dressing like he does, and following him around.
Risk:	You might lose your own identity in your quest to be like someone else.
Defense:	**Projection**—shifting the responsibility for your behavior onto someone or something else.
Example:	You do poorly on a test for which you did not study. You tell your friends that your roommate kept you up all night telling you about all kinds of problems. If your roommate hadn't kept you up, you would have done better.
Risk:	If you continue to deny responsibility for your behavior, you will hinder personal growth.
Defense:	**Rationalization**—giving seemingly good reasons for your behavior, but the reasons are not the real ones.
Example:	You sneak down to the ice-cream store and wolf down a triple banana split. You say you've earned it because you did 15 extra situps in your aerobics class.
Risk:	Rationalizing only puts off the guilt you would normally feel for such behavior. Rationalizing also keeps you from taking appropriate action to stop potentially unhealthy behaviors.

lems on the substance. "I was drunk" or "I was stoned" are common excuses for inappropriate and irresponsible behavior. For a discussion of addictive behaviors, see Chapter 10.

Suicide

Suicide researchers believe that nearly everyone at one time or another has contemplated self-destruction. There are 25,800 reported suicides each year in the United States. Because of the stigma attached to suicide, many more cases no doubt go unreported. Some researchers believe that the annual suicide rate in the United States exceeds 100,000 per year.

People who commit suicide are convinced that existence is intolerable. They feel cut off from the rest of society, alienated, and isolated. Suicide has been called the final step in a progressive failure to adapt to life's circumstances.

Suicide crosses all social and cultural lines. Suicides among young adults and the elderly have been rising steadily during the past decade (see Figure 2.2). Each year a reported 5,000 people between the ages of 15 and 24 take their own lives. Suicide is the second leading cause of death among teenagers and young adults. Each day, over 1,000 people in this age group attempt to destroy themselves. For every one who succeeds, 100 more will try and fail. Self-destruction is also a problem among the elderly. Each year, 10,000 Americans over the age of 60 kill themselves. In many cases, suicide among the elderly is a reaction to the aging process, personal loss, or catastrophic illness.

Who commits suicide? There are certain risk factors that make some of us more susceptible to suicide. Among these risk factors are previous suicide attempts, family history of suicide, drug abuse, clinical depression, marital stress, financial problems, catastrophic illness, and recent bereavement. People with multiple risk factors are more likely to commit suicide than are those with only single risk factors. Members of certain groups that feel alienated, disenfranchised, and frustrated also seem to be more susceptible to suicide.

Promoting Your Health

Suicide Symptoms

Most people who commit suicide give warnings about their intentions. In many cases, people who attempt suicide are asking for help, and they warn others in the hope that someone will hear them and rescue them. The following list of symptoms and hints may help you recognize suicidal intentions in a friend or an acquaintance.

1. Making a direct statement about killing oneself. An example might be, "I can't take it. I don't want to live anymore."

2. Making an indirect statement, such as "Soon this pain will be over," or "I wonder where my father hides his gun."

3. Making "final preparations," such as writing a will, repairing poor relationships with friends or relatives, giving away treasured possessions, or writing long-overdue letters.

4. Showing a preoccupation with themes of death.

5. Withdrawing from friends and family and from activities that were once pleasurable.

6. Demonstrating a rapid and unexplained feeling of happiness or elation following a period of depression. (Sometimes the decision to commit suicide relieves depression and leads to an improved mood.)

If Someone You Know Threatens Suicide

1. Be aware of the danger signs.

2. Believe any threats.

3. Form a relationship; let the person know you care.

4. Listen. Try not to be shocked by what the person says to you.

5. Ask directly: "Are you thinking of hurting or killing yourself?"

6. Do not belittle the person's feelings. Saying "You don't really mean that" often alienates the potential suicide even more.

7. Help the person explore alternatives.

8. Get help. Call your local suicide hotline. If there is none available, call the person's physician, clergy, or the police.

9. Do not leave the suicidal person alone. You may have to transport the person to an emergency room. Remember that all relationships entail responsibilities. Stay with the person until professional help has taken over.

If the person does commit suicide, you will probably feel guilty. It may be difficult for you to realize that the suicide was not your fault, and you may need short-term counseling to help you work through your feelings. Some communities offer support groups for families and friends of people who commit suicide.

Figure 2.2 Changes in suicide rates among young adults and the elderly, 1981–1989.

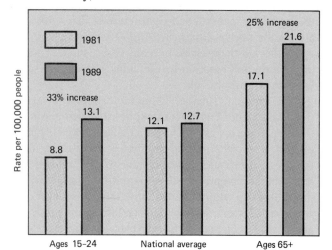

Changes in suicide rates among young adults and the elderly, 1981–1989

The growing incidence of suicide indicates that most of us will be touched by a suicide at some time in our lives. In most cases, the suicide does not occur suddenly or unpredictably. In fact, between 70 and 75 percent of suicides give a warning of their intentions before they kill themselves. Therefore, we must learn to recognize the presuicidal symptoms and find the appropriate help. See the box entitled "Suicide Symptoms" for information on helping to prevent suicide.

▌ MENTAL ILLNESS

The term *mentally ill* is frightening to many people. Movies, books, and magazines often depict mental illness in frightening ways. In some cases, people suffering from a mental illness do act unpredictably or even dan-

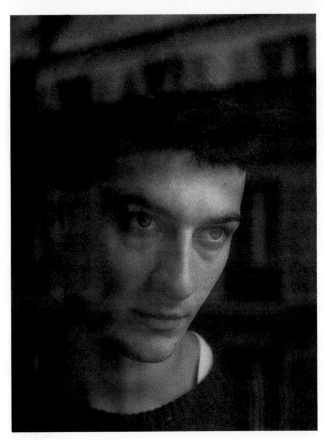
Mental illnesses must be recognized and treated like other diseases.

gerously. In many cases, however, people with mental-health problems are able to function in society. With proper diagnosis and treatment, most of the symptoms of mental disorders can be controlled.

It is tempting to distinguish ourselves from people with mental-health problems. However, there is often a fine line between mental health and mental illness. It is important to understand that mental-health problems vary in their severity. For example, many of us have suffered from various levels of anxiety or depression. Others have suffered from serious mental disorders with biological origins, such as schizophrenia. Education about mental illness is vital for those with mental-health problems as well as for their friends and family.

Obsessive-Compulsive Disorders

Approximately 5 million Americans suffer from obsessive-compulsive disorders. An **obsessive-compulsive disorder** is an illness in which people have obsessive thoughts or perform habitual behaviors that they cannot control. People with *obsessions* often have recurring ideas or thoughts that they cannot control. People with *compulsions* feel forced to engage in a repetitive behavior, almost as if the behavior controls them. Continual handwashing, counting to a certain number while using the toilet, and checking and rechecking all the light

switches in the house before leaving or going to bed are examples of compulsive behaviors. Some compulsive behaviors that are more harmful include pulling out one's hair and other forms of self-mutilation.

The causes of obsessive-compulsive disorders are difficult to isolate. Some theorists believe that sufferers engage in compulsive behaviors to distract themselves from more pressing problems. Until recently, behavioral therapy, which focuses on controlling and changing behaviors, has been the common treatment for sufferers of obsessive-compulsive disorders. However, research now indicates that some of these disorders may be caused by a lack of the neurotransmitter *serotonin* in the limbic system. In early 1990, a drug called clomipramine (Anafranil) was released for prescription use in the United States. Researchers believe that clomipramine alters the way serotonin is used in the brain. When used in conjunction with behavioral therapy, this drug has been found to be helpful in alleviating symptoms of obsessive-compulsive disorder.

Anxiety Disorders

Between 20 and 30 million Americans suffer from panic and anxiety disorders. **Anxiety disorders** are characterized by fatigue, back pains, headaches, feelings of unreality, the sensation of weakness in the legs, and fear of losing control. *Generalized anxiety disorders* last for more than 6 months and typically result in unrealistic and excessive worry about two or more personal problems. Other types of anxiety disorders include phobias, panic attacks, and posttraumatic stress disorder.

A **phobia** is a deep and persistent fear of a specific object, activity, or situation that results in a compelling desire to avoid the source of the fear. Experts estimate that 1 out of 8 American adults suffers from phobias. Phobias are also thought to be more prevalent in women than in men.*

Simple phobias, such as fear of animals (spiders and snakes, for example), fear of flying, and fear of heights, can be treated successfully through behavioral therapy. *Social phobias,* fears that are related to interaction with others, such as fear of public speaking, fear of inadequate sexual performance, and fear of eating in public places, are not as easily treated and require more extensive therapy.

Obsessive-compulsive disorder   A disorder characterized by obsessive thoughts or habitual behaviors that cannot be controlled.
Anxiety disorders   Disorders characterized by fatigue, back pains, headaches, feelings of unreality, and a fear of losing control.
Phobia   A deep and persistent fear of a specific object, activity, or situation.

* Michael S. Gazzaniga, *Mind Matters: How Mind and Brain Interact to Create Our Conscious Lives* (Boston: Houghton Mifflin, 1988), pp. 101–2.

Community Health

Characteristics of Good Communicators

Good communicators are interpersonally aware. When talking with other people, they create feelings of intimacy and fellowship. Without these elements, interpersonal contacts are strained and unsatisfying.

Good communicators are assertive without being aggressive or manipulative. They can accurately and honestly describe their feelings and contribute to conversations and to any resulting decisions. They avoid passivity. If they experience doubts and confusion, they express them rather than dropping out of a conversation. Good communicators share their ideas and opinions without imposing them on others. Their interest in conversations goes beyond themselves. They want to get to know other people and go about this by listening and sharing.

Good communicators are sincere. They focus on the conversation, not on their thoughts about unrelated matters. Good communicators do not say things they do not mean or make promises they cannot keep.

Finally, good communicators are sensitive to the needs of those with whom they communicate. During a conversation, good communicators respond in ways that encourage the speaker: by smiling, laughing, nodding, agreeing, or disagreeing at appropriate times to assure the speaker that he or she is being heard. Furthermore, although honesty is desirable, good communicators appreciate the fine distinction between honesty and total candor. The person who advocates absolute frankness, with no respect for the feelings and thoughts of others, is interpersonally naive.

A phobic's typical reaction is one of intense anxiety, with symptoms such as sweating and dizziness. Researchers believe that these reactions are triggered by certain memories. For example, a person may develop *agoraphobia*, the fear of crowded and public places, as a result of a negative experience that involved or took place in a crowded room. Thereafter, the agoraphobic suffers anxiety in any crowded situation.

A **panic attack** is the sudden, rapid onset of disabling terror. Its symptoms include shortness of breath, dizziness, sweating, shaking, choking, trembling, and heart palpitations. A victim of a panic attack may feel that he or she is having a heart attack.

Panic attacks occur spontaneously and have no obvious link to environmental stimuli. This factor distinguishes them from the natural fear reaction that occurs when we feel threatened by a real danger. Researchers believe that panic attacks are caused by some physiological change or biochemical imbalance in the brain and are still searching for the events that trigger such attacks.

One newly recognized anxiety disorder is **posttraumatic stress disorder.** This syndrome afflicts victims of severely stressful situations such as rape, assault, war, or airplane crashes. Victims suffer terrifying flashbacks in which they relive the traumatic situation.

When correctly diagnosed, anxiety disorders are treatable, usually through a combination of methods. Because undiagnosed diabetes, heart conditions, and endocrine disorders can mimic anxiety disorders, doctors recommend a thorough physical examination to rule out organic causes. When the causes are not physical, treatment usually consists of psychotherapy combined with some type of medication.

Depression

Depression is the most common emotional disorder in the United States. One out of 5 of us will suffer depression at some time in our lives. For reasons that are not well understood, two-thirds of all depressives are women. Three main theories exist to account for this phenomenon. The first is that women seek help for problems more frequently than men. Although this may be true, critics of this theory point out that community studies that measure the number of depressed people based on survey data, whether these people have applied for help or not, also report more female than male depressives. Maggie Scarf of Yale University is among those who consider this theory inadequate. She, along with the late Marcia Guttentag of Harvard University, believes that women are inherently more sensitized to personal losses, particularly losses in relationships. Pointing out that women in the same phase of life were

Panic attack   The sudden, rapid onset of disabling terror.
Posttraumatic stress disorder   An anxiety disorder that affects victims of severely stressful situations.

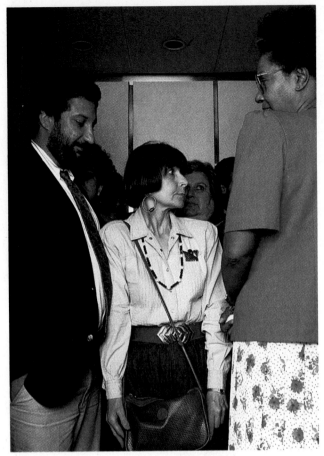
Anxiety disorders affect between 20 and 30 million Americans.

activities, loss of interest in work, diminished or increased appetite, unexplainable fatigue, sleep disorders, including insomnia or early-morning (3 A.M.) awakenings, loss of sex drive, withdrawal from friends and family, feelings of hopelessness and worthlessness, and a desire to die. Depressed people often will not be able to get out of bed in the morning. If they do arise, they may not be able to leave the house and may return to bed.

Depressed people usually suffer from low self-esteem. They often feel alone, separated from and unable to communicate with others. After a while, depression becomes a habit. The feelings of helplessness and entrapment offer no way out. Depressed people may feel their depression is a deserved punishment for real or imagined failings. A person whose self-image has slipped into the realm of utter worthlessness may see suicide as the only way out.

Treating Depression   Depression is not a single condition that can always be treated in the same manner. Rather, different types of treatment are effective for different subtypes of depression. Securing the best treatment involves targeting the type and degree of depression and possible causes.

In many cases, both psychotherapeutic and pharmacological (drug) modes of treatment are recommended. Clinical depression often requires drug therapy. Experts agree, however, that clinicians who rely exclusively on either pharmacological or psychological forms of therapy are not acting in the client's best interest. Drugs are often used to relieve the symptoms of depression such as loss of sleep or appetite, whereas psychotherapy is most helpful in improving social and interpersonal functioning. The treatment may be weighted more toward drugs or psychotherapy depending on the specific situation. In some cases, psychotherapy alone may be the most successful treatment. Psychotherapists in combination with psychiatrists can best make the decisions regarding treatment.

Antidepressant drugs are credited with much success in treating chronic depression. These drugs can help to relieve symptoms in nearly 80 percent of chronic depressives. Several types of antidepressant drugs, known as *tricyclics,* are available for use with chronic depressives. They work by preventing the excessive reuptake of mood-lifting neurotransmitters. Antidepressant drugs can take from 6 weeks to 3 months to become effective. Newer drugs called *tetracyclics* that work in 1 or 2 weeks are also being prescribed.

Electroconvulsive therapy (ECT) is another method of treating depression. A patient given ECT is sedated under light general anesthesia. Electric current is then

depressed about similar sorts of things, Scarf and Guttentag theorized that biological and environmental conditions account for higher rates of depression among women. A third theory, proposed by Phyllis Chesler in her book *Women and Madness,* argues that women are diagnosed as depressed more often simply because it is more socially acceptable for women to be labeled depressed. She believes that men often are not diagnosed as depressed, but rather as "under pressure," "burned out," or "strained."

Two acknowledged forms of depression exist: endogenous and exogenous depression. **Endogenous depression** is of biochemical origin. Neurotransmitters in the brain, those responsible for mood elevation, become unbalanced for unknown reasons. A corresponding decrease in these neurotransmitters gives rise to outward expressions of depression. If not treated, endogenous depression may become ongoing.

Exogenous depression is usually caused by an external event such as the loss of something or someone of great value. Victims of exogenous depression can slide into endogenous depression if they are not able to work through the grieving process necessary for overcoming event-related depression.

Symptoms of both types of depression are similar: lingering sadness, inability to find joy in pleasure-giving

---

Endogenous depression   A type of depression that has a physiological basis, such as a hormonal imbalance.

Exogenous depression   A type of depression that has an external cause, such as the loss of a loved one.

applied to the temples for 5 seconds. The patient's limbs jerk mildly. The entire process takes about 15 to 20 minutes. Between 10 and 20 percent of depressives who do not respond to drug therapy are responsive to ECT. One major risk is that of permanent memory loss. Some therapists do not recommend the use of ECT under any circumstances.

Depression clinics have been established in large metropolitan areas to offer group support for depressed people. Clinics and support groups can treat all types of depressed people or restrict themselves to specific groups, such as widows, adolescents, or families and friends of depressives.

Manic-Depressive Mood Disorder

Endogenous and exogenous depressions are sometimes called *unipolar depressions* because their victims suffer depression only. Conversely, victims of **manic-depressive mood disorder** suffer from violent mood swings. Manic-depressives may be energetic, creative, vivacious, and "happy" for a time and then become severely depressed. Thus, the characteristic mania of happiness followed by the melancholy of depression classifies the disorder as a *bipolar* affliction. Between 10 and 15 percent of the total American population is afflicted with manic-depressive mood disorders.

Manic-depressive disturbances are apparently caused by chemical imbalances of unknown origins within the brain. The antidepressants used to regulate unipolar depressions have no effect upon bipolar depressions. Medications containing **lithium** and related minerals are used in combination with psychotherapy to treat such disorders.

Bipolar mood disorders are known to have hereditary components, but they may be event-related as well. Some victims have low self-esteem. A major problem experienced with treatment of the disorder stems from the patient's actually liking the manic stage. When manic, the person has high energy and creativity and increased capacity for accomplishing major tasks such as artistic or musical endeavors. The depressive phase throws the person into the same inactivity seen in unipolar depression. Drug therapy serves to level out the manic-depressive's moods. The patient does not experience depression but also does not experience the "high" feeling of the mania. Some manic-depressives feel uncomfortable with the lack of mania. They feel an important source of energy has been lost, and they may feel bored. Some go off their medication in order to stop the feelings of stagnation. As soon as the medication is stopped, the bipolar swings resume, and the victim is forced to make a choice between medication and mood swings.

Seasonal Affective Disorder

In 1987, the American Psychiatric Association recognized seasonal affective disorder as a type of depression.

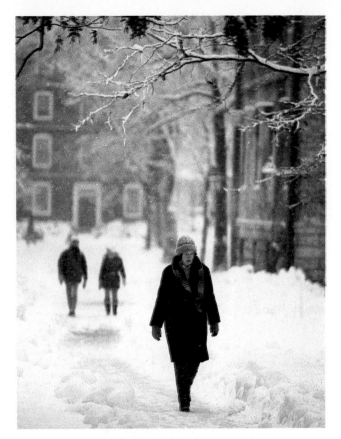

Seasonal affective disorder is a type of depression that affects some people during the winter months, when there is limited sunlight.

Seasonal affective disorder (SAD) occurs during the winter months, primarily from December through March, and is associated with reduced exposure to sunlight. People with this disorder suffer the typical symptoms of depression, including loss of desire to work or to participate in activities, loss of appetite, fatigue, and lingering sadness.

Researchers believe that the disorder is related to a malfunction in the hypothalamus, the gland responsible for regulating responses to external stimuli. In the winter, when sunlight levels are lower, the hypothalamus may be affected by chemical imbalances that affect mood. Stress is also a contributing factor. People under severe stress during the winter have an increased risk of developing SAD.

An estimated 6 percent of the U.S. population suffer from SAD, and an additional 14 percent suffer from a milder form of the disorder known as the "winter blues." Many types of people are vulnerable to SAD. Women are four times more susceptible to SAD than are men. Al-

Manic-depressive mood disorder A disorder in which frantic high mood states alternate with suicidally low states.

Lithium An element used in drugs to control manic-depressive mood disorders.

Seasonal affective disorder (SAD) A type of depression that occurs in the winter months, when sunlight levels are low.

though the disorder occurs in people of all ages, people aged 20 to 40 appear to be the most vulnerable. The disorder also tends to run in families.

People living in northern latitudes are more susceptible to the disorder than are those living in southern areas. During the winter, there are fewer hours of sunlight in northern regions than in southern areas. An estimated 10 percent of the population in northern states, such as Maine, Minnesota, and Wisconsin, experience SAD, whereas less than 2 percent of those living in southern areas, such as Florida and New Mexico, suffer from the disorder.

Effective therapies for sufferers of SAD do exist. The most beneficial appears to be light therapy, in which a patient uses special lighting equipment that mimics sunlight through the use of *broad-spectrum* lighting. These lighting units generate light rays from all colors of the spectrum. The patient is exposed to this light for a certain amount of time each day. Eighty percent of patients experience relief from their symptoms within 4 days of beginning treatment.

Other forms of treatment include dietary changes (eating foods high in complex carbohydrates), exercise, stress-management techniques, sleep restriction (limiting the number of hours slept in a 24-hour period), psychotherapy, and use of antidepressant medications.

Schizophrenia

Perhaps the most frightening of all mental disorders is **schizophrenia,** a disease that affects about 1 percent of the U.S. population. Schizophrenia is characterized by alterations of the senses (including visual and auditory hallucinations), the inability to sort out incoming stimuli and make appropriate responses, an altered sense of self, and radical changes in emotions, movements, and behaviors. Victims of this disease often cannot function in society.

For decades, scientists considered schizophrenia to be an environmentally produced form of madness. Since the mid-1980s, however, scientists have studied schizophrenia more thoroughly, using computerized technologies such as magnetic resonance imaging (MRI) and positron emission tomography (PET). It is now recognized as a disease of the brain, with biological origins.

Schizophrenia primarily affects the limbic system, its connections, and its attendant neurotransmitters. The disease tends to run in families, although no specific carrier gene has been identified. It is also evident that the brain damage involved occurs very early in life, possibly as early as the second trimester of pregnancy. However, the disease most commonly has its onset in late adolescence.

Post-mortem examinations performed on brains of schizophrenics show abnormal development of the hippocampus. The hippocampus in the brain of a schizophrenic is smaller and differently shaped than the hippo-

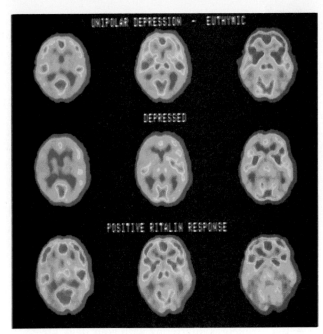

A bipolar PET scan, which detects whether different parts of the brain are functioning properly.

campus in a normal brain. These differences in brain structure are thought to contribute to the chemical aberrations that cause the symptoms of the disease.

Schizophrenia was once attributed to abnormal family interaction or to early childhood traumas. However, these theories have been discarded in favor of biological theories. Nonetheless, a stigma remains attached to the disease.

Schizophrenia is treatable but not curable. Depending on the severity of the symptoms, treatments include some combination of hospitalization, medication, and supportive psychotherapy. Supportive psychotherapy, as opposed to psychoanalysis, helps the patient acquire skills for living in society.

Families of schizophrenics often experience anger and guilt associated with misunderstandings about the causes of the disease. They often need help in the form of information, family counseling, and methods of meeting the schizophrenic's needs for shelter, medical care, vocational training, and social interaction.

SEEKING PROFESSIONAL HELP

Many of us feel that seeking professional help for emotional problems is an admission of failure in our personal lives. Typically, any physical health problem, such as an abscessed tooth or prolonged severe pain, sends us to the

Schizophrenia A mental illness with biological origins that is characterized by irrational behavior, severe alteration of senses (hallucinations), and, often, an inability to function in society.

nearest dentist or physician. Emotional problems, on the other hand, tend to be ignored until they pose a serious threat to our well-being. Even then, we may not seek the help we need.

Despite this tradition, an increasing number of Americans are turning to mental-health professionals for help with emotional problems. Researchers believe that more people are seeking help today because of the hazards associated with "normal" living. Breakdown in support systems, high expectations of society, and dysfunctional family units are cited as the 3 major reasons for seeking assistance.

Successful work with a mental-health professional can be a rewarding and beneficial experience. You should consider seeking help under the following circumstances.

- If you think you need help
- If you experience wild and drastic mood swings
- If a problem is interfering with your daily life
- If your fears or feelings of guilt are beginning to distract your attention
- If you begin to isolate and withdraw yourself from others
- If you have hallucinations
- If you have feelings that life is not worth living
- If you feel inadequate or worthless

One way to cope with emotional or mental health problems is through group therapy.

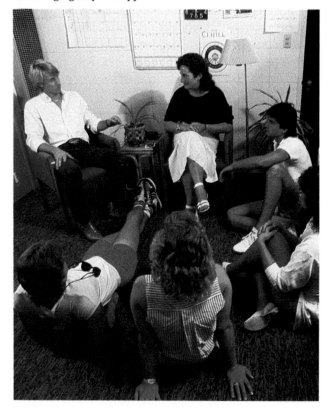

- If your emotional responses are inappropriate to various situations
- If daily life seems to be nothing but repeated crises
- If you feel you can't "get your act together" at all
- If you are seriously considering suicide
- If you turn to drugs or alcohol to escape from your problems.

Types of Mental-Health Professionals

Several types of mental-health professionals are available. The most important aspect of finding a provider is whether you feel you can work well with that particular person, not how many degrees the provider has.

Psychiatrist   A **psychiatrist** is a medical doctor. After obtaining the M.D. degree, the psychiatrist spends up to 12 years studying psychological health and disease. As a licensed physician, a psychiatrist can prescribe medications for various mental or emotional problems.

Psychoanalyst   A **psychoanalyst** is a psychiatrist with special training in psychoanalysis. *Psychoanalysis* is a type of therapy that can take two or more sessions per week for several years. The patient is helped to remember early traumas that have blocked personal growth.

Psychologist   A **psychologist** usually has a Ph.D. degree in counseling or clinical psychology. This degree requires approximately 8 to 10 years of college work. In addition, many states require licensure. Psychologists are trained in various types of talk therapy. Most psychologists are trained to conduct both individual and group counseling. Psychologists may also be trained in family counseling, sexual counseling, or types of counseling related to compulsive behaviors.

Social Worker   A **social worker** with a master's degree in social work (M.S.W.) can counsel patients with emotional problems. Some social workers work in clinical settings, whereas others have private practices. A registered clinical social worker (R.C.S.W.) often works in private practice, and patients are eligible to receive insurance reimbursement.

Counselor   Persons with a variety of academic and experiential training call themselves counselors and do professional counseling. Often the **counselor** will have a

---

Psychiatrist   A licensed physician with specialization in treating emotional disorders.

Psychoanalyst   A psychiatrist with special training in psychoanalysis.

Psychologist   A person with a Ph.D. degree and training in techniques for treating emotional disorders.

Social worker   A person with a M.S.W. degree who counsels patients with emotional problems.

Counselor   A person with an M.S. degree in the treatment of emotional disorders.

master's degree in counseling, psychology, educational psychology, or a related human service. Professional societies recommend at least 2 years of graduate coursework or supervised practice as a minimal requirement. Many are trained to do individual and group counseling. Often they specialize in the type of counseling they provide, such as family, marital, relationship, children, drug, divorce, behavioral, and personal.

Some health and health-education professionals possess counseling skills. In many settings where behavioral change is desired, these individuals can be of assistance.

As with the selection of any service, the credentials, desired outcomes, and expectations of both the counselor and the client should be considered before treatment begins.

Types of Therapy

Over 250 types of **therapy** exist, ranging from "traditional" individual and group therapy to "soap-opera therapy" or "past-lives therapy." Freudian psychoanalysis is probably the best known, yet it is no longer practiced as widely as it once was.

Traditional psychoanalysis requires from 2 to 5 sessions weekly for 2 to 15 years. Because of the extended time involved, many Americans are rejecting psychoanalysis in favor of short-term therapies. In these arrangements, the client meets the provider for 1 to 20 sessions. The provider gives support and helps the client find positive coping devices while keeping time and finances to a minimum. The 4 most popular types of therapy are behavioral, cognitive, family, and psychodynamic.

Behavioral Therapy   Disorders such as compulsions, phobias, and obsessive thinking are types of problems most responsive to **behavioral therapy**. These types of behaviors are learned. Because learning involves chemical and physical changes in the brain, the only way to treat behavioral disorders is through relearning.

Behavioral therapists first ask the client to define the behavior that must be changed. Clients are then required to monitor old behaviors as they substitute new ones. A system of client-made charts to monitor progress, along with a program of rewards and punishments, helps the client make the desired changes. Clients may also be taught methods of deep relaxation and various mind-stopping techniques. Behavioral therapy usually takes from 16 to 17 weeks.

Cognitive Therapy   Cognitive therapists believe that what we feel is a reaction not to the world around us, but rather to our thoughts about what happens. In **cognitive therapy**, the client is taught to recognize and prevent the thoughts and beliefs that stifle growth. For example, a client who feels miserable about a poor test grade will be taught how to prevent these miserable feelings from regressing into an "I don't deserve to live" attitude.

Those who benefit most from this type of therapy are usually bright, verbal people. Cognitive therapists often use humor to refute the client's negative self-feelings. The duration of the therapy is usually 1 session a week for 6 months.

Family Therapy   **Family therapy** focuses on the problems of the entire family system rather than those of one individual. In family therapy sessions, the members of a family play out the dynamics of their relationships. Each member of the family is held accountable for his or her treatment of the others.

Length of therapy is determined by the severity of the problem. For example, a stepfamily attempting to clarify some issues of living together or trying to improve communications might need only 2 or 3 sessions. For more severe problems, therapy must last up to a year. Sessions are often 1½ to 3 hours long. Fees vary according to the qualifications of the therapist and the length of the sessions.

Psychodynamic Therapy   **Psychodynamic therapy** helps the client to scrutinize feelings and memories. The therapist assists the client to unearth and react to repressed memories. The client's reactions can include crying, screaming, and ranting. The client is then helped to understand the experiences and memories. Psychodynamic therapists believe that facing problems and reactions on an intellectual level frees the client from emotional blocks that create maladaptive behaviors. Therapy of this type usually consists of 1 session a week for 1 to 2 years.

What to Expect When You Begin Therapy

The first trip to a therapist can be extremely difficult. Most of us have misconceptions about what therapy is and about what it can do. That first visit is a verbal or mental "sizing up" of each other. You will not accomplish much in the first hour. If you decide that the therapist is not for you, you will at least have learned how to present your problem and what qualities you need in a therapist.

Therapy   Treatment designed to help overcome personal problems.

Behavioral therapy   Therapy aimed at teaching a person to change unwanted behaviors through a system of rewards and punishments.

Cognitive therapy   Therapy aimed at teaching a person to recognize and refute the beliefs that hinder personal growth.

Family therapy   Therapy that focuses on the problems of an entire family system rather than those of one individual.

Psychodynamic therapy   Therapy that allows a person to express emotions dramatically; release comes through catharsis.

1. Before going, *briefly* explain your needs to the therapist or reservations secretary. Ask what the fee is ahead of time. Arrive on time. Wear clothing in which you are comfortable. Expect to spend between 50 and 60 minutes on your first visit.

2. Your therapist will want to take down a history and details on the particular problem or problems that have brought you to therapy. Answer as honestly as possible. Many therapists will ask you how you *feel* about particular things in your life. Do not be ashamed or embarrassed to acknowledge your feelings.

3. Therapists are not mind readers. They cannot tell what you are thinking. Therefore, it is critical to the success of your treatment that you build trust in your therapist.

4. Do not expect the therapist to tell you what to do and how to behave. Very few hand out behavioral prescriptions for their clients.

5. Find out if the therapist will allow you to set your own therapeutic goals and timetables if you wish.

Also, find out if, later in therapy, your therapist will allow you to determine what is and what is not helping you.

6. If, after your first visit (or even after several visits), you feel you cannot work with a particular therapist, you must summon the courage to say so. Do not worry about hurting the therapist's feelings. If there is a personality conflict, or if you do not feel comfortable with a particular person, then therapy will not be effective.

Some of us may believe that our problems are not serious enough to warrant sessions with a mental-health professional. We may decide to heal ourselves with the help of a few good books and a few good friends. Whether we choose to seek professional help or to work out our problems ourselves, we must learn to be open to the advice of others and must take steps to change our behavior and improve our self-esteem. Like physical wounds, emotional wounds can heal with time and proper attention.

▌ SUMMARY

- Emotional health is a dynamic state. Emotionally healthy people deliberately and purposefully devote themselves to facing and adapting to the realities of life.

- Our personalities are the outward expression of how we view life and how our emotions affect our behaviors.

- Personality has four characteristics: emotionality, sociability, level of activity, and impulsiveness.

- There are several ways to maintain self-esteem, including setting realistic expectations, establishing a support group, preparing for successful completion of tasks, enjoying oneself, proper nutrition, and exercise.

- The emotions of sadness, fear, and anger are related to the unmet needs for love, security, and respect. Joy, or happiness, is the emotion that results from meeting those needs.

- Decision making is a five-step process involving identifying the problem, identifying possible solutions, iden-

tifying positive and negative outcomes, selecting alternatives, and evaluating the decision.

- We sometimes choose to avoid resolving problems. In some cases, this avoidance can lead to unsound adaptations to problems, including drug abuse and suicide.

- Some mental illnesses, such as obsessive-compulsive disorders, anxiety disorders, and depression, can vary in severity and can be treated with some combination of therapy and medication. Other mental illnesses are related primarily to biochemical imbalances in the brain. These illnesses include manic-depressive mood disorder, seasonal affective disorder, and schizophrenia.

- When professional help is needed, several types of practitioners are available, including psychiatrists, psychoanalysts, psychologists, counselors, social workers, and pastoral counselors.

3

Stress: The Inevitable Reaction

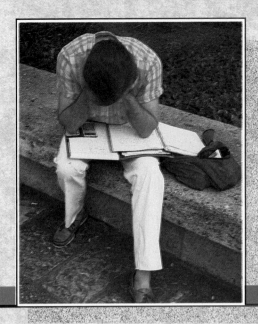

Chapter Outline

- The Dimensions of Stress
- Factors Influencing the Stress Response
- Stress and Special Populations
- Recognition and Assessment of Distress
- Managing Our Reactions to Distress
- Stress and the Consumer

Objectives

- Define "stress" and discuss the connection that exists between mind and body in physiological responses to stress.

- Explain how the psychological and emotional factors that make up the cognitive stress system influence our response to stress.

- Discuss the different effects stress may have on people at different points in their lives and explain why stress is often called the "disease of prolonged arousal."

- Recognize and assess the symptoms of distress.

- Take specific mental and physical action to manage stress and, ultimately, any threats of stress that might arise in your life from day to day.

- Evaluate and judge for yourself the effectiveness of various commercial methods available for the reduction of stress.

S tress is a phenomenon that is almost impossible to live without, although we have difficulty living with it. We are bombarded by a host of subtle and not so subtle internal and external stresses from the moment we awake in the morning until we finally drift into deep sleep at day's end. Even during our sleeping moments, noise, temperature changes, and other activities can be sources of stress. Rarely does a day go by without someone you know talking about being under stress from homework, financial pressures, relationship demands, or other dilemmas. In spite of our best efforts to ignore it, stress cannot be run from, hidden from, or wished away. For some people, stress provides the stimulus for growth and higher levels of achievement. For others, stress increases the likelihood of dysfunctional or abnormal behavior or illness. Although much has been written about stress in contemporary society, understanding the complex physiological and psychological reactions to stress is no easy task. According to Hans Selye, a noted Canadian researcher, "Stress is a scientific concept which has suffered from the mixed blessing of being too well known and too little understood."* What is stress? Why are some people more susceptible to stress than others? What can be done to reduce the negative consequences of stress?

Stress and stressful situations are discussed in virtually every popular periodical. After a time, we may begin to see stress as an adversary against which we must struggle in a never-ending battle. But stress in itself is neither positive nor negative. Rather, our personal reactions to stress can be positive or negative. Whether we are aware of it or not, our reactions to stress can become the habits that lead us either to health-enhancing personal growth or to debilitation in the form of migraines, alcohol and drug addiction, circulatory disorders, asthma, gastrointestinal problems, and hypertension (high blood pressure). In addition, stress can lead to psychological and social problems, including dysfunctional relationships.

THE DIMENSIONS OF STRESS

Multiple factors contribute to stress and our stress responses, including physiological reactions, psychological factors, environmental distressors, and social factors. Each of these elements influences our stress responses in different ways, depending on the stressful circumstances, our general health, our personal health habits, our psychological state, our personality, our attitudes, and the quality of our support system. Thus, responses vary considerably from one person to another. (See Figure 3.1.)

In defining **stress,** we can see many different dimensions of the stress response. The definition of stress has three main components. First, stress is represented by *external* factors that place a demand on our minds and bodies. Second, stress is the *internal* state of emotional tension or arousal that occurs in response to the various demands of living. Finally, stress is represented by the *physiological responses* or *reactions* to the demands placed upon us.** Another way to look at stress is to view it as the mental and physical responses of our bodies to any type of change in our lives.

A **stressor** is any physical, social, or psychological event or condition that triggers a stress reaction. Stressors may be tangible, such as an angry boss or a disgruntled roommate, or indiscernible, like the emotions associated with anticipation or imagination. Our response to stressors causes **strain** to develop in our lives. Strain results from the wear and tear our minds and bodies sustain during the process of resisting or coping with the stressors in our lives.

Stress and strain are associated with most of our daily activities. Generally, stress that presents the opportunity for personal growth and satisfaction is called **eustress.** Included here are such events as getting married, starting school, beginning a career, developing new relationships, and learning a new physical skill. **Distress** is caused by those events that result in debilitative stress and strain, such as financial problems, injury or illness, the death of a loved one, trouble at work, poor grades, and the breakup of a relationship.

In many cases, we cannot prevent the occurrence of distressors. Like eustressors, they are part of life. However, we can train ourselves to recognize distressors and to anticipate the reactions we have to them. We can learn to practice prestress coping skills and to develop poststress management techniques. Development of both types of skills depends on our understanding of the major components of stress.

The Mind-Body Connection: Physiological Responses

All living organisms have innate mechanisms that regulate activity levels and keep physiological functioning in

---

Stress The mental and physical responses our bodies experience in response to any type of change.

Stressor An event or condition that triggers a stress response.

Strain The results of the wear and tear our bodies sustain as we resist or cope with the stressors in our lives.

Eustress Stress the presents positive opportunities for personal growth.

Distress Stress that can have a negative or debilitative effect on health.

---

* Hans Selye, "The Stress Concept Today," in I. Kutash et al., eds., *The Handbook on Stress and Anxiety* (San Francisco: Jossey-Bass, 1989), p. 27.

** Phillip L. Rice, *Stress and Health* (Monterey, Calif: Brooks/ Cole, 1992).

Figure 3.1 Selected Factors That May Contribute to Our Stress Response

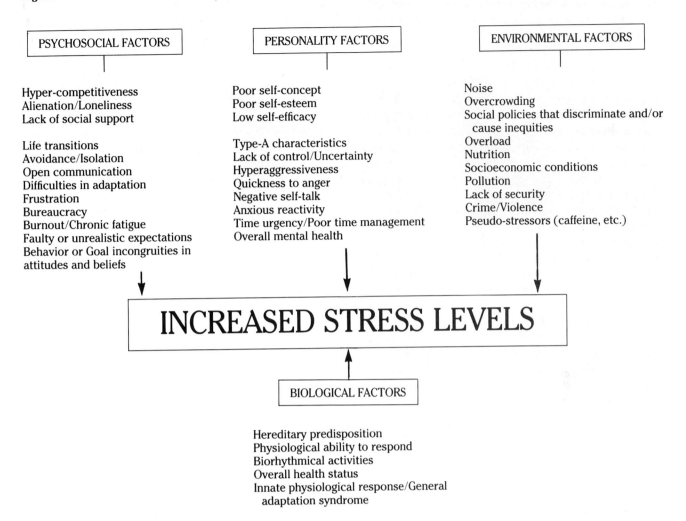

| PSYCHOSOCIAL FACTORS | PERSONALITY FACTORS | ENVIRONMENTAL FACTORS |

Hyper-competitiveness
Alienation/Loneliness
Lack of social support

Life transitions
Avoidance/Isolation
Open communication
Difficulties in adaptation
Frustration
Bureaucracy
Burnout/Chronic fatigue
Faulty or unrealistic expectations
Behavior or Goal incongruities in
attitudes and beliefs

Poor self-concept
Poor self-esteem
Low self-efficacy

Type-A characteristics
Lack of control/Uncertainty
Hyperaggressiveness
Quickness to anger
Negative self-talk
Anxious reactivity
Time urgency/Poor time management
Overall mental health

Noise
Overcrowding
Social policies that discriminate and/or
cause inequities
Overload
Nutrition
Socioeconomic conditions
Pollution
Lack of security
Crime/Violence
Pseudo-stressors (caffeine, etc.)

INCREASED STRESS LEVELS

| BIOLOGICAL FACTORS |

Hereditary predisposition
Physiological ability to respond
Biorhythmical activities
Overall health status
Innate physiological response/General
adaptation syndrome

balance. This state of balance, known as **homeostasis,** refers to the combined attempt of physical and psychological systems to function smoothly and maintain equilibrium. When the body perceives a real or imaginary stressor, it responds automatically to ward off the threat and regain homeostasis. This response to stressors may differ significantly from person to person, depending on the level and intensity of a particular event. However, everyone experiences a similar physiological pattern, which was described in 1936 by Hans Selye. The three-stage response to stress outlined by Selye is called the **general adaptation syndrome (GAS).** The phases of the GAS are alarm, resistance, and exhaustion.*

In the *alarm phase,* homeostasis is disturbed. During this phase, the brain rapidly and subconsciously perceives the stressor and prepares the body either to fight or run away. This response is sometimes called the "fight or flight" response. The subconscious appraisal and perceptions of the stressor stimulate the areas in the brain that

are responsible for emotions. Emotional stimulation in turn starts the physical reactions that we associate with stress. This entire process generally takes only seconds. Diagrams of the pathway involved in the emotional response to stressors are contained in Figures 3.2 and 3.3.

When an event (either real or imaginary) is perceived to have occurred, areas of the *cerebral cortex,* the region of the brain that interprets the nature of the event, are called to attention. If the cerebral cortex consciously or unconsciously perceives a threat, an alarm triggers an instantaneous response by the **autonomic nervous system (ANS)** that prepares the body for action. The ANS is the portion of the central nervous system that regulates bodily functions over which we do not usually have

---

Homeostasis   A balance physical state in which all the body's systems function smoothly.
General adaptation syndrome (GAS)   The pattern formed by our physiological responses to stress, consisting of the alarm, resistance, and exhaustion phases.
Autonomic nervous system   The portion of the central nervous system that regulates bodily functions that we do not consciously control.

---

* Hans Selye, *Stress without Distress* (New York: Lippincott, 1974), pp. 28–29.

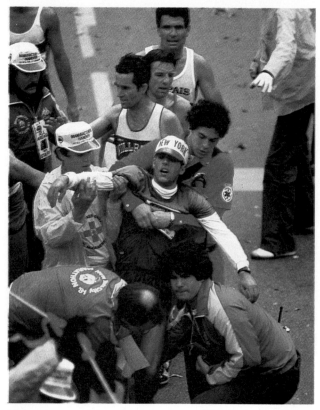

Physical competition can be a source of both eustress and distress.

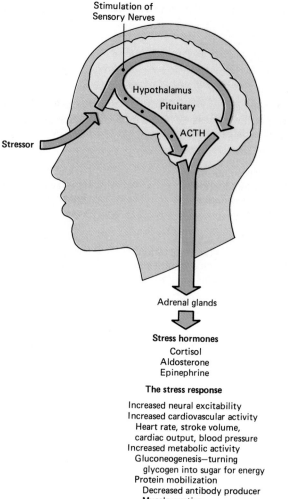

Figure 3.3 How the body responds to stress.

conscious control, such as heart rate, breathing rate, and glandular secretions. A branch of the ANS known as the **sympathetic nervous system** begins to energize the body by signaling the release of several stress hormones that speed the heart rate, increase the breathing rate, and

Figure 3.2 How the body and mind interact in the stress responses.

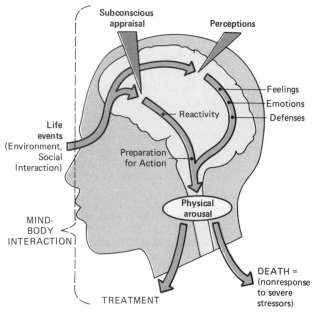

trigger many other stress responses. Another branch of the ANS, known as the **parasympathetic nervous system,** functions to slow down all of the systems that have been stimulated by the stress response. Thus, the sympathetic and parasympathetic branches of the ANS serve as a unique system of checks and balances. In the healthy person, these two systems work to control the negative effects of stress. However, long-term stress can cause this balance to become strained, and chronic physical problems can occur.

Another region of the brain, the *hypothalamus*, functions as the control center of the sympathetic nervous system and determines the overall reaction to the stres-

Sympathetic nervous system The part of the autonomic nervous system responsible for stress arousal.

Parasympathetic nervous system The part of the autonomic nervous system responsible for bringing the stress arousal phase under control.

sors (see Chapter 2). When the hypothalamus perceives that greater-than-average energy will be needed to fight a stressor, it stimulates the adrenal glands, located near the top of the kidneys, to release **epinephrine,** or *adrenaline.* The release of this hormone increases heart action by causing more blood to be pumped with each beat, dilates the bronchioles (air sacs in the lungs) to increase oxygen intake, increases respiration rate, and stimulates the liver to release more glucose for energy for muscular exertion. The pupils of the eyes expand in response to the stimulation, improving visual sensitivity. Other effects of epinephrine secretion are a diversion of blood away from the digestive system, possibly causing nausea and cramping if the distress occurs shortly after a meal, and drying of nasal and salivary tissues, producing a dry mouth.

In addition, the hypothalamus releases a hormone called *corticotropin releasing factor (CRF),* which stimulates the *pituitary gland,* the master gland of hormonal regulation. Once stimulated, the pituitary responds by releasing another powerful hormone, **adrenocorticotropic hormone (ACTH).** This hormone travels through the bloodstream until it reaches the *adrenal glands.* The adrenal glands then release yet another key energy-producing hormone known as **cortisol,** which aids in speeding metabolic activity by making stored nutrients more readily available for energy demands. As the alarm phase continues, the above activities prepare the body to fight or flee from the perceived stressor.

Once the alarm phase is called into action, the second phase, known as the *resistance* phase, of the GAS begins to take effect. In this phase, the body attempts to return to normal, and our body systems adapt to the stress challenge.

As the sympathetic nervous system is working to energize the body via the hormonal action of epinephrine, **norepinephrine** (also known as *catecholamine*), cortisol, and other hormones, the parasympathetic nervous system is helping to keep these energy levels under control. The parasympathetic nervous system acts to slow the system down and return it to normal (see Figure 3.4).

The third phase of the GAS is the *exhaustion phase,* in which physical and psychological energy used to fight the stressors has been depleted and the organism must rest. Chronic distressors, such as some job distressors, create continuous states of alarm and resistance. When the person no longer has the reserves for fighting the distressor, serious illness may result.

Many stress researchers believe that each of us possesses different levels of *adaptation energy stores.** These energy stores are the physical and mental foundations of our ability to cope with stress of any type. Two levels of adaptation energy exist: *superficial* and *deep.* Physically,

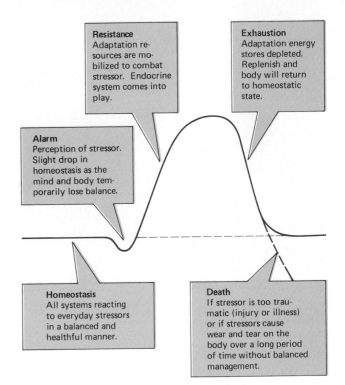

Figure 3.4 The general adaptation syndrome (GAS).

these might be illustrated by showing the deep level encapsulated by the superficial level.

We apparently have little control over our deep-adaptation energy stores. Heredity seems to be the primary influence on these levels. Some scientists speculate that these levels are preset in each of our cells.

Superficial energy stores surround the deep stores. These relatively easy-to-reach stores are renewable and offer protection for the deep energy stores beneath them.

Stress researchers theorize that when deep energy stores are depleted, the organism dies. Stress management, then, is dependent on our ability to replenish superficial stores, thereby conserving the deeper stores. Superficial adaptation energy can be replenished through participating in aerobic exercise (exercise that raises and sustains the heart rate at a predetermined level), balancing work with relaxation, eliminating unnecessary drugs, maintaining a secure home environment, practicing good nutritional habits, finding challenges and adventures instead of threats in stressors, setting realistic goals, and establishing and maintaining supportive relationships.

Epinephrine   Also called *adrenaline,* a hormone secreted by the adrenal glands that is responsible for stimulating the body.

Adrenocorticotropic hormone (ACTH)   A pituitary hormone that stimulates the adrenal glands to secrete cortisol and aldosterone.

Cortisol   Hormone released by the adrenal glands under stress that helps speed up metabolic activity by making stored nutrients more readily available for energy demands.

Norepinephrine   A hormone released by the adrenal glands that energizes the body; also called *catecholamine.*

---

* Daniel A. Girdano, George S. Everly, and Dorothy Dusek, *Controlling Stress and Tension,* 3rd ed. (Englewood Cliffs, N.J.: Prentice Hall, 1990).

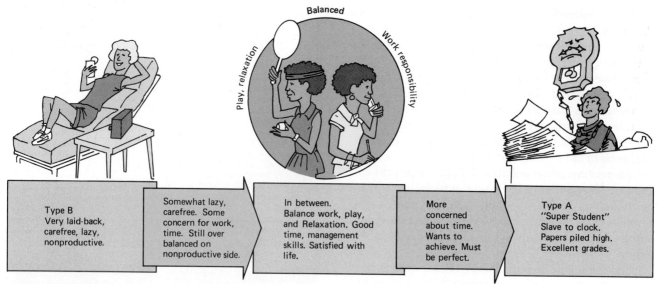

Figure 3.5 Very few of us are "pure" Type A or Type B. Most of us have behavior patterns that fall between the two extremes.

FACTORS INFLUENCING THE STRESS RESPONSE

Self-Concept and Stress

How we feel about ourselves, our attitudes toward others, and our perceptions and interpretations of the stressors in our lives are all part of the psychological component of stress. Also included are the defense, or coping, mechanisms we have learned to use in various stressful situations (see Chapter 2).

The psychological system that governs our responses to stressors is called the **cognitive stress system.*** Our cognitive stress system serves to recognize stressors, evaluate them on the basis of self-concept, past experiences, and emotions, and make decisions regarding how to cope with them.

Our sensory organs serve as input channels for any information reaching the brain. From that point on, attention to the problem, memory, reasoning processes, and problem solving are organized in various parts of the brain before we act on the stressor. Because learning and memory involve the changing of various proteins in brain neurons, the emotions experienced during the stress response also "tickle" the memory storage neurons and contribute to our responses. Behaviorally, we will respond to the stressor in ways consistent with our memories of similar situations.

Self-esteem is closely related to the emotions engendered by past experiences. People with low self-esteem are more likely to become victims of "helpless anger," an emotion experienced by people who have not learned to express their anger in appropriate ways. These people have usually learned that anger is a "negative" emotion

and is therefore bad. Instead of learning to express anger in healthy ways, they turn their anger inward. They may "swallow" their anger in food, alcohol, or other drugs, or they may turn their anger outward in violence or other aggressive behaviors.

Research indicates that self-esteem significantly affects various disease processes. People with low self-esteem create a distressor within themselves that, over a period of time, can impair the immune system's ability to combat disease. Some researchers believe that chronic distress can depress the immune system and thus increase the symptoms of such diseases as acquired immune deficiency syndrome (AIDS), multiple sclerosis, and Epstein-Barr syndrome. The specific effects of stress on health-related problems will be discussed in later chapters.

Personality Types and Hardiness

The effects of personality and stress on diseases of the circulatory system have been the focus of numerous investigations in recent years. The coronary disease-prone personality was first described in 1974 by physicians Meyer Friedman and Ray Rosenman in their book *Type A Behavior and Your Heart.*** Friedman and Rosenman described two stress-related personality types: Type A and Type B. Subsequent study has shown that Types A and B represent different points along a continuum rather than opposite extremes (see Figure 3.5).

Cognitive stress system   The psychological system that governs our emotional responses to stress.

---

* Rice, *Stress and Health*, 1992.

** Meyer Friedman and Ray H. Rosemann, *Type A Behavior and Your Heart* (New York: Knopf, 1974), pp. 193–207.

At one end of the scale, the Type A personality shows "hurry syndrome," which is characterized by a sense of being driven by time, impatience, competitiveness, aggressiveness, insecurity over status, and inability to relax even when on vacation. At the other end of the scale is the Type B-4 personality, who is extremely laid-back and unhurried. In between are the Type A-2 personality, with moderate amounts of the hurry syndrome, and the Type B-3 personality, who is relaxed and free of the hurry syndrome, but not as carefree as Type B-4.†

Research has shown that Type A men in the 39- to-49-year-old age group are at least 6 times more likely to suffer heart attacks than are their less-hurried counterparts. Type A women are 3 to 7 times more likely to suffer from hypertension than are non–Type A women. Both Type A men and Type A women are more likely to smoke more and are less likely to exercise. Lack of exercise and use of cigarettes are two risk factors contributing to the development of heart disease.

Economic status and job responsibility contribute to Type A behavior. As economic status and promotions increase, so does Type A behavior. Type A behavior was once thought to be a strictly male personality characteristic. However, research now shows that more women than men in the 18-to-39-year-old age group exhibit Type A behavior, particularly women who are attempting to manage both a career and a family. Some researchers have labeled this category Type E, in which the woman feels she must be "*everything* to *everybody*."

Not all Type A people suffer negative consequences from their behaviors. Health experts have sought explanations for this. Recently, researchers have shown that some Type A personalities may in fact be more resilient as a result of a lifetime of exposure to stress. Type A people who had suffered from heart attacks appeared to recover more quickly with fewer severe consequences than people with Type B personalities did. Type A people are often better equipped to take charge of their medical situations than Type B people.* Other researchers identify some people as Type C personalities—those who use the Type A behavior and personality traits to their advantage. These people are actually Type A people who have learned to channel their ambition and nervous energy in creative directions.

Over the years, many studies have raised questions about the role of specific behaviors and severe, debilitating consequences. Researchers at Duke University have conducted several studies that indicate that it is not the hurry syndrome often associated with Type A behavior that makes us sick. Instead, they have identified a *toxic core* of the Type A behavior pattern that makes people especially vulnerable to negative effects. People who have this toxic core are distrustful of others and have

Taking time to relax is not "killing time"; it is, in fact, a major component of mental health.

above-average levels of cynicism. Excessive anger seems to be a key element of this type of personality.**

Psychologist Susanne Kobasa identified **psychological hardiness** as a characteristic that has helped some people to negate the potential hazards associated with Type A behavior. The psychologically hardy person has three major traits that contribute to his or her hardiness: control, commitment, and challenge.† People with *control* are able to accept responsibility for their behaviors and make changes in behaviors that they discover to be debilitative. A person with a sense of *commitment* has a good feeling of self-esteem and understands his or her purpose in life. The psychologically hardy person also sees changes in life as challenging, stimulating opportunities for personal growth.

Some modification of Type A behavior is possible because some of this behavior is "learned." Some Type A people are able to reduce their hurried behavior and to become more tolerant, more patient, and better-humored. Unfortunately, many people do not decide to modify their Type A habits until after they have suffered a heart attack or other circulatory-system distress. Prevention of heart and circulatory disorders resulting from stress entails recognizing and changing dangerous behaviors before damage is done (see Chapter 12).

Psychological hardiness A personality characteristic characterized by control, commitment, and challenge.

---

† Rice, *Stress and Health*, pp. 97–98.
* D. Ragland and R. Brand, "Type A Behavior, Aggression and Heart Disease," *New England Journal of Medicine* (January 14, 1988).

** "Distrust, Rage May Be 'Toxic Core' That Puts 'Type A' Person at Risk," *Journal of the American Medical Association*, 261, no. 6 (1989), 813.
† Rice, *Stress and Health*, pp. 97–98.

Self-Efficacy and Control

Whether or not people are able to cope successfully with a stressful situation often depends on their level of *self-efficacy,* or belief in their skills and performance abilities.‡ If people have been successful in mastering similar problems in the past, they will be more likely to believe in their own effectiveness in future situations. Similarly, people who have repeatedly tried and failed may lack confidence in their abilities to deal with life's problems. In some cases, this insecurity may prevent them from even trying to cope.

In addition, those people who feel that they lack *control* in a situation may become easily frustrated and give up. People who feel they have no personal control over anything tend to have an *external locus of control* and a low level of self-efficacy. People who feel that their behavior will influence the ultimate outcome of events tend to have an *internal locus of control* (see Chapter 1). People who feel that they have limited control over their lives tend to have higher levels of stress.

Incongruent Goals and Behaviors

For many of us, negative stress effects become exacerbated when there is a conflict between our *goals* (what we value, or hope to obtain in life) and our *behaviors* (our actions or activities that may or may not lead us to achieving these goals). One of the best examples of this for college students may be related to our quest for superior grades. We may *want* the "A" and our families may *expect* it, but if we party and procrastinate throughout the term, our behaviors are incongruent with our goals, and significant stress in the form of guilt and last-minute frenzy before exams may result. On the other hand, if we wanted to dig in and work, and were committed to getting the "A", much of our negative stress may be eliminated or reduced.

Likewise, a young adult whose goal is to be in a committed, long-term relationship may find that goal seems elusive. This search for the perfect partner may cause significant stress over time, particularly if the young adult who wants the permanent relationship likes to "sleep around" or refuses to prioritize relationships in his or her life. Thus, his or her actions (or the lack of them!) may sabotage any hopes of a solid relationship. Frustration may be the net result of these thwarted goals, and frustration has been shown to be a significant stressor or disrupter of homeostasis (see Figure 3.6).

Determining whether or not our behaviors are consistent with goal attainment is an essential component of our efforts to maintain a balance in our lives. If we consciously strive to attain our goals in a very direct manner, our chances of success are greatly improved. If we deviate from the plan, or if we act in a manner that

‡ Albert Bandura, "Self-Efficacy Mechanism in Human Agency," *American Psychologist,* 37 (1982), 122–47.

STRESS AFFECTS HOMEOSTATIC BALANCE

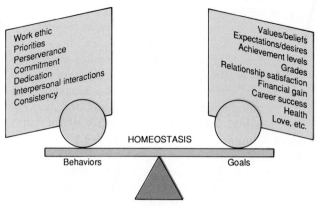

Figure 3.6   Stress affects homeostatic balance

makes our goals impossible, goals may become negative sources of stress.

Environmental Distressors

Environmental distressors include natural disasters such as floods, earthquakes, hurricanes, and forest fires. Other environmental distressors include chemical spills, accidents at nuclear power plants, and other one-time catastrophes that occur infrequently and generally affect a more local population. **Background distressors** such as noise, air, and chemical pollution, crowding, and urban commuting can be just as damaging as one-time disasters, although their effects may not become apparent for decades. As with other distressors, our bodies respond to disasters through the general adaptation syndrome. People who cannot escape background distressors might suffer from a constant state of resistance that could contribute to the development of stress-related disorders. For more information on environmental distressors, see Chapter 15.

Psychosocial Distressors

Psychosocial distressors result from living, working, and associating with others. They include problems with *adaptation,* or difficulty in adapting to life's changes; *frustration,* the thwarting or inhibiting of natural or desired behaviors or goals; *overcrowding,* or having too many people in a space that is too small; *discrimination,* or the unfavorable actions taken against others based on factors such as race, religion, social status, gender, lifestyle, national origin, or physical characteristics; and *socioeconomic factors,* such as inflation, unemployment, low income, or economic recession. These psychosocial distressors may lead to violent reactions, racially-oriented crime, bigotry, and a host of negative social responses.

Background distressors   Everyday sources of stress that we tend to take for granted: noise, air, and chemical pollution, crowding, urban commuting.

Communication

Controlling Your Anger: Communicating Effectively to Reduce Stress

"Fighting fairly" and expressing anger constructively are important skills in learning to cope with the inevitable pressures of intimate relationships, family interactions, and other stressful situations in our lives. Fighting fairly assumes that you are battling to come to a constructive, "no winner" type of resolution to a problem, rather than trying to batter someone else's ego so that you can feel better. Below are suggestions for constructive expression of anger:

1. *Determine the real reason that you are angry.* Is it because of a *real* event (for example, someone you trusted is spreading malicious gossip) or a *perception* you have about the situation (friends are avoiding you, so you *think* someone has done something wrong)?

2. *Don't let your anger build.* When you become angry, take *control*, and decide what actions you need to take. Try not to act rashly, but don't sit and stew for a long time. If you choose to write a letter expressing your anger, sit down and do it, but don't mail the letter immediately. Put the letter away, wait a few days, and then reread it. Often you will find that you no longer want to say the same things. However, the letter writing itself has been *cathartic* and has helped you relieve stress.

3. *If you decide to confront the person, select an appropriate time and place for the meeting.* Try not to attack the other person unexpectedly or in the presence of others so that the person becomes defensive. Give the other person a general idea of what you want to discuss ahead of time.

4. *Stick to the major or most recent reason for your anger.* Bringing up a whole list of things that have made you angry over the last year will just complicate the issue and make the other person want to create his or her own list of things that you have done. Plan in advance which issue you want to discuss.

5. *Attack the problem rather than the person.* Don't get into a battle over personal characteristics. Use "I" statements to communicate resentment or disappointment. "You" statements often put the person on the defensive (see Chapter 3).

6. *Listen carefully to what the other person has to say.* If the other person starts wandering from the issue, gently try to bring them back. If the person attacks you personally, stay in control and don't allow yourself to fight back if at all possible. Assume personal responsibility for your anger by speaking to the "I feel" mode.

7. *Treat the other person with respect.* Even though you may say the right things, gestures and body language can reveal that you don't value what the other person has to say, that you are hostile, or that you are losing patience. Drumming your fingers, sighing, rolling your eyes, or staring off into space while the other person is talking can often increase friction.

8. *Recognize when to quit.* Sometimes even the best-laid plans go awry. No matter what you do, the situation may appear impossible to resolve. In such situations, knowing when to quit, either temporarily or permanently, is a key factor in controlling stressful anger levels.

9. *When it's over, let it be over.* After you have done all that you can do, learn to let go of your anger. Don't dwell in the past. Acknowledge your right to be angry, recognize it for what it was, and move on.

Most psychosocial distressors are treatable, but usually a strong combination of social-policy revision, economic assistance, and individual and community support is necessary.

Overload and Burnout

Have you ever felt that you had so many responsibilities that you couldn't possibly begin to fulfill them all? Have you longed for a weekend when you could just curl up and read a good book, or take time out with friends and not feel guilty? These feelings typically occur when we have been under continued stress for a period of time and are suffering from **overload**, or overstimulation. Overload occurs when we suffer from (1) excessive time pres-

Overload A condition in which we feel overstimulated by the demands made on us.

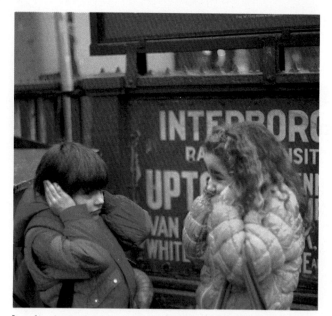

Loud noises can cause physical and psychological distress.

sure, (2) excessive responsibility, (3) lack of support, and (4) excessive expectations of ourselves and those around us.

Students suffering from overload and pressure from their families to succeed may experience anxiety over tests, poor self-concept, a desire to drop classes or to drop out of school, and other problems. In severe cases, in which students are unable to see any solution to problems, they may suffer more severe mental disturbances such as depression, or turn to substance abuse. Recognizing these potential problems, many colleges have expanded counseling and mental-health services.

People who suffer from overload, frustration, and disappointment on a regular basis may eventually begin to experience **burnout,** a state of physical and mental exhaustion. People involved in "helping professions," such as teachers, social workers, drug counselors, nurses, and psychologists, appear to experience high levels of burnout, as do people working in high-pressure, dangerous jobs, such as police officers and air-traffic controllers.

Occupations that have unclear work objectives, ambiguous responsibilities and management expectations, poor lines of communication, long periods of inactivity or boredom, and lack of job security are among the most stressful. We can reduce the effects of burnout by recognizing the warning signs early. Practicing prestress coping behaviors such as good nutrition, regular aerobic exercise, planned relaxation, effective communication skills, and a strong social-support network can be important factors in stopping the progress of burnout. Occupational burnout can be reduced by improved relations between workers and management, clear job descriptions, regular evaluations, and other actions designed to make workers feel that what they do is important and valued.

STRESS AND SPECIAL POPULATIONS

Stress and the Life Span

Each stage of the life span offers different stresses and challenges. Successfully meeting these tasks is a form of growth-producing eustress. Failure to meet the tasks is a distressor with multiple effects. If we fail to meet a certain task at one stage of development, we cannot move ahead. If we try to move ahead without the necessary foundation for the next step, we compound the distressor and doom ourselves to additional failure and loss of self-esteem.

The distress experienced by infants whose parents are urging them to be "super babies" has gained media attention. Research in this area is not yet complete, but it is known that excessive pressure from parents to achieve success contributes to childhood depression and may be a factor in later childhood or teenage suicide. Our mental and physical capacities develop according to natural timetables. Infants and toddlers need time to explore the world and develop their skills on individual timetables, not the timetables of overanxious parents who want a child prodigy.

Distress among children between the ages of 5 and 12 is also gaining media attention. Children raised in dysfunctional families where parental problems are often a part of the daily living experience often have high levels of distress. Families where one or both parents have substance-abuse problems, where the home environment may be unpredictably volatile, or where physical or sexual abuse occurs often have difficulties in coping with life's stresses. When their main avenue of support and security is disrupted from a very early age, children often have difficulty in trusting others and coping with adversity for the rest of their lives. Suicide rates in this age group are increasing for unknown reasons. Mental-health experts estimate that more than half the children in this age group think about killing themselves.*

The stresses that lead to suicidal depression among children are generally related to a major loss. The greatest stressor for any child is the death of a parent, followed by parental divorce and the death of a sibling.

"Latchkey kids"—children whose parents or guardians work or are not able to be home with them before or after school—also face stresses. Many of them are responsible for the care of younger siblings, for making meals, and for completing household chores, in addition to doing their own schoolwork.

Burnout The physical and mental exhaustion resulting from excessive stress.

* Ben Allen, "Youth Suicide," *Adolescence,* 23, no. 86 (1987), 271–90; Brad Neiger and Rodney Hopkins, "Adolescent Suicide: Characteristic Traits," *Adolescence,* 23, no. 90 (1988), 468–75.

Although the responsibilities associated with gaining independence are healthful for some, many adolescents suffer distress and depression because of low self-esteem, confusion about sexual identity, peer pressure, and lack of supportive family and peer relationships. Adolescence is a time for establishing self-identity, but many teenagers have trouble with this task. More than 12 out of every 100,000 people aged 15 to 20 kill themselves each year. As with younger children, loss-related distressors are the major causes of suicide.

Adults also face loss-related distressors, with the possibility of loss of employment becoming more of a factor. In addition, career stresses and other social distressors often become prominent in adult lives.

When adults are responsible for others in their families, distress can be multiplied. Parenthood is distressful to some, as is evidenced by the 652,000 reported cases of physically abused children (2,000 deaths) and 329,000 reported cases of emotionally abused children each year.** Loss of jobs, job insecurity, and potential economic threats during a recession may significantly increase stress levels. Patterns of violence, crime, and abuse increase dramatically in such cases.

Parents of newborns often find that their lifestyles have been disrupted in ways they had not anticipated. Although they realize that having a baby involves night feedings, diapering, and major modifications in social life, the experience does not become real until after the baby arrives. Parents of toddlers may be stressed by the inquisitiveness shown by these children. As children grow, the distress to their parents increases primarily at adolescence, when children begin to assert their independence. Parents who cannot tolerate the feeling that they are "losing control" of their children may resort to abuse to try to regain control. Letting go of children when they reach adulthood is also difficult for many parents.

Adults who are responsible for the care of their aging

_____
** Rice, *Stress and Health*, p. 42.

Loneliness is a major source of stress, especially among the elderly.

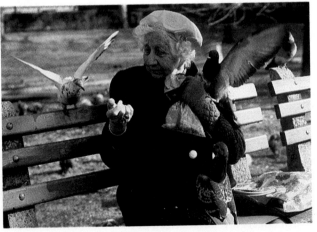

parents also experience distress at this added responsibility. Cases of parent abuse appear to be growing.

Older adults moving from the work force to retirement also encounter distressors. Loneliness and boredom may be present in those who do not have a social-support network. Loss of the ability to care for themselves, lapses of memory, physical deterioration, and the death of old friends are the primary losses that older people experience.

The distresses that accompany any stage of life can be life-threatening or life-enhancing, depending on how we choose to see them. If we are taught at an early age to recognize the symptoms of distress, we can take steps to reduce the distress. Stress-management skills and coping skills are available to all of us.

Stress and the College Student

College-related stress may seem to be caused only by the pressure to excel in the academic arena. In fact, college students experience numerous distressors, including changes caused by being away from home for the first time, possible climatic differences between home and school environments, pressure to make friends in a new and perhaps intimidating setting, the feeling of anonymity imposed by large classes, and the pressures related to time management. Some students are stressed by athletic team requirements, dormitory food, roommate habits, expectations of peers, questions about personal values and beliefs, relationship problems, fraternity or sorority demands, or financial worries. For older students, worries about not being able to compete with 18-year-olds may also be distressful. Most colleges offer stress-management workshops through their health centers or student counseling departments.

Stress: The Disease of Prolonged Arousal

Although much has been written about the negative effects of stress, researchers have only recently begun to unlock the complex web of physical and emotional interactions that actually cause the body to break down over time. As a result, stress is often described generically as a "disease of prolonged arousal" that often leads to other negative health effects. Nearly all systems of the body become potential targets for this onslaught, and the long-term effects may be devastating.

Much of the initial impetus for studying the health effects of stress came from seemingly indirect observations. Social scientists and epidemiologists noted that mortality rates for individuals who were single or who had few close relationships were often significantly higher than for those who were married or who had high levels of support.* Cardiologists in the Framingham

_____
* J. Lynch, *The Broken Heart: Medical Consequences of Loneliness* (New York: Basic Books, 1977).

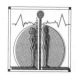

When Stress Responses Are Aroused Again and Again

- **Cardiovascular Effects/Hypertension**
  - Hormone aldosterone is secreted.
  - Increased sodium retention causes increased fluid retention.
  - Increased blood volume results in decreased urination.
  - Hormone epinephrine is secreted. Blood vessels constrict, heart rate increases and stroke volume intensifies, blood pressure rises.
  - Cortisol levels increase, raising levels of fatty acids in blood and increasing risk of atherosclerosis.

- **Kidney Effects**
  - Negative effects result from prolonged hypertension.
  - Vasoconstriction occurs. Blood flow and normal kidney function are inhibited as blood supply is redirected to other areas of the body. Damage may result if chronic.

- **Hyperglycemic States**
  - Cortisol - Delays or interferes with insulin availability which may lead to subsequent difficulties with insulin utilization. If so, blood sugar levels will rise and diabetes develop.

- **Immunological Effects**
  - Cortisol brings glucose, fatty acids, and amino acid stores into bloodstream to be used for energy.
  - Depletion of protein reserves occurs. These reserves are needed for formation of white blood cells.
  - Helper T and B cells are depleted or damaged, causing difficulty in fighting invading organisms. Infections or diseases such as cancer may be able to gain a foothold.
  - As immunological competence is impaired, cancer risk increases due to difficulties in tissue repair.
  - Possible arthritislike conditions may develop.

- **Gastrointestinal Effects**
  - Blood flow and digestive activity in GI tract are slowed as body channels vital energy to essential organs.
  - Food remains in stomach for longer periods. Indigestion and nausea may occur; chemicals in food in contact with stomach lining for longer time may lead to cancer development.
  - Hormone thyroxine causes increases in gastric juices, resulting in bad breath and indigestion.
  - Fluid imbalance may lead to diarrhea or constipation.
  - Ulcer development may occur as well as irritable bowel syndrome and colitis.

- **Skin**
  - Constriction of capillaries and vessels in outer layers and disruption of sebaceous-gland activity may lead to dryness, itching, hives, and acne.

- **Nervous-System Effects**
  - Hormonal imbalances may affect emotional homeostasis, leading to depression, emotional volatility, and so forth.
  - Thyroxine may cause increased agitation and mental arousal, producing insomnia.
  - Muscular twitching and contraction due to irregular nerve-fiber activity may occur; hyperexcitability may also result.

- **Other Distress Effects**
  - Tension headaches due to inappropriate muscular activity.
  - Migraine headaches due to changes in blood-vessel flow patterns.
  - Muscle spasms.
  - Increased use of drugs.
  - Dysfunctional relationships.
  - Poor productivity.
  - Increased proneness to accidents.

Heart Study and other research projects noted that highly stressed individuals seemed to experience significantly greater risks of cardiovascular disease and hypertension.** While the battle over the legitimacy of these observations continues to be waged in research labs across the country, certain factors relating too much stress over long periods of time to selected ailments has gained in credibility. What does too much stress actually do to the body? Why are health experts so concerned about stress in contemporary American society? These health effects are summarized in the box entitled "Stress and Your Health."

** Walt Schafer, *Stress Management for Wellness*, 2nd ed. (New York: Harcourt Brace Jovanovich, 1992).

RECOGNITION AND ASSESSMENT OF DISTRESS

We must recognize the physical and emotional symptoms of distress before undertaking a stress-management program. If we know where our stresses are coming from, we can anticipate them in ways that will reduce their impact. Typically, there are three types of daily stress situations:

1. *Stresses that are foreseeable and avoidable.* These types of stressors are those that you should be able to anticipate and avoid. For example, if you have just had a painful breakup and your boyfriend or girlfriend is dating someone else, putting yourself in a position where you have to watch them together does not make sense. Going to a dance where you will see the two of them together would undoubtedly cause you needless pain and anxiety. Going to a movie with other friends instead would be a means of avoiding the inevitable confrontation.

2. *Stresses that are neither foreseeable nor avoidable.* Whether because of a serious car accident, being stuck in a freak snowstorm and missing an appointment, or inclement weather canceling your plane flight, some forms of stress are unavoidable. Recognition of this fact and calm acceptance of those things over which you have no control are key factors in stress management. Swearing, screaming, or yelling at close friends and strangers in these situations will not help you get through them more effectively.

3. *Stresses that are foreseeable but not avoidable.* Knowing that you have an exam on Monday morning might seriously affect your weekend social life. However, the fact remains that you cannot avoid the exam. If you party all weekend and begin studying at 10 P.M. on Sunday, trying to cram a week's worth of studying into a few short hours, you will face enormous pressure. By planning ahead and studying a little bit each day during the previous week and saving Sunday night for review only, you would undoubtedly have a much better "time off" and significantly reduce the stress you would face by waiting until the last minute.

Distressors can consist of typical everyday happenings or larger catastrophic events. The cumulative effects of multiple daily stresses may be just as damaging as a single catastrophic event. Noted stress researcher Richard Lazarus points out that the seemingly trivial problems that each of us faces daily may add up to a serious "stress load" when each problem is added to the previous one.* Although standing in line for an hour to buy books may not make you sick, finding that your parked car has been damaged, or that your roommate has invited guests when you wanted some time alone, or that there is a pile of dirty dishes in the sink waiting for you may add to more than a "bad day." These seemingly minor stressors added together over extended periods of time may have serious consequences. Typical distressors found among college students are listed in the box entitled "Assess Your Distress."

Regardless of the type of distressor, our first step is to examine the problem thoroughly. Inevitably, we will be "stuck" in classes that bore us and for which we find no application in real life. We feel powerless when a loved one has died. The facts themselves cannot be changed. Only our reactions to the distressors in our lives can be changed.

MANAGING OUR REACTIONS TO DISTRESS

After recognizing a distressor, we should examine the situation. Can the circumstances be altered in any way to reduce the amount of distress we are experiencing, or must we change our behavior and reactions to reduce distress?

If five term papers from five different courses are due during the semester, we know we cannot persuade our professors to withdraw the assignments. We can, however, begin those papers early, spacing them out over a period of time to avoid the last-minute rush. If the boss is vague about directions, we cannot change bosses. We can, however, ask him or her to clarify in writing the things that are expected of us.

Changing responses requires practice and emotional control. If a roommate is habitually messy, we can choose among several responses. We can express our anger by yelling, we can pick up the mess and leave a nasty note, or we can defuse the situation with humor. The quickest response is not always the best response. Taking a moment to say "Stop!" before reacting can help give us the time needed to find the appropriate response. Asking yourself "What is to be gained from my (anger, notewriting, humor, moving out?)" is the next step. In changing our responses to stressful situations, we act mentally to change attitudes or physically to combat the physical effects of stress.

---

* R. Lazarus, "The Trivialization of Distress," in J. C. Rosen and L. J. Solomon, eds., *Preventing Health Risk Behaviors and Promoting Coping with Illness*, vol. 8, Vermont Conference on the Primary Prevention of Psychopathology (Hanover, N.H.: University Press of New England, 1985), pp. 279–98.

Health in Your Community

Working with Others to Overcome Stress

One of the many ironies associated with stress is that it is often easier to recognize in *other* people. Another irony is that even when you recognize obvious symptoms of stress in another person, that person may—for reasons of pride or embarrassment—wholeheartedly deny that she or he is suffering from stress. Observing stress in other people can help make you more aware of the way you deal with specific stressors in your life. However, the material you have learned in this chapter should enable you to help other people—friends, classmates, family members, and other people in your community—cope with their stress symptoms, too. The very least you can do is offer your help. If you find that the person denies any stress-related problems, don't contribute to his or her stress by forcing the issue. Express your willingness to help—and then back off! Examine the following lists of stress symptoms. The questions that follow them are intended to help you develop a stress-reduction program for yourself or for someone you know. (We'll refer to that someone as "your friend," even though she or he may be a "family member" or "classmate.")

Physical Symptoms

Excessive sweating
Persistently dry mouth
Rapid heartbeat
Flushed face, chills
Recurring shortness of breath
Frequent headaches or migraine
Recurring nausea, queasiness
Diarrhea, constipation, gas
Difficulty swallowing, choking
Trembling, nervous tics
Restlessness, insomnia
"Wired" feeling, jumpiness
Fatigue
Loss of or increase in appetite
Gnashing or grinding of teeth
Claustrophobia or smothered feeling
Constant frowning or lip-biting

Emotional and Behavioral Symptoms

Forgetfulness
Inability to concentrate, mental blocks
Feelings of emptiness, sadness, emotional numbness
Short temper
Apprehensiveness, irrational fear
Urge to escape
Impatience, cynicism
Lack of motivation, frustration
Speech difficulties
Increased gesturing
Fast or loud talking, inappropriate laughing
Lack of concentration and focus
Use of television, sleep, or drugs as escape
Increased consumption of foods, coffee, soft drinks
Excessive complaining, gossiping, worrying
Lack of interest in personal and sexual relationships
Short attention span
Chronic distrust, feeling out of control

How many of these emotional and behavioral symptoms have you or your friend experienced recently? Which of these symptoms appear to you or your friend as most damaging to relationships with other people? Which ones would be easiest to change? Which would be most difficult to change? What actions could you or your friend take right now to cope with these problems? What long-term plans can you or your friend make to cope with these problems?

Taking Mental Action: Developing Awareness

Healthy stress management demands that we adopt mental coping styles in two areas. First, we may need to change our attitudes and beliefs in order to meet present and future stressors in facilitative ways. Feeling good about ourselves gives us the foundation to meet stressful situations with confidence and assertiveness rather than passivity. Confidence comes from learned habits. Developing and practicing the positive self-esteem and communication skills necessary to prepare us to cope with future stressors take time. Many of these skills were discussed in Chapter 2.

Promoting Your Health

Assess Your Distress

All changes cause stress. If we are able to recognize the situations that cause distressful emotional reactions for us, we can better prepare ourselves to combat negative feelings and actions. Think about the following situations. Put a check mark in the left-hand column of each stressor you have experienced in the last 12 months. When you are finished, add your total points. A scale for evaluating your responses appears at the end of the assessment.

Stressor	Point Values
_____ Death of a close family member	100
_____ Jail sentence	80
_____ First year or final year in college	63
_____ Pregnancy (to you or caused by you)	60
_____ Severe personal illness or injury	53
_____ Marriage	50
_____ Any interpersonal problems	45
_____ Financial difficulties	40
_____ Death of a close friend	40
_____ Arguments with your roommate or housemate (more than 3 times a week; points for each)	40
_____ Major disagreements with your family	40
_____ Major change in personal habits	30
_____ Change in living environment	30
_____ Beginning or ending a job	30

Stressor	Point Values
_____ Problems with your boss or professor (each)	25
_____ Outstanding personal achievement	25
_____ Failure in a course	25
_____ Final exams	20
_____ Increased or decreased dating	20
_____ Change in working conditions	20
_____ Changing your major	20
_____ Changing your sleeping habits	18
_____ Vacation	15
_____ Change in eating habits	15
_____ Family reunion	15
_____ Change in recreational activities	15
_____ Minor violations of the law	11

If your point total was lower than 150, your stress levels are low. Maintain your prestress coping strategies at current intensity. If your total was between 151 and 299 points, you have experienced moderate stress. Try to reduce the rate of change in your life and pay more attention to prestress and poststress coping strategies. If your total was higher than 300 points, you have been subjected to high stress levels and must plan a vigorous poststress coping routine. Try to eliminate or reduce drastically the changes in your life.

SOURCE: Daniel A. Girdano, George S. Everly, and Dorothy Dusek, _Controlling Stress and Tension,_ 3rd ed. (Englewood Cliffs, N.J.: Prentice Hall, 1990), p. 67.

Second, because we can never completely anticipate what our next distressor will be, we need to develop the communication skills necessary to manage our reactions to stresses after they have occurred. The ability to think and react "on our feet" comes with time, practice, experience with a variety of stressful situations, and patience. Most of all, we must strive to become more _aware_ of potential threats to our stress levels and act quickly to avoid or deal with potential stressors.

Rather than seeing our stressors as adversaries, we should learn to view them as exercises in life. Stress management also requires that we learn to deal with _irrational beliefs_, attitudes about the self that have no basis in fact. Irrational beliefs often cause us to react to stressors in negative ways, thus adding to distress rather than alleviating it. For a discussion of how to recognize, control, and refute irrational beliefs, see Chapter 2.

Managing Emotional Responses

Irrational beliefs are not the only factors that cause emotional responses to distress. In many cases, emotional responses are the naturally occurring outcomes of distressful situations. However, you should remember to examine your emotions as you experience them to determine whether they arise from irrational beliefs. For example, the stress we feel when we speak in front of a class often produces a state of anxiety and fear. A _rational_ fear would be a fear of making mistakes, forgetting your speech, or doing a poor job and receiving a lower grade than you hoped for. An _irrational_ fear would be the fear that everyone in the class thinks you are stupid and that if you do poorly, they will dislike you even more. Allowing your irrational fear to control you could cause you to panic, to become easily frustrated, and to fail. Recogniz-

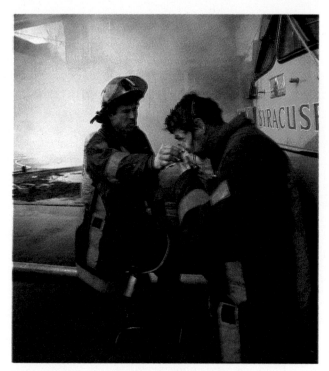

Certain occupations, such as firefighting, involve tremendous physical stress.

ing that everyone in your class is probably nervous, that your speech really does not determine your competence, and that you do not need the approval of others will help you adopt a more positive response to the situation.

With any emotional response to a distressor, we are responsible for the emotion and the behaviors elicited by the emotion. Learning to tell the difference between normal emotions and those based on irrational beliefs can help us either stop the emotion or express it in a healthy and appropriate way. Admitting your feelings and allowing them to be expressed through either communication or action is a stress-management technique that can help you get through many difficult situations.

Learning to Laugh and Cry

For some people, learning to express emotions freely is a difficult task. However, it can help reduce tension. Laughter stimulates cardiovascular responses, aids in digestion, and ultimately serves to relax tired muscles. Some researchers believe that prolonged stress causes changes in the immune system that can limit its effectiveness in recognizing and destroying cancer cells. Despite the many unanswered questions about the actual role of stress in cancer development, it is generally accepted that emotions influence individual recuperative powers. Laughter and a positive mental attitude have been found to be important variables in cancer recovery.* Taking

---

* Anthony Audier, "Determination of a Constitutional Neuroendocrine Factor Influencing Tumor Development in Man: Prophylactic and Therapeutic Aspects," *Cancer Detection and Prevention*, 11 (1988), 203–8; Bernard Siegel, *Love, Medicine, and Miracles* (New York: Harper & Row, 1986).

life too seriously may be more detrimental to our health than was previously thought. The ability to laugh at our mistakes and cry over our disappointments is probably an underestimated form of stress relief.

Taking Physical Action

Adopting the attitudes necessary for effective stress management may seem to have little effect. However, developing successful emotional coping skills is actually a satisfying accomplishment that can help us gain confidence in ourselves. Learning to use physical activity to alleviate stress helps support and complement the emotional strategies we employ in stress management.

Aerobic Exercise *Aerobic exercise* is a significant contributor to stress management. Each of us needs a planned aerobic exercise program tailored to meet our individual tastes (see Chapter 8). Engaging in 25 minutes of aerobic exercise three to four times a week will help to reduce the effects of distress. Exercise offers an excellent way to fight stress not only before it happens but also during stressful times. Exercise may also serve as a stress reducer by raising levels of *endorphin* in our bloodstream. Endorphins are mood-elevating, painkilling chemicals that have a morphinelike action in the body (see Chapter 12). As a result, exercise is believed to increase energy, reduce hostility, improve mental alertness, and, in general, make people more efficient at coping with stress.

Most of us have experienced relief from distress at one time or another through engaging in some aggressive physical activity; chopping wood when we are angry is one example. Exercise performed as part of an immediate response to a distressor can help alleviate the symptoms by offering a poststress-management technique. However, you should be careful to observe the proper safety precautions for your chosen activity. (Strong emotions may inhibit your judgment.) A continuous and regular exercise program usually has more substantial results than does exercise performed as an immediate reaction to a distressor. Not only do fitness levels improve but our body's ability to adapt to and resist the stress is enhanced, thus conserving and replenishing adaptive energy stores and adding to our prestress coping strategies.

Relaxation Like aerobic exercise, relaxation techniques can be used on the spot to help cope with stressful feelings and as part of a continuous program to preserve adaptation energy and dissipate the chemicals associated with distress. Relaxation also helps us refocus our energies.

Several methods of relaxation can be used. You might listen to a soothing instrumental or "sound effect" record or tape. (Albums and tapes specifically labeled "relaxation music" are available. These might include music

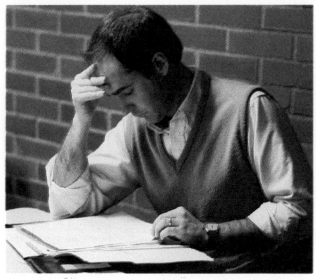

Long hours of studying can be stressful for even the most organized student.

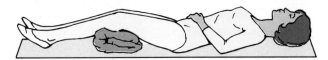

Figure 3.7 Many relaxation techniques require you to lie down with neck and knees supported (more relaxing to the back).

or sounds like falling rain, light breezes, or ocean waves.) Find a quiet time to listen, and sit or lie down and let your mind float along with the sound. Using the sounds to "paint" a mental picture of the soothing environment of your choice, try to "travel" to that place, concentrating on allowing the music to do the work.

Six-Second Quieting Response—Deep Breathing

This technique is very simple and extremely effective. Do it several times a day on a routine basis. It is particularly useful when you need a "quick fix" tension reliever.

1. Draw in a long, deep breath.
2. Hold for 2–3 seconds.
3. Exhale slowly and completely.
4. As you exhale, let your jaw and shoulders drop. Feel the relaxation of your arms, hands, and jaw.

Breath control is an essential part of learning to relax. There are many variations in technique. However, most methods employ conscious inhaling through the mouth, or the nose and mouth, until the abdominal muscles expand outward, followed by slow, controlled exhaling.

Deep-muscle (progressive) **relaxation** is another technique used to help reduce stress. In this exercise, you lie down and begin alternately to tense and relax the muscles of the face, head, neck, shoulders, arms, hands, chest, abdomen, buttocks, thighs, calves, and feet. The progression may go from head to toe or vice versa, or may focus on just one tense area, such as the neck. Concentration should be focused on the feeling of relaxation following deliberate tensing of the muscles.

Meditation is another way to relax. You can learn meditation in a special class or on your own, depending on time and financial considerations. Meditation gener-

ally focuses on deep breathing, allowing tensions to leave the body on each exhalation.

Once relaxation techniques have been learned, they can be used at any time during the day. If faced with a tough exam, you might choose to relax before the test or at intervals during the test. You can also use relaxation techniques when you face stressful confrontations or assignments. When you begin to feel your body respond to distress, make time to relax, both to give yourself added strength and to help alleviate the negative physical effects of stress.

Autogenics is a type of meditation that involves focusing self-suggestions of warmth and heaviness in successive body parts, such as the hands, arms, feet, and legs.

Visualization is a relaxation technique in which you re-create a calming, peaceful place in your mind and place yourself in the middle of it, in an effort to gradually bring your tension level down.

Changing Responses to School or Occupational Stress

Stress at school and on the job is related to social stress. Poor planning skills, poor time-management skills, and inadequate interpersonal skills are the major causes of school or occupational stress.

Some job-related distress is related to unrealistic expectations grounded in irrational beliefs. Many of us pretend to have skills that we do not have. In so doing, we create additional work-related strain and pressure. Realizing that progress takes time and setting reasonable goals for ourselves are the beginnings of stress management at work. Time-management skills are also important if we are to meet deadlines for projects and reports.

College students face distress during final examinations in particular. Some students engage in all-night study marathons, using stimulant drugs to help them through their exams. Others decide that the effort is not worth the trouble and decide to either sleep or drink their worries away. Use of drugs to avoid a distressor is unhealthy regardless of the type of distressor. Stimulant drugs only contribute additional adrenaline to an already stressed system.

Some problems during exam week can be avoided by

Deep-muscle relaxation A stress-reduction technique that involves alternate tensing and relaxing of muscles.

Meditation A relaxation technique that involves deep breathing and concentrating on an object.

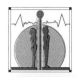

Breathing and Muscle Relaxation Techniques

Learning to Relax

Learn to Breathe

Learning to become aware of and to control your breathing patterns can help you relax. Deep breathing techniques, controlled breathing, and other breathing exercises are often used to help reduce stress levels.

Example

1. Sit in a comfortable position with hands folded over your abdomen, just over your navel.
2. Keeping your eyes open, imagine a balloon lying beneath your hands.
3. Begin to slowly inhale through your nose, concentrating on the warm air entering your nose and slowly filling the balloon. When the balloon is full (this should take 3 to 4 seconds initially), slowly exhale to empty the balloon, feeling your chest and abdomen relaxing.
4. Repeat the entire process 2 to 3 times. When finished, sit quietly for a few minutes before rising. If you feel dizzy at any point, stop the procedure.

Learn to Relax

Learning to relax certain muscle groups trains your muscles as well as the nerve centers that control muscles. Depending on the body part you want to work on, significant body tension can be relieved. (Be cautious if you have a chronic injury or disability in any area.)

Example

Because your head, neck, and facial muscles may become very tense after you have been sitting and reading or working at a computer for a long time, relaxation of these parts can be very important.

SOURCE: Adapted from Daniel A. Girdano, George S. Everly, and Dorothy Dusek, *Controlling Stress and Tension,* 3rd ed. (Englewood Cliffs, N.J.: Prentice Hall, 1990), p. 219.

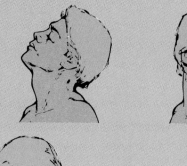
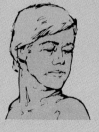
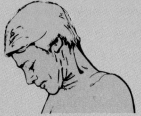
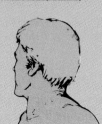

Rotation of the Head and Neck

1. Close your eyes.
2. Roll your head slowly forward and back and then side to side. Repeat this motion.
3. When your head begins to feel heavy, stop, tilt your head forward, and rest.

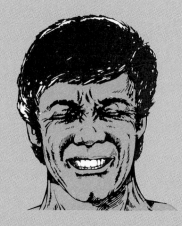

Facial Relaxation

1. Clench your teeth.
2. Contract the facial muscles tightly.
3. Relax.

planning at registration time. Most college course lists include a finals-week schedule. Many students are able to arrange their class schedules so that, come exam week, their major examinations are not back-to-back on the same day. This strategy takes a little more work, but it can be an effective prestress coping strategy.

Managing Time

Anyone who has ever been faced with the rush of traffic in a major city is familiar with the term "gridlock," a point where traffic is so snarled that nothing can move. Recently, the term "timelock" has been used to describe a state that many of us experience on a regular basis.* Timelock occurs when demands on our time become so overwhelming that it feels impossible to wring one more second out of a crowded schedule. Can you already identify with this? It's the feeling you get after making a list of "must do" items for the weekend, working night and day, and finding that, come Sunday night, you have only gotten through half of the items on your list. A 1990 Gallup Poll indicates that timelock is a pervasive element in American life:

1. Nearly 8 of 10 Americans report that time moves too fast for them.

2. The lower the age, the greater the struggle with time. For example, 68 percent of those 50 and older say they have enough time compared with 44 percent of those younger than 50. Baby boomers with a college education struggle the most: only 33 percent say they have enough time.

3. Responses clearly suggest that work has a negative impact on people's experiences with time. Monday is by far the least favorite day of the week; Friday, Saturday, and Sunday are most preferred. The least favorite hours of the day are 6:00 A.M. and 7:00 A.M.

Although most of us are strapped for time on any given day, following a few simple guidelines may help you not only enjoy more guiltfree time but become more productive during work hours:

Plan life, not time. Determining what we want from life rather than what we can "get done" may help change the way we use time. To do this, we must evaluate all our activities, even the most trivial, to determine whether they add to that life. If they don't, get rid of them.

Decelerate. Rushing can be addictive. It is also part of our American work ethic and a mind-set that says that "busy is better." When rushed, ask yourself if you really need to rush. What's the worst thing that could happen if you slowed down? Learn to con-

sciously slow your pace in talking, walking, eating, and so on. Tell yourself at least once each day that failure seldom results from doing a job slowly or too well. Failures happen when attention to detail is lacking and mistakes result.

Learn to delegate and share. Our need to feel in control and in charge is a powerful one. If you are unusually busy, leave details to someone else. Don't be afraid to ask others to help or to share the work load and responsibilities. Probably no one will remember who did what in a few days.

Learn to say no. Prioritize those things that are most critical to your life, your job, or your current situation. Decide what things you *can* do, what things you *must* do, and what things you *want* to do and delegate the rest to someone else, either permanently or until you complete some of your priority tasks. Before you take on a *new* responsibility, finish or drop an old one.

Schedule time alone. Find time each day for quiet reflecting, reading, exercising, playing piano, or other enjoyable activities. Avoid "stress-producing" competitive people or Type A individuals who push you in many different ways.

Reduce your awareness of time. Rather than being a slave to the clock, try to ignore it. Get rid of your watch and try to listen more to your body in deciding if you need to eat, sleep, and so on. When you feel *awake,* do something productive. When you are too tired to work, take time out to sleep, or relax and try to energize yourself.

Remember that time is precious. Many people only learn to value their time when they are forced to face a few short weeks during a terminal illness. Then they try to cram a lifetime into a few short moments. Try to place value in each day. A day wasted is a significant loss. Time wasted in not enjoying life and taking time for yourself is a tremendous waste of potential.

Become aware of your own time patterns. For many of us, our hours and minutes drift by without our even noticing them. Chart your daily schedule, hour by hour, for one week. Note the time that was wasted and the time spent in productive work, or restorative pleasure. Assess what areas you could change to be more productive and to make more time for yourself.

Support Groups and Stress

Our support groups can also help us to respond to stress in positive ways. We need friends, family members, and coworkers who can provide us with emotional and phys-

---

* R. Keyes, *Timelock: How Life Got So Hectic and What You Can Do About It* (New York: HarperCollins, 1992).

Promoting Your Health

Are Your Goals Causing You Stress?

Completing this simple questionnaire may help you analyze your own tendencies to cause unnecessary stress in your life.

1. What are the 3 most important goals that you would like to achieve in the next year?
   a.
   b.
   c.

2. What would you have to do to achieve these goals (changes in lifestyle or behaviors, personal sacrifices, etc.)?
   a.
   b.
   c.

3. Within your current resources (time, energy, money, etc.) how likely is it that you *can achieve these goals?*

	Very unlikely	Unlikely	Likely	Very likely
a. Goal A				
b. Goal B				
c. Goal C				

4. What is your greatest *obstacle* in achieving each goal?
   a. Goal A
   b. Goal B
   c. Goal C

5. How *motivated* are you right now to do what is necessary to achieve these goals?

	Unmotivated	Somewhat motivated	Very motivated
a. Goal A			
b. Goal B			
c. Goal C			

Answering the above questions should cause you to examine whether or not you are really ready or able to achieve these goals at this point in your life. You might also consider whether what you might have to sacrifice in achieving these goals is really worth the effort. If your ultimate goals are unrealistic or not enough of a priority, a half-hearted attempt may actually cause you more negative hours than it would have taken to make an honest assessment of (1) what you want to achieve, (2) the potential barriers, (3) the efforts necessary to reach your goals, and (4) your willingness to do what it takes to achieve these goals.

ical support. Although the "ideal" support group differs for each of us, you should have two or three close friends in whom you are able to confide, several neighbors with whom you can trade favors, and the opportunity to participate in community activities at least once a week. The establishment and maintenance of a committed relationship also provide support for you.

If you do not have a close support network, it is important that you know where to turn when the pressures of life seem overwhelming. Family members are often a steady base of support on which you can rely. But if friends or family are unavailable, most colleges and universities have counseling services available at no cost for short-term crises. Clergy members, instructors, and dorm supervisors may also be excellent resources. When university services are unavailable, or if you are concerned about confidentiality, most communities offer low-cost counseling through mental-health clinics.

STRESS AND THE CONSUMER

The popularity of stress management as a topic in the media has also increased the amount of advertising for various "stress fighters." We have been made aware of consumer products and services designed to fight stress: vitamin tablets, massage therapies, cassette tapes, biofeedback devices, and hypnosis techniques. Some of these are not worth the money spent on them.

Hypnosis

Hypnosis, whether induced by oneself of by another person, is a method of reducing certain types of stress.

Hypnosis A process that allows people to become responsive to suggestions given to them; helpful in breaking habits such as overeating.

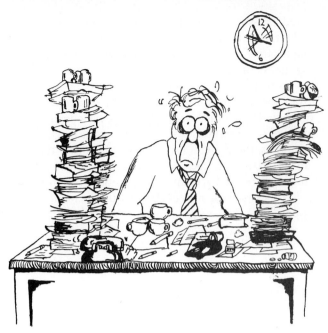

If you can identify with this cartoon, you may need to reconsider your lifestyle.

structure and function of body systems and can lead to addiction and serious side effects. The term *drugs* includes alcohol, caffeine, nicotine, and over-the-counter medications as well as prescription medications and illegal substances.

Various over-the-counter products designed to relieve stress are of questionable benefit. In particular, so-called "stress vitamins," which consist of megadoses of fat- and water-soluble vitamins, are of little real benefit in reversing the detrimental effects of excessive stress. In fact, such large doses of vitamins may be harmful in the long run, and they are expensive (see Chapter 13).

Certain foods have also come under scrutiny in recent years as possible culprits in making people more stress-prone. During the 1970s, research indicated that dietary sugar acted as a stressor. Although early studies appeared to indicate that excessive sugar intake caused a physiological response characterized by hyperactivity, particularly in children, most authorities today question those findings. Carefully controlled studies currently show no significant relationship between the two.* In healthy people, the body apparently quickly adjusts to such changes to maintain homeostasis.

Hypnosis is a process that allows people to become responsive to suggestions given to them. By requiring the subject to focus on one thought, object, or voice, hypnosis frees the right hemisphere of the brain (see Chapter 2) to become more active. Thus, spatial perception and imagination are more accessible under hypnosis than at other times.

The most easily hypnotized people are those who can briefly "escape" from reality through such activities as reading, music, and fantasy. Hypnosis can be used to eliminate bad habits, such as overeating and nail biting. Hypnosis can also be used to reduce tension and anxiety, alleviate headaches, or reduce the effects of other signs of stress. Contrary to popular myths, hypnotized people will not do anything that goes against their basic value system. If something contrary to their beliefs is suggested, they will wake up immediately.

Self-hypnosis must be learned from a qualified professional. Some mental-health professionals are trained to teach self-hypnosis to their clients.

Nutrition, Drugs, and Stress

The foods and substances we put into our bodies can help or hinder our stress-management efforts. Overeating or undereating, eating the wrong kinds of foods, and taking dangerous or unnecessary drugs can create distress by upsetting the body's homeostasis.

Diets that contain too many of the wrong kinds of foods can cause distress by overtaxing different body systems. Included are processed foods and foods high in fats, calories, and sodium. Likewise, drugs affect the

Massage as Therapy

If you have ever had someone massage your stiff neck or aching feet, you know that massage is an excellent means of relaxation. Massage therapists and stress clinics have become a growing part of our quest for stress relief. Therapists use massage techniques that vary from the more aggressive methods typical of Swedish massage to the gentler methods associated with acupressure and Esalen massage. Before selecting a private therapist, check his or her credentials carefully. Certified massage therapists should have training from reputable programs that teach scientific principles for anatomic manipulation.

Biofeedback

Biofeedback is a technique that involves self-monitoring of physical responses to stress. Such factors as perspiration, heart rate, respiration, blood pressure, surface body temperature, and muscle tension can be measured. Many communities have stress-management clinics associated with community mental-health facilities. Some of these clinics use biofeedback instruments.

Clients using biofeedback techniques must first learn to read the measurements given by the machine. Once they have learned this, they are taught to lower their

---

Biofeedback A technique involving self-monitoring of physical responses to stress.

---

* H. Guthrie, *Introductory Nutrition*, 7th ed. (St. Louis: Times Mirror/Mosby, 1989), p. 342.

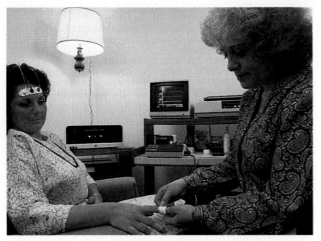
Biofeedback machines can help people control their responses to stress.

blood pressure, respiration rate, perspiration, surface body temperature, and muscle tension through conscious effort. Using the measurements illustrated by the machines, on graphs and charts, the client gradually learns which mental and physical responses actually lower his or her stress responses. After a time (which varies with the individual), the client develops the ability to lower stress responses at will without the machines. At this point, the client is usually able to transfer the techniques learned at the stress clinic to real life. When taught correctly by reliable professionals, biofeedback techniques provide an effective means to reduce stress responses.

SUMMARY

■ Stress is an inevitable part of our daily lives. Although the term *stress* is often used, it is seldom understood.

■ Stress consists of our mental and physical responses to any type of change.

■ Multiple factors contribute to stress and to the stress response, including physiological responses, psychological factors, social factors, and environmental distress.

■ Stress may be healthy (eustress) or unhealthy (distress).

■ Stressors pose threats to homeostasis by causing an organism to become unbalanced as it tries to overcome physical strain.

■ The general adaptation syndrome describes the typical physiological response to stress. It includes three phases: alarm, resistance, and exhaustion.

■ In the first phase of the stress response, the higher centers of the brain interpret the degree of real or imaginary threat. In the second phase, the body prepares itself to fight a real or perceived threat. In the third phase, the victim begins to relax, and the body slowly begins to return to its original state.

■ Self-concept, personality type (A, B, C, or E), and hardiness levels are important factors in determining our vulnerability to stress.

■ Anger and a "toxic core" personality are important factors in susceptibility to stress.

■ Our sense of self-efficacy and control often influences our coping abilities.

■ Time management is an essential aspect of stress reduction.

4

Intimate Relationships and Sexuality

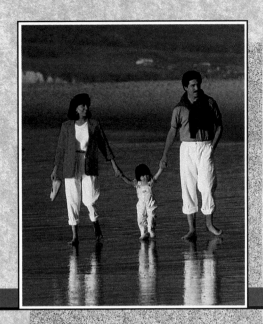

■ Objectives

- Explain why intimate relationships are important, identify some sources of intimate relationships, and discuss the reasons why intimacy may be difficult to achieve for some people.
- Describe several types of committed relationships and discuss how they may be created and maintained.
- Discuss some of the warning signs of troubled relationships and how relationships end.
- Define sexual identity and sexual maturity and outline male and female reproductive anatomy and physiology.
- Identify the three basic sexual orientations and discuss the various ways that we can express our sexuality.
- Discuss the incidence and treatments of the basic sexual problems males and females may encounter.
- List and discuss sexual activities that are illegal.

During recent years, psychosocial researchers, health professionals, and therapists have shown tremendous interest in the nature of our interpersonal interactions. Our relationships with our friends, our families, our intimate partners, people we work with, and complete strangers have been the subject of numerous articles, television programs, and a wide variety of self-help books, workshops, and counseling sessions.

Intense scientific investigations have attempted to unlock the mysteries of our relationships, the effects of these relationships on our self-esteem, our health, our happiness, our individual successes and failures as human beings, and a host of other areas. We have been analyzed genetically, biologically, socially, and psychologically in an effort to determine why we behave as we do and whether there might be a better "recipe" for influencing later interpersonal behaviors.

Each of these studies acknowledges the importance of our casual and intimate interactions in our development into well-adjusted, healthy adulthood. Friendship, close family bonds, and loving intimate and nonintimate relationships are viewed as significant factors in achieving overall health. The eternal quest to be loved and to love others appears to be one of our most basic human needs.

For many, the motivation to seek and receive love appears to be a natural result of previous life experiences and our development as sexual beings. For others, the struggle to find, develop, and maintain relationships becomes a difficult, often painful and frustrating experience, punctuated by unhappy sexual and nonsexual interactions. What makes one person more successful in his or her relationships than another? What effect, if any, does one's sexual identity have on one's ability to form healthy relationships? Taking a look at the nature of relationships (intimate and nonintimate) and our development as sexual beings may help provide the answers to these questions.

INTIMATE RELATIONSHIPS

There are many possible definitions of **intimate relationships.** One classic definition defines these relationships as "close relationships with another person in which you offer, and are offered, validation, understanding, and a sense of being valued intellectually, emotionally, and physically."* In this context, friends, family, lovers, partners, and even people we work with or interact with at the grocery store may be included in the sphere of intimate interactions. However, most experts today tend to focus more on family, close friends, and romantic relationships when they discuss intimate relationships.

For the purposes of this chapter, we will define intimate relationships in terms of three characteristics: behavioral interdependence, need fulfillment, and emotional attachment. Each of these three characteristics may be related to interactions with family, close friends, and romantic relationships.**

Behavioral interdependence refers to the mutual impact that people have on each other as their lives become intertwined. What one person does may have an impact on what the other person may want to do and can do. Such interdependence may become stronger over time, until the point that each person would find a great void in his or her life if the other person were gone.

Another characteristic of intimate relationships is that they *serve to fulfill psychological needs*. These needs may often only be met through relationships with others:

- the need for intimacy—requiring someone with whom we can share our feelings freely
- the need for social integration—requiring someone with whom we can share our worries and concerns
- the need for being nurturant—requiring someone we can take care of
- the need for assistance—requiring someone to help us
- the need for reassurance of our own worth—requiring someone who will tell us that we matter

In close, rewarding, intimate relationships, partners meet each other's needs. They disclose feelings and share confidences and discuss practical concerns, helping each other and providing reassurance.

In addition to behavioral interdependence and need fulfillment, intimate relationships involve strong bonds of *emotional attachment* or feelings of love and attachment.

The intimacy level experienced by any two people cannot easily be judged by those outside the relationship. Individuals share their inner selves so differently that it is impossible to assign a certain meaning to any given action. Friendship relationships can be very intimate and contribute essential elements to a person's sense of inclusion and well-being. Love relationships may be very intimate and include many aspects of intimacy in addition to sexual sharing. Sex is not synonymous with intimacy, although it may be an important part of an intimate relationship. Important relationships with high levels of intimacy may be either sexual or nonsexual.

Intimate Relationships Behavioral interdependence, need fulfillment, and emotional attachment between individuals.

---

* Janet D. Woititz, *Struggle for Intimacy* (Pompano Beach, Fla: Health Communications, 1985).

** Sharon S. Brehm, *Intimate Relationships* (New York: McGraw Hill, 1992), pp. 4–5.

Parental Influences on Intimacy Potential

Balanced intimacy is a goal most people pursue either directly or indirectly. The chances of obtaining balanced intimacy are greater for people who were raised in an environment where close relationships were valued and nurtured. Children's role models are the influential component, be they in a two-parent or single-parent family.

In addition to watching adults relate to one another, children also learn relating patterns from the way a parent interacts with them. Parents who are not afraid to be close to their children when sharing feelings and affection with them generally raise children who can in turn be emotionally connected with others.

The concept of **emotional availability** is important in developing intimacy. Emotionally available people can give and receive emotionally from other people without being inhibited by the fear of being hurt. At times, however, such people may need to protect themselves psychologically by being unavailable emotionally.

Sources of Intimate Relationships

Family of Origin The people present in the household during a child's first years of life are considered to be the **family of origin,** or family of orientation. This group may include a parent or parents, a stepparent, siblings or stepsiblings, lovers or significant others involved with a parent, grandparents, or even aunts and uncles. The family of origin has a tremendous impact on the psychological development of a child. If the home environment provides stability and support for the child and a safe place to express emotion, children will learn intimacy skills.

Friendship In a mobile society such as modern-day America, the family of origin may not be geographically accessible to provide primary support for older children once they leave the parent's home. Even if the family of origin provided intimacy and support during the growing-up years, other forms of social contact are important. Equal relationships with other adults in the form of **friendship** can fill these needs. At any age, having people who care about and appreciate you is important. During our late teen years and twenties, it is especially important for us to establish meaningful contact with others. Depression and suicidal tendencies often stem from isolation. A society that stresses the sexual liaison as the ultimate goal of intimacy may downplay the value of nonsexual friendship. Rarely do the media highlight a friendship relationship, and yet these relationships can provide unconditional and lasting support during the years when both sexual and romantic experimentation are creating emotional turmoil. The skills necessary to develop and maintain a good friendship are the same skills that are valuable in developing a committed partnership: trust, self-disclosure, negotiation, and compromise.

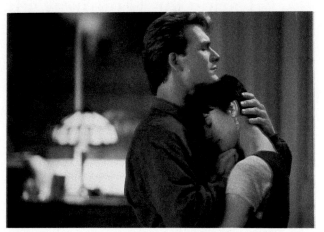

The media often romanticize intimate relationships.

Psychologist Dan McAdams points out that most of us are fortunate to develop one or two lasting friendships in a lifetime. McAdams notes that the two major components of friendships are self-disclosure and support.* Close friendships are based on the ability of the friends to confide in one another and to offer emotional support during the bad as well as the good times.

Significant Others, Partners, Couples Most people choose at some point in their life to enter into an intimate sexual relationship with another person. Over the years numerous studies have analyzed the many ways in which couples form significant partnering relationships. Most couples fit into four categories of significant sexual or committed relationships. These categories are married heterosexual couples, cohabiting heterosexual couples, lesbian couples, and gay male couples. These groups are discussed in the "Types of Committed Relationships" section.

Emotional Availability The ability to give and receive emotionally with another person without the fear of being hurt.
Family of Origin The family in which a person spends the first years of life.
Friendship A close relationship between two people involving high degrees of trust and mutual support.

---

* Dan P. McAdams, *Intimacy: The Need to Be Close* (New York: Doubleday, 1989), pp. 87–91.

The Family of the Future

Caring for Tomorrow's Babies

In 1987, over 57 percent of mothers with children under the age of 5 worked outside the home. While their mothers are away, 41 percent of these children are cared for in someone else's home, 30 percent are cared for in their own homes, 15 percent go to day-care centers, 7 percent go to preschools, and another 7 percent are cared for at work by company-sponsored programs. The average cost of day care exceeded $100 per week per child in 1988, with considerably higher costs in certain regions of the country. The burden of finding alternative means of child care, particularly on very young parents from low-income families, may be very serious.*

The Family of the Future

The likelihood that a child born today will be raised in the traditional "mom and pop" family of past generations is small. Consider the following issues:

- Of all marriages begun since 1970, 50 percent are likely to end in divorce. For second marriages, the estimated divorce rate is 60 percent.
- Stepchildren make up 20 percent of all children in families headed by a married couple. As many

as one-third of all children born in the 1980s will live with a stepparent by the age of 18.
- Single women are opting to bear children "alone" in the 1990s. The typical single woman pursuing pregnancy is a middle-class professional in her mid-thirties or older.
- As more and more parents find it impossible to raise their children because of drug and alcohol problems or financial woes, increasing numbers of grandparents are being asked to step in and help raise their grandchildren.**

The decline in the traditional family structure forces society to examine alternative means of raising our children. Day-care centers, extended families, and live-in babysitters will all become important alternatives to the traditional parental unit. The question then becomes, What effect do these alternative methods of child rearing have on today's children? What are the implications for future generations?

The 21st Century Family, Newsweek special issue (Winter/Spring 1990), pp. 92–93, 104.
** Ibid., p. 34.

Barriers to Intimacy

Obstacles to intimacy include lack of personal identity, emotional immaturity, and a poorly developed sense of responsibility. The fear of being hurt, low self-esteem, mishandled hostility, chronic "busyness" (and its attendant lack of emotional presence), a tendency to "parentify" loved ones, and a conflict of role expectations may be equally detrimental. In addition, individual insecurities and difficulties in recognizing and expressing our emotional needs can lead to an intimacy barrier. These barriers to intimacy may have many causes, including the different emotional development of men and women and an upbringing in a dysfunctional family.

Emotional Development   Although there are various theories regarding the way males and females relate, one that is often quoted is that of author Lillian Rubin, who has proposed a serious barrier to intimacy based on what she considers a basic difference in the development patterns of men and women.** According to Rubin, men

** Lillian B. Rubin, *Intimate Strangers* (New York: Harper & Row, 1983).

are less able to express emotions and achieve intimacy than women due to the process of identity development in infancy, which she sees as more difficult for males than for females.

The disparity in the ability to express emotions may account for common female complaints about male attitudes toward sex. Rubin feels that emotion generates sexual feelings in women, whereas sexual feelings may generate emotion in men. In fact, sexual activity carries the major burden of emotional expression for many men and may explain the urgency with which some men approach sex.

Dysfunctional Families   As we noted earlier, our ability to sustain genuine intimacy is largely developed in our family of origin. Unfortunately, sharing, trust, and openness do not always occur in the family. A **dysfunctional family** is one in which the interaction between family members inhibits psychological growth rather

Dysfunctional Family   A family in which the interaction between family members inhibits rather than enhances psychological growth.

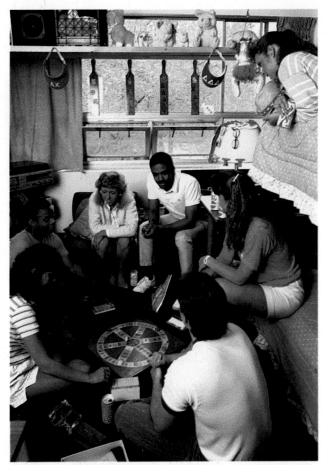
Friendship is one of the most valuable yet overlooked of all intimate relationships.

than encouraging self-love, emotional expression, and individual growth. For example, children who grow up in alcoholic homes, often called *adult children of alcoholics (ACOA)*, may have severe problems creating and maintaining intimate relationships. The family messages that these children live with are typically very contradictory, as the family tries to hide the presence of alcohol abuse in the home.

The Nature of Love

What is love? Finding a definition of love may be more difficult than defining what an intimate relationship is. The term *love* has more entries in *Bartlett's Familiar Quotations* than any other word except *man*.* The word has been written about and engraved on walls, and has been the theme of countless novels, movies, and plays. There is no one definition of love, and the word may mean different things to people of different cultural values, age, gender, and situations.

Many social scientists maintain that all love is divided into two parts: *companionate* and *passionate*. In com-

panionate love, there is a secure, trusting attachment, similar to what we may feel for family members or close friends. Passionate love is a state of high arousal, filled with the ecstasy of being loved by the partner and the agony of being rejected.**

In his article "The Triangular Theory of Love," R. J. Sternberg isolates three key ingredients of love:

- *Intimacy,* the emotional component, which involves feelings of closeness
- *Passion,* the motivational component, which reflects romantic, sexual attraction
- *Decision/Commitment,* the cognitive component, which includes the decisions people make about being in love and the degree of their commitment to their partner.

According to Sternberg's model, the higher the levels of intimacy, passion, and commitment, the more likely a person is to be involved in a healthy, positive relationship. (See Table 4.1.)

▌MAKING A COMMITMENT

Feelings of love or sexual attraction do not always equate with commitment in a relationship. There can be love without commitment and there can be sex without commitment. The concept of **commitment** in a relationship with another person means there is an intent to act over time in a way that perpetuates the well-being of the other person, yourself, and the relationship. A committed relationship involves tremendous diligence on the part of both partners. Over the years, partners learn about one another and constantly adjust the direction of their rela-

Table 4.1 The Triangular Theory of Love: Types of Relationships

	Intimacy	Passion	Decision and Commitment
Nonlove	Low	Low	Low
Liking	High	Low	Low
Infatuated Love	Low	High	Low
Romantic Love	High	High	Low
Empty Love	Low	Low	High
Companionate Love	High	Low	High
Fatuous Love	Low	High	High
Consummate Love	High	High	High

SOURCE: R. J. Sternberg, "The Triangular Theory of Love," *Psychological Review,* 93 (1986), pp. 119–35.

Commitment An intent to act over time in a way that perpetuates the well-being of the other person, the self, and the relationship.

---

* G. Levinger, "Can We Picture 'Love'?" in R. J. Sternberg and M. L. Barnes, eds., *The Psychology of Love* (New Haven, Conn.: Yale University Press, 1988), pp. 139–58.

** E. Hatfield, "Passionate and Companionate Love," in Sternberg and Barnes, *The Psychology of Love,* pp. 191–217.

Promoting Your Health

Assessing Your Intimacy Level

How well do you and your partner know each other? Complete this exercise to find out.
DIRECTIONS: Respond to each of the following questions by writing YES or NO in the blank to the right.

1. Do you feel that your partner does not understand you? _____
2. Do you know how to dress to please your partner? _____
3. Are you able to give constructive criticism to each other? _____
4. In appropriate places, do you openly show your affection? _____
5. When you disagree, does the same person usually give in? _____
6. Are you able to discuss money matters with each other? _____
7. Are you able to discuss religion and politics without arguing? _____
8. Do you often know what your partner is going to say before he/she says it? _____
9. Are you afraid of your partner? _____
10. Do you know where your partner wants to be in five years? _____
11. Is your sense of humor basically the same as your partner's? _____
12. Do you have the persistent feeling you do not really know each other? _____
13. Would you be able to relate an accurate biography of your partner? _____
14. Do you know your partner's secret fantasy? _____
15. Do you feel you have to avoid discussion of many topics with your partner? _____
16. Does your partner know your biggest flaw? _____
17. Does your partner know what you are most afraid of? _____
18. Do you both take a genuine interest in each other's work? _____

19. Can you judge your partner's mood accurately by watching his/her body language? _____
20. Do you know who your partner's favorite relatives are and why? _____
21. Do you know what it takes to hurt your partner's feelings deeply? _____
22. Do you know the number of children your partner would like to have after getting married? _____

Scoring
Look over your responses and give yourself one point for each YES response for numbers 2, 3, 4, 6, 7, 8, 10, 11, 13, 14, and 16 to 22 and one point for each NO response to 1, 5, 9, 12, and 15.

1–5: This indicates a low intimacy level between you and your partner. However, you are together, so you must be fulfilling some need through your relationship. Perhaps the two of you simply need to develop better communication.

6–9: This indicates your intimacy level is rather low but perhaps you are trying to strengthen the relationship.

10–14: This indicates a moderate intimacy level with some room for improvement. Just keep working on the development of open and honest communication.

15–18: You have a great relationship as it is, but you do have your differences. With open communication you are learning to deal with your differences, which will strengthen the relationship.

19–22: You seem to have a great understanding of each other and what it takes to make a successful relationship.

REACTIONS: Now write what you have learned about yourself from this exercise.

---

tionship. What separates committed from uncommitted relationships is the willingness of committed partners to dedicate themselves to acquiring and using the skills that will ensure a lasting relationship. National polls have shown that as many as 96 percent of the American population strives to develop some form of a committed relationship at some time in their lives.

Types of Committed Relationships

Marriage Marriage is the traditional committed relationship in many societies around the world. When two Americans marry, they enter into a legal agreement that

Marriage Legal, and often religious, union of two people intending to spend their lives together.

includes shared financial plans, property, and responsibility in raising children. For religious people, marriage is also a sacrament that stresses the spirituality, rights, and obligations of each person. Close to 90 percent of all Americans eventually marry at least once. However, the United States Census Bureau reports that in recent years Americans have become more particular about commitment and more reluctant to marry young. In 1990 the median age for first marriage was higher than ever before, at 26.1 years for men and 23.9 years for women, compared with 22.5 and 20.6 respectively in 1970.*

Most Americans believe that marriage also involves **monogamy,** or exclusive sexual involvement with one partner. The lifetime pattern for many American heterosexuals appears to be **serial monogamy,** which means that a person has a sexual relationship with one partner for the duration of a relationship before moving on to another monogamous relationship. Some people prefer to have an *open relationship,* or open marriage, in which the partners agree that there may be sexual involvement for each person in addition to the primary partner. Unlike some other species, humans are not naturally monogamous; that is, most of us are capable of loving more than one person at a time. However, sexual infidelity remains an extremely common factor in divorces and breakups. Perhaps only those with strong self-images and a dedication to the principles of open relationships are able to maintain nonmonogamy over a period of time.

As with all relationships, there are marriages that work well and bring much satisfaction to the partners, and there are marriages that are unhealthy for the people involved. A good marriage can yield much support and stability not only for the couple but also for those involved in the couple's life. Because marriage is socially sanctioned and highly celebrated in our culture, there are numerous incentives to stay together and improve the relationship. Behavioral scientists agree that couples who make some type of formal commitment are more likely to stay together and develop the fulfilling relationship they initially sought than those who do not commit.

Cohabitation For various reasons, many people prefer to live together without the bonds of matrimony. Commonly called **cohabitation,** this type of relationship is defined as two people who have an intimate connection with each other living together in the same household. The relationship can be very stable with a high level of commitment between the partners. Cohabitation lasting a designated number of years (usually 7) constitutes a **common-law marriage** for purposes of real estate and other financial obligations in some states.

It is believed that increasing numbers of Americans will opt to cohabit in the 1990s, because of loneliness, soaring housing costs, and a variety of "practical" reasons. Elderly and college-age cohabitors, for example, share the costs of housing, utilities, and food.

The disadvantage of cohabitation lies in the lack of societal validation for the relationship and, in some cases, societal disapproval. The couple usually does not experience the social incentives to stay together that they would if they were married. If they decide to separate, however, they also do not experience the legal problems of going through a divorce. Today, several states are considering legislation to legally validate the relationship between committed partners who live together but do not marry. Eligiblity for tax deductions, health-insurance benefits, and other issues are among those being considered for cohabiting adults.

Lesbian Couples An estimated 10 percent of all women are involved in intimate relationships with other women.** Lesbians are socialized like other women in the culture and tend to place high value on relationships. Lesbians seek the same things in their primary relationships as do heterosexual partners: communication, validation, companionship, and a sense of stability. Most of the lesbians interviewed by Blumstein and Schwartz were in relationships. These women indicated their willingness to work toward creating a partnership to meet their personal and mutual needs. Many lesbians do achieve long-term and even lifelong relationships. Because of the social, legal, and religious restrictions against homosexual people, it is more difficult for lesbian couples to create and maintain a balanced, long-lasting relationship than for heterosexual couples. There is no validation for the lesbian relationship in the form of a wedding with gifts and honeymoon, mutual invitations to gatherings, inclusion at holidays, or even mention of the partner's name. In addition, lesbian couples are often expected to hide their intimate relationship.

Homosexual Male Couples Media attention given to gay men often centers around their sexual behavior, especially since the onset of the AIDS epidemic. Although it is true that young homosexual men generally have more sexual partners than heterosexual men and women or lesbians, it is also true that gay men form committed, long-lasting relationships. As with the data for lesbian couples, reports on numbers of partners and length of relationships are varied. The literature indicates that some male homosexuals enter lifelong, monogamous relationships whereas others have many sexual partners, similar to heterosexual males. Among both homosexuals

---

Monogamy Sexual involvement exclusively with one partner.
Serial Monogamy A series of committed, one-to-one sexual relationships.
Cohabitation Living together outside of marriage.
Common-law Marriage Cohabitation lasting a designated number of years (usually 7) that is considered as binding as marriage in terms of legal and financial obligations.

---

* U.S. Census Bureau statistics, as reported in "Breaking the Cycle of Divorce," *Newsweek,* January 13, 1992, p. 49.

** *Facts on File,* 1985.

Communication

Premarital Contracts

Although it remains the most popular form of cohabitation in American culture, many aspects of marriage are more complicated now than ever before. Many dual-career couples have fears and concerns about legal and financial interests that they should openly communicate before marriage —which does, after all, involve a legal contract. For some couples, a premarital contract may help reduce concerns by establishing guidelines to be followed in the event the marriage does not last. They are more likely to be used in second marriages. Some of the components generally included in premarital contracts are described below:

1. **Daily functions and responsibilities:** Aggrements regarding household tasks, employment expectations, and parenting obligations.
2. **Alimony:** Relinquishing previous alimony payments for marriage but retrieving them from the new spouse should a second divorce occur. Statements of expectations for alimony payments in the event of a divorce.

3. **Estate rights:** Acknowledging that the new spouse will have no claims on money or property to be inherited by partner's children from previous relationship.
4. **Divorce litigation:** Stating what is separate property (owned by one partner before marriage or inherited during it) and marital property (accumulated during the marriage) and agreeing on the division of assets can avoid legal battles should a divorce occur. The divisions may be changed if the couple has children.
5. **Individual property:** Exempting businesses or major possessions owned prior to the marriage from joint ownership and rights. Assets belonging to parents but under children's names may be exempted under agreement.

Lawyers with experience in matrimonial law should be consulted in drawing up the premarital contract to ensure its validity. Premarital contracts are not binding in all states.

---

and heterosexuals, younger men express a greater need for independence and freedom from a partner, whereas older men place more emphasis on companionship and commitment. Gay men who form partnerships in their thirties or forties tend to stay together for many years or for a lifetime.

Challenges to a successful gay male relationship stem from the discrimination they face as homosexuals and from socialization into the male cultural role. Homophobia and invalidation of relationships parallel those experienced by lesbian couples.

Creating and Maintaining Healthy, Committed Relationships

Accountability and Self-Nurturance It is often stated that you must love yourself before you can love someone else. What does this mean? Learning how you function emotionally and how to nurture yourself through all of life's situations is a lifelong task. Certainly you should not postpone intimate connections with others until you have achieved this state. There does, however, seem to be a certain level of individual maturity

that needs to be reached before a successful intimate relationship becomes possible. In the case of marriage relationships, divorce rates are much higher for couples under the age of 30 than for older couples (see Table 4.2). It appears that people who have had a chance to experience and react to a variety of life experiences are better able to sustain a relationship.

Two concepts that are especially important in knowing yourself and maintaining a good relationship are accountability and self-nurturance. **Accountability** means that both partners see themselves as responsible for their own decisions and actions. The other person is not held responsible for the positive or negative experiences in life. This eliminates the very common feeling of being "used" in a relationship. Each and every choice is one's own responsibility. When two people are accountable for their own emotional states, partners can be angry, sad, or frustrated without the other person "taking it personally." Accountable people might even say something like, "This has nothing to do with you; I just happen to be angry right now."

Accountability Accepting responsibility for personal decisions, choices, and actions.

Table 4.2 Divorce Rates by Sex and Age*

Age	Men	Women
15–19	42.9	45.5
20–24	48.2	44.4
25–29	37.6	35.0
30–34	31.7	28.1
35–39	27.1	23.5
40–44	22.0	18.5
45–49	16.1	11.8
50–54	10.7	7.4
55–59	6.4	4.3
60–64	4.0	2.7
65 years & over	1.9	1.4

* Rates per 100 married couples.
SOURCE: National Center for Health Statistics, *Monthly Vital Statistics Report,* June 1990.

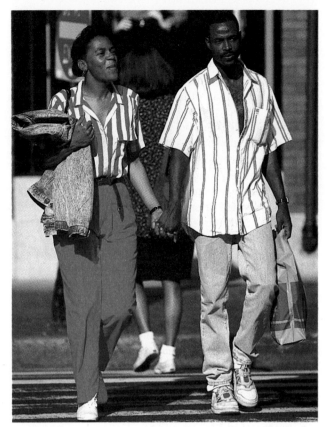
A true commitment involves far more than just youthful attraction.

Self-nurturance goes hand-in-hand with accountability. In order to make good choices in life, you need to maintain a balance of sleeping, eating, exercising, working, and socializing. It is a lifelong process to live in a balanced and healthy way. Two people who are on a path of accountability and self-nurturance together have a much better chance of maintaining satisfying relationships.

Elements of Good Relationships Relationships that are satisfying and stable share certain elements. Some of these are achieved through conscious efforts and communication; others evolve over time. People in healthy, committed relationships trust one another. Without trust, intimacy will not develop, and the relationship will experience trouble and possible failure. **Trust** can be defined as the degree of confidence felt in a relationship. Psychologists John Rempel and John Holmes define trust to include three fundamental elements: predictability, dependability, and faith.*

The first element is *predictability*—the ability to predict your partner's behavior, based on the knowledge that your partner acts in consistently positive ways.

The second aspect of trust is *dependability*. Dependable partners can be relied on to give support in all situations, particularly in those in which you feel threatened with hurt or rejection.

Faith is the third component of trust. When you have faith in your partner, you feel absolutely certain about his or her intentions and behavior.

One study cited sexual intimacy as a major part of healthy relationships, but sex was not recognized as a major reason for the existence of the relationship.* Some

couples even admitted to sexual dissatisfaction within their relationships but felt the relationship was more important than sexual satisfaction. Rather than seek an outlet in an extramarital affair, those who were dissatisfied with their sex lives adjusted and spent little energy worrying about it because the relationship was satisfying in other, more important ways.

Couples valued flexibility and openness to change in their partners. Some couples made periodic decisions to "stay married." An assumption of permanence underlay these relationships. Each couple's beliefs in commitment were strong. To all couples, commitment meant a willingness to experience periodic unhappiness, because troubled times cannot be avoided in the course of human life. Furthermore, happily married couples refused to see divorce or separation as a viable option when problems did arise.

Shared values, life goals, and interests were also characteristic of contented couples. At the same time, each partner pursued interests and activities individually and with other people. Happily married people seem to be secure enough in their relationships that jealousy over outside friendships is nonexistent.

One important quality of successful relationships was a shared and cherished history, including private jokes,

* John K. Rempel and John G. Holmes, "How Do I Trust Thee?," *Psychology Today,* (February 1986), pp. 28–34.
** Jeanette Lauer and Robert Lauer, "Marriages Made to Last," *Psychology Today* (June 1985), pp. 22–34.

Self-nurturance Developing individual potential through a balanced and realistic appreciation of self-worth and ability.
Trust The degree of confidence felt in a relationship.

nicknames, rituals, emotions, and significant shared time and activities. Equally important was luck. Luck in choosing a partner was first, followed by luck in life events. Certain events such as major illnesses, unemployment, career failures, family feuds, and the death of a child can derail an otherwise good marriage.

Having Children The presence of children in the home necessarily changes the lives of the adults around them. When a couple decides to raise children, the relationship changes. Resources of time, energy, and money are split many ways and the partners no longer have each other's undivided attention. Babies and young children do not time their requests for food, sleep, and care to the convenience of the adults.

Therefore, individuals or couples whose own basic needs for security, love, and purpose are already met make better parents. Any stresses that are already in a relationship are only accentuated when parenting is added to the list of responsibilities. Having a child does not save a bad relationship and in fact only seems to compound the problems that already exist. A child cannot and should not be expected to provide the parents with self-esteem and security.

Changing patterns in family life affect the way children are raised. In modern society, it is not always clear which partner will adjust his or her work schedule to provide primary care of children. According to a recent poll, nearly 18 percent of parents are single parents.* Nearly half a million children per year become part of a "blended" family when their parents remarry. Remarriage creates a new family of stepparents and stepsiblings. For a discussion of the changing family structure, see the box entitled "The Family of the Future."

In addition, an increasing number of individuals and couples are choosing to have children in a family structure other than a heterosexual marriage. Single women can choose adoption or alternative (formerly "artificial") insemination as a way to create a family. Lesbian couples can also choose to have children through a specified donor or alternative insemination. Single men can choose to adopt, or they can obtain the services of a surrogate mother. Regardless of the structure of the family, certain factors remain important to the well-being of the unit: consistency, communication, affection, and mutual respect.

ENDING A RELATIONSHIP

Warning Signs of a Declining Relationship

The symptoms of a troubled relationship are relatively easy to recognize. Many couples choose to ignore them, however, until the situation erupts into some type of emotional confrontation. By then, the relationship may be beyond salvaging.

Breakdowns in relationships usually begin with a change in communication, however subtle. Either partner may stop listening, ceasing to be emotionally present for the other. In turn, the other feels ignored, unappreciated, or unwanted. Unresolved conflicts may increase. In turn, unresolved anger can cause problems in sexual relations, with one partner not wanting sex and perhaps "giving in" and subsequently feeling used.

When a couple who previously enjoyed spending time alone together find themselves continually in the company of others or spending time apart, it may be a sign that the relationship is in trouble. Of course, individual privacy and **autonomy** (the ability to care for oneself emotionally, socially, and physically) are important.

People with a good sense of their own identity and the ability to nurture themselves will not allow themselves to be treated poorly in a relationship. Emotional abuse is often unidentified in a relationship and yet has devastating effects on the self-esteem of both the abused and the abuser. Physical abuse or unwanted sexual advances are reasons enough to end a relationship.

Seeking Help: Where to Look The first place some people look for help when there are problems in a relationship is a trusted friend. Although friends can offer needed support during trying times, few have the training and detachment necessary to resolve problems.

Most communities have private practitioners trained to counsel married or committed couples. Community mental-health centers usually have trained counselors as well. These practitioners might be psychiatrists, licensed psychologists, social workers, or counselors with advanced degrees. Couples might also wish to consult clergy members for advice.

Trial Separations Sometimes a relationship becomes so dysfunctional that even counseling cannot bring about significant change. Moving apart for a period of time may allow some preliminary healing and give both parties an opportunity to reassess themselves and their commitment to the relationship. Trial separations do not guarantee that the situation will improve, nor do they mean the relationship is ending. If both people are involved in counseling or have other support systems and mutually agree on the need for a trial separation, it may be a way to regroup and save a failing relationship.

The Decision to Break Up The decision to end the relationship is usually difficult, even for couples whose relationship was "over" long before the decision.

For married couples, wading through divorce or dissolution proceedings, as they decide child-custody issues, alimony questions, and division of property, may be

---

* Mark Tager, "Work and Family Issues: A New Frontier in Health Promotion," *American Journal of Health Promotion*, January/February, 1990.

Autonomy The ability to care for oneself emotionally, socially, and physically.

painful. Finding legal assistance may be difficult, because painful emotions usually affect judgment. Friends or counselors may be able to recommend lawyers who understand the emotions that follow the ending of a relationship.

Couples who choose not to marry also experience difficulty in separating. Legal problems involving property, children, and alimony are often more ambiguous than in a marriage. Some couples expend much time, money, and energy working out settlements with lawyers who specialize in problems following the breakup of a nonmarried committed relationship.

Aside from legal worries, many newly separated or divorced people experience painful emotions of anger, guilt, rejection, and unworthiness. Newly single people may experience great loneliness and an intense desire for new relationships. They may deal with their loneliness through such behaviors as frantic activism, superficial socializing, a string of sexual affairs, workaholism, or abuse of drugs, alcohol, or food. People who acknowledge the difficulty of what they are going through, share their feelings with others, and seek counseling will heal faster and more completely than those who are isolated. Cycles of anger–sadness–resolution diminish with time until the resolution stage becomes dominant.

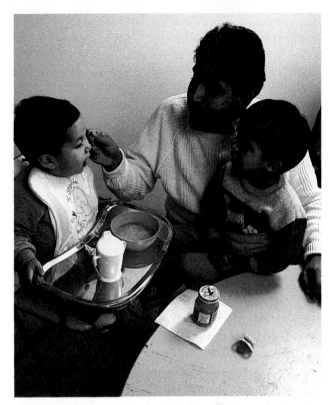
Gender identity is influenced by the roles of parents in the family.

SEXUALITY IN MIND AND BODY: PSYCHOLOGICAL AND PHYSICAL ASPECTS OF SEX

Perhaps no area of human activity invites as much curiosity, conjecture, and controversy as does sexuality. Certainly no human function is surrounded by as many taboos, mores, laws, and myths as are our reproductive roles and activities.

Our era is permeated with sexual concerns: AIDS, abortion, incest, prostitution, pornography, rape, premarital sex, and teenage pregnancy, among others. The Information Age provides us with more information than we can possibly process. Sadly, possession of information does not automatically promote sexual maturity. The development of a mature sexuality requires a system of values and a knowledge of our individual personalities.

Sexual Identity and Sexual Maturity

Although we are born as sexual creatures with the potential to reproduce, we are not born with our sexual identities. Our sexual identities develop just as do our familial, social, religious, political, professional, and ethnic identities. Like these other identities, our sexual identities reflect many influences: our parents' attitudes toward sex, personal and cultural definitions of masculinity and femininity, sexual orientation, personal body image, our sexual experiences, and the meanings, implications, and effects of sexual relationships in our lives.

The development of our **sexual identity**—a composite of our sex (biological gender), social gender roles, sexual preference, body image, and sexual scripts—begins at birth. Our *sex* simply refers to our biological condition of being male or female based on physiological and hormonal differences. Our *gender,* on the other hand, refers to our sense of masculinity or femininity—a certain set of established behaviors and expectations for each sex. For example, in our society, men have traditionally been expected to be more aggressive, whereas women have been expected to be more sensitive. **Gender identity,** then, refers to our personal sense of being masculine or feminine. Our gender identity is determined in large part by our contact with others, our upbringing, and society as a whole.

As we grow into adulthood, our sexual identity is also reflected in our **sexual maturity.** Sexual maturity refers to the manner in which we express ourselves through our sexual behavior. Unlike physical maturity, sexual maturity is not something we achieve automatically. Rather, the process of achieving sexual maturity, although

---

Sexual Identity   Our recognition of ourselves as sexual creatures; a composite of gender, gender roles, sexual preference, body image, and sexual scripts.

Gender Identity   The recognition of ourselves as masculine or feminine.

Sexual Maturity   The manner in which we express ourselves through sexual behavior.

loosely linked to physical age (we need to be physically capable of reproduction in order to manage our sexual growth process), involves intentional effort on the part of the individual. We must desire to grow up sexually in order to begin the process. Sexual growth follows a different timetable for each person. Achieving sexual maturity is not limited to one group of people; heterosexuals, bisexuals, and homosexuals are all capable of sexual maturity.

Sexually mature people exhibit the following behaviors or beliefs:

- They understand and accept the mental, physical, spiritual, and social aspects of human sexuality.
- They carefully explore and continually examine their personal values regarding sexual behavior.
- They can discuss sexuality with little or no embarrassment and can discuss sexual concerns tactfully and sensitively with their partners.
- They do not use sexual behavior to manipulate or injure other human beings.
- They accept responsibility for the consequences of their sexual activity.
- They take steps to prevent unwanted pregnancies and the spread of sexually transmitted diseases.

- They are able to recognize and seek help for sexually related problems.
- They assume active responsibility for the health of their reproductive systems.
- They are able to integrate their choice of sexual expression into their lives.
- They do not allow their desires for sexual gratification to rule their lives. Rather, they balance sexual gratification with other pleasures, values, and rewards.

The journey to sexual maturity begins at birth and continues into our adult lives. It is a long process that involves pitfalls, heartbreaks, alternate setbacks and successes, positive self-examination, problem resolution, and the desire for personal growth.

Reproductive Anatomy and Physiology

Sexual activity is a physical activity that depends upon anatomical and physiological characteristics and conditions. A thorough understanding of the functions of the male and female reproductive systems helps sexually mature people derive pleasure and satisfaction from their sexual relationships.

 # Promoting Your Health

Testing Your Sexual IQ

Take a few minutes to examine your knowledge about selected aspects of human sexuality. Circle the correct answer.

1. The size of a man's penis is directly related to his ability to satisfy a woman sexually. T F
2. More than one out of four (25 percent) of American men have had a sexual experience with another male during their teens or adult years. T F
3. It has been estimated that 70–80 percent of all rapes are committed by men the victim knows. T F
4. Petroleum jelly (e.g., Vaseline) and baby oil are *not* good lubricants to use with a condom or diaphragm. T F
5. Many researchers have reported that approximately 90 percent of adult males and slightly more than 60 percent of all females have masturbated. T F

6. It is not healthy to engage in sexual intercourse during the woman's menstrual cycle. T F
7. Sex should be avoided during pregnancy. T F
8. It is easy to recognize homosexuals by the way they walk or talk. T F
9. Homosexuals can be cured by having sexual relationships with the right persons of the opposite sex. T F
10. Both men and women have erectile tissue in their reproductive organs. T F

Answers:
(1) F   (6) F
(2) T   (7) F
(3) T   (8) F
(4) T   (9) F
(5) T   (10) T

Female Reproductive Anatomy and Physiology

Most of the female's reproductive system lies within the pelvic girdle. The external female genitalia extend from the **mons veneris** over the public bones to the anal opening. (See Figures 4.1 and 4.2.)

The mons divides into two thick fleshy folds called the **labia majora.** These "outer lips" are covered with pubic hair. The labia majora protect two inner folds of thin tissue known as the **labia minora,** or inner lips. The tissues found inside the two sets of labia are called the **vulva.** Nestled at the apex of the "V" formed by the labia is the **glans clitoris,** a highly sensitive nodule of **erectile tissue.** (When erectile tissue becomes suffused with blood, it becomes stiff and *erect.*)

Below the clitoris is the tiny **urethral opening** through which urine leaves the body. Just below the urethra is the **vagina** (birth canal), a hollow, muscular tube capable of expanding to accommodate the passage of an infant during birth. The vaginal opening may be partially covered with a thin piece of tissued called the **hymen.** The hymenal membrane serves no anatomical purpose and is usually stretched or broken through physical activity, use of tampons, masturbation, or sexual intercourse.

Below the vaginal opening, the vulvar tissue tapers to a flat section of skin called the **perineum.** Just below the perineum is the **anus,** the opening through which fecal wastes leave the body. Although not part of the reproductive system, the anus is surrounded by sensitive tissue and is sometimes stimulated as part of sexual activity.

The internal female reproductive organs are located at the interior end of the vagina. At their upper end,

Figure 4.1 The female reproductive organs.

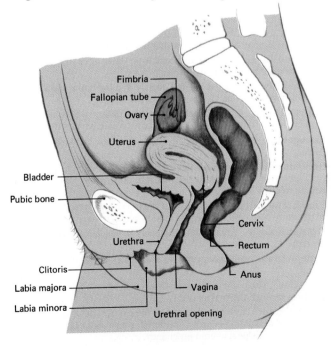

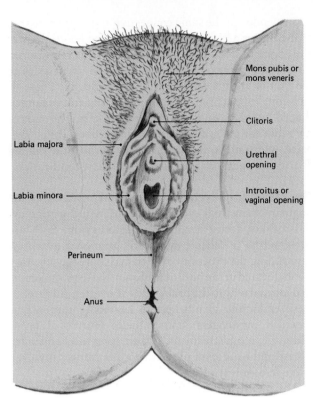

Figure 4.2 Female external genitals.

the vaginal walls flare out and end up to join with the **cervix**—the opening to the uterus. The **uterus** (womb) is normally tipped slightly forward over the top of the urinary bladder. A hollow, pear-shaped organ, the uterus is composed of alternating layers of muscle. In a nonpregnant woman, it is about the size of a fist. An intricate system of ligaments supports the organ. As with the ligaments that attach bones to other bones, the ligaments in the reproductive system are made of tough, fibrous tissue with minimal capacity to stretch and maximum capacity to support weight.

Mons Veneris (mons pubis) Fatty tissue covering the pubic bones in females; in physically mature women, the mons is covered with coarse pubic hair.

Labia Majora The "outer lips" or folds of tissue covering the female sexual organs.

Labia Minora The "inner lips" or folds of tissue just inside the labia majora.

Vulva The female's external genitalia.

Glans Clitoris A pea-sized nodule of tissue located at the apex of the labia minora.

Erectile Tissue Any tissue capable of becoming engorged with blood; usually extremely sensitive to stimulation.

Urethral Opening (urethral meatus) The opening through which urine leaves the body.

Vagina The hollow, muscular tube through which menstrual flow leaves the body and through which babies are delivered.

Hymen Thin tissue covering the vaginal opening.

Perineum Tissue extending from the labia minora to the anus.

Anus Opening through which fecal wastes leave the body.

Cervix Lower end of the uterus that opens into the vagina.

Uterus (womb) Hollow, pear-shaped, muscular organ whose function is to contain the developing fetus.

Suspended in the same connective and support tissues as the uterus are the **ovaries,** two organs about the size and shape of almonds, designed to serve as repositories for developing eggs. Extending from the upper sides of the uterus are the **fallopian tubes** (oviducts). These 4-inch-long tubes curve from the uterus and end in funnel-shaped openings that arch over the ovaries. The ends of the tubes are fringed with tiny hairlike fibers called *fimbriae,* which move continuously, thus aiding the pulling of released eggs into the tubes for possible fertilization.

The Menstrual Cycle Commonly referred to as the singular "menstrual cycle," the ovarian and uterine cycles are key factors in human reproduction. Both are governed by a delicate system of hormonal interplay. Controlling the processes of both cycles are the **pituitary gland,** located at the base of the brain, the **hypothalamus,** also located within the brain, and the ovaries. All three of these endocrine glands secrete hormones that act as chemical messengers among them. Hormonal levels within the bloodstream act as the trigger mechanism for release and regulation of the various hormones involved in the female reproductive cycle.

The menstrual cycle occurs in three distinct phases that are characterized by different hormonal secretions. The length of the cycle varies with individuals, with 28 days used as a point of reference to explain the cycle. The first day of menstrual bleeding is called the *first day* of the cycle. (See Figure 4.3.)

Hormones called **estrogens** are produced in the ovaries. In addition to regulating the reproductive cycle, estrogens also assist in the development of **secondary sex characteristics** such as breasts, fat deposits on hips, higher voice, and fine-textured skin and body hair. When estrogen levels drop below a certain point, as during menstruation, the hypothalamus releases another hormone called *gonadotropin-releasing hormone (GnRH).* This function in turn signals the pituitary to release *follicle-stimulating hormone (FSH).*

The release of these hormones moves the body into the second phase of the cycle, the **proliferatory phase.** During this stage, FSH stimulates the maturation process of from 10 to 20 **ovarian follicles** (egg sacs). In turn, the follicles secrete estrogens.

At the same time, the lining of the uterus, the **endometrium,** begins to grow in response to hormonal secretions from the developing follicles. The inner walls of the uterus become coated with a thick, spongy lining composed of blood and mucus. In the event of fertilization, the endometrial tissue will serve as a nesting place for the developing embryo.

Of all the follicles maturing in the ovaries, only one each month normally reaches complete maturity. (The others disintegrate gradually but continue to secrete vital estrogens.) At about the fourteenth day of the proliferatory phase, the one egg destined to mature bursts from the ovary in a process called **ovulation.** Just prior to ovulation, the mature egg's follicle secretes a hormone called **progesterone,** the first function of which is to add further nutrients to the developing endometrium.

Increases in estrogen that accompany the release of progesterone signal the hypothalamus to release GnRH, which signals the pituitary to release *luteinizing hormone (LH).* The combination of these two hormones causes the follicle to release its mature egg.

After ovulation, the ovarian follicle—the *corpus luteum,* or yellow body—continues to secrete estrogen and progesterone, but in decreasing amounts. In addition, FSH also falls back to its preproliferatory levels. Essentially, the woman's body is waiting to see whether fertilization will occur. During this time after ovulation, LH declines and progesterone levels begin to rise slightly, causing additional tissue growth in the endometrium. This phase of the cycle is called the *secretory phase.*

If fertilization takes place, the developing embryo releases a hormone called *human chorionic gonadotropin (HCG).* Chemically identical to LH, HCG is also similar in function: it produces increased levels of progesterone secretion.

When fertilization does not occur, the egg gradually disintegrates within approximately 72 hours. The corpus luteum gradually becomes nonfunctional, causing levels of progesterone and estrogen to decline. As hormonal levels decline, the endometrial lining of the uterus loses its nourishment, dies, and is sloughed off as menstrual flow. *Menstruation* is the third phase of the reproductive cycle. See Figure 4.3 for a representation of a complete menstrual cycle.

Male Reproductive Anatomy and Physiology While obviously not capable of carrying a developing infant, the male reproductive system is far from simple. Men do not experience monthly uterine/ovarian cycles, but some of the processes involved in manufacturing sperm are similar to the ova-producing processes in the female.

Ovaries Almond-shaped organs that house developing eggs.

Fallopian Tubes Tubes that extend from the ovaries to the uterus and through which mature eggs pass.

Pituitary Gland A gland located deep within the brain; controls reproductive functions.

Hypothalamus A gland located near the pituitary; works in conjunction with the pituitary to control reproductive functions.

Estrogens Female sex hormones that control the menstrual cycle.

Secondary Sex Characteristics Characteristics that make us outwardly male or female such as vocal pitch, degree of body hair, and location of fat deposits.

Proliferatory Phase First stage of the menstrual cycle; the lining of the uterus builds up and eggs begin to ripen in the ovary.

Ovarian Follicle Areas within the ovary in which individual eggs develop.

Endometrium Soft spongy matter that makes up the uterine lining.

Ovulation The point of the menstrual cycle when a mature egg ruptures through the ovarian wall.

Progesterone Hormone secreted by the ovaries; helps keep the endometrium building in order to nourish a fertilized egg; also, the hormone that helps maintain pregnancy.

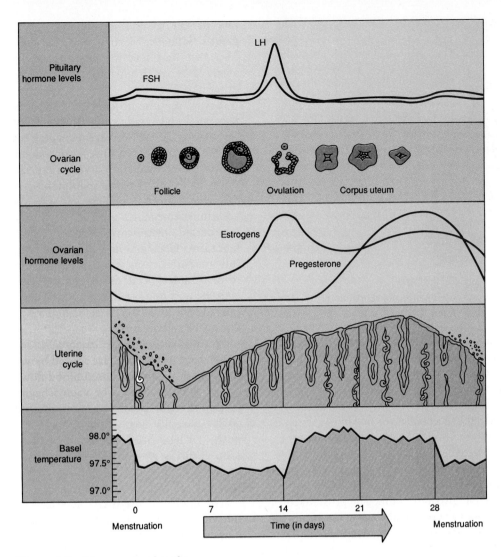

Figure 4.3 The menstrual cycle.

Most of the major male sex organs lie outside the body (see Figure 4.4). The most prominent of these is the **penis.** Penile tissue is separated into three cylinders of spongy *erectile tissue* having the capacity to become engorged with blood during erection. The end of the penis, the *glans,* is coned-shaped and in the uncircumcised male is covered with a flap of skin called the **foreskin.** A tiny central opening of the penis, the *meatus,* allows both urine and semen to pass from the body.

Also situated outside the body and behind the penis is a sack called the **scrotum.** The scrotum contains two **testes,** egg-shaped structures in which sperm are manufactured. The testes also contain cells responsible for the manufacture of **testosterone,** the hormone responsible for the development of male secondary sex characteristics. These characteristics include growth of facial and body hair, deepening of the voice, broadening of the shoulders, and narrowing of the hips. Within each testis are thousands of tiny, coiled *seminiferous tubules.* In some 300 sections of these tubules, sperm are manufactured.

Spermatogenesis is the term used to describe the development of sperm. Like the production of ova in the female, this process is governed by the pituitary gland. Follicle-stimulating hormone (FSH) is secreted into the bloodstream to stimulate the testes to manufacture sperm. Beginning as tiny specks in the walls of the seminiferous tubules, the sperm cells mature and divide through three stages, moving ever closer to the center of the testis. When fully developed, the sperm are released into a comma-shaped structure on the back of the testis called the **epididymis.**

Penis Male sexual organ designed for releasing sperm into the vagina.

Foreskin Flap of skin covering the end of the penis; it is removed by circumcision.

Scrotum The sack of tissue that hangs behind the penis.

Testes Two organs located in the scrotum; responsible for manufacturing sperm.

Testosterone The male sex hormone manufactured in the testes.

Epididymis A comma-shaped structure inside the testes in which sperm are stored for a short period of time.

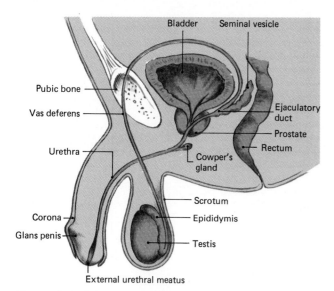

Figure 4.4 Side view of male internal reproductive organs.

Labels in figure: Bladder, Seminal vesicle, Pubic bone, Vas deferens, Ejaculatory duct, Prostate, Urethra, Rectum, Cowper's gland, Corona, Scrotum, Epididymis, Glans penis, Testis, External urethral meatus

The epididymis also contains coiled tubules that gradually "unwind" and straighten out to become the **vas deferens.** The vas deferens arches forward, upward, and backward to circle the urinary bladder. These two tubes (one for each testicle) end in oblong organs called the **seminal vesicles.** In the receptacles formed by the seminal vesicles, the sperm are provided with nutrients and other fluids that compose **semen.**

Both vas deferens empty into a single tube called the *ejaculatory duct.* Surrounding the upper end of this duct is the pyramid-shaped **prostate gland.** The prostate contributes more fluids to the semen, including chemicals to aid the sperm in fertilization of an ovum, and, more important, a chemical that neutralizes the acid in the vagina to make its environment more conducive to sperm motility (ability to move) and potency (potential for fertilizing an ovum).

Just below the prostate gland are two pea-shaped nodules called the *Cowper's glands* (bulbo-urethral glands). Their primary function is to secrete a fluid that lubricates the urethra and neutralizes any acid that may remain in the urethra after urination. Urine and semen do not come into contact with each other. During ejaculation of semen, the tube to the urinary bladder is closed off by a small valve.

During sexual arousal, the spongy tissue in the penis becomes filled with blood, making the organ stiff, or *erect.* Further sexual excitement leads to **ejaculation,** a series of rapid spasmodic contractions that propel semen out of the penile meatus.

Human Sexual Response   Sexual response is a physiological process that involves different stages. The biological goal of the response process is the reproduction of the species. Because of the intense pleasure involved in sexual relations, sexual activity transcends procreation. As emotional and spiritual creatures, human beings find the sexual experience to be a powerful factor in bonding one person to another. Human psychological traits greatly influence sexual response and sexual desire. Thus, we may find the relationship with one partner vastly different from those we might experience with other partners.

Sexual reponse generally follows a pattern. Laboratory research has delineated four or five stages within the response cycle, and researchers agree that each individual has a personal response pattern that may or may not conform to the stages observed in experimental research. Both males and females exhibit four common stages: excitement/arousal, plateau, orgasm, and resolution. In addition, some males experience a fifth stage, the refractory period. Identification of these stages was achieved in laboratory situations in which genital response was carefully measured using specially designed instruments. The response stages occur during masturbation, heterosexual activity, and homosexual activity. Changes in the genitalia during the first three sexual response stages are illustrated in Figure 4.5.

During the first stage, *excitement/arousal*, male and femal genital responses are caused by **vasocongestion** in the genital region. Increased blood flow to these organs causes them to swell. The vagina begin to lubricate in preparation for penile penetration, and the penis becomes partially erect. Both sexes may exhibit a "sex flush," or light blush all over their bodies. Excitement/arousal can be generated by touching other parts of the body, by kissing, through fantasy, viewing films or videos, or reading erotic literature.

The *plateau phase* is characterized by an intensification of the initial responses. Voluntary and involuntary muscle tensions increase. The female's nipples and the male's penis become erect. A few drops of semen, which contain sperm, may be secreted from the meatus.

During the *orgasmic phase,* vasocongestion and muscle tensions reach their peak, and rhythmic contractions occur through the genital regions. In females these contractions are centered in the uterus, the outer vagina, and the anal sphincter. In males the contractions occur in two stages. First, contractions within the prostate gland begin propelling semen through the urethra. In the second stage, the muscles of the pelvic floor, the urethral bulb, and the anal sphincter contract. Semen usually, but not always, is ejaculated from the penis. In both sexes, spasms in other major muscle groups also occur, particularly in the buttocks and abdomen. Feet and hands may

---

Vas Deferens   Two tubes that carry sperm toward the penis.
Seminal Vesicles   Additional storage areas for sperm where nutrient fluids are added to the sperm.
Semen   Fluid containing sperm and nutrient fluids that increase sperm viability and neutralize vaginal acid.
Prostate Gland   Gland that secretes nutrient and neutralizing fluids into the semen.
Ejaculation   The propelling of semen from the penis.
Vasocongestion   The engorgement of the genital organs with blood.

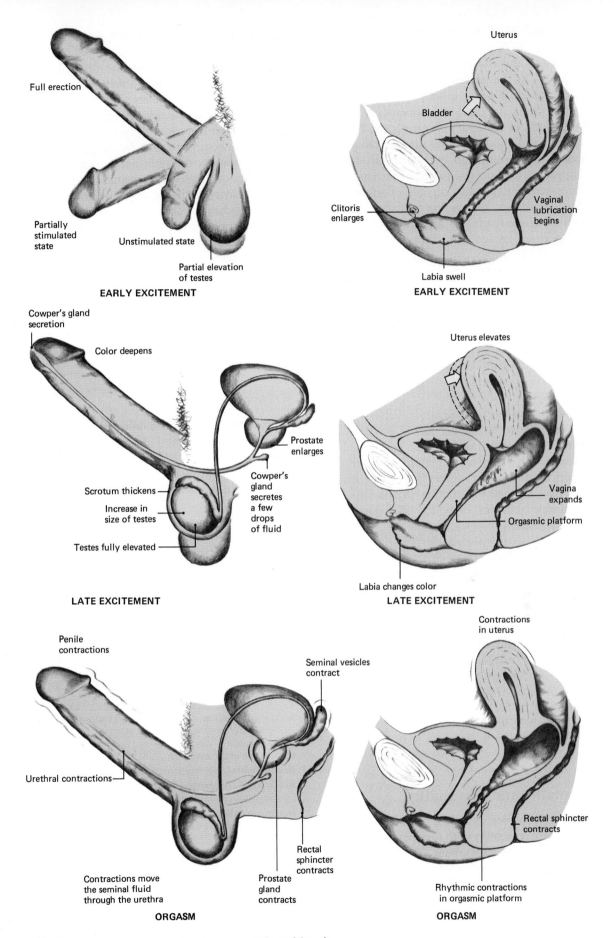

Figure 4.5 Sexual response comparison between male and female.

also contract, and facial features often contort into a grimace.

Muscle tension and congested blood subside in the *resolution phase,* as the genital organs return to their prearousal states. Both sexes usually experience deep feelings of well-being and profound relaxation.

In males, a fifth, or *refractory phase,* occurs. Following orgasm and resolution, many females are capable of being aroused and brought to orgasm again. Males, however, appear to experience a period of time in which their systems rest before being capable of subsequent arousal. Some males are able to skip this refractory, or resting, period. These males can achieve erection soon after ejaculation and can continue through the cycle to another orgasm. This ability diminishes with age.

Males and females experience the same stages in the sexual-response cycle; however, the length of time spent in any one stage is variable. Thus, one partner may be in the plateau phase while the other is in the excitement or orgasmic phase. Such variations in response rates are entirely normal. Some couples believe simultaneous orgasm is desirable for sexual satisfaction. Although simultaneous orgasm is pleasant, so are orgasms achieved at different times.

Sexual pleasure and satisfaction are possible without orgasm or intercourse. Achieving sexual maturity includes learning that sex is not a contest with a real or imaginary opponent. The sexually mature person enjoys sexual activity whether or not orgasm occurs. Expressing love and sexual feelings for another person involves many pleasurable activities, of which intercourse and orgasm are only a part.

SEXUAL ORIENTATION AND EXPRESSION

An important part of our sexuality is our **sexual orientation.** Sexual orientation refers to our preference or choice of sexual partners. We may be attracted to and interested in members of the opposite sex (heterosexual), the same sex (homosexual), or both sexes (bisexual). Our sexual orientation is established during the first few years of life and is not usually subject to change.*

Homosexuality and Bisexuality

Homosexuality is defined as sexual attraction to, and preference for, sexual activity with members of the same sex. Researchers believe that about 25 percent of the population engages in homosexual activity at some time in their lives. Between 5 and 10 percent of men are

homosexual, or *gay,* and 3 to 5 percent of women are homosexual, or *lesbian.***

The AIDS (acquired immune deficiency syndrome) epidemic has added a new dimension or fear regarding homosexuals in our society. **Homophobia** is the term given to irrational hatred or fear of homosexuals. In some parts of the country, incidents of "gay bashing" (attacks on homosexuals) have escalated.

Bisexuality is the term used to describe the sexual preference of people who are attracted to, and engage in sexual activity with, members of both sexes. Because bisexuality has not been studied as thoroughly as homosexuality and heterosexuality, we cannot accurately estimate the number of bisexual people in the U.S. population. However, some researchers believe that 8 to 12 percent of men and 6 to 8 percent of women in the United States are bisexual.†

Psychosociologist Judd Marmor estimates that about 15 percent of married men are either bisexual or gay. Between 40 and 100 percent of these men keep their bisexuality a secret from their wives.‡

Heterosexuality

Heterosexuality is the sexual orientation of between 75 and 80 percent of the U.S. population, and was long considered the only "normal" sexual orientation. Heterosexuals are attracted to members of the opposite sex. Their sexual contacts are exclusively with members of the opposite sex.

Origins of Sexual Orientation

Opinions concerning the development of sexual orientation are diverse. Most researchers argue that sexual orientation is "programmed" during the first 5 to 7 years of life; some even believe that it is established by the time a person is born.§

The origins of heterosexuality and homosexuality have not been identified. No proof exists that homosexu-

---

Sexual Orientation Attraction to and interest in members of the opposite sex, the same sex, or both sexes.

Homosexuality Attraction to, and preference for, sexual activity with people of the same sex.

Homophobia The irrational hatred or fear of homosexuals.

Bisexuality Attraction to and preference for sexual activity with people of both sexes.

Heterosexuality Attraction to, and preference for, sexual activity with people of the opposite sex.

** Mary S. Calderone and Eric W. Johnson, *The Family Book about Sexuality,* rev. ed. (New York: Harper & Row, 1989), pp. 106–112.

† Ivan Hill, ed., *The Bisexual Spouse* (McLean, Va.: Barlina Books, 1987), p. 255.

‡ Hill, *The Bisexual Spouse,* p. 260.

§ Calderone and Johnson, *The Family Book about Sexuality,* p. 106.

* Elizabeth Thompson Ortiz, *Your Complete Guide to Sexual Health* (Englewood Cliffs, N.J.: Prentice Hall, 1989), pp. 42–44.

Finding healthy ways to express our sexuality is an important part of developing sexual maturity. With the many avenues of sexual expression open to us, discovering one that will bring us satisfaction can be very difficult. We should begin by understanding how the chemistry of sexual attraction works.

Developing Sexual Relationships

Perhaps the most important part of developing mature sexuality is learning to develop rewarding sexual relationships. Like all skills, developing relationships takes time, patience, and practice. Our sexual education begins with our family. We watch the significant adults in our lives and pattern our behaviors after theirs. At puberty, when extrafamilial elements, peers, and the media become more important, we adapt some of their standards to our behaviors. Our shyness, aggressiveness or assertiveness, passivity, and levels of comfort with our sexuality come from our own personalities and from what we have learned from others.

Not only do we bring our history to our sexual relationships, but we also bring our peculiar chemistry. The human potential for passionate sexual love has been defined as **limerence**. In a book titled *Love and Limerence: The Experience of Being in Love,* Dorothy Tennov discusses the issue of passionate or romantic love based on sexual attraction. The word *limerence* is derived from the name of the portion of the brain that controls sexual response, the *limbic cortex.* Limerence is what makes us feel sexually "turned on" by a person. This powerful feeling can overshadow common sense. Sexual relationships based on limerence may or may not develop into long-lasting or committed relationships. Tennov believes that limerence only lasts 2 years at most. Relationships based upon a love that has taken time to mature are much more likely to last. Following are some of the "symptoms" of limerence:

- Intrusive thoughts about the object of desire
- Dependency of mood on love object's actions
- Relief from unrequited passion through fantasy
- Fear of rejection, along with almost incapacitating shyness
- Sharp capacity to interpret desired person's actions favorably, and ability to interpret *any* signs from the other as hidden passion
- An "aching of the heart" (a physical tightening of the chest or stomach) when uncertainty is intense

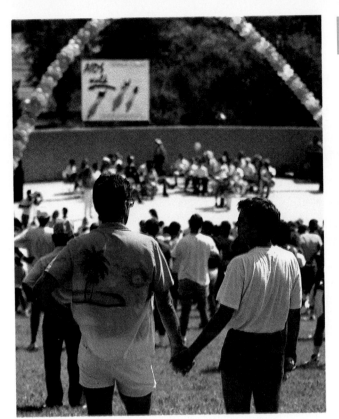

Public displays of affection between homosexuals are far more common today than in past decades.

ality can be inherited. Homosexuality is not a sign of emotional illness or maladjustment. Psychiatric theory once blamed homosexuality on overly possessive mothers and passive fathers, but there is no research evidence to support this idea. Seduction by an older homosexual also does not seem to be a factor.** Indeed, the determinants of sexual orientation simply cannot be identified at this time.

Nature versus Nurture The interplay between biological and environmental factors has not been sufficiently studied to yield concrete conclusions regarding the development of sexual preference. Research does suggest, however, that such interplay exists. For example, some researchers believe that hormone imbalances during fetal development may predispose a person to homosexuality. This biological factor, coupled with some environmental factors, such as lack of nurturing by a parent, *might* contribute to a homosexual orientation.

Researchers have concluded that sexual orientation is not a matter of choice. People who try to change their sexual orientation through therapy rarely succeed. Patterns of sexual orientation appear to be patterns for life.

** Hill, *The Bisexual Spouse,* p. 254.

Limerence The quality of sexual attraction based on chemistry and gratification of sexual desire.

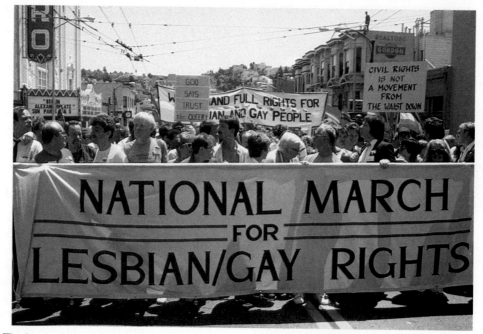

The issue of gay rights has received support from many heterosexuals as well as homosexuals.

- Intensity of feelings that leaves other concerns in the background
- Ability to emphasize what is admirable in the love object and to avoid dwelling on the negative, or even to reconceptualize the negative into a positive attribute.*

In developing our sexual relationships, we must look beyond limerence. To do this, we must begin slowly, learning to recognize limerence, and realizing that the weak-kneed, heart-palpitating feelings do not have to be acted upon immediately. Taking the time to know another person helps reduce the risks involved with sexual activity. Although risk-free sex can never be guaranteed, sex between two people who are comfortable with each other (because they have taken the time to get to know one another) is likely to be more satisfying.

Am I Normal?

The range of human sexual expression is virtually infinite. What we like in one circumstance we may not like in another. What we enjoy on one particular day may not suit us on another. The following are among the most common sexual acts performed by couples.

Missionary position—a sexual position in which the male is on top of the female, each one facing the other.

Rear entry—a sexual position in which the male penetrates the vagina from a kneeling position behind the female.

Female on top—a sexual position in which the female is on top of the male, each one facing the other.

Fellatio—the act of sucking or licking the male genitalia.

Cunnilingus—the act of sucking or licking the female genitalia. Performed simultaneously, fellatio and cunnilingus are called "69."

Anal intercourse—the act of penetrating the anus with the penis. During anal intercourse, men should wear condoms to prevent the spread of AIDS and other diseases.

Foreplay—the actions and behaviors performed during the arousal phase of the sexual-response cycle. Includes kissing, licking, nibbling or sucking various parts of the body, hugging, stroking, and talking.

In *The Joy of Sex*, Alex Comfort provides a classic definition of "normality": "any sex behavior . . . which (1) you both enjoy, (2) hurts nobody, (3) isn't associated with anxiety, (4) doesn't cut down your scope. . . . 'Normal' implies there is something which sex ought to be. There is. It ought to be a wholly satisfying link between two affectionate people, from which both emerge unanxious, rewarded and ready for more."*

Many couples worry that they don't have sex often enough. Popular magazines frequently give the "average" number of times couples engage in sex every week. Such numbers are meaningless. Rather than compare ourselves to these statistics, we would be wise simply to follow our own feelings.

---

* Dorothy Tennov, *Love and Limerence* (Chelsea, Mich.: Scarborough House, 1989), pp. 45–50.

* Alex Comfort, *The Joy of Sex* (New York: Simon & Schuster, 1972), p. 14.

Masturbation

Masturbation is the act of self-manipulation of the genital organs, usually to achieve orgasm. Practiced by an estimated 90 percent of males and 70 percent of females, masturbation is a normal and enjoyable activity. Partners involved in committed relationships often masturbate to provide variety or to relieve sexual tension when their partner is unable or unavailable to engage in sexual activity.

Masturbation becomes abnormal only when it assumes inordinate emphasis in a person's life. The person who stays home to masturbate rather than engaging in social activities might have a problem that needs to be examined. In addition, people who grow up under parental or religious systems that forbid masturbation might experience guilt or shame if they do masturbate.

Celibacy

Celibacy is a state of being uninvolved in a sexual relationship. Many people experience periods of celibacy throughout their lives—following the breakup of a long-term relationship, for example, or after the death of a spouse or during times of depression. Some people who feel that their sex lives are not fulfilling may choose celibacy. In addition, certain religious orders take vows of celibacy because the bonding involved in sexual relationships could distract them from their selfless vocations.

Drugs and Sexuality

Because psychoactive drugs (discussed in Chapter 12) affect our entire physiology, it is only logical that they affect our sexual behavior. Promises of increased pleasure make drugs very tempting to those seeking greater sexual satisfaction. Too often, however, drugs become central to sexual activities and damage the relationship.

Alcohol is notorious for reducing inhibitions and giving increased feelings of well-being and desirability. At the same time, alcohol inhibits sexual response; thus, the mind may be willing, but not the body.

Perhaps the greatest danger associated with the use of drugs during sex is the tendency to blame the drug for negative behavior. "I can't help what I did last night because I was stoned" is a response that demonstrates sexual immaturity. A sexually mature person carefully examines risks and benefits and makes decisions accordingly. Good sex should not be dependent on chemical substances.

Variant Sexual Behavior

Although attitudes toward sexuality have changed radically since the Victorian era, some people believe that any sexual behavior other than heterosexual intercourse is abnormal, deviant, or perverted. Rather than using these negative terms, people who study sexuality prefer to use the nonjudgmental term **variant sexual behavior** to describe sexual behaviors that are not engaged in by most people. The following list of variant sexual behaviors includes behaviors that are illegal in some states and some behaviors that could be harmful to others.

GROUP SEX   Sexual activity involving more than two people. Participants in group sex run a high risk of exposure to AIDS and other sexually transmitted diseases.

TRANSVESTISM   The wearing of clothing of the opposite sex. Most transvestites are male, heterosexual, and married.

TRANSSEXUALISM   Strong identification with the opposite sex, in which men or women feel that they are "trapped in the wrong body." In some cases, transsexuals undergo sex-change operations. Since the 1960s, 4,000 of these operations have been performed in the United States.

FETISHISM   A condition in which a person experiences sexual arousal by looking at or touching inanimate objects, such as underclothing or shoes.

EXHIBITIONISM   The exposure of one's genitals to strangers in public places. Most exhibitionists are seeking a reaction of shock or fear from their victims. Exhibitionism is a minor felony in most states.

VOYEURISM   Observing other people for sexual gratification. Most voyeurs are men, who attempt to watch women undressing or bathing. Voyeruism is an invasion of privacy and is illegal in most states.

SADOMASOCHISM   Sexual activities in which gratification is received by inflicting pain (verbal or physical abuse) on a partner or by being the object of such pain. A *sadist* is a person who receives gratification from inflicting pain, and a *masochist* is a person who receives gratification from being the object of pain.

DETERRENTS TO REALIZING SEXUAL POTENTIAL

From time to time, each of us experiences sexual problems. **Sexual dysfunction** is the label given to the various problems that interfere with sexual pleasure. In most

---

Masturbation   Deliberate manipulation of one's own genitals for sexual pleasure.
Celibacy   The state of not being involved in a sexual relationship.
Variant Sexual Behavior   A sexual behavior that is not engaged in by most people.
Sexual Dysfunction   Problems associated with achieving sexual satisfaction.

cases, sexual dysfunction can be treated successfully if the partners involved are willing to work together to solve the problem.

Impotence and Premature Ejaculation

Impotence is the inability to attain or maintain an erection or sufficient penile rigidity for intercourse. At some time in his life, every man experiences impotence. The causes are varied and include underlying diseases, such as diabetes or prostate problems; reactions to some medications (for example, medication for high blood pressure); depression; fatigue; stress; alcohol; performance anxiety; and guilt over real or imaginary problems (such as when a man compares himself to his partner's past lovers).

Impotence generally becomes more of a problem as men age. Statistics indicate that 2 percent of men at age 40 and 25 percent of men over age 65 experience the problem occasionally. At any given time, 10 million American men suffer from impotence.*

For impotence related to physical causes, new treatments are being explored. These include hormone therapy, treatment with vasoactive drugs (drugs that work on the circulatory system), and vascular surgery to correct abnormalities in the blood vessels that supply the penis. Impotence due to psychological factors can be treated with psychotherapy. Such treatment is effective in 90 percent of cases.

Premature ejaculation is ejaculation that occurs prior to or almost immediately after penile penetration of the vagina. Premature ejaculation is estimated to affect 50 percent of the male population at some time.

Therapy for the premature ejaculator involves a physical examination to rule out organic causes. If the cause of the problem is not physiological, a therapist can help the man learn to control the timing of his ejaculation. First, he will be taught to recognize the sensations that precede ejaculation. He is then taught to control the timing of his ejaculation through two techniques: the *squeeze technique* and the *pause*, or *Semans*, technique.

Both techniques rely upon the man and his partner to cease penile stimulation before ejaculation. In the pause technique, the partners stop and wait until the preejaculatory feelings subside. In the squeeze technique, the man or his partner is required to squeeze just below the coronal ridge (base of the head) on the penis for 20 seconds, or until the urge to ejaculate disappears. In most cases, therapy succeeds in 6 to 10 weeks.

The Preorgasmic Woman

When a woman is unable to achieve orgasm with her partner, she often blames herself and learns to fake or-

gasm in order to preserve her partner's ego. Until recently, our society dictated that women were not supposed to enjoy sex, but were to engage in it only to fulfill the "marital duty." The Kinsey reports in the 1950s and Masters and Johnson's findings in the 1960s and 1970s raised questions about these female sexual myths. We recognize today that women enjoy sexual experiences when their partners are genuinely interested in the female's enjoyment, when there is open communication about likes and dislikes, and when the sexual act occurs in a nonthreatening, comfortable environment. In the past, women who did not experience orgasm were called *frigid*. This term is no longer used because it implies that the woman is at fault. Instead, the terms *preorgasmic* and *sexually unresponsive* have been substituted, since most women can be taught to become orgasmic. Therapy is available for women whose sexual pleasure is hampered.

Dyspareunia

Pain experienced by a female during intercourse can be a deterrent to sexual pleasure. Called **dyspareunia**, such pain may be caused by diseases such as endometriosis, uterine tumors, chlamydia, gonorrhea, or urinary-tract infections. Damage to tissues during childbirth and insufficient lubrication during intercourse may also cause pain or discomfort. Dyspareunia can also be psychological in origin. As with other problems, dyspareunia can be treated, with good results. The first step in treatment is a thorough pelvic examination to rule out physical disease.

Diseases or disorders can usually be cured with either medication or surgery. Vaginal lubricants can be purchased to help with inadequate lubrication. Psychologically caused dyspareunia is much more difficult to treat. A condition called **vaginismus** is the most frequently recognized psychologically related disorder. In vaginismus, the vaginal muscles contract involuntarily, making intercourse difficult or impossible. In most cases, vaginismus is related to fear or unresolved sexual conflicts.

Treatment of dyspareunia involves teaching the woman to achieve orgasm through nonvaginal stimulation. Becoming orgasmic is important because research has indicated that treatment for vaginismus is more successful in orgasmic women. The woman and her partner are then taught methods for dilating the vagina, either with fingers or a vibrator. As dilation is achieved, the woman is taught to relax in order to effect penetration. Cure rates are close to 100 percent.

Impotence   The inability to attain or maintain an erection or sufficient rigidity for intercourse.
Premature Ejaculation   Ejaculation that occurs prior to or almost immediately following penile penetration of the vagina.
Dyspareunia   Painful intercourse experienced by women.
Vaginismus   A state in which the vaginal muscles contract so forcefully that penetration cannot be accomplished.

---

* Robert J. Krane, Irwin Goldstein, and Inigo Saenz de Tejada, "Impotence," *New England Journal of Medicine*, December 14, 1989, pp. 1648–57.

SEX AND THE LAW

Although many people feel free to engage in various sexual acts behind closed doors, not all sexual activity is legal. Many states have laws forbidding sodomy (anal sex, bestiality, or fellatio) or homosexual activity. In 1991 and 1992, Congress and the judicial system had to deal with the issues of sexual harassment (Anita Hill vs. Supreme Court nominee Clarence Thomas) and date rape (the cases of Mike Tyson and William Kennedy Smith). Televised coverage moved these issues out of the closet and into the homes of millions of Americans.

Sexual Assault

Rape is the crime of forcing an individual to have sex without his or her consent. *Statutory rape* is a special category of unlawful sexual intercourse with a female minor. Between 1.5 million and 2 million women are raped in the United States each year. Less than 50 percent of rape cases are reported. Just over another 1 million women are victims of attempted rape, and half of these cases go unreported. Not all rape victims are female; in 1985, 123,000 men were reported to have been raped. Approximately 75 percent of apprehended rape suspects are brought to trial, but less than 13 percent of these suspects are convicted.*

Although rape is often thought of as a sexually aggressive crime, it is usually a form of assault performed to hurt or demean the victim rather than to achieve sexual gratification. No profile of a "typical" rapist exists; however, the majority of arrested rapists are between the ages of 15 and 25. Alcoholism or problem drinking are common among convicted rapists. Some studies have found that rapists have higher levels of testosterone than do other offenders and that they score high on measures of hostility.

Acquaintance Rape and Date Rape Acquaintance rape and date rape have received increased media attention in recent years. **Acquaintance rape** is forced sexual intercourse between two people who know each other. **Date rape** is forced sexual intercourse by one's dating partner. It is estimated that between 70 and 80 percent of all rapes are committed by people known to the victim.**

In 1988, *Ms.* magazine and the National Institute of Mental Health conducted a survey of 32 college campuses across the nation. Twenty-five percent of women interviewed reported having been raped. Eight-four percent of the victims knew their attackers, and 57 percent

of the rapes occurred while the couple were on a date. The average age of female victims was 18.5 years.***

The William Kennedy Smith and Mike Tyson date-rape cases caused colleges and universities across the country to focus on these issues. Programs to increase awareness and prevent occurrences typically are designed to: (1) educate men about rape and the pain and suffering it causes, (2) teach them to respect the fact that when a woman says no she means it, (3) inform men of possible legal consequences, (4) inform women of their legal rights, and (5) educate men and women about prevention. See the box titled "Dealing with Rape" for more information.

Child Sexual Abuse

Child sexual abuse also appears to be widespread in the United States. Approximately 27 percent of women and 16 percent of men are sexually molested before they reach their eighteenth birthday. Eighty percent of these crimes are committed by people whom the child knows.† Sexual-abuse-prevention programs in schools focus on distinguishing between appropriate and inappropriate touching, saying no to an adult, and reporting abuse or threatened abuse to trusted authorities.

Two classifications of child sexual abuse exist. The first, **pedophilia,** is abuse of a child by an adult in search of sexual excitement. Genital fondling of prepubescent (preteenaged) children is the most common form of pedophilia. Most child victims know their abuser; it is almost always a male and may be a neighbor or friend of the family. In most cases, the child is induced to participate through mild forms of intimidation or offers of gifts. Violence is seldom used. Pedophiles are likely to be men who have problems with their adult sexuality. Treatment is generally imprisonment combined with therapy. As with therapy for rapists, the success rate for this therapy is directly related to the person's willingness to change.

Incest is the other form of child sexual abuse. Incest is sexual relations between close blood relatives. A common form of incest is between brothers and sisters. Father–daughter incest is believed to be the most psychologically damaging type of incest. In most incestuous relationships, the girl is postpubescent. Intercourse is more likely to occur as the daughter matures.

Rape Sexual intercourse or activity forced upon another person against his or her will.
Acquaintance Rape A type of rape that occurs between two people who know each other; usually forced intercourse on a date.
Date Rape A type of rape consisting of forced intercourse by a person's dating partner.
Pedophilia A condition in which an adult has a sexual desire for children.
Incest Sexual relations between close adult blood relatives.

---

* Ortiz, *Your Complete Guide to Sexual Health,* p. 100.
** Andrea Parrot, *Coping with Date Rape and Acquaintance Rape* (New York: Rosen, 1988), pp. 4–5.

*** Robin Warshaw, *I Never Called It Rape* (New York: Harper & Row, 1988), p. 11.
† Calderone and Johnson, *The Family about Sexuality,* p. 161.

Dealing with Rape

Although there are no measures that can guarantee protection against rape, there are certain steps that you can take to decrease the likelihood of its occurrence.

1. At home, be sure that all doors and windows can be locked securely. When you leave home, be sure that all entrances are secured.

2. Keep emergency telephone numbers in accessible places near the telephone and, if possible, commit them to memory.

3. Do not admit strangers to your home. If someone claims to be from a utility company, keep the door locked and call the company to verify the stranger's identity. If you have any doubts, refuse to admit the person. Tell the stranger that you will call the company to arrange for service at a more convenient time.

4. Avoid informing telephone callers that you are home alone.

5. Walk or jog with a companion rather than by yourself. If you must walk alone, do so in populated areas where there is access to telephones. Walk briskly and with purpose. Remember that rape can occur at any time of the day.

6. If you are returning from a friend's home, arrange to call your friend when you arrive home, with the understanding that if you do not call within a reasonable time, your friend will check on your whereabouts.

7. If you are traveling alone by car at night, be aware that stopping for vehicle problems can be hazardous. If you have to stop, stay in your car with the windows rolled up and the doors locked until somebody stops for you. Roll down the window a crack and ask the stranger to call for help. Above all, keep your vehicle in good repair.

8. Develop assertiveness skills to avoid date rape.

9. Take a self-defense class designed specifically for preventing physical assault.

10. If you are approached, remember that there are methods of warding off an attack. The following strategies are listed in descending order of effectiveness: run away; physically resist the attack; scream or blow a whistle in the assailant's ear; reason with the attacker. Pleading with the assailant is the least effective method. Researchers have found that women using physical force are more likely to be injured but, if force is used early in the attack, are more likely to prevent the rape and escape.

Unfortunately, rape can occur in spite of the best precautions. If you or someone you know has been raped, knowing what to do can help the healing process that needs to follow the violation.

1. Call your community rape-hotline center. Keep the number with your other emergency numbers. The counselors at the center are trained to help victims through the legal processes necessary for rape cases. Because their presence can ease the difficulties surrounding this experience, call them before you call the police.

2. After you have called the hotline, or if no hotline exists, call the police and report the crime. The police will want to know your name, address, and age, the location at which the rape took place, and a description of the assailant and the events that occurred before and during the assault. You will undoubtedly be emotionally upset, angry, and hurt after the attack. Try to remain assertive and give law-enforcement officers as much information as you can. Be prepared to answer what may seem to be unnecessary questions.

3. If you have sustained physical injuries, you will need to go to a hospital emergency room. Some large hospitals have personnel available to help rape victims. Law-enforcement agencies often need laboratory analysis of semen. Many will ask you not to bathe or douche prior to examination at the emergency room. Medical personnel can obtain the desired evidence at the time you are admitted to the emergency room.

4. Arrange for counseling for yourself and those members of your support system who will be able to give you the most help. No one survives a rape without emotional scars of some type. Your ability to heal will depend upon both your own resources and the help of your family, friends, and others.

5. Above all, remember that *you* are not at fault in any way for what happened. You did not provoke the assault. You did not cause it. The person who assaulted you needs help, but that person is responsible for the crime, not you.

The causes of incest are unknown. Fathers and step-fathers who engage in incestuous relationships with their daughters are likely to believe that their homes and families are their private property and that they have the right to do as they please with them. They tend to be domineering, possibly to compensate for their weakness outside the home.

Various programs exist to help abusive parents break the cycle of violence. Organizations such as Parents Anonymous as well as community parenting resource centers provide counseling and group support for abusive parents.

In many cases, the child is placed in temporary foster care until the parent receives the help necessary to stop the abuse. Victims of incest often resort in promiscuity in adolescence, and their adult lives may be hampered by sexual dysfunction.

Pornography

Pornography includes literature, photographs, drawings, videos, and films designed to produce sexual arousal. Many American communities are fighting against what they perceive as a plague of pornography. Several franchise grocery stores have been persuaded to remove erotic magazines from their shelves. Others are only allowed to sell such wares at the counter. In some cases, liberal feminists are joining conservative groups in the battle against pornography.

Pornographic items featuring sexual abuse or exploitation of children have come under attack by many church and civic organizations. Some people contend that pornography contributes to the growing rate of sexual violence. Others equate the banning of pornography with censorship. Disputes surrounding pornography are long-standing, and the controversy continues.

Sexual Harassment

Sexual harassment is any unwanted verbal or physical sexual advance that involves a threat to the business or educational career of the person being harassed. Legally, the definition refers only to employment situations in which an employee is threatened with not being hired, not receiving a promotion, or being fired if he or she will not submit to the harasser's sexual demands. Sexual harassment occurs in educational institutions as well, in situations in which students may be threatened with failing grades, poor evaluations, or refusal of letters of reference. Sexual harassment may be of either a heterosexual or a homosexual nature.

Studies have shown that between 42 and 60 percent of women and between 9 and 15 percent of men report having been harassed on the job. Studies also estimate that 20 percent of women in college experience sexual harassment by a professor.[*]

Sexual harassment is extremely serious and can ruin a person's career, reputation, or educational success. Although few states have enacted sexual-harassment laws, such cases are often prosecuted under sexual discrimination laws. No one should have to submit to unwanted sexual demands. For some basic steps for avoiding or preventing sexual harassment, see the box entitled "Sexual Harassment."

Pornography   Literature, films, pictures, or other media designed to produce sexual stimulation.

---

[*] Ortiz, *Your Complete Guide to Sexual Health*, p. 104.

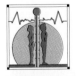

Sexual Harassment

Preventing Unwanted Advances

1. Remember that sexual harassers like to prey on helpless people. Show confidence in your work and avoid acting or looking helpless, weak, or vulnerable.

2. Be assertive with anyone who uses inappropriate language or touch. Set limits early and clearly to let the person know that these behaviors are offensive.

3. Some sexual harassers have a history of engaging in this behavior. Listen to friends' and coworkers' warnings about sexual harassers.

4. Do not allow yourself to be alone with or under the direct supervision of a suspected sexual harasser.

5. If someone harasses you, keep a detailed log of dates and specific behaviors and statements.

6. Investigate sources of legal help and counseling in your college, place of employment, or community. Know your rights and responsibilities.

SOURCE: Adapted from Elizabeth Thompson Ortiz, *Your Complete Guide to Sexual Health* (Englewood Cliffs, N.J.: Prentice-Hall, 1989), pp. 105–6.

- There are many different levels and types of intimate relationships.

- Family, friends, and partners or lovers provide the most common opportunities for intimacy.

- Barriers to intimacy include the different emotional needs of men and women and emotional wounds from being raised in a dysfunctional family.

- Committed relationships usually take the form of legally sanctioned marriage.

- Cohabitation is not legally sanctioned as a committed relationship but can be socially sanctioned.

- Lesbians and gay men do form lasting, committed relationships despite societal invalidation of their experience.

- Greater levels of individual maturity and personal accountability enhance a couple's chances for a rewarding, long-term relationship.

- Each year more than a million couples in the United States are divorced.

- Communication and cooperation in an atmosphere of intimacy and trust are vital to successful relationships.

- Other factors that contribute to successful relationships include commitment to permanence, ability to change, ability to accept what cannot be changed, genuine liking and respect for your partner, balance of dependencies, a shared history, and luck.

- Counseling from a psychiatrist, psychologist, social worker, counselor, or clergy can help repair and strengthen relationships.

- When all attempts to save a relationship fail, divorce, dissolution, or separation may be the only alternatives.

- Our sexual identity is a composite of characteristics, manifested in our sexual behavior. Sexual identity is based on our parents' attitudes toward sex, our biological sex, personal and cultural definitions of masculinity and feminity, our sexual preference, our body image, our sexual experiences, and the meanings, implications, and effects of sexual relationships in our lives.

- Sexually mature people exhibit certain behavioral characteristics, including an understanding of human sexuality, acceptance of their responsibilities regarding sexual behavior, and integration of sexual choices into lifestyle. Sexually mature people also have a thorough understanding of human sexual anatomy and human sexual response. They are able to recognize problems in sexual expression and to seek help.

- Human sexual response comprises four stages: excitement, plateau, orgasm, and resolution. Men experience a fifth, refractory stage.

- Theories abound regarding the origin of sexual preference. At the present time, no one is sure whether environmental or biological factors, or some combination of these, are responsible for the development of sexual preference.

- Because the range of human sexual expression is broad, many sexual activities are considered "normal."

- Sexual dysfunction includes any problems in sexual response that inhibit sexual activity. Most cases of sexual dysfunction can be successfully treated with therapy.

- Each of us must learn to communicate with a potential partner regarding sexually transmitted disease and contraception.

- The incidence of sexually related crimes, including rape and child sexual abuse, appears to be increasing in the United States.

- Sexually related crimes have been under study for some time. However, we do not yet have concrete answers as to their cause. Prevention of sexual crimes involves both individual and community effort.

5

Pregnancy, Childbirth, and Birth Control

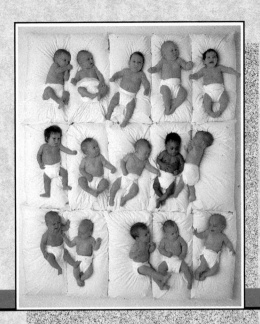

Objectives

- Discuss parenthood in terms of your own life goals and expectations, including some of the most important things you and your spouse or partner should consider before becoming pregnant.

- Discuss what is meant by prenatal care and describe the process of pregnancy.

- Describe the basic stages of childbirth as well as some of the things that can go wrong during labor and delivery.

- List permanent and reversible contraceptive methods in order of their effectiveness against pregnancy and STDs and describe how these methods are used.

- Summarize both the social and political issues surrounding abortion and the various types of abortion procedures used today.

- Discuss some of the primary causes of and possible solutions to infertility.

Human beings are the only species that has the power to understand the ramifications of reproduction. Not only do we have the ability to understand this process but we also have the technology to control our own fertility. Along with this understanding and technology comes the significant responsibility to manage our reproductive capacities.

Today, the decision to have children has become a choice rather than an obligation, and is influenced by a variety of factors. Couples contemplating having children must ultimately face the possibility of upheavals in their lives. For example:

- The divorce rate has doubled since 1965, and demographers project that half of all first marriages today will end in divorce.
- Six out of 10 second marriages now end in divorce.
- One-third of all children born in the past decade will probably live in a stepfamily before they reach age 18.
- One out of 4 children today is raised by a single parent.
- One out of every 5 children lives in poverty; the rate is twice as high among blacks and Hispanics.
- Over two-thirds of all mothers are forced to work to support their families.*

Whereas women in the 1940s bore an average of 3 to 4 children, the modern woman bears an average of 2 children. Nearly one-third of all married couples choose not to have children.** Those choosing to have children must consider the following questions: Is this new life truly wanted? Can this new human being be cared for in a loving and nurturing manner? Is there adequate financial support for prenatal care and for the raising of this child? Are we (am I) ready to make all the sacrifices necessary to bear and raise a child? Do we (I) even know the magnitude of the sacrifices in terms of time, money, and emotional well-being? Finally, prospective parents should carefully examine their reasons for wanting a child. Do they want a child to fulfill an inner need, to carry on the family genes, out of loneliness, or for other reasons?

In our culture we are taught from birth that human life is sacred and that the creation of a new life should not be taken lightly. Unfortunately, the possibilities and consequences associated with sexual activity are often ignored because we are swept along by the powerful and pleasurable feelings of the moment. Responsible and mature people are able to control their desire for sexual gratification long enough to make rational decisions regarding their intended behavior.

One measure of maturity is the ability to discuss reproduction and fertility control with one's sexual partner before giving in to sexual urges. This type of discussion should not be any more difficult than discussing sexually transmitted disease. Embarrassment-free discussion is best achieved through obtaining objective information regarding human reproduction and contraception and by considering individual attitudes prior to getting into compromising situations.

THE DECISION TO BECOME A PARENT

The technological ability to control our fertility gives us choices that our parents did not have. The loosening of social restrictions in the area of marriage and parenting also affords single men and women the opportunity to become parents. Regardless of a person's lifestyle, the preparation to become a parent involves similar considerations and decisions.

The first step in deciding to have a child is to set goals for yourself as a parent. Without goals, you have no direction, even at the outset of your relationship with the child. Once the child is born, setting goals can become clouded with the day-to-day responsibilities of caring for the child.

The second step is to evaluate the parenting skills of both you and your partner. A quick test of parenting readiness is found in the box entitled "Am I Parent Material?"

You should also evaluate your finances. In 1990, the cost of raising a child from birth to 21 years of age was estimated to be over $250,000. This amount does not include the cost of a college education. Medical care during pregnancy and birth can cost from $1,500 to $5,000, depending upon the medical practitioner, the nature of the pregnancy, complications, and the geographical location. Some insurance companies provide pregnancy benefits, and others provide limited benefits or none at all. A review of your insurance policy is important before planning a pregnancy.

Related to finances is the question of maternity or paternity leave from your place of employment. The length of leave available, as well as the conditions for returning to work, are things to consider carefully before becoming pregnant.

Another factor to consider is maternal health. Before becoming pregnant, a woman should have a thorough medical examination in order to rule out any possible problems that could complicate the pregnancy. Women with chronic medical problems such as diabetes should also carefully discuss their intentions with their physician.

The availability of high-quality child care should also be considered. Many young parents assume that nearby relatives will be happy to take the baby at any time, even

---

* Jerrold Footlick, "What Happened to the Family," *Newsweek*, special issue (Winter/Spring 1990), p. 16.

** Ibid.

Communication

Am I Parent Material?

The decision to have children should never be taken lightly. Even the best prenatal classes do not fully teach us how to cope with the reality of having a child. Before decisions about parenthood are made, partners should answer the following set of questions. After each of you answers the questions, you should discuss your responses.

1. What do I want out of life for myself? What do I think is important?

2. Could I handle a child and a job at the same time? Would I have time and energy for both?

3. Would I be willing to cut back my social life and spend more time at home? Would I miss my free time and privacy?

4. Can I afford to support a child? Do I know how much it takes to raise a child?

5. Do I want to raise a child in the neighborhood where I live now? Would I be willing and able to move?

6. How would a child interfere with my growth and development?

7. Would a child change my educational plans? Do I have the energy to go to school and raise a child at the same time?

8. Am I willing to give a great part of my life, at least 18 years, to be responsible for a child? And spend a large portion of my life being concerned about my child's well-being?

9. Do I like children? When I'm around children for a while, what do I think or feel about having one around all the time?

10. Does my partner want to have a child? Have we talked about our reasons?

11. Could we give a child a good home? Is our relationship a happy and strong one?

12. Are we both ready to give our time and energy to raising a child?

13. Could we share our love with a child without jealousy?

14. What would happen if we separated after having a child, or if one of us should die?

15. Do my partner and I understand each other's feelings about religion, work, family, child raising, and future goals? Do we feel pretty much the same way? Will children fit into these feelings, hopes, and plans?

16. Suppose one of us wants a child and the other doesn't? Who decides?

17. Would I want a child to be "like me"?

18. Would I expect my child to keep me from being lonely in my old age? Will I do that for my parents? Do my parents do that for my grandparents?

19. Would having a child show how mature I am?

20. Will I prove I am a man or woman by having a child?

21. Do I expect my child to make my life happy?

22. How would I take care of my child's health and safety? How do I take care of my own?

23. What if I have a child and find out I made the wrong decision?

24. Would I want my child to achieve things that I wish I had, but didn't?

SOURCE: *Am I Parent Material?* (Santa Cruz, Calif.: Network Publications.

on a moment's notice. Expectations of family assistance with a new baby as well as the availability of nonfamily child care should also be considered. Although the federal government makes provisions for child-care allowances on income-tax forms, the provision may not be enough to cover child-care expenses. For this reason, the quality and cost of child care in the community should be researched prior to the pregnancy.

A final consideration is that of providing for the child should something happen to his or her parents. Although unpleasant to consider, a couple planning a pregnancy should think about what would happen to the child if both of them were to die while the child is young. Are there relatives or close friends who could take the child? If there is more than one child, can they be split up or would it be better to keep them together? Planning for this contingency will ease the problems involved with shuffling children after parents' deaths. Children who lose their parents are usually confused enough, and a prearranged plan of action may help to smooth the transition of the children into new families.

Once the decision to become a parent is made, preparation for parenthood takes several forms. Reading about parenthood, taking classes, talking to parents of children of all ages, or joining a support group can all be helpful preparation. For those choosing to adopt, various types of support groups exist, including groups for adopters of foreign children, handicapped children, abused children, or mentally retarded children.

PREGNANCY

Prenatal Care

Given our present knowledge and technology, pregnancy should occur by choice. We know how pregnancy occurs. We know how to prevent it. We should allow ourselves and our partners the time necessary to examine and explore all the issues concerning pregnancy, childbirth, and parenting before deciding to conceive.

A successful pregnancy goes beyond asking the question, "Can I (we) afford to have this child?" Financial issues are important, but equally important are the mother's physical condition, her level of nutrition, her confidence in her ability to give birth, her use of drugs and medications, and the availability of a skilled practitioner who can oversee the pregnancy and delivery. (See the box titled "Choosing a Childbirth Practitioner.") Women planning a pregnancy also need to examine their human support systems. Are there members of that support system (spouse or partner, family, friends, community groups) willing to give her and her child the love and emotional support she will need during and after her pregnancy?

Pregnancy and Drugs A woman should avoid all types of drugs during pregnancy. Even common over-the-counter medications such as aspirin, and beverages such as coffee and tea, can damage a developing fetus.

During the first 3 months of pregnancy, the fetus is especially subject to the **teratogenic** (birth-defect-causing) effects of some chemical substances (see Table 5.1). The fetus can also develop an addiction to or tolerance for drugs the mother is using.

Of particular concern to medical professionals is the use of tobacco and alcohol during pregnancy. Women who are heavy drinkers may have normal babies with their first pregnancy but deliver children with fetal alcohol syndrome with subsequent pregnancies. The symptoms of **fetal alcohol syndrome** include mental retardation, slowed nerve reflexes, and small head size. The exact amount of alcohol necessary to cause the syndrome is not known. Researchers doubt that any level of alcohol consumption is safe, and they recommend total abstinence during pregnancy. Fetal alcohol syndrome is discussed in more detail in Chapter 10.

Smoking cigarettes during pregnancy has more predictable effects than drinking alcohol. Studies have shown a 25 to 50 percent higher rate of fetal and infant deaths among women who smoke during pregnancy

Table 5.1	Teratogenic Effects of Drugs
Drug	Effect
Alcohol	Mental retardation, growth retardation, increased spontaneous abortion rate
Amphetamines	Suspected nervous-system damage
Aspirin	Newborn bleeding
Cocaine	Uncontrolled jerking motions, paralysis, depressed interactive behavior, poor organizational response to environmental stimuli
Opiates	Immediate withdrawal in newborns, permanent learning disability
Tetracycline	Tooth discoloration
Sulfa drugs	Facial and skeletal abnormalities
Barbiturates	Congenital malformations
Streptomycin	Deafness
Accutane	Small or absent ears, small jaws, heart defects
Valium	Possible congenital anomalies

SOURCE: M. Samuels, M.D., and N. Samuels, *The Well Pregnancy Book* (New York: Summit Books, 1986), p. 131.

than among those who do not.* Women who continue to smoke more than 10 to 15 cigarettes a day have higher rates of miscarriage, stillbirth, premature birth, and low-birth-weight babies than do nonsmokers. Research regarding the effects of "secondhand," or sidestream, smoke (smoke produced by others) is inconclusive. But infants whose parents smoke can be twice as susceptible to pneumonia, bronchitis, and other related illnesses.

X-rays X-rays present a clear danger to the fetus. Although most diagnostic tests produce minimal amounts of radiation, even low levels may cause birth defects or other problems, particularly if several low-dose X-rays are taken over a short time period. Pregnant women are advised to avoid X-rays unless absolutely necessary.

Nutrition Pregnant women must pay special attention to nutrition. They have additional needs for protein, calories, and certain vitamins and minerals, and their diets should be carefully monitored by a qualified practitioner. Folic acid (found in dark leafy greens), iron (dried fruits, meats, legumes, liver, egg yolks), calcium (nonfat or lowfat dairy products, some canned fish), and fluids all require special consideration. Babies born to mothers whose nutrition has been poor run high risks of

Fetal Alcohol Syndrome A collection of symptoms, including mental retardation, that can appear in infants of women who drink too much alcohol during pregnancy.

Teratogenic Causing birth defects; may refer to drugs, environmental chemicals, X-rays, or diseases.

* U.S. Department of Health and Human Services, *The Health Benefits of Smoking Cessation: A Report of the Surgeon General, 1990, Executive Summary* (1990).

substandard mental and physical development (see Table 5.2).

Weight gain during pregnancy has been a controversial subject. As recently as the 1960s, physicians were recommending that a woman gain no more than 20 pounds during her pregnancy. In the early 1980s, the medical establishment revised this number to closer to 30 pounds. Generally, the recommended weight gain is from 20 to 30 pounds and varies from woman to woman (see Table 5.3).

Exercise during pregnancy is an important factor in weight control as well as in overall maternal health. A balanced, 45-minute exercise session 3 days per week has been associated in one study with heavier-birthweight babies, fewer surgical births, higher Apgar scores (discussed later in this chapter), and shorter hospital stays after birth.* Pregnant women should consult with their physician before taking on any exercise program.

Other Factors A pregnant woman should avoid exposure to toxic chemicals. She should not clean cat-litter boxes because cat feces can contain organisms that cause a disease called *toxoplasmosis.* If a pregnant woman contracts the disease, damage to the infant can occur, including stillbirth, mental retardation, and birth defects.

Prior to becoming pregnant, a woman should be tested to determine if she has had rubella (German measles). If she has not had the disease, she should get an immunization for it and wait the recommended length of time before becoming pregnant. A rubella infection can kill a fetus or can cause blindness or hearing disorders in the infant. If she has ever had genital herpes, she should inform her physician. The physician may want to deliver the baby by cesarean section, especially if the woman has

Table 5.2 How the Mother's Nutrients Correspond to Her Infant's Potential Deficiencies

Nutrient	Deficiency Effect
Protein	Low infant birthweight, reduced infant head circumference
Folate	Miscarriage and neural-tube defect
Vitamin D	Low infant birthweight
Calcium	Decreased infant bone density
Iron	Low infant birthweight and premature birth
Iodine	Varying degrees of mental and physical retardation in the infant
Zinc	Congenital malformations

SOURCE: L. K. Debruyne and S. R. Rolfes, *Life Cycle Nutrition: Conception Through Adolescence,* ed. E. N. Whitney (St. Paul: West, 1989).

* D. Hall and D. Kaufmann, "Effects of aerobic and strength conditioning on pregnancy outcomes," *American Journal of Obstetrics and Gynecology,* 157 (1987), 1199–1203.

Table 5.3 Components of Mother's Weight Gain During Pregnancy

Development	Mother's Weight Gain (lbs.)
Infant at birth	7 1/2
Placenta	1
Increase in the mother's blood volume to supply placenta	4
Increase in size of mother's uterus and muscles to support it	2 1/2
Increase in size of mother's breasts	3
Fluid to surround infant in amniotic sac	2 to 8
Total	20 to 26

active lesions. Contact with an active herpes infection during birth can be fatal to the infant.

Age and Motherhood

Today a woman over 35 who is pregnant has plenty of company. While births to women in their twenties are declining, the rate of first births to women between the ages of 30 and 39 has doubled in the past decade, and births to women over 39 have increased by more than 50 percent. Many women who wait till their thirties might find themselves asking "Am I too old to have this baby?" Researchers believe that there is a decline in both the quality and viability of eggs produced after age 35. Statistically, the chance of having a baby with birth defects does rise after the age of 35. **Down's syndrome,** a condition in which a child is mildly to severely retarded with varied prognoses, is the most common birth defect among babies born to mothers after the age of 35. The incidence of Down's syndrome in babies born when the mother is 20 years old is 1 in 10,000 births and rises to 1 in 365 by the time the mother is 35. After that the risk increases to 1 in 100 at 40 and 1 in 32 at age 45.

Women choosing to delay motherhood until their late thirties often worry about their physical ability to carry and deliver their babies. For these women, a comprehensive exercise program will assist in maintaining good posture and promoting a successful delivery. Many doctors are encouraging older women to go ahead with plans to become pregnant because these women tend to be more conscientious about following medical orders during pregnancy and often make outstanding parents. Psychologically, older women may be more settled and more ready to include an infant in their family.

Down's Syndrome A type of mental retardation occurring most frequently in babies whose mothers were over 35 at the time of pregnancy.

Choosing a Childbirth Practitioner

Trusting Someone With Your—and Your Baby's—Life

A woman should carefully choose a practitioner to attend her pregnancy and delivery. If possible, she should choose the practitioner before she becomes pregnant. Recommendations from friends who were satisfied with the care they received during pregnancy may be a good starting point for a woman in her search for a practitioner. Her family physician may also be able to recommend a specialist. Regardless of the decision, the pregnant woman needs a practitioner she can trust with both her own life and that of the infant and with whom she can communicate freely.

In choosing a practitioner, a woman should ask a number of questions concerning the practitioner's credentials and professional qualifications. In addition to this information, however, a pregnant woman must ask questions specific to her condition. She should inquire as to the practitioner's attitudes toward normal deliveries, birth control, abortion, and alternative birth procedures. The practitioner's approach toward nutrition and medication during pregnancy should be similar to her own. Finally, she must be aware of the circumstances under which the practitioner would perform a cesarean section.

Two types of physicians can attend the mother. The *obstetrician-gynecologist* (ob-gyn) is an M.D. who specializes in obstetrics (pregnancy and birth) and gynecology (women's reproductive organs). These practitioners are trained to handle all types of pregnancy and delivery-related emergencies.

A *family practitioner* is a licensed M.D. who provides comprehensive care for people of all ages. The majority have obstetrical experience but will refer a patient to a specialist if necessary. Unlike the ob-gyn, a family practitioner can attend the birth and afterward serve as the baby's physician.

Midwives are also experienced practitioners who can attend pregnancies and deliveries. *Certified nurse-midwives* are registered nurses with specialized training in pregnancy and delivery. Most midwives work in private practice or in conjunction with physicians. The latter have access to traditional medical facilities to which they can turn in an emergency. *Lay midwives* may or may not have extensive training in handling an emergency. They may have taught themselves or learned through experience rather than through formal certification procedures.

Pregnancy Testing

A woman may suspect she is pregnant before any type of pregnancy tests are taken. A typical sign is a missed menstrual period, yet this is not always an accurate indicator. A woman can miss her period for a variety of reasons, including stress, exercise, and emotional upset. Other symptoms of pregnancy include nausea, breast tenderness, weight gain, and fatigue.

Women wishing to know immediately whether or not they are pregnant can purchase home pregnancy kits. These kits are sold over the counter in drug stores, and they are about 85–95 percent reliable. A positive test is based on the secretion of human chorionic gonadotropin (HCG) in the woman's urine. Home test kits come equipped with a small sample of red blood cells coated with HCG antibodies to which the user can add a small amount of urine. If the concentration of HCG is great enough, it will clump together with the HCG antibodies, indicating the user is pregnant.

Problems with the home kits are associated with the accuracy of the tests. Taking the test too early in the pregnancy may produce a false negative. Other causes of false negatives are unclean test tubes, ingestion of certain drugs, and vaginal or urinary infections. The accuracy of the test also depends on the quality of the test and the user's ability to perform the test and interpret the test results. Blood tests administered and analyzed by a medical laboratory give more accurate results.

The Process of Pregnancy

Pregnancy begins at the moment a sperm fertilizes an ovum in the fallopian tubes. From there, the single cell multiples and curves into a sphere-shaped cluster of cells as it travels toward the uterus, a journey that may last 3 to 4 days. Upon arrival, the embryo burrows into the thick spongy endometrium and is nourished from this carefully prepared lining.

Pregnancy typically lasts from 240 to 300 days. The due date is calculated from the expectant mother's last menstrual period. Because only 5 percent of women deliver on their due dates, pregnancy is divided into three phases, or **trimesters,** of 3 months each.

During the first trimester, few noticeable maternal body changes occur. The expectant mother may urinate more frequently and experience morning sickness, swollen breasts, or undue fatigue. She may not even know she is pregnant at this time unless she has had a pregnancy test. Pregnancy tests can be given in medical offices, birth-control clinics, and at home.

During the first 2 months after conception, the **embryo** differentiates and develops its various organ systems, beginning with the nervous and circulatory systems. At the start of the third month, the embryo becomes a **fetus,** indicating that all organs systems are in place. For the rest of the pregnancy, growth occurs in each major body system, refining all structures so that they can function independently yet together at birth. Figure 5.1 illustrates physical changes during fetal development.

At the beginning of the second trimester, physical changes in the mother become more visible. Her breasts swell and her waistline thickens. During this time, the fetus makes greater demands upon the mother's body. In particular, the **placenta,** the network of blood vessels that carry nutrients and oxygen to the fetus and fetal waste products to the mother, is well established.

The third trimester extends from the end of the sixth month through the ninth month, the period of the greatest fetal growth. Although it is possible for a baby born in the sixth or seventh month to survive, survival rates are low because the infant's body systems are not yet prepared to handle life independently from the mother.

Prenatal Testing and Screening

Modern technology has enabled medical practitioners to detect major health defects in a fetus as early as the fourteenth to twentieth weeks of pregnancy. One common testing procedure, **amniocentesis,** involves inserting a long needle through the mother's abdominal and uterine walls into the *amniotic sac,* the protective pouch surrounding the baby (see Figure 5.2). The needle draws out 3 to 4 teaspoons of fluid, which is analyzed for genetic information about the baby. This test reveals the presence of 40 genetic abnormalities, including Down's syndrome, Tay-Sachs disease—a fatal disorder of the nervous system common among Jewish people of Eastern European descent—and sickle-cell anemia, a debilitating blood disorder found primarily among blacks. Amniocentesis can also reveal the sex of the child, a fact many parents choose not to know until the birth. Although widely used, amniocentesis is not without risk.

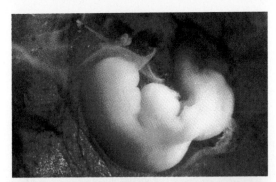

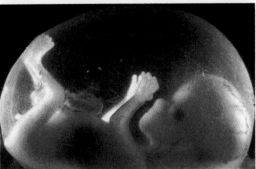

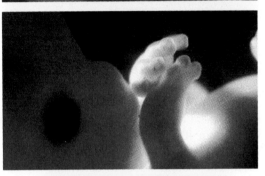

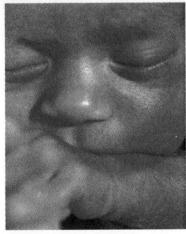

Figure 5.1 The fetus at 28 days, at 15 weeks, at 5 months, and at 7 months.

Trimester A 3-month segment of pregnancy, during which specific developmental changes occur in the embryo or fetus.

Embryo The fertilized egg from conception until the end of 2 months' development

Fetus The developing baby from the third month of pregnancy until birth.

Placenta The network of blood vessels that carry nutrients to the developing infant and carry wastes away; it connects to the umbilical cord.

Amniocentesis A medical test in which a small amount of fluid is drawn from the amniotic sac as early as the fourteenth to twentieth week of pregnancy; it tests for Down's syndrome and genetic diseases.

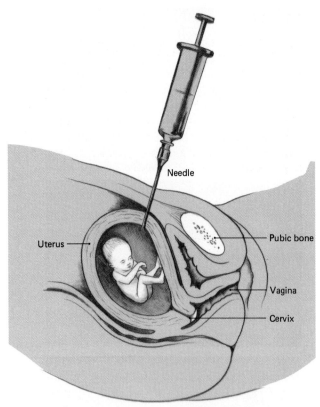

Needle

Uterus

Pubic bone

Vagina

Cervix

Figure 5.2 The process of amniocentesis can detect certain congenital problems as well as the sex of the fetus.

Chances of fetal damage and miscarriage as a result of testing are 1 in 400.

Another procedure, *ultrasound,* or *sonography,* uses high-frequency sound waves to determine the size and position of the fetus. Ultrasound can also detect defects in the central nervous system and digestive system of the fetus. Knowing the position of the fetus can also assist practitioners in performing amniocentesis and in delivering the child. In 1985, a National Institutes of Health panel found ultrasound safe for mother and

child, although it cautioned that the procedure should be employed only for diagnostic purposes.

A third procedure, *fetoscopy,* involves making a small incision in the abdominal and uterine walls and then inserting an optical viewer into the uterus to view the fetus directly. This method is still experimental and involves some risk. It causes miscarriage in approximately 5 percent of cases.

If these tests reveal serious birth defects, parents are advised to undergo genetic counseling. In the case of a chromosomal abnormality such as Down's syndrome, the parents are usually offered the option of a therapeutic abortion. Some parents choose this option; others research their unborn child's disability and choose to go ahead and offer the baby the love and support all children deserve.

▎CHILDBIRTH

Labor and Delivery

Labor begins sometime between day 240 and day 300 of the pregnancy. The exact mechanisms that signal the mother's body that the baby is ready to be born are unknown. During the few weeks preceding delivery, the baby normally shifts and turns into a head-down position, and the cervix begins to dilate (expand). The junction of the pubic bones also loosens to permit expansion of the pelvic girdle during birth.

As labor begins, the amniotic sac (bag containing fluid) breaks, causing a rush of fluid from the vagina commonly referred to as "breaking of the waters." Contractions in the abdomen and lower back also signal the beginning of labor. Early contractions push the baby downward, putting pressure on the cervix, causing it to dilate further. The first stage of labor may last up to 40

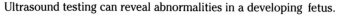

Ultrasound testing can reveal abnormalities in a developing fetus.

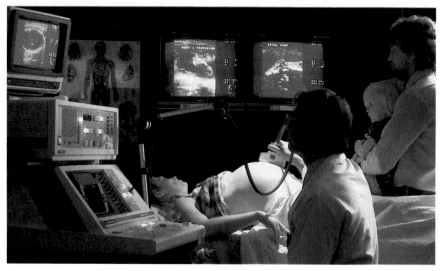

Table 5.4 Apgar Scale

Criterion	Score: 0	1	2
1. Color	Blue, pale	Body pink, extremities blue	All pink
2. Heart rate	Absent	Less than 100	Greater than 100
3. Respiration	Absent	Irregular, slow	Breathing and crying
4. Reflex irritability	No response	Weak (grimace)	Vigorous (sneeze or cough)
5. Muscle tone	Completely flaccid	Limp, some flexion of extremities	Active, resilient

hours for a first birth, but is usually much shorter during subsequent births.

When the cervix is sufficiently dilated, the contractions become rhythmic, stronger, and more painful as the uterus works to push the baby through the birth canal. The second stage of labor (called the expulsion stage) may last between 1 and 4 hours and concludes when the infant is finally pushed out of the mother's body. In some cases, the attending practitioner will do an *episiotomy,* a straight incision in the perineum, to prevent tearing of tissues and to assist the baby in entering the world. Sometimes women can avoid an episiotomy by good nutrition throughout pregnancy, exercise, and trying different birth positions, or having an attendant massage the perineal tissue; but the skin's elasticity and the baby's size are also limiting factors.

After delivery, the attending practitioner cleans the baby's mucus-filled breathing passages, and the baby takes its first breath, generally accompanied by a loud wail. (The traditional slap on the baby's buttocks, often romanticized in old movies, is no longer a common practice because of the trauma associated with it). An attendant then cleans the baby, weighs it, and assesses its general condition, usually using the Apgar Scale (see Table 5.4). The baby is scored 0, 1, or 2 for skin color, heart rate, respiration, reflex irritability, and muscle tone. A score of 10 indicates the baby is in the best possible condition. In the meantime, the mother continues to labor to expel the placenta, or **afterbirth,** usually within 30 minutes following delivery. The umbilical cord is then tied and severed. The stump attached to the baby's navel dries up and drops off within a few days.

Alternatives

Today's prospective mothers have many options available to them for pregnancy, labor, and delivery. These range from the traditional hospital birth to home birth. When considering birthing alternatives, parental values are important. Many couples feel the modern medical establishment has dehumanized the birth process. Thus, they choose to deliver at home or at a "birthing center." Financial considerations are also important, and the couple's income and insurance coverage will often dictate their choice.

Expectant parents have several options for their infant's birth and their participation in the delivery. Childbirth is no longer a matter of turning the process over to a physician in the labor room. The most popular birth alternative is the *Lamaze method.* The husband (or labor coach) assists by giving emotional support, comfort through massage, and coaching during the contractions for proper breathing control. The *Leboyer method* allows the mother to deliver in a dark and quiet setting. Immediately after delivery, the infant is placed in a warm bath, minimizing the trauma of birth. Studies have shown that women who have gone through childbirth preparation have fewer complications and require fewer drugs.

Breast-Feeding and the Postpartum Period

Most mothers prefer to have their new infants placed next to them following the birth. Together with their spouse or partner, they feel a need to share this time of bonding with their infant. Although the mother's milk will not begin to flow for 2 or more days, her breasts secrete a thick yellow substance called *colostrum.* Because this fluid contains vital antibodies to help fight infection, the newborn baby should be allowed to suckle.

As a result of recent scientific findings, the American Academy of Pediatrics has made strong recommendations that full-term newborn infants be breast-fed. Breast milk is perfectly suited to the baby's nutritional needs. However, this does not mean that breast milk is the only adequate method of nourishing a baby; prepared formulas can provide nourishment that allows the baby to grow and thrive.

There are many advantages to breast-feeding. Breast-fed babies have fewer illnesses and a much lower hospitalization rate. Breast milk provides maternal antibodies and immunological cells that stimulate the infant's immune system. When breast-fed babies do get sick, they recover more quickly. Breast-fed babies are less likely to be obese and have fewer allergies.

Afterbirth   The placenta that is expelled from the womb following childbirth.

The Ethics of Fertility

Made-to-Order Babies

Modern technology, with all of its advances, may present ethical dilemmas for the prospective parents of the future. Along with the ability to probe the genetic makeup of offspring for possible strengths and weaknesses comes the opportunity to decide which babies to carry to term and which ones to abort because of the possibility of future disease, undesired gender, a predisposition toward obesity, or low IQ.

According to George Annas, a professor of health law at Boston University's School of Medicine, "The whole definition of normal could well be changed in the decades ahead. The issue becomes not the ability of the child to be happy, but rather our ability to be happy with the child."

In the past, *amniocentesis,* a technique that is used to detect hereditary defects such as Down's syndrome, Tay-Sachs disease, and cystic fibrosis, has been the typical method of detecting early problems. However, amniocentesis will not detect such defects until the fourteenth to twentieth week of pregnancy. Today, thanks to a new procedure called *chorionic villus sampling,* tissue snipped from the developing fetal sac can detect these defects as early as the ninth week. According to Dr. John Buster, a pioneer in reproductive technology, we will eventually be able to detect these defects as early as 5 days after fertilization, before the embryo is even implanted in the uterine wall. Because we cannot correct the majority of these defects, parents often must choose between aborting the fetus or accepting responsibility for the affliction, no matter how severe it may be.

Although aborting on the basis of serious diseases or defects has become more commonplace, a growing fear of the consequences for other "less than perfect" babies has surfaced. It may be just as easy to screen for genetically marked imperfections such as stuttering, reading disorders, and obesity as it is to screen for more serious problems.

Conceiving children of "undesired gender" has always been an issue for parents. However, more and more parents today consider abortion an option if they feel they have too many children of one gender or too few of another. Although abortion is not typically used in the United States to control the number of boys and girls born to a family, the practice is more common in other countries where one sex is culturally preferred over another. For example, Asian and East Indian cultures have a preference for males and consider abortion a means of ensuring a greater number of male births over female births. Right or wrong, prenatal testing and the decisions that result will pose ethical questions for future generations. An important precedent may already have been set. Results of a preliminary study of 200 New England couples indicated that although only 1 percent would abort on the basis of gender, 11 percent would abort to save a child from obesity!

What do you think about prenatal screening for diseases and defects? For gender? What do you think about the idea of aborting a fetus on the basis of possible problems identified during these screening procedures? Should health insurance pay for such tests?

Adapted from Geoffrey Cowley, "Made to Order Babies," *Newsweek,* special issue (Winter/Spring 1990), pp. 94–100.

When deciding whether to breast- or bottle-feed, the mother needs to consider her own desires and preferences. Both methods provide the physical and emotional closeness so important to the parent-child relationship.

The *postpartum period* lasts from 4 to 6 weeks following the delivery. During this time, the reproductive organs revert to a nonpregnant state. Many women experience symptoms of energy depletion, anxiety, mood swings, and depression. This experience, known as *postpartum depression,* appears to be a normal result of the birth process. For most women, these symptoms gradually disappear as the body begins to return to normal. For others, the effects of this depression, coupled with the stresses of managing a new family, can cause more severe depressive symptoms for several months.

If Something Goes Wrong

Problems and complications during labor and delivery can occur even with a successful pregnancy. Such possibilities should be discussed with the practitioner prior to labor so the mother has a chance to understand what medical procedures may be necessary for her safety and that of her child. Although pregnancy may involve a certain amount of risk, the risks from other activities are usually much greater.

If labor is too long or if the baby is presenting wrong (anything but head first), a **cesarean section** (C-section) may be necessary. This surgical procedure involves making an incision across the abdomen and through the uterus to remove the baby. This operation is also performed in cases where labor is extremely difficult, maternal blood pressure falls rapidly, the placenta separates from the uterus too soon, the mother has diabetes, or in several other circumstances.

A cesarean section can be extremely traumatic for the mother if she is not prepared for it. Over the past two decades, the rate of delivery by cesarean section in the United States increased from 1 in 20 births in the mid-1960s to more than 1 in 4 by 1988.* Risks to the mother are the same as those with any major abdominal surgery, and recovery time is lengthened after a C-section. Although a cesarean section may be necessary in certain cases, some physicians and critics feel the option is used too frequently.

Present-day surgical techniques allow some cesarean patients to have vaginal delivery with later children, depending upon the reasons for the original cesarean. Formerly, the adage was "once a cesarean, always a cesarean." Now, guidelines published by the American College of Obstetricians and Gynecologists allow an estimated 50 to 80 percent of women the option of a vaginal birth after cesarean (VBAC).

Slowing of the fetal heartbeat is another common problem during delivery. If the umbilical cord becomes entangled or if the baby's oxygen supply is otherwise cut off, the baby may be stillborn or may suffer from serious medical problems such as **cerebral palsy,** a brain disorder that causes uncontrollable spasms in various parts of the body. Fetal heart function is normally monitored with a machine called a fetal heart monitor, which is attached to the mothers' abdomen during labor.

Pregnancy Loss

One in 10 pregnancies does not end in delivery. Pregnancy loss before fetal viability is called a **miscarriage** (also referred to as *spontaneous abortion*). An estimated 70 to 90 percent of women who miscarry eventually become pregnant again.

Reasons for pregnancy loss vary. In some cases the egg and sperm have failed to divide correctly. In others, genetic abnormalities, maternal illness, or infections are responsible. Maternal hormonal imbalance may also cause pregnancy loss, as may a weak cervix or toxic chemicals in the environment. In most cases the cause is not known.

A blood incompatibility between mother and father occurs when **Rh factors** are not the same. *Rh* is a blood protein named after the rhesus monkey, in which it was first studied. Rh problems occur when the mother is

Rh-negative and the fetus is Rh-positive. During a first birth, some of the baby's blood passes into the mother's bloodstream. An Rh-negative mother may manufacture antibodies to destroy the Rh-positive blood introduced into her bloodstream at the time of birth. Her first baby will be unaffected, but subsequent babies with positive Rh factor are in danger of contracting a severe anemia called *hemolytic disease* while in the uterus, because the Rh antibodies attack the fetus's red blood cells.

Medical advances now offer prevention and treatment. The mother and fetus can be tested. If Rh incompatibility is found, intrauterine transfusions are possible, as are early deliveries by cesarean section, depending upon the individual case. Prevention of the problem is preferable to treatment. All women with Rh-negative blood should be injected with a medication called Rho-GAM within 72 hours of any birth, miscarriage, or abortion. This injection prevents the woman from developing the Rh antibodies.

Ectopic pregnancy takes place outside the uterus. A fertilized egg may implant itself in the fallopian tube or occasionally in the pelvic cavity. Because these structures are not capable of expanding and nourishing a developing fetus, the pregnancy cannot continue. Such fetuses are surgically removed. Most often, the affected fallopian tube is also removed.

Ectopic pregnancies have tripled over the past 12 years, and no one understands why. Ectopic pregnancy is generally accompanied by pain in the lower abdomen or aching in the shoulders as the blood flows up toward the diaphragm. If bleeding is significant, blood pressure drops and the woman can go into shock. If the pregnancy is not detected before the fallopian tube ruptures, the woman is at great risk of hemorrhage, *peritonitis* (infection in the abdomen), and death.

Women who have had one ectopic pregnancy run a higher risk of having another. Ectopic pregnancy is a potential side effect of *pelvic inflammatory disease (PID)* due to scarring or blockage of the tubes.

Stillbirth is one of the most traumatic events a couple can face. A stillborn baby is one that is born dead, often for no apparent reason. The void and loneliness experienced following this type of pregnancy loss is worse than with a miscarriage. Nine months of happy anticipation have been thwarted. Family, friends, and other children

---

Cesarean Section   A surgical procedure in which the baby is removed through an incision made in the abdominal and uterine walls.

Cerebral Palsy   A central-nervous-system disorder characterized by uncontrolled muscle spasms; may or may not be associated with mental retardation; can result from lack of oxygen at birth.

Miscarriage   Loss of pregnancy before fetal viability.

Rh Factor   A blood protein related to the production of antibodies. If an Rh-negative mother is pregnant with an Rh-positive fetus, the mother will manufacture antibodies that kill the fetus, causing miscarriage.

Ectopic Pregnancy   A pregnancy with the fertilized egg developing outside the uterus in the fallopian tube or occasionally in the pelvic cavity.

Stillbirth   A baby born dead.

---

* Gregory Goyert, et al., "The Physician Factor in Cesarean Births," *New England Journal of Medicine* 320 (1989), 706.

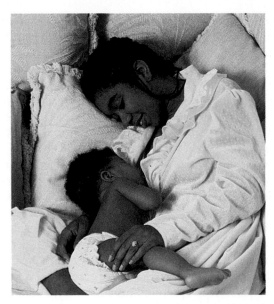
Breast-feeding can be an important source of intimacy between mother and child.

may be in a state of shock, needing comfort and not knowing where to turn. The mother's breasts produce milk, and there is no infant to be fed. A room with a crib and toys is left empty.

Grief associated with stillbirths can last for years, and both partners may blame themselves or each other at some time. In many cases, no amount of reassurance from the attending physician, relatives, or friends can help assuage the grief or guilt. Well-intended comments such as "Oh, you'll have another baby someday" may create uncomfortable feelings.

Some communities have groups called the Compassionate Friends to help parents and other family members through the grieving process. This nonprofit organization is for parents who have lost a child of any age for any reason.

METHODS OF FERTILITY CONTROL

Conception refers to the fertilization of an ovum by a sperm. At the time of conception, the fertilizing sperm enters the ovum. Its tail breaks off, and a protective chemical barrier is secreted by the ovum to surround it and prevent other sperm from entering.

The following conditions are necessary for conception:

1. A viable egg
2. A viable sperm
3. Access to the egg for the sperm.

Contraception refers to the methods involved in preventing conception. Ever since people first began to asso-

ciate sexual activity with pregnancy, society has searched for simple, infallible, and risk-free methods to prevent pregnancy. We have not yet succeeded. Our present methods of contraception work by interfering with one or more of the three conditions necessary for conception.

Contraceptive methods fall into two categories: *reversible methods,* such as the Pill, condoms, and abstinence, and *permanent methods,* such as vasectomy (for men) and tubal ligation (for women). Let's discuss some of the methods in each category in detail.

Reversible Contraception

A number of methods of reversible contraception are listed in Table 5.5.

Abstinence and "Outercourse"   Strictly defined, abstinence means that a person or couple deliberately shuns sexual contact. This strict definition often does not include forms of sexual intimacy such as massage, kissing, and solitary masturbation. However, many people substantially broaden their definition of abstinence to include *any* sexual contact that does not culminate in sexual intercouse. Couples who go a step further than massage and kissing and engage in such activities as oral-genital sex and mutual masturbation are sometimes said to be engaging in "outercourse." Like strict abstinence, outercourse can be 100 percent effective as birth control as long as the male does not ejaculate near the vaginal opening. Strict abstinence is 100 percent effective against sexually transmitted diseases (STDs). Depending on the types of activities engaged in, outercourse may not be quite as effective against STDs. Safer oral-genital contact may be achieved by using a condom on the penis or a dental dam on the vaginal opening.

The Condom   The **condom** is a strong sheath of latex rubber of other material designed to fit over an erect penis. The condom catches the ejaculate in its end, thereby preventing sperm migration toward the egg. At the present time, the condom is the only temporary means of birth control available for men. Originally used as decorative garments by Egyptian men, condoms come in a wide variety of styles: colored, ribbed for "extra sensation," spermicide-treated, lubricated, nonlubricated, with or without reservoirs at the tip. All may be purchased in pharmacies, some supermarkets, some public bathrooms, and many health clinics. A new condom must be used for each act of intercourse.

ADVANTAGES   Condoms help prevent the spread of some sexually transmitted diseases, including genital herpes and HIV. They are easy to purchase and do not

---

Conception   The fertilization of an ovum by a sperm.
Contraception   Methods of preventing conception.
Condom   A sheath of thin material designed to fit over an erect penis and catch semen upon ejaculation.

Table 5.5 Contraceptive Advantages, Disadvantages, and Effectiveness Ratings (When Properly Used)

Type	Advantages	Disadvantages	Effectiveness
Permanent			
Sterilization			
Vasectomy	Convenient; fewer surgery-related risks than tubal ligation; effective	Irreversible; does not prevent STDs	99.8%
Tubal ligation	Convenient; effective	Surgical-related risks; irreversible; does not prevent STDs	99.6%
Reversible			
"Strict" Abstinence	No risk of STDs or pregnancy	Lack of some aspects of sexual intimacy	100%
"Outercourse"	Relatively small risk of STDs or pregnancy	Requires high degree of self-control	90–100%(?)
Norplant	Convenient; cost-effective; no serious side effects known; 5 years of protection	Does not prevent STDs; implantation and removal process	>99%
Condom used with foam, jelly, or cream	Helps prevent sexually transmitted disease; inexpensive; easy to carry; requires no prescription	Decreased sensations in males; less spontaneity	98%
The Pill (combination progesterone and estrogen)	Convenient; effective; decreased risks of endometrial and ovarian cancer	Daily medication easy to forget; risk of serious side effects; does not prevent STDs	97%
Progestin-only Pill	Convenient; fewer side effects than combination pill; less risk of blood clotting complications	Menstrual irregularities; slightly higher risk of pregnancy; does not prevent STDs	96%
IUD	Convenient; does not interfere with spontaneity	Higher risks of tubal pregnancy; pelvic infections; infertility; heavy menstrual flow; painful to insert; increased menstrual cramps; does not prevent STDs	94%
Condom only	See above	See above; also, less effective than condom used with foam, jelly, or cream	88%
Diaphragm with cream or jelly	May help prevent sexually transmitted disease; inexpensive after initial fitting	Requires prescription and fitting	82%
Sponge	Easy to obtain; does not interfere with spontaneity; subsequent intercourse possible	Less effective than some other methods	82% (if woman has never had a child) 72% (if woman has given birth)
Cervical cap	Does not interfere with spontaneity	May be dislodged; requires prescription and fitting	82%
Cervical-mucus test	No chemicals	Requires abstinence for 7–10 days every month; does not prevent STDs	80%
Body-temperature test	No chemicals		80%
Calendar	No chemicals; does not interfere with spontaneity Can be used to get pregnant when desired	Requires daily record keeping; Less effective; does not prevent STDs	80%
Foams, suppositories, jellies, and creams	Easy to obtain; inexpensive; may help prevent some sexually transmitted diseases	Timing can interfere with spontaneity; allergic reactions possible; less effective	79%
Chance (no method)	No restrictions	High pregnancy rate; does not prevent STDs	10%

require a medical prescription. They are small and easy to carry. There are no age restrictions on buying condoms. Some men find they help maintain an erection longer.

DISADVANTAGES The theoretical effectiveness rate for the condom is 98 percent, meaning that *if used correctly,* 2 women out of 100 whose partners used condoms would become pregnant in 1 year. In actuality, however, the effectiveness rate is about 88 percent, since condoms are often used incorrectly. (For greatest efficacy, a condom can be used with a spermicide that contains nonoxynol-9.) Some couples don't use the condom at certain times during the woman's cycle because they think the woman cannot get pregnant at those times. This belief is incorrect, and the practice greatly increases the chance of pregnancy. Condoms must be rolled onto the penis before the penis touches the vagina and held in place when the penis is removed from the vagina after ejaculation (see Figure 5.3). Condoms can break during intercourse. They must be stored in a cool place (not in a wallet or hip pocket) and should be inspected before use for small tears.

For some people, a condom ruins the spontaneity of sex; stopping to put on the condom breaks the mood for them. These feelings of inconvenience contribute to improper use of the device. Some people report a decrease in sensation. Other couples put on the condom together as a part of foreplay.

The Female Condom A new contraceptive device for internal use by women has been tentatively approved by the FDA for use in the United States. The **female condom** is a soft, loose-fitting, single-use, polyurethane sheath. It is designed as one unit with two diaphragmlike rings. One ring lies inside the sheath and serves as an insertion mechanism and internal anchor; the other ring remains outside the vagina once the device is inserted and protects the labia and the base of the penis from infection. Exact effectiveness rates have not been established.

ADVANTAGES Many women feel the condom gives them increased control of their reproductive freedom. Some women disagree and believe that women are being offered a device that eliminates any male responsibility at all. Regardless of one's stance on the female condom, it does provide additional protection against STDs because it allows less skin-to-skin contact than the male condom.

Female Condom A polyurethane sheath designed for insertion into the vagina in order to catch semen upon ejaculation.

* W. L. Drew and M. Conant, *For Virus Permeability* (San Francisco: Mount Zion Hospital and Medical Center

Figure 5.3 The Basics of Using a Condom

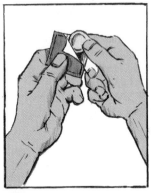 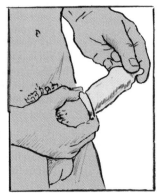 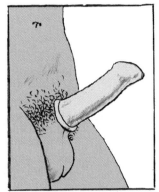

When the male has achieved an erection, carefully open the condom package and determine which way the condom rolls open. If you don't know which way the condom will roll open, you may place the wrong side of the unrolled condom on the tip of the penis and have to discard the condom (remember, there may be a few drops of Cowper's gland secretion at the tip of the penis soon after erection).

Next, unroll the condom onto the penis as far down as it will unroll. Leave some room– about half an inch- -at the tip of the condom to catch the semen when the male ejaculates. You should leave a little room at the tip of the condom even when the condom has a built-in tip; this will help avoid breaking the condom. After ejaculation, and before the male loses erection, the penis should be withdrawn from the vagina while the

rim of the condom is held tightly against the male's body. Then the condom should be grasped at the tip and the rim and carefully taken off the penis and discarded. A new condom must be used for each new act of intercourse. For safest results, the male should also thoroughly wash his penis and genital area with warm water and soap before each new act of intercourse.

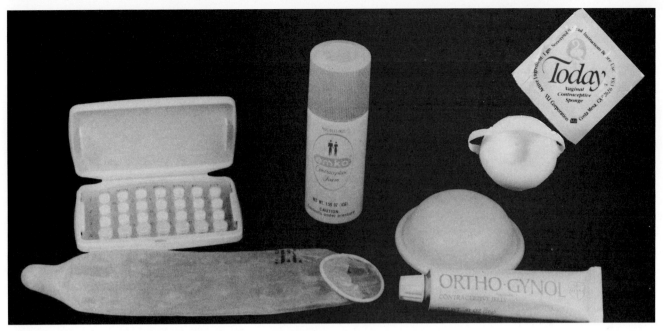

The birth-control devices pictured above include the vaginal sponge, the condom, oral contraceptives, and a diaphragm with foam and jelly.

DISADVANTAGES As with the traditional condom, decreased sensation and interference with spontaneity are common complaints.

Foams, Suppositories, Jellies, and Creams Like condoms, these contraceptive preparations are available without a prescription. Chemically, they are called **spermicides**—substances designed to kill sperm.

Jellies and creams are packaged in tubes, and foams are available in aerosol cans. All have tubes designed for insertion into the vagina. They must be inserted far enough to cover the cervix, providing both a chemical barrier that kills sperm and a physical barrier that stops sperm from continuing toward an egg.

Suppositories are waxy capsules that are placed deep in the vagina and melt once inside. Suppositories must be inserted 10 to 20 minutes before intercourse (to have time to melt) but no more than 1 hour prior to intercourse. Additional contraceptive chemicals must be applied for each subsequent intercourse (see Figure 5.4).

ADVANTAGES Jellies, creams, suppositories, and foam are easy to obtain. When used in conjunction with a condom, their effectiveness rate is nearly 98 percent. They help prevent the spread of certain sexually transmitted diseases. Recent research has shown nonoxynol-9 to be the active ingredient in some spermicides that helps decrease the transmission of sexually transmitted viruses and bacteria. However, it should be pointed out that some of these products may create an environment in which bacteria may actually multiply.

DISADVANTAGES Jellies and creams are designed to be used with a diaphragm. By themselves, their effectiveness rate is 79 percent. Foam, designed to be used alone, also has an effectiveness rate of 79 percent. Some people experience allergic reactions to these products. Timing of insertion may interfere with lovemaking. Some people find the taste of these substances disagreeable, thus interfering with oral sex.

The Diaphragm with Spermicidal Jelly or Cream Invented in the mid-nineteenth century, the **diaphragm** was the first widely used birth-control method for women. Prior to that time, most women had to rely upon their male partners to use a condom or withdraw the penis before ejaculation.

The diaphragm is a soft, shallow cup made of thin latex rubber. Its flexible rubber-coated ring is designed to fit snugly behind the pubic bone in front of the cervix and over the back of the cervix on the other side. Diaphragms are manufactured in sizes and must be fitted to the woman by a trained practitioner. The practitioner should also be certain that the user can insert her diaphragm correctly before she leaves the office.

Diaphragms must be used in conjunction with spermicidal cream or jelly. The spermicide is applied to the inside of the diaphragm before insertion. The jelly or cream is held in place by the diaphragm, creating a physical and chemical barrier for sperm. Additional spermicide must be applied for subsequent intercourse, and the diaphragm must be left in place for 6 to 8 hours after

Spermicide A chemical substance that kills sperm.

Diaphragm A latex rubber saucer-shaped device designed to cover the cervix and block access to the uterus; should always be used with spermicide.

Promoting Your Health

Choosing a Method of Birth Control

It is important to choose a method of birth control that works well to prevent pregnancy. Whichever method you choose to use, you must use it carefully. It is also important to choose a method you will like. Ask yourself the following questions so you can judge carefully.

What type of birth control are you thinking about?

_____

Have you ever used it before? _____ yes _____ no.

If yes, how long did you use it? _____

Circle Your Answers

Are you afraid of using this method?   yes   no   don't know

Would you rather not use this method?   yes   no   don't know

Will you have trouble remembering to use this method?   yes   no   don't know

Have you ever become pregnant while using this method?   yes   no   don't know

Will you have trouble using this method carefully?   yes   no   don't know

Do you have unanswered questions about this method?   yes   no   don't know

Does this method make menstrual periods longer or more painful? yes   no   don't know

Does this method cost more than you can afford?   yes   no   don't know

Does this method ever cause serious health problems?   yes   no   don't know

Do you object to this method because of religious beliefs?   yes   no   don't know

Have you already had problems using this method?   yes   no   don't know

Is your partner opposed to this method?   yes   no   don't know

Are you using this method without your partner's knowledge?   yes   no   don't know

Will using this method embarrass you?   yes   no   don't know

Will using this method embarrass your partner?   yes   no   don't know

Will you enjoy intercourse less because of this method?   yes   no   don't know

Will this method interrupt lovemaking?   yes   no   don't know

Has a nurse or doctor ever told you not to use this method?   yes   no   don't know

Do you have any "don't know" answers? If so, you should seek more information.

Do you have any "yes" answers? If you have several, the chances are that you might not like this method and may need to think about another.

Source: *Contraceptive Technology, 1988–1989* (New York: Irvington Publishers, 1989).

---

intercourse to allow the chemical to kill any sperm remaining in the vagina (see Figure 5.5).

ADVANTAGES Diaphragm users experience very few side effects. Most adverse reactions involve allergies to the cream or jelly. The diaphragm can be inserted several hours prior to intercourse, so there is no reason for it to interfere with spontaneity. Because of the spermicide, the diaphragm also appears to be helpful in the prevention of sexually transmitted disease.

DISADVANTAGES The effectiveness rate of the diaphragm is 82 percent. Using the diaphragm during the menstrual period or leaving the diaphragm in place beyond the recommended time increases the user's risk of developing **toxic shock syndrome.** This condition results from the multiplication of a type of bacteria that spreads

Toxic Shock Syndrome A potentially life-threatening disease that occurs when specific bacterial toxins are allowed to multiply unchecked in wounds or through improper use of tampons or diaphragms.

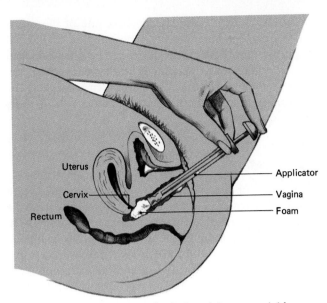

Figure 5.4 The proper method of applying spermicide within the vagina.

micide and designed to be inserted into the vagina. A small cord is attached to the sponge to aid in removal. Like condoms, creams, jellies, and foams, sponges are available in pharmacies. They come in only one size.

The sponge must be dampened with water to activate the spermicide and must be inserted prior to intercourse. Once in place, it fits over the cervix, blocking the entrance, and releases a spermicide. (See Figure 5.6).

The sponge is effective for 24 hours once inserted. It must be left in place for 6 to 8 hours after intercourse. When removed, it is thrown away.

ADVANTAGES The sponge is easy to obtain. Because it expands to fit after insertion, it does not have to be fitted by a medical practitioner. Spontaneous and continuous intercourse is permissible with no interruptions or need for additional spermicide for 24 hours.

DISADVANTAGES Some women experience difficulty in removing the sponge and an unpleasant odor if the sponge is left in for more than 18 hours. Some users may have an allergic reaction to the spermicide, especially since the overall dose is significantly higher than other spermicide products. Because of the dangers of toxic shock syndrome, the sponge should not be used during the menstrual period nor should it be left in place for longer than 30 hours. The sponge is less effective for women who have had children. For couples who have frequent intercourse, the sponge may be expensive.

to the bloodstream and causes sudden high fever, rash, nausea, vomiting, diarrhea, and a sudden drop in blood pressure. If not treated, toxic shock syndrome can be fatal. The diaphragm, as well as tampons left too long in place, creates conditions conducive to the growth of these bacteria.

When in place, the diaphragm can put undue pressure on the urethra, blocking urinary flow and predisposing the user to bladder infections. Insertion of the device can be awkward, especially if the woman is rushed. When inserted incorrectly, the effectiveness rate of the diaphragm declines.

Cervical Cap **Cervial caps** are one of the oldest methods used to prevent pregnancy. Early caps were made from beeswax, silver, and copper. They have been available in Europe for several years, and were approved

Contraceptive Sponge A doughnut-shaped device moistened with water and placed in the vagina to block access to the uterus; the sponge is saturated with spermicide.

Cervical Cap A small diaphragmlike device designed to be worn internally over the cervix.

The Contraceptive Sponge The **contraceptive sponge** was first marketed in the United States in 1983. Shaped like a miniature doughnut with a depression in the center, these polyurethane devices are saturated with a sper-

Figure 5.5 Proper use and placement of a diaphragm.

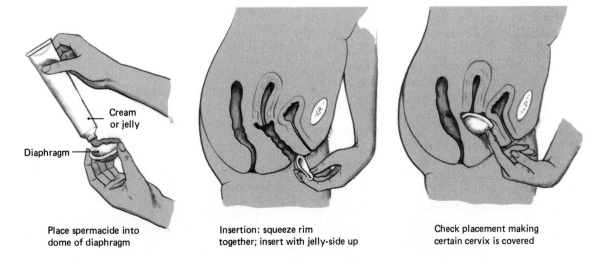

Place spermacide into dome of diaphragm

Insertion: squeeze rim together; insert with jelly-side up

Check placement making certain cervix is covered

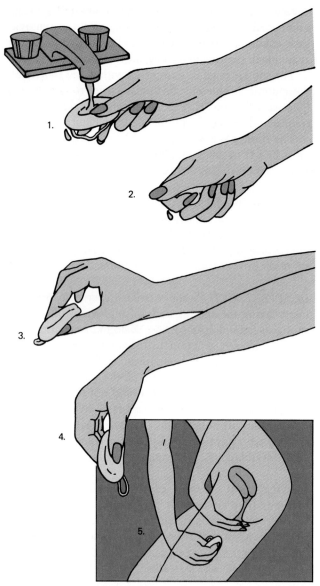

Figure 5.6 Steps in proper use of the contraceptive sponge.

for use in the United States by the Food and Drug Administration (FDA) in 1988.

The cervical cap is a small cap made of latex rubber and is designed to fit snugly over the cervix. It must be fitted by a practitioner and is somewhat more difficult to insert than a diaphragm because of its smaller size. It is designed for use with contraceptive jelly or cream.

The cap keeps sperm out of the uterus. It is held in place by suction created during application. Insertion may take place anywhere up to 2 days prior to intercourse, and the device must be left in place for 6 to 8 hours after intercourse. The maximum length of time the cap can be left on the cervix is 48 hours. It is then cleaned and can be reinserted immediately.

ADVANTAGES The cervical cap does not interfere with spontaneity in lovemaking. Because the cap fits tightly, it does not require the reapplication of a spermicide.

DISADVANTAGES The effectiveness rate of the cap is only 82 percent. Some women report unpleasant vaginal odors after use. Because the device can become dislodged during intercourse, placement must be checked frequently. It cannot be used during the menstrual period or for longer than 48 hours because of the risk of toxic shock syndrome.

Norplant

Approved for use by the FDA in 1990 and marketed since February 1991 in the United States, Norplant is the most recent form of hormonal contraceptive. It has been tested by more than 1 million women in 45 countries, and is now approved for use in 14 countries. Increasing numbers of women in the United States are now considering this option because of its convenience, effectiveness, and safety.

Norplant is one of the most effective methods of birth control, approaching the effectiveness rate of sterilization.* It has a greater than 99 percent success rate in preventing pregnancy.

Six silicon-rubber capsules that contain progestin are surgically inserted under the skin of a woman's arm. For five years small amounts of progestin are continuously released. The progestin in Norplant works the same way as oral contraceptives, by suppressing contraception and thickening of cervical mucus.

Norplant can be inserted by a specially trained doctor, nurse, or nurse practitioner in 10 to 15 minutes. A local anesthetic is administered to the upper arm, a small incision is made, and with a special needle the six capsules are placed just under the skin in a fan shape. The capsules are similarly removed after five years or, if necessary, at any point after their insertion.

The capsules usually cannot be seen, nor do they leave a scar in most women. At this time there are no serious side effects known. The use of Norplant can result in irregular bleeding and menstrual periods. Other possible side effects include acne, weight gain, breast tenderness, headaches, nervousness, and nausea.

ADVANTAGES An effectiveness rate greater than 99 percent, making it the most effective reversible method of fertility control. In addition to being very convenient, the implant method is simple; therefore, there is little chance of error. Implants cost approximately half as much as birth-control pills (about $550 compared with $1180 over 5 years).** The cost has been approved by medical-assistance programs in many states.

DISADVANTAGES The small surgical procedure appears to be the greatest disadvantage with Norplant. In addition, some users will not have regular periods, and

---

* P. Silva and K. E. Glasser, "Update on Subdermal Contraceptive Implants," *The Female Patient*, 17 (1992), 34–45.
** Ibid.

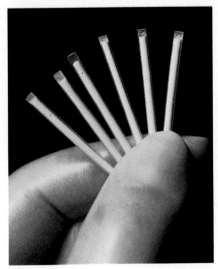

Norplant

some will experience persistent spotting, which is unacceptable to some women. Serious risks are less than with regular combination birth-control Pills because there is no estrogen and the amount of hormones is smaller.

Oral Contraceptives   Contraceptive pills were first marketed in the United States in 1960. Their convenience quickly made them the most widely used reversible method of fertility control.

Most **oral contraceptives** work through the combined effects of synthetic estrogen and progesterone. Because the levels of estrogen in the Pill are higher than those produced by the body, the pituitary gland is never signaled to produce follicle-stimulating hormone (FSH), without which ova will not develop in the ovaries (see Chapter 4). Progesterone in the Pill prevents proper growth of the uterine lining and thickens the cervical mucus, forming a barrier against sperm.

Pills are meant to be taken in a cycle of some type. At the end of each 3-week cycle, the user discontinues the drug or takes a placebo pill for 1 week. The resultant drop in hormones causes the uterine lining to disintegrate, and the user will have a menstrual period, usually within 1 to 3 days. The same cycle is repeated every 28 days. Flow is generally lighter than in a non-Pill user because the hormones in the Pill prevent thick endometrial buildup.

The most serious risk with the Pill is an increased tendency to form blood clots in the blood vessels. Clotting can lead to strokes or heart attacks. The risk increases with age and especially with cigarette smoking. This risk is low for most healthy women under 35 who do not smoke. A few women may develop high blood pressure while on the Pill.

Today's Pill is different from the one first introduced in the 1950s. The original Pill contained large amounts of estrogen and carried increased risks to the user, whereas the current Pill contains the minimal amount of estrogen necessary to prevent pregnancy.

Recent studies indicate that use of the Pill actually protects some women from endometrial and ovarian cancer. Women who use the Pill are less likely than nonusers to develop fibrocystic breast disease. Pill users also have decreased incidences of ectopic pregnancies, ovarian cysts, and pelvic inflammatory disease.[*] At this time, the Pill is not thought to protect against or increase the chance of breast cancer.

Because the chemicals in oral contraceptives change the way the body metabolizes certain nutrients, all women using them should check with the prescribing practitioner regarding dietary supplements. The nutrients in question include vitamin C and the B-complex vitamins—B_2, B_6, and B_{12}. A nutritious diet that includes whole grains, fresh fruits, and vegetables, lean meats, fish and poultry, and nonfat dairy products is advised.

Oral contraceptives can interact negatively with other drugs. Some antibiotics diminish the Pill's effectiveness. Medications to treat tuberculosis and seizure disorders may also reduce effectiveness. Women in doubt should check with their prescribing practitioner, their pharmacist, or other knowledgeable health professionals.

Fertility may be delayed after discontinuing the Pill, but the Pill is not known to cause infertility. Women who had irregular menstrual cycles before going on the Pill are more likely to have problems conceiving regardless of Pill use.

ADVANTAGES   The effectiveness rate of oral contraceptives is 97 percent, making them an effective method of fertility control. Use of the Pill is convenient and does not interfere with lovemaking. Menstrual difficulties such as cramps and premenstrual syndrome (PMS) may be lessened. Women using oral contraceptives have lower risks of developing endometrial and ovarian cancers and benign breast disease. Oral contraceptives may also help protect women against pelvic inflammatory disease and iron-deficiency anemia.

DISADVANTAGES   There are possible serious health problems—clotting and high blood pressure. In addition to the risk factors and side effects associated with the Pill, the greatest disadvantage is that it must be taken every day. If one Pill is missed, it is advisable for the user to use an alternative form of contraception for the remainder of the cycle. Cost of the pills may be a problem for some women.

The Morning-after Pill   The term **morning-after pill** refers to drugs that can be taken up to 3 days after

---

Oral Contraceptives   Pills taken daily to prevent ovulation through regulation of hormones.

Morning-after Pill   Drugs that are taken within 3 days after intercourse to prevent fertilization or implantation

[*] University of Southern California School of Medicine, *Dialogues in Contraception*, 3, no. 2 (1990), p. 2.

unprotected intercourse to prevent fertilization or implantation. The most common drug prescribed is a combination of estrogen and progesterone. Other preparations include large doses of progesterone or a large dose of estrogen called *diethylstilbesterol (DES)*. Of all the drugs available to prevent pregnancy, DES is the most risky. Between 1941 and 1970, DES was given to pregnant women to prevent miscarriage. Babies born to these women are today at increased risk of developing a rare vaginal cancer (in women) or genital abnormalities (in men).

Nausea or vomiting is the most likely side effect of these drugs. The risks are the same as those associated with combination Pills.

The morning-after pill is intended for emergency use only—it is not a method to be used every month. Women using morning-after preparations stand a 3 percent chance of becoming pregnant. The FDA has not approved any of these drugs as "morning-after" medications.

The morning-after pill should not be confused with RU 486, a recently developed drug that safely induces abortion during the first 9 weeks of pregnancy. We will consider RU 486 in the discussion of abortion.

Methods of fertility control that rely upon the alteration of sexual behavior are called **natural methods** of birth control. These methods include observing female "fertile periods" through the examination of cervical mucus and/or keeping track of internal temperature and then abstaining from sexual intercourse (penis-vagina contact) during these fertile times.

Two decades ago, the "rhythm method" was the object of much ridicule because of its low efficacy rates. However, it was the only method of birth control available to women belonging to religious denominations that forbade the use of oral contraceptives, barrier methods, and sterilization. Our present reproductive knowledge enables women and their partners to use natural methods of birth control with fewer risks of pregnancy, although these methods remain far less efficient than others.

Natural methods of birth control rely upon basic physiology. A released ovum can survive for up to 48 hours after ovulation. Sperm can live for as long as 5 days in the vagina. Natural methods of birth control teach women to recognize their fertile times. Changes in cervical mucus prior to and during ovulation and a rise in basal body temperature are two indicators frequently used in natural contraceptive techniques. Another method involves charting a woman's menstrual cycle and ovulation times on a calendar. Any combination of these methods may be used at the same time to determine fertile times more accurately.

In the first method, the **cervical-mucus method,** women are taught to examine the consistency and color of their normal vaginal secretions. Prior to ovulation, the mucus becomes gelatinous and stringy in consistency, and normal vaginal secretions may increase. Sexual ac-

tivity involving penis-vagina contact must be avoided while this "fertile mucus" is present and for several days following the mucus changes.

The second, the **body temperature method,** relies on the fact that the female's basal body temperature rises between 0.4 and 0.8 degrees after ovulation has occurred. For this method to be effective, the woman must chart her temperature for several months to learn to recognize her body's temperature fluctuations. Abstinence from penis-vagina contact must be observed from before the temperature rises until several days afterwards.

The third method, the **calendar method,** requires the woman to record the length of her menstrual cycle in days, with the first day of flow being day 1. This method assumes that ovulation occurs at the midpoint of the cycle. Abstinence from penis-vagina contact must be observed during the fertile time.

Women interested in natural methods of birth control are advised to take supervised classes in their use. The risks of an unwanted pregnancy are great for the untrained woman. Reading a book, talking to the proprietor of the local health-food store, or watching a film will not provide the necessary training to ensure maximum effectiveness. Information on these methods can also be used to help couples who are trying to conceive.

ADVANTAGES None of the natural methods of fertility control involves chemical or physical intervention with the reproductive process or with lovemaking.

DISADVANTAGES All three methods have comparatively low efficiency rates. Accurate record keeping is necessary on a continuous basis. Women with irregular menstrual cycles have difficulty using these methods, because indicators may change from month to month, making accurate record keeping difficult at best. Finally, many couples do not like to abstain from sexual intercourse for 7 or more days during the month.

Withdrawal

The least effective method of birth control is most commonly used by people who have not taken the time to consider alternatives. The **withdrawal** method involves withdrawing the penis from the vagina just prior to ejac-

---

Natural Methods Several types of contraception that require alteration of sexual behavior

Cervical-mucus Method A natural method of contraception relying upon observation of changes in cervical mucus (in normal vaginal secretions); abstention required during fertile times.

Body-temperature Method A natural method of contraception that involves monitoring the rise of female body temperature prior to ovulation; abstention during fertile times is required.

Calendar Method A natural method of contraception that requires mapping the menstrual cycle on a calendar and abstaining from penis-vagina contact during "fertile" times.

Withdrawal Withdrawing the penis from the vagina before ejaculation.

ulation. Because there can be up to 500,000 sperm in the drop of fluid at the tip of the penis before ejaculation (see Chapter 4), this method is not reliable. Timing withdrawal is also difficult; males concentrating on accurate timing may not be able to relax and enjoy intercourse. The efficacy rate for the withdrawal method is 82 percent.

Intrauterine Devices   Widespread use of **intrauterine devices (IUD)** for contraception began in the mid-1960s when these devices were advertised as less risky and more convenient than the Pill.

The devices began to fall out of favor in the mid-1970s following the negative publicity surrounding the Dalkon shield, a device associated with pelvic inflammatory disease and sterility. The manufacturer stopped making Dalkon shields in 1975.

We are not certain how IUDs work. Although people once thought that IUDs act by preventing implantation of a fertilized egg, most experts now believe they interfere with the sperm's fertilization of the egg.

Two IUDs are currently available. The first, the Progestasert, is a T-shaped plastic device that contains synthetic progesterone (one of the female hormones). The progesterone is released slowly. The practitioner must remove this IUD and insert a new one every year. The second, the ParaGuard, is also a T-shape, but it has copper wrapped around the shaft and does not contain any hormones. It can be left in place for 4 years before it needs to be replaced.

For insertion, the device is folded and placed into a long, thin plastic applicator. The practitioner measures the depth of the uterus with a special instrument and then uses the measurements for accurate placement of the IUD. When in place, the arms of the "T" open out across the top of the uterus. One or two strings extend from the IUD into the vagina so that the user can check to see that her IUD is in place. The device is removed by a practitioner when desired.

ADVANTAGES   IUDs are very effective. Users have a 5 percent chance of becoming pregnant. The device does not interfere with the spontaneity of sex.

DISADVANTAGES   A physician must fit and insert the device. The Progestasert IUD must be removed and a new one inserted every year. The discomfort and cost of the process may be a disadvantage for some. When in place, the device can cause heavy menstrual flow and severe cramps. There is a risk of uterine perforation. Women using IUDs have higher risks of ectopic pregnancy, pelvic inflammatory disease, infertility, tubal infections, and congenital abnormalities in infants conceived while the device is in place. If a pregnancy occurs, the chance of a miscarriage is 25 to 50 percent. Removal of the device as soon as the pregnancy is known is advised. Because IUDs increase the risk of pelvic infections and infertility, they are not suitable for most women.

Women who have more than one sexual partner are at increased risk of catching a sexually transmitted disease. However, the IUD may be a very suitable method for older women who have completed childbearing and have only one sexual partner.

Permanent Contraception

In the late 1980s, **sterilization** became more common among married couples in the United States. Perfection of the procedures has made this method increasingly popular ever since the 1970s. Although some of the newer surgical techniques make potential reversal of sterilization possible, anyone considering sterilization should assume that the operation is *not* reversible. A person should consider such possibilities as remarriage or a future improvement in financial status before becoming sterilized.

Tubal Ligation   Sterilization in females is called **tubal ligation**. Achieved through a surgical procedure called *laparoscopy*, this technique involves tying the fallopian tubes closed or cutting them and cauterizing (burning) the edges to seal the tubes, blocking access to released eggs.

The operation is usually done in a hospital on an outpatient basis. First, the abdomen is inflated with carbon-dioxide gas through a small incision in the navel. The surgeon then inserts a *laparoscope* into another incision just above the pubic bone. This specially designed instrument has a fiber-optic light source that enables the physician to see the fallopian tubes clearly. Once located, the tubes are cut and tied or cauterized (see Figure 5.7).

Intrauterine Device (IUD)   A T-shaped plastic device that is implanted in the uterus to prevent conception.
Sterilization   Permanent fertility control achieved through surgical procedures
Tubal Ligation   Sterilization that involves the cutting and tying of the fallopian tubes.

Figure 5.7   Two methods of tubal ligation.

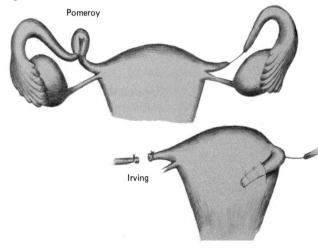

Ovarian and uterine functions are not affected. The woman's menstrual cycle continues. Released eggs simply disintegrate and are absorbed by the lymphatic system. As soon as her incision is healed, the woman may resume sexual intercourse with no fear of pregnancy.

As with any kind of surgery, risks exist. In some cases, the patient is given general anesthesia, although other women receive local anesthesia. The procedure itself usually takes less than an hour, and the patient is generally allowed to return home within a short time after waking up. All risks should be thoroughly discussed with the physician prior to the operation.

Vasectomy Sterilization in males is less complicated than in females. The procedure, called a **vasectomy,** is usually done on an outpatient basis using a local anesthetic. The surgeon (generally a urologist) makes an incision on each side of the scrotum. The *vas deferens* on each side is then located, and a piece is removed from each. The ends are usually tied or sewn shut (see Figure 5.8).

Because sperm are stored in other areas of the reproductive system, couples must use alternative methods of birth control for at least 1 month after the vasectomy. The man must check with his physician (who will do a

semen analysis) to determine when unprotected intercourse can take place.

Many men are reluctant to consider sterilization because they fear the operation will affect their sexual performance. Such fears are unfounded (although not abnormal) and can be alleviated by talking to men who have already been vasectomized.

A vasectomy in no way affects sexual response. Because sperm constitute only a small percentage of the semen, the amount of ejaculate is not changed significantly. The testes continue to produce sperm, but the sperm are prevented from entering the ejaculatory duct because of the surgery. After a time, sperm production may diminish, and any sperm manufactured will disintegrate and be absorbed into the lymphatic system.

ABORTION

In 1973, the landmark Supreme Court decision in *Roe v. Wade* ruled that the "right to privacy . . . founded on the Fourteenth Amendment's concept of a personal lib-

---

Vasectomy Sterilization that involves the cutting and tying of both *vas deferens.*

Figure 5.8 Vasectomy.

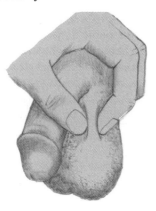
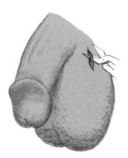
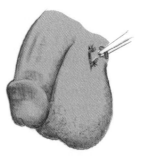

(1) Locating vas deferens

(2) Vas deferens exposed by small incision in scrotum

(3) A small section of vas deferens removed and ends tied and/or cauterized

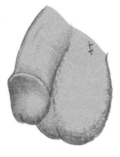
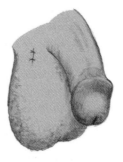

(4) Incision in scrotum closed

(5) Steps 1–4 repeated on right side

erty . . . is broad enough to encompass a woman's decision whether or not to terminate her pregnancy."* The decision maintained that during the first trimester of pregnancy, a woman and her practitioner have the right to terminate the pregnancy through **abortion** without legal restrictions. Individual states retained the right to restrict second-trimester abortions, and third-trimester abortions were declared illegal unless the mother's life was clearly in danger.

In July 1989, in *Webster v. Reproductive Health Services,* a landmark decision by the Supreme Court gave states the right to impose sharp new restrictions on abortions. In a vote of 5 to 4, the Court upheld a restrictive Missouri abortion law, giving states the authority to restrict abortion. This decision, in addition to three other rulings, has paved the way for individual state interpretations of abortion acceptability.

As of 1990, strict abortion laws have been proposed in many states. There is intense political debate now occurring in many states; antiabortion proponents are putting pressure on state and local governments to pass laws and ordinances that would restrict the availability of abortions. For example, some states have passed laws that prohibit the use of public funds for abortion as well as for abortion counseling. Abortions cannot be performed in publicly funded clinics in some states. Other states have passed laws that would require parental notification before a teenager could obtain an abortion. Although *Roe v. Wade* has not been overturned, it faces many future challenges.

Prior to the legalization of first- and second-trimester abortions, women wishing to terminate a pregnancy resorted to traveling to a country where the procedure was legal, consulting an illegal abortionist, or performing their own abortions. The last two methods led to death from hemorrhage or infection in some cases and to infertility from internal scarring in others.

Prior to the 1973 Supreme Court ruling, approximately 480,000 illegal abortions were performed in the United States each year.** One-third of these abortions were performed on married women. Since the 1973 decision, the law has been continually challenged by groups that believe the termination of a pregnancy is murder. Those who oppose abortion believe the embryo or fetus is a human being with rights that must be protected. Although many opponents work through the courts and the political process, attacks on abortion clinics are increasing.

The best birth-control methods can fail. Women may be raped. Pregnancies can occur despite every possible precaution. When an unwanted pregnancy does occur, the decision whether to terminate, to carry to term and keep, or to carry to term and give the baby away must be

made quickly. Hasty decisions are not always easy to make, and the potential for maternal guilt is immeasurable.

More than 1.6 million abortions are performed in the United States every year. Three of every 100 American women between the ages of 15 and 44 choose to end a pregnancy every year. Sixty-three percent of these women obtaining abortions are single. The majority of abortions, 52 percent, are performed after less than 8 weeks gestation.

The type of abortion procedure used is determined by how many weeks pregnant a woman is. Pregnancy length is calculated from the first day of a woman's last menstrual period.

If performed during the first trimester of pregnancy, *therapeutic abortion* presents a relatively low risk to the mother. The most commonly used method of first-trimester abortion is **vacuum aspiration.** The procedure is usually performed with local anesthetic. The cervix is dilated with instruments or by placing *laminaria,* a sterile seaweed product, in the cervical canal. The laminaria is left in place for a few hours or overnight and slowly dilates the canal. After it is removed, a long tube is inserted into the uterus and through the cervix. Gentle suction is then used to remove the pregnancy tissue from the uterine walls.

Pregnancies that progress into the second trimester can be terminated through **dilation and evacuation (D & E),** a procedure that combines vacuum aspiration with a technique called *dilation and curettage (D & C).* For this procedure, the cervix is dilated with laminaria for 1 to 2 days and a combination of scraping and vacuum aspiration is used to empty the uterus (see Figure 5.9).

Second-trimester abortions are frequently done under general anesthetic. Both procedures can be performed on an outpatient basis (usually in the physician's office) with or without pain medication. Generally, however, the woman is given a mild tranquilizer to help her relax. Both procedures may cause moderate to severe uterine cramping and blood loss.

The risks associated with abortions include infection, incomplete abortion (parts of the placenta remain in the uterus), missed abortion (still pregnant after abortion), excessive bleeding, and cervical and uterine trauma. Follow-up and attention to dangerous signs decrease the chance of any long-term problems.

The mortality rate for first-trimester abortions averages out to 0.8 per 100,000. The rate for second-trimester abortions is higher, 4.3 per 100,000. This higher rate is due to the increased risk of uterine perforation, bleeding, infection, and incomplete abortion be-

---

* Boston Women's Health Collective, *The New Our Bodies, Ourselves* (New York: Simon & Schuster, 1984), p. 218.

** John J. Burt and Linda Brower Meeks, *Education for Sexuality* (Philadelphia: Saunders, 1975).

Abortion   The medical means of terminating a pregnancy.

Vacuum Aspiration   The use of gentle suction to remove pregnancy tissue during the first trimester of pregnancy.

Dilation and Evacuation (D & E)   An abortion technique that combines vacuum aspiration with dilation and curettage; pregnancy tissue is both sucked and scraped out of the uterus.

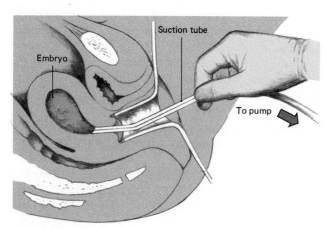

Figure 5.9 Vacuum aspiration abortion.

cause the uterine wall becomes thinner as the pregnancy progresses.

Two other methods used in second-trimester abortions are *prostaglandin* or saline **induction abortions.** In these methods, prostaglandin hormones or saline is injected into the uterus. The saline solution kills the fetus and causes labor contractions to begin. After a time, the dead fetus is delivered vaginally. The D & C procedure is more commonly used.

Finally, recent technological discoveries have yielded a promising method of abortion called RU 486. The drug, which may be taken as a pill, safely induces abortion during the first 9 weeks of pregnancy. Some authorities consider RU 486 to be "birth control" and refuse to call it an "abortion pill" because of the social and political debates over abortion. However, the purpose of RU 486 is clearly to abort pregnancy rather than stop it before it ever happens. In any case, RU 486 was developed in Europe and has not been approved for use in the United States. See the box titled "Abortion in a Pill" for more information about RU 486.

The decision to have an abortion is rarely made lightly. Each woman contemplating an abortion must weigh not only the medical risks but also the moral, religious, and social implications. As long as abortion remains a viable choice, the questions will continue. There are no simple answers.

INFERTILITY

An estimated 15 percent of American couples (1 in 6) experience difficulties in conceiving. The reasons for this phenomenon include the trend toward delaying childbirth (as a woman gets older, she is less likely to conceive) and the use of IUDs.

Pelvic inflammatory disease (PID) is a serious infection that scars the fallopian tubes and prevents conception by blocking sperm migration, resulting in sterility. Women often develop PID as a result of a gonorrhea or chlamydial infection that progresses to the fallopian tubes and the ovaries. The risk of infertility after 1 bout of PID is 12 percent. After 2 bouts it doubles to nearly 25 percent, and following 3 bouts it jumps to more than 50 percent.[*]

Endometriosis is another cause of infertility in women. In this disorder, parts of the endometrial lining of the uterus implant themselves outside the uterus in the fallopian tubes, lungs, intestines, outer uterine walls, ovarian walls, and on the ligaments that support the uterus. The disorder can be treated surgically or with hormonal preparations. Success rates vary. More information about endometriosis is contained in Chapter 14.

Among men, the single largest fertility problem is **low sperm count.** Although only one viable sperm is needed for fertilization, research has shown that all the other sperm in the ejaculate aid in the fertilization process. Normally there are 60 to 80 million sperm per milliliter of semen. When that count drops below 20 million, fertility begins to decline.

Low sperm count may be attributable to environmental factors such as exposure of the scrotum to intense heat or cold, radiation, altitude, or even wearing excessively tight underwear or outerwear. Some men are afflicted with the mumps virus, which damages the cells that make sperm, and some have varicose veins above one or both testicles, rendering them infertile. Male infertility problems account for around 40 percent of infertility cases.

For the couple desperately wishing to conceive, the road to parenthood may be frustrating. The efforts to conceive, the countless tests, and the invasion of privacy can all adversely affect an otherwise strong and healthy relationship. Prior to engaging in fertility tests, the wise couple redefines their priorities. Some undertake counseling to help them clarify their feelings about the fertility process. A good physician or fertility team also takes time to ascertain the couple's level of motivation.

Fertility workups may be very expensive and are not usually covered by insurance companies. Fertility workups for men include a sperm count, a test for sperm motility, and analysis of any disease processes present. Such procedures should only be undertaken by a qualified urologist. Women are thoroughly examined by an obstetrician/gynecologist for the composition of cervical mucus, extent of tubal scarring, and evidence of endometriosis.

Induction Abortion A type of abortion in which chemicals are injected into the uterus through the uterine wall; labor begins and the woman delivers a dead fetus.

Pelvic Inflammatory Disease (PID) A serious infection that scars the fallopian tubes and prevents conception by blocking sperm migration, resulting in sterility.

Endometriosis A disorder in which uterine lining tissue establishes itself outside the uterus; the leading cause of infertility in the U.S.

Low Sperm Count A sperm count below 60 million sperm per milliliter of semen; it can prevent conception from occurring.

[*] University of Southern California School of Medicine, *Dialogues in Contraception*, 3, no. 4 (1991), p. 2.

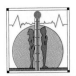

Abortion in a Pill

RU 486, A European Postconception Drug

The abortion debate has recently heated up with the development of RU 486, a drug that safely induces abortion during the first 9 weeks of pregnancy. ("RU" refers to Roussel-Uclaf, a French pharmaceutical company that is a subsidiary of the German pharmaceutical company Hoechst.) Antiabortion protests have helped restrict the production and availability of RU 486. Proponents of the drug are pushing for global distribution. Both sides agree on the extreme effectiveness of RU 486 in inducing abortion in early pregnancy.

RU 486 is a steroid hormone that induces abortion by blocking the action of progesterone, a vital hormone produced by the ovaries and placenta, which maintains the lining of the uterus. Similar in structure to progesterone, RU 486 binds to cell receptor sites normally occupied by progesterone, causing the breakdown of the uterine lining. The embryo and the uterine lining are expelled from the uterus and the pregnancy is terminated.

Treatment consists of the oral ingestion of three pills of RU 486. A dose of prostaglandins must be administered 48 hours later to encourage contractions of the uterus. Ninety-six percent of the women who take these two drugs during the first 9 weeks of pregnancy will experience a complete abortion. The side effects of this treatment are similar to those reported during heavy menstruation and include cramping, minor pain, and nausea. Approximately 1 in a 1000 women require a blood transfusion due to severe bleeding. The procedure does not require hospitalization; women may be treated on an outpatient basis.

Anti-abortion groups view RU 486 with alarm. The easier and less painful method of a drug-induced abortion may increase the total number of abortions obtained. In the future, RU 486-induced abortions may occur in the privacy of a doctor's office. Abortion clinics, often the target of protestors, could become obsolete.

Proponents of RU 486 believe that the treatment could save lives, particularly in developing countries. The World Health Organization (WHO) estimates that 200,000 women die every year from unsafe surgical abortions. In some countries, this figure amounts to half of the maternal death rate. In poverty-stricken countries with overextended medical facilities, RU 486 could be used on an outpatient basis. Only 4 percent of the women would need skilled medical intervention for complications. Drug-induced abortions would reduce the risks of infection and perforation common with surgical abortions performed in poor countries.

British doctors fear that pressure will keep RU 486 out of England. At a conference in London in November 1989, doctors urged Roussel-Uclaf's British subsidiary to apply for a product license to begin distribution in England. It does not seem likely that the drug will be available in the United States in the near future. Anti-abortion groups, such as the National Right to Life Coalition, have lobbied sympathetic legislators into making access to RU 486 as difficult as possible. The drug has not been approved by the FDA, and it is illegal for the National Institutes of Health to finance research on RU 486. In addition, the United States has used political means to try to slow testing of the drug by WHO.

China has approved the use of RU 486, but so far Roussel-Uclaf has refused to distribute it outside of France. Some scientists feel that China may begin to manufacture its own supply of the drug. Chemists from other countries have the capabilities to produce RU 486 and may start manufacturing a black market supply. A substantial demand for RU 486 almost guarantees it will be utilized, legally or not, outside the borders of France.

SOURCES: "Abortion Pill to Be Subsidized," *The Register-Guard,* February 28, 1990; "Drug Company Holds Back Abortion Pill," *New Scientist,* (November 4, 1989), p. 24; "The Pill of Choice," *Science,* 245 (September 22, 1989), pp. 1319–23).

Complete fertility workups may take 4 to 5 months and can be unsettling for the couple. A couple may be asked to have sex "by the calendar" to increase chances of conceiving.

In some cases, surgery can correct structural problems such as tubal scarring. In others, administering hormones can increase the health of ova and sperm. Some pregnancies can begin by collecting the husband's sperm and inseminating the wife at a later time.

When all surgical and hormonal methods fail, the

couple has some options. Use of **fertility drugs** such as Clomid and Pergonal has gained publicity because of the numbers of multiple births they seem to cause. These drugs stimulate ovulation in women who are not ovulating. Ninety percent of women using these drugs will begin to ovulate, and half will become able to conceive.

Fertility drugs are associated with a great number of side effects, including headaches, irritability, restlessness, depression, fatigue, edema (fluid retention), abnormal uterine bleeding, breast tenderness, vasomotor flushes (hot flashes), and visual difficulties. Women using fertility drugs are also at increased risk of multiple ovarian cysts (fluid-filled growths) and liver damage. The drugs sometimes trigger the release of more than one egg. A woman treated with one of these drugs has a 2 in 20 chance of having multiple births. Most such births are twins.

Alternative insemination of a woman with her husband's sperm is an option. If this procedure fails, the couple may choose to be inseminated by an anonymous donor through a "sperm bank." Many men sell their sperm to such banks, where the sperm are classified according to the characteristics of the donor (for example, blonde hair or blue eyes) and then frozen for future use. Sperm can survive in the frozen state for up to 5 years. The woman being inseminated usually chooses sperm from a man whose physical characteristics resemble those of her partner or according to her own personal preference.

In the last few years, concern has been expressed over the possibility of transmitting the AIDS virus (see Chapter 14 through alternative insemination. As a result, donors are routinely screened for the disease before they donate.

In-vitro fertilization, often referred to as "test tube" fertilization, involves collecting a viable ovum from the prospective mother and transferring it to a nutrient medium in a laboratory where it is fertilized with sperm from the woman's partner or a donor. After a few days, the embryo is transplanted into the mother's uterus, where, it is hoped, it develops normally.

Until 1984, in-vitro fertilization was classified as "experimental." Since then, it has moved into the mainstream of standard infertility treatments. About 500 "test tube" babies are born each year.

Nonsurgical embryo transfer is another treatment for infertility in which a donor egg is fertilized by the husband's sperm and then implanted in the wife's uterus. This procedure may also be used in cases involving the transfer of an already-fertilized ovum into the uterus of another woman.

Embryo transfer may also be used. In this procedure, an ovum from a donor's body is artifically inseminated by the husband's sperm, allowed to stay in the donor's body for a time, and then transplanted into the wife's body.

Some laboratories are experimenting with **embryo freezing,** in which a fertilized embryo is suspended in a solution of liquid nitrogen. When desired, it is gradually thawed and implanted into the prospective mother. The first U.S. birth of a frozen embryo was reported in June 1986. In the future, this technique may be available for young couples to use through the fertilization of younger eggs and saved for later implantation when the couple is ready to have a child, thus reducing the risks of fertilization of older eggs.

Cloning has been successfully used with lower

Fertilization labs will probably become more common as our technology progresses.

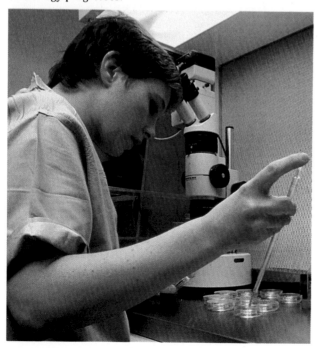

Fertility Drugs   Hormones that stimulate ovulation in women who are not ovulating; often responsible for multiple births.

Alternative Insemination   Fertilization by depositing partner or donor semen into a woman's vagina through a thin tube; always done in a doctor's office.

In-vitro Fertilization   Fertilization of an egg in a test tube followed by transfer to a nutrient medium and subsequent transfer to the mother's body.

Nonsurgical Transfer   A treatment for infertility in which a donor egg is fertilized by the husband's sperm and then implanted in the wife's uterus.

Embryo Transfer   A treatment to infertility in which an ovum from a donor's body is inseminated by the husband's sperm, allowed to stay in the donor's body for a time, and then transplanted into the wife's body.

Embryo Freezing   An experimental treatment for infertility in which a fertilized embryo is suspended in liquid nitrogen, then gradually thawed and implanted in the prospective mother.

Cloning   A possible treatment for infertility in which the nucleus of an in-vitro-fertilized egg is replaced with the nucleus of a body cell from a donor of the mother's choice; cloning has be used only on lower animals such as toads, and the possibilities of human cloning are still remote.

animals such as toads and salamanders. In cloning, the nucleus of an in-vitro-fertilized egg is replaced with the nucleus of a body cell from a donor of the mother's choosing. Resulting offspring will be genetically identical to the donor. The possibilities of human cloning are still remote.

The ethical and moral questions surrounding experimental methods of infertility treatments are staggering. Would it be possible for a nation or a group of people to attempt the development of a "super race" through cloning or through embryo freezing? What about homosexuals who wish to have children? Will cloning be an option for them, allowing homosexuals to produce their own child using one another's cells? What would happen if cell nuclei from certain people were frozen for later use? Will humans use these techniques to gain immortality?

The expense of any of these procedures can be staggering. Alternative insemination costs approximately $1,500 for 5 monthly attempts. In-vitro fertilization costs $5,000 per attempt. Fewer than 50 percent of these cases succeed on the first try.

Surrogate Motherhood

Between 60 and 70 percent of infertile couples are able to conceive after treatment. The rest decide to live without children, to adopt, or to attempt *surrogate motherhood*. In this option, the couple hires a woman to be alternatively inseminated by the husband. The surrogate then carries the baby to term and surrenders it upon birth to the parents. Surrogate mothers are paid for their services and are reimbursed for medical expenses. Surrogates are reportedly paid about $10,000. Legal and medical expenses may be as high as $30,000. Couples considering surrogate motherhood are advised to consult a lawyer regarding contracts.

Most legal documents drawn for childless couples and surrogate mothers stipulate that the surrogate must undergo amniocentesis. If the fetus is defective, she must consent to an abortion. Should this occur, or if the surrogate miscarries, she is reimbursed for part of her expenses. The prospective parents must also agree to take the baby if it is carried to term, even if it is unhealthy or deformed.

▌ SUMMARY

■ Parenting is a demanding job for which few of us are truly prepared. The decision to become a parent requires careful planning.

■ The most important aspect of parenting is providing a secure place for a child to grow, including adequate nourishment, touch, communication, support, and an atmosphere that encourages self-esteem.

■ Prior to becoming parents, we must assess our abilities to be parents and also set goals for ourselves as parents.

■ Each of us is responsible for managing our personal fertility.

■ A pregnant woman has certain responsibilities, including adequate nutrition, abstinence from drugs, and proper medical supervision.

■ A mother may choose from many pregnancy and birthing options including traditional hospital delivery, home delivery, the Lamaze method, and the Leboyer method.

■ Complications during the birth process often force the attending physician to perform a cesarean section, removing the baby through an incision in the abdominal and uterine walls. The number of cesarean births in the United States has increased in recent years.

■ Modern medical practices make vaginal birth after cesarean (VBAC) a possibility for 50 to 80 percent of women with previous cesareans.

■ Miscarriage and stillbirth are types of pregnancy losses that can devastate new parents or parents-to-be. Many communities have support groups to help the parents and other family members adjust.

■ Devices, procedures, or drugs designed to prevent conception are called contraceptives.

■ Norplant is the most effective reversible means of preventing pregnancy. Six capsules are placed in a fan-like pattern just under the skin, in the upper arm. Norplant provides contraceptive protection for 5 years, with minimal side effects.

■ Oral contraceptives are one of the most effective reversible means of preventing pregnancy. Although the side effects and risk factors associated with the drug frighten some women, the Pill has been found to decrease risks of various cancers and nonmalignant breast disease.

■ An abortion is a medical means of terminating a pregnancy. The right to have an abortion continues to be a volatile political issue in the United States.

■ Abortions conducted during the first trimester of pregnancy are safer than those conducted later.

■ One in 6 couples wishing to have a baby suffers from infertility.

■ The options available to couples with fertility problems are varied and expensive. Overall success rates for infertile couples are below 50 percent.

■ The issue of surrogate motherhood has surfaced as a controversial political and emotional issue in the United States.

6

Nutrition: Eating for Optimal Health

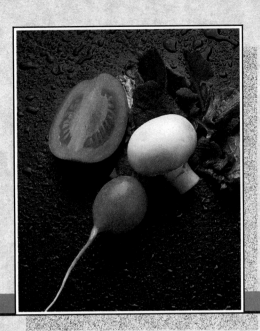

Objectives

- Name some of the most significant factors that influence what we eat and when, and explain why we may actually do ourselves harm through food consumption.

- Describe how the human body obtains essential nutrients from the foods we eat.

- Discuss exactly what is meant by "proper nutrition" in terms of the basic food nutrients.

- Name three dietary patterns that differ from the standard, recommended American diet and describe some of the special dietary needs that people who abide by these patterns may have.

Finding the proper balance between food intake (diet) and energy expenditure (exercise) has become a major concern for many Americans. Caught in a barrage of advertised claims by the food industry and advice provided by health and nutrition experts, consumers of all ages find it difficult to make decisions.

Television advertisements subtly attempt to influence us to buy "cholesterol-free" products, "high-fiber" oat bran, "stress vitamins," and a variety of items that promise to make us healthier. Newsstands overflow with books and magazines promoting certain health foods, weight-loss aids, and the next "super" diet. Many of these articles and books are written by people who have no educational background in nutrition but who claim to be nutritional experts. Their theories are based on results obtained with poorly designed research techniques and provide questionable or controversial recommendations. The ability to sift through the untruths, half-truths, and scientific realities and to select a nutritional plan designed to meet our individual needs is an essential health-promoting skill. Understanding the reasons for our nutritional choices may help us change negative dietary patterns and enhance positive behaviors.

INFLUENCES ON DIETARY PATTERNS

Eating is one activity that the majority of Americans take for granted. We assume that we will have sufficient food to get us through the day. We assume, too, that we will have choices in deciding the types of food that we eat. Although we have all undoubtedly experienced **hunger** a few hours before mealtime, few of us have ever experienced the type of hunger that continues for days and threatens our survival. Most of us do not eat because we *need* to eat at a given moment for physical survival. Instead, we eat because we *feel* like eating or because some type of inner signal tells us that "it's time to eat."

Many factors influence when we eat, what we eat, and how much we eat. Sensory stimulation, such as smelling, seeing, and tasting foods, can entice us to eat. Social pressures, including family traditions, social events that involve eating, and busy daily work schedules, can also influence our diets. Our economic status may determine what types of foods we purchase. Certain foods or food groups may be too expensive for some people. However, if we have access to healthy and affordable foods, many of us will make educated choices in our purchases.

If our **appetite** for food is stimulated, we may want to eat something because it looks or smells good, even though we are not actually hungry. Finding the right balance between eating to maintain body functions (eating to live) and eating to satisfy our appetites (living to eat) is a problem for many of us. The problems that result

from failing to achieve this balance are detailed in Chapter 7.

With our overabundance of food, our vast number of choices, and our easy access to almost every nutrient, Americans should have few nutritional problems. Because we do not have to eat whatever happens to be available but can choose our foods, it would seem that the likelihood of poor choices would be minimal.

If we were like most other species and ate only for survival, the likelihood of excessive food consumption would be small. We would also be unlikely to suffer from nutrient deficiencies. However, humans learn from their earliest moments that eating is an enjoyable experience, to be associated with warmth, pleasure, and sensory delights. Infants cry and are fed; children are rewarded with food for doing well; weddings, births, and other special occasions center on eating. We learn to enjoy and reward ourselves with rich foods.

Thus, with all our wealth and vast reserves of food, Americans suffer from numerous nutrition-related diseases. Although America does not have large numbers of people dying from starvation, a condition that characterizes other regions of the world, nutritionists believe that our "diets of affluence" are responsible for many diseases and disabilities, including heart disease, certain types of cancer, hypertension (high blood pressure), cirrhosis of the liver, tooth decay, and chronic obesity. The food choices that Americans make have changed over the past three decades. Some of these changes are outlined in Table 6.1.

Responsible Eating: Changing Old Habits

On the average, Americans consume more **calories** per person than any other group of people in the world. A calorie is a unit of measure that indicates the amount of energy we obtain from a particular food. These calories are eaten in the form of *proteins, fats,* and *carbohydrates,* three of the basic nutrients necessary for life. Three other nutrients, *vitamins, minerals,* and *water,* are necessary for bodily function but luckily do not contribute any calories to our diets.

Excessive calorie consumption is a major factor in our tendency to be overweight. However, it is not so much the quantity of food that is likely to cause weight problems (and resultant disease) as it is the relative proportion of nutrients in our diets and a lack of physical activity. Out of a typical daily diet of 2,000 calories, Americans are likely to consume about 840 calories of fat, 240 calories of protein, 440 calories of complex carbohydrates, and 480 calories of simple sugar (see Figure 6.1).

Hunger   The physiological need to eat.
Appetite   The desire to eat; normally accompanies hunger and is more psychological.
Calorie   A unit of measure of the amount of energy derived from food.

Table 6.1 Changes in Annual Food Consumption of Americans, 1960–1987

The following table illustrates changes in annual food consumption per person during the last 3 decades. Unless otherwise indicated, the amounts are presented in pounds. Are these trends generally healthy or unhealthy?

Food Product	1960	1970	1984	1987
Red meat	173.7	162.8	151.9	144.0
Fish and shellfish	10.3	11.8	13.7	15.4
Poultry	34.0	48.2	66.5	77.8
Eggs (number)	334.	309.	259.	249.
Whole milk	263.9	219.1	126.6	109.9
Lower-fat milk (1% and 2%)	—	50.0	99.1	113.6
Nonfat milk	10.7	11.6	11.5	14.0
Fats and oils	—	52.6	58.6	62.7
Flour (white, whole-wheat)	—	110.8	118.1	128.0
Pasta	—	7.7	11.3	17.1
Breakfast cereals	—	10.8	14.0	15.2
Sugar and corn sweeteners	111.5	121.	125.1	130.
Saccharin	—	5.8	10.0	5.5
Aspartame	—	—	5.8	13.5
Fruits (fresh)	—	76.9	87.8	98.6
Fruits (canned)	—	14.4	8.9	8.7
Vegetables (fresh)	—	64.0	78.8	78.6
Coffee (gallons)	—	33.4	26.5	26.5
Soft drinks (gallons)	—	20.8	27.2	30.3
Beer (gallons)	—	30.6	35.0	34.4
Wine (gallons)	—	2.2	3.4	3.4
Distilled spirits (gallons)	—	3.0	2.6	2.3

− = data not available

SOURCE: U.S. Department of Commerce, Bureau of the Census, *Statistical Abstracts of the United States, 1989.*

This high concentration of fats, particularly *saturated fats* (those coming from animals), appears to increase our risk for heart disease. High concentrations of highly processed sugars also appear to increase our risk for certain diseases, particularly tooth decay. In response to what they perceived as an epidemic of poor dietary habits, several scientific organizations received funding to conduct research in the area of nutritional habits of Americans. In 1977, the Senate Select Committee on Nutrition and Human Needs reviewed much of this research information and developed a set of dietary rules for health and nutrition titled *Dietary Goals for the United States.* These goals were established with the objective of reducing risks for nutritionally related disorders. After nearly a decade of implementation, these dietary goals were updated in 1986 to reflect current beliefs about the way we eat (see Table 6.2). In 1988, in *The Surgeon General's Report on Nutrition and Health,* a list of key recommendations based on accumulated research, was presented. These recommendations include the following:

- Reduce consumption of fat (especially saturated fat) and cholesterol.
- Achieve and maintain a desirable body weight by balancing calorie intake with energy expenditure.
- Increase consumption of complex carbohydrates and fiber.
- Reduce sodium intake.
- Drink alcohol only in moderation (no more than two drinks per day).*

---

* *The Surgeon General's Report on Nutrition and Health* (Washington, D.C.: USDA, USDHHS, 1988), p. 3.

The heavy use of fast-food restaurants has had a negative effect on the eating habits of Americans.

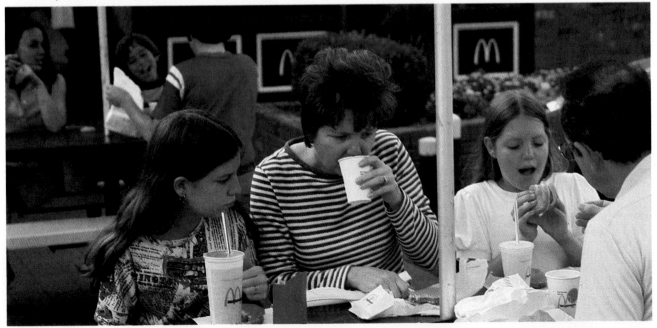

Rating Your Nutritional IQ

1. Eating foods that are "cholesterol-free" will eliminate cholesterol from your diet.
   _____ True   _____ False

2. Hydrogenated oils are essentially equivalent to saturated fat.
   _____ True   _____ False

3. Fruit sugar is less fattening than table sugar.
   _____ True   _____ False

4. Athletes need significantly more protein than nonathletes.
   _____ True   _____ False

5. Potatoes are a good source of vitamin C.
   _____ True   _____ False

6. Saturated fat is found only in animal products.
   _____ True   _____ False

7. People who eat a lot of sugar tend to be heavier than others.
   _____ True   _____ False

8. Red meats are better protein sources than poultry or fish.
   _____ True   _____ False

9. Rice and flour are good sources of the B vitamins.
   _____ True   _____ False

10. Cottage cheese, like all dairy products, is an excellent source of calcium.
    _____ True   _____ False

KEY

1. False. Cholesterol levels in the body are not totally based on dietary intake. Your body produces a certain amount of cholesterol each day, regardless of what you eat. Also, just because a product is "cholesterol-free" does not mean that it is low in saturated fats. High saturated-fat levels may be as important in influencing your body's production of cholesterol as actual intake of cholesterol.

2. True. *Hydrogenation* is another name for "hardening," a process in which hydrogen atoms are readded to unsaturated-fat molecules to make a new saturated fat, with all the same potential for causing cardiovascular disease as regular saturated fats.

3. False. Fruit sugar and table sugar have the same number of calories per serving.

4. False. Although an athlete may need slightly more protein during the initial stages of

training or competition, that need is not very great. Since most Americans already consume more than enough protein, chances are that the increased need has already been met by a normal diet.

5. True. White potatoes in particular are a good source. One medium potato offers about one-third of the daily requirement for vitamin C. However, the more potatoes are whipped, the more vitamin C is lost.

6. False. Animal foods are the primary, but not the only source, of saturated fats. Saturated fat is also present in products made with coconut oil, palm-kernel oil, and palm oil, all of which come from plants. In fact, the fat in coconut and palm-kernel oil is actually more saturated than that found in animals. These oils are most often found in snack products and other highly processed foods.

7. False. Overweight people, according to epidemiological studies, actually eat less sugar than thin people. Moreover, the amount of sugar someone eats is not necessarily a determinant of whether one will gain weight. Obesity results from a variety of factors, including lifestyle, genetics, and overall eating and activity patterns.

8. False. Red meats tend to be higher in fat, so the percentage of protein on an ounce-for-ounce basis is lower than in fish or poultry.

9. True. But since milling and polishing remove so much of the vitamins, flour and rice in the United States are usually enriched with thiamin, riboflavin, and niacin.

10. False. Cottage cheese is only a modest source of calcium, supplying 60 to 70 mg in a half-cup. In contrast, half a cup of plain yogurt has, on average, 200 mg. An ounce of most hard cheese contains 150 to 200 mg. Most of milk's calcium is whey, which is drained off when cottage cheese is made.

SCORING
8–10 correct: Excellent. You do not believe some of the common nutrition misconceptions.
6–7 correct: Okay. You have some beliefs that are incorrect, but you have a good foundation.
0–5 correct: Improvement needed. You should increase your nutritional awareness.

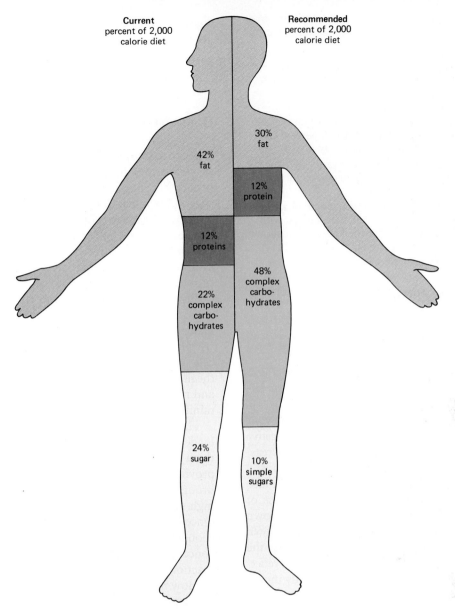

Current
percent of 2,000
calorie diet

Recommended
percent of 2,000
calorie diet

30%
fat

42%
fat

12%
protein

12%
proteins

48%
complex
carbo-
hydrates

22%
complex
carbo-
hydrates

24%
sugar

10%
simple
sugars

Figure 6.1 This figure contrasts a recommended, nutritionally balanced diet with a typical American diet.

To use this information, you must first understand the role of specific nutrients in the body, how the body utilizes these nutrients, nutrient sources, and most important, proper eating behaviors. Once you have acquired this knowledge, you can incorporate this information into your everyday life. You will also realize that changing bad dietary habits into reasonable ones does not mean becoming a "nutritional purist" who never deviates from the optimal nutritional path.

THE DIGESTIVE PROCESS

The foods that we eat provide us with chemicals necessary for energy and body maintenance. Because our bodies cannot synthesize or produce certain essential nutri-

ents, we must obtain them through the foods we eat. Even though we may take in adequate amounts of foods and nutrients, if our body systems are not functioning properly, much of the nutrient value in the foods may be lost. Before foods can be utilized properly, the digestive system must break the larger food particles down into smaller, more usable, forms.

The process by which foods are broken down and either absorbed or excreted by the body is known as the **digestive process.** Although many of us think of digestion as occurring only in the stomach and intestines, the digestive system actually begins in the mouth and ends in the anus. Along the 30-odd feet of pathway that food

Digestive Process Process by which foods are broken down and either absorbed for bodily use or eliminated.

Table 6.2 U.S. Dietary Goals

1. To avoid becoming overweight, consume only as much energy (calories) as is expended; if overweight, decrease energy intake and increase energy expenditure.
2. Increase the consumption of complex carbohydrates and "naturally occurring" sugars from about 28 percent of energy intake to about 48 percent of energy intake.
3. Reduce the consumption of refined and processed sugars by about 45 percent to supply about 10 percent of total energy intake.
4. Reduce saturated-fat consumption to account for about 10 percent of total energy intake, and balance that with polyunsaturated and monounsaturated fats, which should account for about 10 percent of energy intake each.
6. Reduce cholesterol consumption to about 300 mg per day.
7. Limit the intake of sodium by reducing the intake of salt to about 5 g per day.

SOURCE: Select Committee on Nutrition and Human Needs. *Dietary Goals for the United States,* 2nd ed. (Washington, D.C.: U.S. Senate Select Committee, 1986).

must travel inside the body, numerous chemical conversions occur that convert food into energy.

Even before you take your first bite of pizza, your body has already begun a series of complex digestive responses. The mouth prepares for the food by increasing production of **saliva.** This saliva contains mostly water that aids in chewing and swallowing, but it also contains important enzymes that begin the process of food breakdown, including *amylase,* which breaks down carbohydrates. From the mouth, the food passes down the **esophagus,** a 9- to 10-inch tube that connects the mouth and stomach. A series of contractions and relaxations by the muscles lining the esophagus gently moves food to the next digestive organ, the **stomach.** Here food mixes with enzymes and stomach acids. Hydrochloric acid begins to work in combination with *pepsin,* an enzyme, to break down proteins. For most people, the stomach secretes enough mucus to protect the actual stomach lining from the harsh digestive juices. However, when there are problems with the lining, ulcers can occur.

The major portion of the remaining digestive activity takes place in the **small intestine,** a 20-foot coiled tube containing three sections: the *duodenum,* the *jejunum,* and the *ileum.* Each of these sections secretes digestive enzymes that, when combined with enzymes from the liver and the pancreas, further contribute to the breakdown of proteins, fats, and carbohydrates. Once broken down, foods are absorbed into the bloodstream to supply body cells with energy. The *liver* is the major organ that determines whether nutrients are stored, sent to cells or organs, or excreted. Solid wastes consisting of fiber, water, and salts are dumped into the large intestine, where the water and salts are reabsorbed into the system and the fiber is passed out through the anus. The entire

digestive process takes approximately 24 hours (see Figure 6.2).

PROPER NUTRITION

Basic Nutrients

Water: A Crucial Nutrient If you were to go on a survival trip, which would you take with you, food or water? You might be surprised to learn that you could survive for much longer periods without food than you could without water. Even in severe conditions, the average person could go for weeks without certain vitamins and minerals before experiencing serious deficiency symptoms. **Dehydration,** however, can cause serious problems within a matter of hours.

Just what function does water serve in the body? To begin with, water is a major component of our structural makeup. In fact, between 50 and 60 percent of our total weight is water. It is the water in our system that bathes cells and transports fluids throughout the body. Water is the major component of the blood, which carries oxygen and nutrients to the tissues and is responsible for maintaining cells in working order.

Have you ever noticed that after eating a huge pizza loaded with sausage, cheese, and anchovies, you are thirsty? Careful analysis of what you just ate would provide a startling overview of sodium bombardment, brought on by high-salt cheeses, high-salt tomato sauce, high-salt meats, and special seasonings (see Figure 6.3). Once this salt overload hits the system, the body responds by craving fluids, which serve to dilute a high concentration of salt within the body and avoid toxic reactions by body organs.

How much water do you need? Actual amounts vary dramatically according to dietary factors, age, size, environmental temperature and humidity levels, exercise, and the effectiveness of your own system. Certain diseases, such as diabetes and cystic fibrosis, cause victims to lose fluids at a rate necessitating a high volume of fluid intake.

Perhaps you have heard that to be "regular" in bowel habits and other functions you should drink eight glasses of water per day. Eight glasses may sound like a lot. However, because of the amount of water in most of the foods we consume, the actual number of glasses needed each day is somewhat less than this for the average person.

Saliva Fluid secreted by the salivary glands; aids in the breakdown of certain foods for digestion.

Esophagus Tube that transports food from the mouth to the stomach.

Stomach Large muscular organ that temporarily stores, mixes, and aids in digestion of foods.

Small Intestine Muscular, coiled organ that aids in the digestion of foods; consists of the duodenum, jejunum, and ileum.

Dehydration Excessive water loss from the body.

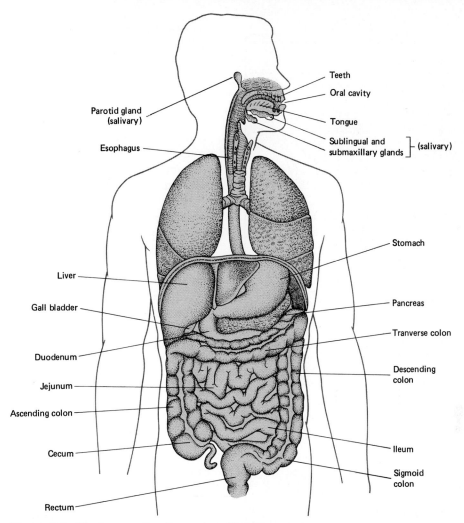

Figure 6.2 The human digestive system. Digestion occurs throughout this system, from the mouth through the rectum.

Parents should impress on their children the importance of good dietary habits.

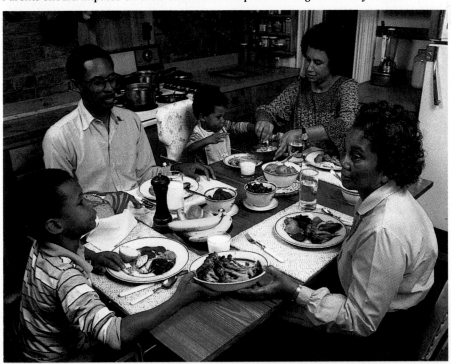

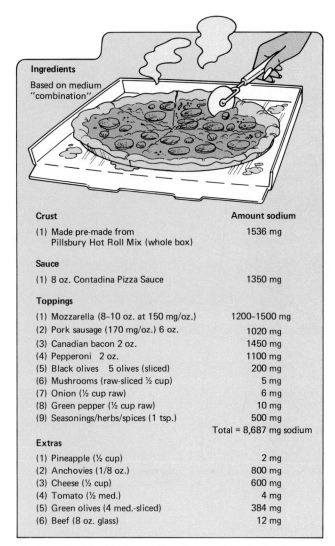

Ingredients

Based on medium "combination"

Crust	Amount sodium
(1) Made pre-made from Pillsbury Hot Roll Mix (whole box)	1536 mg
Sauce	
(1) 8 oz. Contadina Pizza Sauce	1350 mg
Toppings	
(1) Mozzarella (8–10 oz. at 150 mg/oz.)	1200–1500 mg
(2) Pork sausage (170 mg/oz.) 6 oz.	1020 mg
(3) Canadian bacon 2 oz.	1450 mg
(4) Pepperoni 2 oz.	1100 mg
(5) Black olives 5 olives (sliced)	200 mg
(6) Mushrooms (raw-sliced ½ cup)	5 mg
(7) Onion (½ cup raw)	6 mg
(8) Green pepper (½ cup raw)	10 mg
(9) Seasonings/herbs/spices (1 tsp.)	500 mg
	Total = 8,687 mg sodium
Extras	
(1) Pineapple (½ cup)	2 mg
(2) Anchovies (1/8 oz.)	800 mg
(3) Cheese (½ cup)	600 mg
(4) Tomato (½ med.)	4 mg
(5) Green olives (4 med.-sliced)	384 mg
(6) Beef (8 oz. glass)	12 mg

Figure 6.3 The hidden sodium in your favorite foods.

Proteins Next to water, **proteins** are the most abundant substances in the human body. Proteins are major components of nearly every cell and have been called the "body builders" because of their role in developing bone, muscle, skin, and blood. Proteins also are the key elements of the antibodies that protect us from disease, of enzymes that control chemical activities in the body, and of hormones that regulate bodily functions. They also aid in the transport of iron, oxygen, and nutrients to all of the body's cells and supply energy to body cells when fats and carbohydrates are not readily available. In short, adequate amounts of protein in the diet are vital to our survival.

Few Americans suffer protein deficiencies. In fact, the typical American consumes nearly twice as much protein as the body requires. Proteins themselves are made up of smaller molecules known as **amino acids**, the building blocks of proteins. These acids are composed of chains that link together like beads on a necklace in differing combinations. There are over 22 different types of amino acids found in animal tissue, and humans cannot synthe-

size all of them. The 9 amino acids that the body cannot synthesize in adequate amounts are referred to as **essential amino acids**. These nutrients must be supplied through our food. It is therefore essential that we obtain these amino acids from proteins in our diet. **Complete,** or **high-quality, proteins** are those proteins that naturally contain all of the essential amino acids necessary to supply the body's needs. If we consume a food that contains protein but is deficient in some of the amino acids, the total amount of protein that can be synthesized by the other amino acids is decreased. It is important to remember that the mere presence of the essential amino acids does not ensure adequate synthesis. Quality of protein depends on the presence of amino acids in digestible form and in amounts proportional to body requirements.

The most common sources of dietary protein in the United States are red meats, poultry, fish, and dairy products. In addition to providing complete, high-quality proteins, these animal sources of protein (with the exception of fish) also contain high levels of saturated fat and cholesterol. Selecting leaner cuts of meat, removing the fat and skin from chicken, and choosing low-fat dairy products will enable you to get high-quality proteins without the excess calories and fat.

What about plant sources of protein? Many myths exist about the "whole-grain goodness" and relative completeness of these foods. Proteins from plant sources are often **incomplete proteins** in that they contain all but one or two of the essential amino acids. Nevertheless, it is relatively easy for the non–meat eater to combine plant foods effectively and eat complementary sources of plant protein (see Table 6.3). An excellent example of this is eating peanut butter on whole-grain bread. Although each is deficient in essential amino acids, eating them together provides high-quality protein. Plant sources of protein fall into three general categories: *legumes,* including dried beans and peas, peanuts, and soy products; *grains,* which include whole grains, corn, and pasta products; and *nuts and seeds,* including of a variety of different types and sizes. Mixing 2 or more foods from each of these categories during the same meal will provide all of the essential amino acids necessary to ensure appropriate protein absorption. People who are not interested in obtaining all of their protein from plants can combine incomplete plant proteins with complete animal proteins that are low in fat. Excellent meals can be prepared by combining plant proteins and low-fat meats

Proteins Substances made up of amino acids that are major components of cells.

Amino Acids Building blocks of protein.

Essential Amino Acids Eight of the basic nitrogen-containing building blocks of protein that one must obtain from foods to ensure personal health.

Complete, or High-quality, Proteins Proteins that contain all of the eight essential amino acids.

Incomplete Proteins Proteins that are lacking in one or more of the essential amino acids.

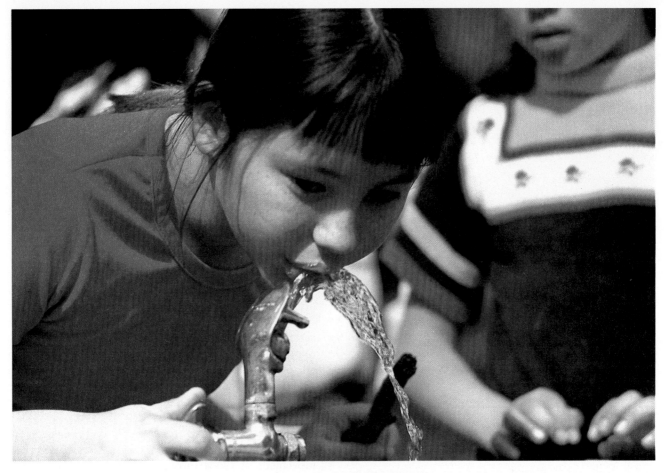

Although we take water for granted, it is one of the most essential of all nutrients.

such as chicken, turkey, fish, and lean cuts of red meat. Low-fat cottage cheese, skim milk, egg whites, and non-fat dry milk all provide high-quality proteins and are low in calories and dietary fat.

Carbohydrates: Energy Providers　Although the importance of proteins in the body cannot be underestimated, **carbohydrates,** and not proteins, supply us with the energy to sustain normal daily activity. Long maligned by weight-conscious people, carbohydrates actually can be metabolized more quickly and efficiently than can proteins. The demand for low-calorie, high-energy foods created by the "fitness craze" in America has reestablished carbohydrates as an integral part of a healthy diet. To many people, a plate of pasta represents an attractive alternative to a fatty steak.

There are two major types of carbohydrates: **simple sugars,** which are found primarily in fruits, and **complex carbohydrates,** which are found in grain, fruits, and the stems, leaves, and roots of vegetables. Simple sugars provide us with quick bursts of short-term energy, but it is the more complex form of carbohydrates (starches) that provide us with sustained energy.

SIMPLE SUGARS　On a typical day, our diet contains large amounts of simple sugars. The most common form is *glucose* (dextrose). Eventually, the human body converts all types of simple sugars to glucose to provide energy to cells. In its natural form, glucose is obtained from substances such as corn syrup, honey, molasses, vegetables, and fruits. *Fructose* is another simple sugar, found in fruits and berries. Glucose and fructose are **monosaccharides** and contain only one molecule of sugar.

Disaccharides are combinations of two monosaccharides. Perhaps the best-known example is common granulated table sugar (known as *sucrose*), which consists of a molecule of fructose chemically bonded to a molecule of glucose. *Lactose* is another form of disaccharide formed by the combination of glucose and *galactose* (another simple sugar). Lactose is found in milk and milk products.

Carbohydrates　Nutrients containing carbon, hydrogen, and oxygen; supply an efficient form of body energy.

Simple Sugars　The basic building blocks of carbohydrates; also known as monosaccharides, consisting of glucose, fructose, and galactose.

Complex Carbohydrates　A carbohydrate consisting of three or more simple-sugar molecules. Fiber, starch, and glycogen are the most common forms.

Monosaccharides　Form of simple sugar.

Disaccharides　Combination of two monosaccharides; table sugar is the most common form.

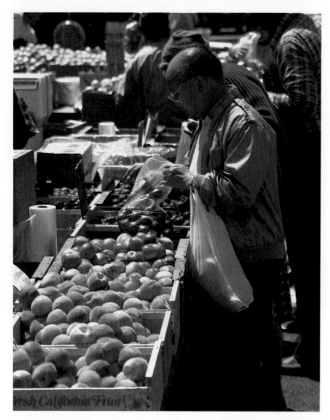

A healthy diet should include large amounts of fresh fruits and vegetables.

Controlling the amount of sugar in our diets can be difficult because sugar, like sodium, is often present in food products where we would not expect to find it. Such diverse items as ketchup, Russian dressing, CoffeeMate, and Shake'n Bake contain between 30 and 65 percent sugar. Therefore, you should read labels carefully before purchasing food products.

COMPLEX CARBOHYDRATES **Polysaccharides** are complex carbohydrates formed by the combining of long chains of saccharides. Like disaccharides, they must be

---

Table 6.3 Complementary Protein Combinations

Choose from two or more of these columns at one meal to obtain complete protein.

GRAINS	LEGUMES	SEEDS AND NUTS
Barley	Dried beans	Sesame seeds
Bulgur	Dried lentils	Sunflower seeds
Cornmeal	Dried peas	Walnuts
Oats	Peanuts	Cashews
Rice	Soy products	Other nuts
Whole-grain breads		Nut butters
Pasta		

Examples of possible meals: black beans and rice, lentil curry on rice, spilt-pea soup and rye bread, tofu dishes with sesame seed, bean chili with whole-wheat toast.

---

broken down into simple sugars before they can be utilized by the body. There are two major forms of complex carbohydrates: *starches* and *fiber,* or **cellulose.**

Starches make up the majority of the complex carbohydrate group. They are found in various grains and vegetables and provide us with the bulk of our energy needs. Starches in our diets come from whole-grain flours, breads, pasta, and related foods. They are stored in body muscles and the liver, in a polysaccharide form called **glycogen.** When the body requires a sudden burst of energy, it breaks down glycogen into glucose. Marathon runners and other people who require reserves of energy for demanding tasks attempt to increase stores of glycogen in the body by a process known as *carbohydrate loading*. This process involves dramatically increasing carbohydrate intake after several days of low carbohydrate intake.

The role of fiber in promoting nutrition and health has been the topic of a great deal of controversy in recent years. What is fiber? How effective is fiber in reducing certain health risks? Are certain types of fiber more effective than others? Recent controversies about oat bran and other sources of fiber have increased confusion. Even those health claims that seem reliable may in fact be questionable. (See the box entitled "Fiber: The Positive Side of the Dietary Battle.")

Fiber, often referred to as "bulk" or "roughage," is the indigestible portion of plant foods. Fiber aids in the movement of foods through the digestive system and softens stools by absorbing large quantities of water. *Insoluble* fiber, which is found in bran, whole-grain breads and cereals, and most fruits and vegetables, is associated with these gastrointestinal benefits and has been found to reduce the risk for several forms of cancer (see Chapter 13). *Soluble* fiber appears to be a factor in lowering blood-cholesterol levels, thereby reducing risks for cardiovascular disease.

Fats Fats (or *lipids*), another group of basic nutrients, are perhaps the most misunderstood of the body's required energy sources. Most people do not realize that fats play a vital role in the maintenance of healthy skin and hair, insulation of the body organs against shock, maintenance of body temperature, and the proper functioning of the cells themselves. Fats make our foods taste better and carry the fat-soluble vitamins A, D, E, and K to the cells. They also provide a concentrated form of energy in the absence of sufficient amounts of carbohydrates. If fats perform all these functions, why are we constantly urged to reduce our intake of these substances?

Polysaccharides Complex carbohydrates formed by combining long chains of saccharides.
Cellulose A plant polysaccharide that is indigestible by humans.
Glycogen A storage form of glucose found in liver and muscle cells.
Fats Nutrients that serve as the body's second major source of energy.

Although moderate consumption of fats is essential to health maintenance, overconsumption can be dangerous. The most common form of fat circulating in the blood is the **triglyceride,** which makes up about 95 percent of the total fat in your body. When you consume too many calories, the excess is converted into triglycerides in the liver, which are stored in the all-too-obvious places on our bodies. As Figure 6.4 shows, choosing foods in terms of their fat content can be somewhat tricky. If you are trying to "fill up" and avoid fat, for example, you're certainly better off eating a large bowl of pasta (depending on the sauce) than an ounce of cheddar cheese.

The remaining 5 percent of body fat is comprised of substances such as **cholesterol,** which can accumulate on the inner walls of arteries, causing a narrowing of the channel through which blood flows. This buildup, called **plaque,** is a major cause of atherosclerosis (hardening of the arteries). At one time, the amount of circulating cholesterol in the blood was thought to be crucial. Current thinking is that the actual amount of circulating

cholesterol itself is not as important as the ratio of total cholesterol to a group of compounds called **high-density lipoproteins (HDLs).** Lipoproteins are the transport facilitators for cholesterol in the blood. High-density lipoproteins are capable of transporting more cholesterol than are **low-density lipoproteins (LDLs).** Whereas LDLs transport cholesterol to the body's cells, HDLs apparently transport circulating cholesterol to the liver for metabolism and elimination from the body. People with a high percentage of HDLs therefore appear to be at lower risk for development of cholesterol-clogged arteries. Regular vigorous exercise plays a part in reduction of cholesterol by increasing high-density lipoproteins.

Fat cells consist of chains of carbon and hydrogen atoms. Those that are unable to hold any more hydrogen in their chemical structure are labeled as **saturated fats.** They generally come from animal sources and are solid at room temperature. **Unsaturated fats** are generally liquid at room temperature and have room for additional hydrogen atoms in their chemical structure. The terms *monosaturated fat* and *polyunsaturated fat* refer to the relative number of hydrogen atoms that are missing. Canola and olive oils are high in monounsaturated fats, whereas corn, sunflower, and safflower oils are high in polyunsaturated fats. Currently there is a great deal of controversy over which type of unsaturated fat is most beneficial. Although polyunsaturated fats were favored by nutritional researchers in the early 1980s, today many researchers prefer monounsaturated fats. For a breakdown of the types of fat found in common vegetable oils and animal-fat products, see Figure 6.5.

Both cholesterol and saturated fats in our diet can contribute to cardiovascular disease. For more information on cholesterol and cardiovascular disease, see Chapter 13. Some foods that are high in cholesterol may be relatively low in saturated fats (shrimp, for example). It is therefore important to consider both components when choosing healthy foods (see the box entitled "The Cholesterol/Saturated-Fat Index."

Figure 6.4 Not all fat is created equal. Each of the foods shown here contains 10 grams of fat.
1.1 OUNCE OF CHEDDAR CHEESE
7 HERSHEY'S KISSES
1.19 TABLESPOONS OF PEANUT BUTTER
14.3 CUPS OF SPAGHETTI

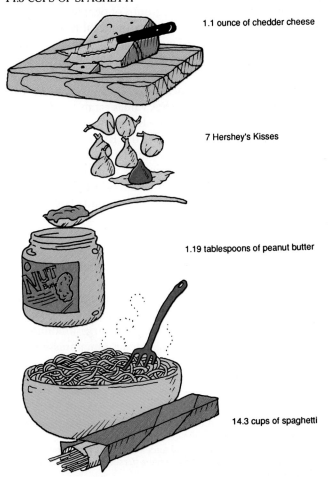

1.1 ounce of chedder cheese

7 Hershey's Kisses

1.19 tablespoons of peanut butter

14.3 cups of spaghetti

Triglyceride   The most commonly occurring fatty substance within the blood.

Cholesterol   A fatty substance manufactured by the body and found in animal fats; associated with risk of cardiovascular disease.

Plaque   A combination of cholesterol, calcium and other minerals that accumulates on the walls of blood vessels, obstructing blood flow.

High-density Lipoproteins (HDLs)   Compounds consisting of a protein and a lipid that carry cholesterol to the liver for breakdown and excretion.

Low-density Lipoproteins (LDLs)   Compounds consisting of a protein and a lipid that carry cholesterol to body cells.

Saturated Fats   Fats derived from animal sources; they are chains of carbon and hydrogen atoms that are unable to hold any more hydrogen atoms.

Unsaturated Fats   Fats derived primarily from nonanimal sources. They are liquid at room temperature and can absorb additional hydrogen atoms.

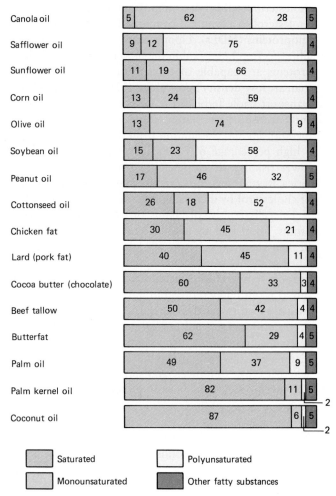

Canola oil	5	62	28	5
Safflower oil	9	12	75	4
Sunflower oil	11	19	66	4
Corn oil	13	24	59	4
Olive oil	13	74	9	4
Soybean oil	15	23	58	4
Peanut oil	17	46	32	5
Cottonseed oil	26	18	52	4
Chicken fat	30	45	21	4
Lard (pork fat)	40	45	11	4
Cocoa butter (chocolate)	60	33	3	4
Beef tallow	50	42	4	4
Butterfat	62	29	4	5
Palm oil	49	37	9	5
Palm kernel oil	82	11	5	2
Coconut oil	87	6	5	2

Legend:
- ▨ Saturated
- ☐ Polyunsaturated
- ▨ Monounsaturated
- ▨ Other fatty substances

Figure 6.5 Percentage of saturated, polyunsaturated, and monounsaturated fats in common vegetable oils and animal-fat products.

Vitamins Vitamins are essential components of our daily diets (see Table 6.4). Although they are required only in small doses, they play a major role in meeting our everyday needs. Rather than serving as actual structural components of our bodies, vitamins work with various enzymes to help the body use other nutrients.

Vitamins are organic in nature, and age, heat, and other environmental conditions can destroy them over time. Vitamins can be classified as either *fat-soluble*, meaning that they are absorbed through the intestinal tract with the help of fats and stored in the body, or *water-soluble*, meaning they are easily dissolved in water. Vitamins A, D, E, and K are fat-soluble; B-complex vitamins and vitamin C are water-soluble. Fat-soluble vitamins tend to be stored in the body, and toxic accumulations in the liver may cause cirrhosislike symptoms to occur. Water-soluble vitamins are generally excreted and cause few toxicity problems.

In spite of all of the media attention to the contrary, few Americans suffer from true vitamin deficiencies if they eat a diet containing all of the food groups at least

part of the time. Nevertheless, Americans continue to purchase large numbers of vitamin supplements. For the most part, vitamin supplements are unnecessary and, in certain instances, may even be dangerous. Overuse of vitamin supplements can lead to a toxic condition known as **hypervitaminosis**. How much of each vitamin is necessary? Although many countries have developed standards for vitamin requirements, United States standards, set by the National Research Council and the National Academy of Sciences, also include other nutrients, such as protein and minerals. Known as **recommended dietary allowances (RDAs)**, these flexible guidelines propose a wide range of recommended nutrient levels for 17 population groups based on age and gender. These recommendations establish an average level of nutrition. They also include a substantial safety margin, so that consuming two-thirds of the RDA is often enough for the majority of healthy people. Individual nutrition requirements may vary depending on age, gender, size, state of health, activity level, and environment.

Many people confuse the RDA with the U.S. RDA, the U.S. Recommended *Daily* Allowance. The U.S. RDAs are guidelines established by the Food and Drug Administration and found on nutritional labeling (see the box entitled "Differences between Old and New FDA Food-Label Requirements"). The U.S. RDAs provide the daily amounts of nutrients needed by adults and children age 4 and older. Although there are actually four different sets of U.S. RDAs for different groups of people, the one that is commonly listed on your box of cereal is for a typical adult male. This may be misleading for women, children, the elderly, and other groups who have different nutritional needs.

Currently, the U.S. RDA recommendations on food labels are still based on RDA values established in 1968, even though the National Research Council (NRC) agreed to several revisions to the RDA in 1989. These changes included increasing the RDA for calcium from 800 to 1,200 milligrams; lowering requirements for zinc, magnesium, iron, vitamin B_{12}, and folicin; and introducing RDAs for vitamin K and selenium. For the most recent RDAs, see Table 6.5.

Minerals Minerals are the inorganic, indestructible elements that aid physiological processes within the body. Without minerals, vitamins could not be absorbed. Minerals are readily excreted, do not build up in the body, and are usually not toxic. **Macrominerals** are those minerals that the body needs in fairly large amounts. Sodium, calcium, phosphorus, magnesium, potassium, sul-

---

Hypervitaminosis A toxic condition brought on by excessive vitamin consumption.
Recommended Dietary Allowances (RDAs) Guidelines for the recommended amounts of nutrients a person should consume for optimal health.

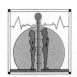

FIBER: The Positive Side of the Dietary Battle

Mixing Research with Common Sense

Although most of the dietary advice given today relates to cutting back on certain types of food and completely eliminating others from our daily menus, fiber is one of those rare substances that we seem to be able to eat more and more of.

A few years ago, oat bran was thought by some to be the remedy for just about everything that ailed the average person. Even though research has proven that much of the oat-bran hype was premature and that it probably wasn't as great for us as they originally told us, our preoccupation with fiber itself continues to be high. Current research supporting the benefits of fiber is promising, the evidence concerning its protective effects remains inconclusive. The following are among the most often cited benefits:

- **Protection against Colon and Rectal Cancer:** One of the leading causes of cancer deaths in the United States, colo-rectal cancer is much rarer in countries with diets high in fiber and low in animal fat. Several studies have supported the theory that fiber-rich diets, particularly those with *insoluble* fiber, prevent the appearance of precancerous growths. Whether this occurs because more fiber helps to move foods through the colon faster, thereby reducing its contact time with cancer-causing substances, or for some other reason remains unknown.

- **Protection against Breast Cancer:** Research into the effects of fiber on breast-cancer risks is very inconclusive. However, some studies have indicated that wheat bran (rich in insoluble fiber) reduces blood-estrogen levels, which may affect the risk of breast cancer. Another theory indicates that when people eat more fiber, their diets have less fat proportionally, thereby reducing overall risk. The jury is still very much out in this area.

- **Constipation:** Insoluble fiber, consumed with adequate fluids, is the safest, most effective way to prevent or treat constipation. The fiber acts like a sponge, absorbing moisture and producing softer, bulkier stools that are easily passed. Fiber also helps produce gas, which in turn, may initiate a bowel movement.

- **Diverticulosis:** About 1 American in 10 over the age of 40 and at least 1 in 3 over 50 suffers from diverticulosis, a condition in which tiny bulges or pouches form on the intestinal wall. These bulges become irritated and cause chronic pain. Insoluble fiber helps to reduce constipation and added pain from straining to defecate.

- **Protection against Heart Disease:** Many studies have indicated that soluble fiber (as in oat bran, barley, and fruit pectin) helps reduce blood cholesterol, primarily by lowering LDL ("bad") cholesterol. Whether this reduction is a direct effect, or occurs instead through the displacement of fat calories with fiber calories in a high-fiber diet, remains in question.

- **Diabetes:** Some studies have suggested that soluble fiber improves control of blood sugar and can reduce the need for insulin or medication in people with diabetes. Exactly why isn't clear, but soluble fiber seems to delay the emptying of the stomach and slow the absorption of glucose in the intestine.

- **Obesity:** Because most high-fiber foods are high in carbohydrates and low in fat, they help control caloric intake. Many take longer to chew, which slows you down at the table and makes you feel full sooner.

How Much Is Enough?

Although eating large amounts of fiber in a short time can result in gas, bloating, and cramps, adding fiber gradually to your diet usually causes few problems. We don't know for sure how much fiber may be needed to produce significant benefits, or if it provides these benefits at all, but it is generally assumed that a high-fiber, low-fat diet makes good sense.

Most experts believe that Americans should double their current consumption of dietary fiber—to *20–30 grams per day* for most people, and perhaps to *40–50 grams* for others. To do this, the following are recommended:

1. Eat a variety of foods.
2. Eat at least 5 servings of fruits and vegetables and 3 to 6 servings of whole-grain breads, cereals, and legumes per day.
3. The less processed the food, the better.
4. Eat the skins of fruits and vegetables.
5. Get your fiber from foods rather than pills or powders.
6. Spread out your fiber intake.
7. Drink plenty of liquids.

(continued)

FIBER: The Positive Side of the Dietary Battle *(Continued)*

Good Source of Insoluble Fiber	Good Source of Soluble Fiber
More than 5 grams total fiber	
High-fiber wheat-bran cereal (1 oz)	Pinto, kidney, navy beans (1/2 oz)
Lentils (1/2 cup)	

More than 5 grams total fiber

Good Source of Insoluble Fiber
High-fiber wheat-bran cereal (1 oz)
Lentils (1/2 cup)

Good Source of Soluble Fiber
Pinto, kidney, navy beans (1/2 oz)

2–5 grams total fiber

Whole-wheat crackers (6)
Banana (medium)
Potato (medium, with skin)
Shredded-wheat cereal (1 oz)
Brown rice (cooked, 1/2 cup)
Brussels sprouts, broccoli, spinach (cooked, 1/2 cup)
Wheat germ (3 Tbsp)
Whole-wheat flour (1 oz)

Oat bran, oatmeal (1 oz)
Barley (1 oz)
Berries (1/2 cup)
Apple, pear (with skin)
Orange, grapefruit (medium)
Figs, prunes, dates (3)
Okra, cabbage, peas, sweet potato (1/2 cup)
Chickpeas, split peas, lima beans (1/2 cup)

1–2 grams total fiber

Whole-wheat bread (1 slice)
Pasta (1 cup)
Rye bread (1 slice)
Corn (1/2 cup
Cauliflower (1/2 cup)

Carrots (1/2 cup)
Peach, nectarine (medium)

Apricots (2)

Adapted from *University of California at Berkeley Wellness Letter,* 8, no. 7 (April 1992), pp. 4–6.

Table 6.4   Vitamins: Where You Get Them and What They Do

Vitamin	Best Sources	Main Roles	Deficiency Symptoms	Risks of Megadoses
Fat Soluble				
A	Liver; eggs; cheese; butter; fortified margarine and milk; yellow; orange, and dark-green vegetables and fruits (e.g., carrots, broccoli, spinach, cantaloupe).	Assists in the formation and maintenance of healthy skin, hair, and mucous membranes; aids in the ability to see in dim light (night vision); needed for proper bone growth, teeth development, and reproduction.	Night blindness; rough skin and mucous membranes; infection of mucous membranes; drying of the eyes; impaired growth of bones and tooth enamel.	Blurred vision, loss of appetite, headaches, skin rashes, nausea, diarrhea, hair loss, menstrual irregularities, extreme fatigue, joint pain, liver damage, insomnia, abnormal bone growth, injury to brain and nervous system.
D	Fortified milk; egg yolk; liver; tuna; salmon; cod-liver oil. Made on skin in sunlight	Aids in the formation and maintenance of bones and teeth; assists in the absorption and use of calcium and phosphorus.	In children, rickets; stunted bone growth, bowed legs, malformed teeth, protruding abdomen. In adults, osteomalacia; softening of the bones leading to shortening and fractures, muscle spasms, and twitching.	In infants, calcium deposits in kidneys and excessive calcium in blood; in adults, calcium deposits throughout body, deafness, nausea, loss of appetite, kidney stones, fragile bones, high blood pressure, high blood cholesterol.

	Important Sources	Major Physiological Roles	Results of Deficiency	Results of Excess
E	Vegetable oils; margarine; wheat germ; whole-grain cereals and bread; liver; dried beans; green leafy vegetables.	Aids in the formation of red blood cells, muscles, and other tissues; protects vitamin A and essential fatty acids from oxidation.	Prolonged impairment of fat absorption.	None definitely known. Reports of headache, blurred vision, extreme fatigue, muscle weakness. Can destroy some vitamin K made in the gut.
K	Green leafy vegetables; cabbage; cauliflower; peas; potatoes; liver; cereals. Except in newborns, made by bacteria in human intestine.	Aids in the synthesis of substances needed for the blood to clot; helps maintain normal bone metabolism.	Hemorrhage, especially in newborn infants.	Jaundice in babies; anemia in laboratory animals.
Water Soluble **Thiamin** (B$_1$)	Pork (especially ham); liver; oysters; whole-grain and enriched cereals, pasta, and bread; wheat germ; oatmeal; peas; lima beans.	Helps release energy from carbohydrates; aids in the synthesis of an important nervous-system chemical.	Beriberi: mental confusion, muscular weakness, swelling of the heart, leg cramps.	None known. However, since B vitamins are interdependent, excess of one may produce deficiency of others.
Riboflavin (B$_2$)	Liver; milk; meat; dark-green vegetables; eggs; whole-grain and enriched cereals, pasta, and bread; dried beans and peas.	Helps release energy from carbohydrates, proteins, and fats; aids in the maintenance of mucous membranes.	Skin disorders, especially around nose and lips; cracks at corners of mouth; sensitivity of eyes to light.	None known. See Thiamin.
Niacin (B$_3$, Nicotinamide, Nicotinic acid)	Liver; poultry; meat; fish; eggs; whole-grain and enriched cereals, pasta, and bread; nuts; dried peas and beans.	Participates with thiamin and riboflavin in facilitating energy production in cells.	Pellagra: skin disorders, diarrhea, mental confusion, irritability, mouth swelling, smooth tongue.	Duodenal ulcer, abnormal liver function, elevated blood sugar, excessive uric acid in blood, possibly leading to gout. See Thiamin.
B$_6$ (Pyridoxine)	Whole-grain (but not enriched) cereals and bread; liver; avocados; spinach; green beans; bananas; fish; poultry meats; nuts; potatoes; green leafy vegetables.	Aids in the absorption and metabolism of proteins; helps the body use fats; assists in the formation of red blood cells.	Skin disorders; cracks at corners of mouth; smooth tongue; convulsions; dizziness; nausea; anemia; kidney stones.	Dependency on high dose, leading to deficiency symptoms when one returns to normal amounts.
B$_{12}$ (Cobalamin)	Only in animal foods; liver; kidneys; meat; fish; eggs; milk; oysters; nutritional yeast.	Aids in the formation of red blood cells; assists in the building of genetic material; helps the functioning of the nervous system.	Pernicious anemia; anemia, pale skin and mucuous membranes, numbness and tingling in fingers and toes that may progress to loss of balance and weakness and pain in arms and legs.	None known. See Thiamin.
Folacin (Folic acid)	Liver; kidneys; dark-green leafy vegetables; wheat germ; dried beans and peas. Stored in the body, so daily consumption is not crucial.	Acts with B$_{12}$ in synthesizing genetic material; aids in the formation of hemoglobin in red blood cells.	Megaloblastic anemia; enlarged red blood cells, smooth tongue, diarrhea; during pregnancy, deficiency may cause loss of the fetus or fetal abnormalities. Women on oral contraceptives may need extra folacin.	Body stores it, so it is potentially hazardous. Can mask a B$_{12}$ deficiency. Diarrhea, insomnia.

continued

Table 6.4   Vitamins: Where You Get Them and What They Do *(Continued)*

Vitamin	Best Sources	Main Roles	Deficiency Symptoms	Risks of Megadoses
C (Ascorbic acid)	Citrus fruits; tomatoes; strawberries, melon; green peppers; potatoes; dark-green vegetables.	Aids in the formation of collagen; helps maintain capillaries, bones, and teeth; helps protect other vitamins from oxidation; may block formation of cancer-causing nitrosamines.	Scurvy: bleeding gums, degenerating muscles, wounds that don't heal, loose teeth, brown, dry, rough skin. Early symptoms include loss of appetite, irritability, weight loss.	Dependency on high doses, possibly precipitating symptoms of scurvy when withdrawn (especially in infants if megadoses taken during pregnancy); kidney and bladder stones; diarrhea; urinary-tract irritation; increased tendency for blood to clot; breakdown of red blood cells in persons with certain common genetic disorders.

SOURCE: Adapted from *Jane Brody's Nutrition Book* (New York: Bantam, 1982), pp. 159–64.

fur, and chloride are included in this group. **Trace minerals** include iron, zinc, manganese, copper, iodine, and cobalt. Although only trace amounts of these minerals are needed, serious problems may result if excesses or deficiencies occur. Specific types of minerals are listed in Table 6.6.

Although minerals are necessary for body function, limits exist in the amounts of each that we should consume. There are certain minerals that Americans tend to overuse or underuse.

SODIUM   The average American consumes between 6,000 and 12,000 milligrams of sodium per day. Some of this is consumed as table salt, but much of it is found in such diverse products as soups, frozen foods, lunch meats, fast foods, salted snacks, and condiments. Although sodium is necessary for the regulation of blood and body fluids, the successful transmission of nerve impulses, heart activity, and certain metabolic functions, the average American consumes 30 times more sodium than the body requires. How much sodium should the average person consume? The National Research Council recommends a limit of 2,400 milligrams of sodium per day as adequate for proper body functioning in adults. This amount is the equivalent of perhaps one-tenth of a teaspoon of salt (sodium chloride), well under the amount we actually consume. Why all the fuss about the extra consumption? Many experts believe that a link exists between excessive sodium intake and hypertension (high blood pressure). However, this theory is controversial. Although a great deal must still be determined about the effects of sodium in the body, many organizations, including the American Heart Association, have recom-

mended sodium reduction as an aid in reducing risk for cardiovascular disorders.

CALCIUM   As will be discussed in Chapter 14, the issue of calcium consumption has gained national attention with the rising incidence of *osteoporosis* among elderly women. Although calcium plays a vital role in building strong bones and teeth as well as in blood clotting, nerve-impulse transmission, heart activity, and fluid balance within cells, most Americans do not consume the 1,200 milligrams of calcium per day established by the RDA.

IRON   Iron is a problem mineral for millions of people. Although it is found in every cell of all living things, many humans have difficulty getting enough iron in their daily diets. Iron deficiencies can lead to **anemia,** a problem resulting in the body's inability to produce hemoglobin, the bright-red oxygen-carrying component of the blood. Generally, women are the most likely to suffer from iron-deficiency problems. Because women typically eat less than men, their diets may contain less iron. Also, because blood loss is the major reason for iron depletion, women with heavy menstrual flow may be more prone toward iron loss. Blood donors and pregnant women need to increase their iron intake. A less common problem, iron toxicity, is caused by too much iron in the blood.

Food Groups and the "Eating Right Pyramid"

For many people, obtaining the right amounts of nutrients is not a serious problem. Most Americans have

Anemia   A condition resulting from iron deficiency, lack of hemoglobin in the blood, and depleted oxygen suppliers.

Table 6.5   Recommended Dietary Allowances (Revised 1989)*

Age (years) & gender	Reference Weight (kg)	Reference Weight (lbs)	Reference Height (cm)	Reference Height (in)	Protein (g)	Vitamin A (RE)	Thiamin (mg)	Riboflavin (mg)	Niacin (NE)	Vitamin B6 (mg)	Folacin (µg)	Vitamin B12 (µg)	Vitamin C (mg)	Vitamin D (µg)	Vitamin E (αTE)	Vitamin K (µg)	Calcium (mg)	Iodine (µg)	Iron (mg)	Magnesium (mg)	Phosphorus (mg)	Selenium (µg)	Zinc (mg)
Infants																							
0.0–0.5	6	13	60	24	13	375	0.3	0.4	5	0.3	25	0.3	30	7.5	3	5	400	40	6	40	300	10	5
0.5–1.0	9	20	71	28	14	375	0.4	0.5	6	0.6	35	0.5	35	10	4	10	600	50	10	60	500	15	5
Children																							
1–3	13	29	90	35	16	400	0.7	0.8	9	1.0	50	0.7	40	10	6	15	800	70	10	80	800	20	10
4–6	20	44	112	44	24	500	0.9	1.1	12	1.1	75	1.0	45	10	7	20	800	90	10	120	800	20	10
7–10	28	62	132	52	28	700	1.0	1.2	13	1.4	100	1.4	45	10	7	30	800	120	10	170	800	30	10
Males																							
11–14	45	99	157	62	45	1000	1.3	1.5	17	1.7	150	2.0	50	10	10	45	1200	150	12	270	1200	40	15
15–18	66	145	176	69	59	1000	1.5	1.8	20	2.0	200	2.0	60	10	10	65	1200	150	12	400	1200	50	15
19–24	72	160	177	70	58	1000	1.5	1.7	19	2.0	200	2.0	60	10	10	70	1200	150	10	350	1200	70	15
25–50	79	174	176	70	63	1000	1.5	1.7	19	2.0	200	2.0	60	5	10	80	800	150	10	350	800	70	15
51+	77	170	173	68	63	1000	1.2	1.4	15	2.0	200	2.0	60	5	10	80	800	150	10	350	800	70	15
Females																							
11–14	46	101	157	62	46	800	1.1	1.3	15	1.4	150	2.0	50	10	8	45	1200	150	15	280	1200	45	12
15–18	55	120	163	64	44	800	1.1	1.3	15	1.5	180	2.0	60	10	8	55	1200	150	15	300	1200	50	12
19–24	58	128	164	65	46	800	1.1	1.3	15	1.6	180	2.0	60	10	8	60	1200	150	15	280	1200	55	12
25–50	63	138	163	64	50	800	1.1	1.3	15	1.6	180	2.0	60	5	8	65	800	150	15	280	800	55	12
51+	65	143	160	63	50	800	1.0	1.2	13	1.6	180	2.0	60	5	8	65	800	150	10	280	800	55	12
Pregnant					60	800	1.5	1.6	17	2.2	400	2.2	70	10	10	65	1200	175	30	320	1200	65	15
Lactating																							
1st 6 mo.					65	1300	1.6	1.8	20	2.1	280	2.6	95	10	12	65	1200	200	15	355	1200	75	19
2nd 6 mo.					62	1200	1.6	1.7	20	2.1	260	2.6	90	10	11	65	1200	200	15	340	1200	75	16

* National Academy of Sciences, *Recommended Dietary Allowances*, 10th rev. ed. (Washington, D.C.: National Academy Press, 1989).

Definitions:

mcg or µg = micrograms; 1000 mcg = 1 mg; 1000 mg = 1 gram. Thiamin = Vit B₁; Riboflavin = Vit B₂; Niacin = Vit B₁.
RE (Retinol equivalents) = 1 µg Vitamin A from animal sources, or 6 µg of Vitamin A from β-carotene (plant sources).
Vitamin D: 10 µg of Vitamin D (as cholecalciferol) = 400 IU (International Units). IUs are an older measure.
Vitamin E: 1 mg of d-α tocopherol = 1 α-TE (TE = tocopherol equivalent).
Niacin (Vitamin B₃); NE (niacin equivalent) is 1 mg of niacin or 60 mg of dietary tryptophan. Also referred to as mg-NE.

SOURCE: ESHA Research, Salem, Ore.

Table 6.6 Minerals: Where You Get Them and What They Do

Best Sources	Main Roles	Deficiency Symptoms	Risks of Megadoses
Macrominerals			
Calcium			
Milk and milk products; sardines; canned salmon eaten with bones; dark-green, leafy vegetables; citrus fruits; dried beans and peas.	Building bones and teeth and maintaining bone strength; muscle contraction; maintaining cell membranes; blood clotting; absorption of B_{12}; activation of enzymes.	In children: distorted bone growth (rickets). In adults: loss of bone (osteoporosis) and increased susceptibility to fractures.	Drowsiness; extreme lethargy; impaired absorption of iron, zinc, and manganese; calcium deposits in tissues throughout body, mimicking cancer on X-ray.
Phosphorus			
Meat; poultry; fish; eggs; dried beans and peas; milk and milk products; phosphates in processed foods, especially soft drinks.	Building bones and teeth; release of energy from carbohydrates, proteins, and fats; formation of genetic material, cell membranes, and many enzymes.	Weakness, loss of appetite, malaise, bone pain. Dietary shortages uncommon, but prolonged use of antacids can cause deficiency.	Distortion of calcium-to-phosphorus ratio, creating relative deficiency of calcium.
Magnesium			
Leafy, green vegetables (eaten raw); nuts (especially almonds and cashews); soybeans, seeds; whole grains.	Building bones; manufacture of proteins; release of energy from muscle glycogen; conduction of nerve impulse to muscles; adjustment to cold.	Muscular twitching and tremors; irregular heartbeat; insomnia; muscle weakness; leg and foot cramps; shaky hands.	Disturbed nervous-system function because the calcium-to-magnesium ratio is unbalanced; catharsis; hazard to persons with poor kidney function.
Potassium			
Orange juice; bananas; dried fruits; meats; bran; peanut butter; dried beans and peas; potatoes; coffee; tea; cocoa.	Muscle contraction; maintenance of fluid and electrolyte balance in cells; transmission of nerve impulses; release of energy from carbohydrates, proteins, and fats.	Abnormal heart rhythm; muscular weakness; lethargy; kidney and lung failure.	Excessive potassium in blood, causing muscular paralysis and abnormal heart rhythms.
Sulfur			
Beef; wheat germ; dried beans and peas; peanuts; clams.	In every cell as part of sulfur-containing amino acids; forms bridges between molecules to create firm proteins of hair, nails, and skin.	None known in humans.	Unknown.
Chlorine			
Table salt and other naturally occurring salts.	Regulation of balance of body fluids and acids and bases; activation of enzyme in saliva; part of stomach acid.	Disturbed acid-base balance in body fluids (very rare).	Disturbed acid-base balance.

Adapted from *Jane Brody's Nutrition Book* (New York: Bantam, 1982), pp. 184–88.

grown up with the basic nutritional idea of the 4 food groups, which was first published in 1956 and included

1. Milk and milk products
2. Meat and meat alternatives
3. Fruits and vegetables
4. Breads, cereals, and grains

Today, many nutritionists add to this list a fifth group of foods consisting of

5. fats, sweets, and alcohol

Although often referred to as "junk foods," some of the foods in this last group are capable of supplying essential dietary fats. Nevertheless, you can assume that the "junk" factor will be far greater than any benefit factor in most of these foods.

In the spring of 1991, the U.S. government planned to replace the 4- (or 5-) food group plan with the "Eating Right Pyramid" in order to show people that grains,

Table 6.6 Minerals: Where You Get Them and What They Do

Best Sources	Main Roles	Deficiency Symptoms	Risks of Megadoses
Trace Minerals			
Iron			
Liver kidneys; red meats; egg yolk; green, leafy vegetables; dried fruits; dried beans and peas; potatoes; blackstrap molasses; enriched and whole-grain cereals.	Formation of hemoglobin in blood and myoglobin in muscles, which supply oxygen to cells; part of several enzymes and proteins.	Anemia, with fatigue, weakness, pallor, and shortness of breath.	Toxic buildup in liver, pancreas, and heart.
Copper			
Oysters; nuts; cocoa powder; beef and pork liver; kidneys; dried beans; corn-oil margarine.	Formation of red blood cells; part of several respiratory enzymes.	In animals: anemia; faulty development of bone and nervous tissue; loss of elasticity in tendons and major arteries; abnormal lung development; abnormal structure and pigmentation of hair.	Violent vomiting and diarrhea. Cooking acid foods in unlined copper pots can lead to toxic accumulation of copper.
Zinc			
Meat; liver; eggs; poultry; seafood; followed by milk and whole grains.	Constituent of about 100 enzymes.	Delayed wound healing; diminished taste sensation; loss of appetite. In children: failure to grow and mature sexually. Prenatally: abnormal brain development.	Nausea, vomiting; anemia; bleeding in stomach; premature birth and stillbirth; abdominal pain; fever. Can aggravate marginal copper deficiency. May produce atherosclerosis.
Iodine			
Seafood; saltwater fish; seaweed; iodized salt; sea salt.	Part of thyroid hormones; essential for normal reproduction.	Goiter (enlarged thyroid with low hormone production). Newborns: cretinism, retarded growth, protruding abdomen, swollen features.	Not known to be a problem, but could cause iodine poisoning or sensitivity reaction.
Fluorine			
Fish; tea; most animal foods; fluoridated water; foods grown with or cooked in fluoridated water.	Formation of strong, decay-resistant teeth; maintenance of bone strength.	Excessive dental decay; possibly osteoporosis.	Mottling of teeth and bones; in larger doses, a deadly poison.
Magnesium			
Nuts; whole grains; vegetables and fruits; tea; instant coffee; cocoa powder.	Functioning of central nervous system; normal bone structure; reproduction; part of important enzymes.	None known in human beings. In animals: poor reproduction; retarded growth; birth defects; abnormal bone development.	Masklike facial expression; blurred speech; involuntary laughing; spastic gait; hand tremors.

Adapted from *Jane Brody's Nutrition Book* (New York: Bantam, 1982), pp. 184–88.

fruits, and vegetables should be a more prominent part of their diets. As you can see in Figure 6.6, bread, pasta, and rice make up the broad base of the pyramid, and fruits and vegetables rank just above them. Notice that meats, poultry, and dairy foods are placed near the upper, narrower part of the pyramid, illustrating that proportionally less of these foods are needed in the diet. As of this writing, the government had not yet officially released the pyramid plan, explaining that it was not known how readily children and adults in lower-income groups would be able to understand and use the pyramid.

ALTERNATIVE NUTRITIONAL CHOICES

For aesthetic, economic, personal, cultural, or religious reasons, many people have chosen very specialized diets. Some of these alternatives provide basic nutrition and

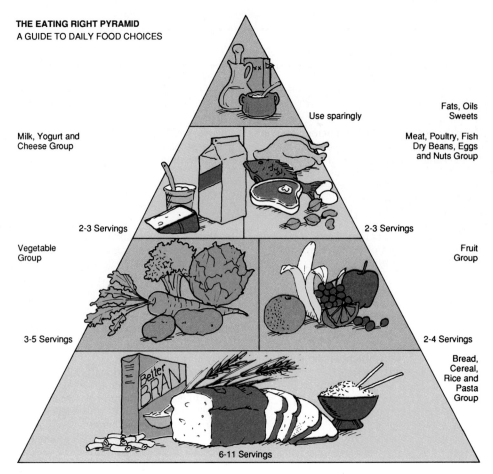

THE EATING RIGHT PYRAMID
A GUIDE TO DAILY FOOD CHOICES

Use sparingly — Fats, Oils Sweets

Milk, Yogurt and Cheese Group

Meat, Poultry, Fish Dry Beans, Eggs and Nuts Group

2-3 Servings

2-3 Servings

Vegetable Group

Fruit Group

3-5 Servings

2-4 Servings

Bread, Cereal, Rice and Pasta Group

6-11 Servings

Figure 6.6   The "Eating Right Pyramid."

assist weight control, but others can cause significant health risk.

The Vegetarian Alternative

For a variety of reasons, many Americans have elected to cut down on their meat consumption. Some people have done so to avoid what they believe to be a contaminated meat supply. Others refuse to eat other animals. Although **vegetarianism** has never been widely practiced in American culture, most other cultures include large numbers of non–meat eaters. During the past decades, vegetarians have come to be regarded in a much more positive light in our country. An emphasis on low-fat, low-calorie, low-protein, and high-fiber diet in the American lifestyle has been largely responsible for this new image. Also, a better understanding of proper nutrition makes it much less likely that today's vegetarian will suffer from dietary deficiencies.

There are three major types of vegetarian diets: vegan, lactovegetarian, and ovolactovegetarian. The *vegan* diet includes only fruits, vegetables, and grains and has the greatest risk for dietary deficiency. The *lactovegetarian* diet includes milk and milk products. The *ovolactovegetarian* diet includes all of the foregoing plus eggs. Because dairy products and eggs are eaten, these two diets are associated with less risk of protein deficiency.

Generally, people who follow a balanced vegetarian diet have lower weights, better cholesterol levels, fewer problems with regularity in bowel movements, and less risk for hypertension and certain forms of cancer and heart disease. Their food bills are also usually lower.

Along with the many benefits of the vegetarian diet come some major risks. Vegetarian diets are often deficient in vitamins, including B_{12}; minerals, including zinc and iron; and amino acids. Knowledge of both basic nutrient sources and the appropriate combinations of food groups to obtain adequate nutrition is vital. The vegetarian diet that effectively combines protein sources should prevent deficits in essential amino acids. Careful attention should be paid to getting adequate amounts of vitamin B_{12}, vitamin D, iron, calcium, and riboflavin from nonmeat sources.

Vegetarianism   The practice of not eating meat and, in some cases, eggs or dairy products.

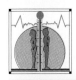

A New Way of Determining Risk

The Cholesterol/Saturated-Fat Index

Dietitian Sonia Connor and her husband, cardiologist William Connor, of the Oregon Health Sciences University in Portland, Oregon, have come up with a unique means of assessing your risk from high-fat, high-cholesterol foods. Their index, known as the *cholesterol/saturated-fat index (CSI)*, provides a numerical value for food choices that indicates how much of a good thing is really too much. In their index, they compare the amount of saturated fat in a given food with the amount of cholesterol, and effectively rate the cardiovascular risk factor. The lower the amount of saturated fat in the food and the lower the amount of cholesterol, the lower the CSI. For example, potatoes, fruits, pastas, rice, and vegetables have

CSIs of zero, for an overall healthy CSI profile. If a food is high in cholesterol but low in saturated fat, it would have an intermediate CSI value. For example, shrimp, with 182 milligrams of cholesterol but virtually no saturated fat has a CSI of 6. In contrast, lean hamburger, with approximately 95 milligrams of cholesterol and 6.3 grams of fat, would have a higher health risk and carries a CSI value of 10. When all CSIs are added together during a typical day, a healthy total CSI would be about 22 for men and 16 for women. Part of the variance relates to body size and general food-intake needs. Naturally, with greater food intake, the CSI will increase.

	Cholesterol (mg)	Saturated Fat (g)	CSI
Fish, shellfish, cooked (3.5 oz)			
Sole	50	3	4
Salmon	74	1.5	5
Shrimp, crab, lobster	182	.2	6
Poultry, no skin	84.7	1	6
Beef, pork, lamb (3.5 oz)			
15 percent fat (ground round)	94.6	6.3	10
30 percent fat (ground beef, chops)	88.6	11.4	18
Cheeses (3.5 oz)			
1–2 percent fat (low fat, cottage cheese)	7.9	1.2	1
5–10 percent (cottage cheese)	15.1	2.8	6
32–38 percent (cheddar, cream cheese)	104.7	20.9	26
Eggs			
Whites (three)	0	0	0
Whole (one)	246	2.41	15
Fats (1/4 cup, 4 tbsp., or 55 g)			
Most vegetable oils	0	7	8
Soft vegetable margarines	0	7.8	10
Stick margarines	0	8.5	15
Butter	124	28.7	37
Frozen desserts (1 serving)			
Frozen low-fat yogurt	*	*	2
Ice milk	13.6	2.4	6
Ice cream (10 percent fat)	60.6	9	13
Specialty ice cream (22 percent fat)	*	*	34

* varies according to brand.
Adapted from Sonia Connor and William Connor. *The New American Diet* (New York: Simon & Schuster, 1989).

Special precautions should be taken by pregnant women, the elderly, the sick, or those who have extra demands placed on them from exercise or work. In each of these situations, total calories, RDAs, and energy expenditure should be considered. Athletes must be careful to take in adequate amounts of nutrients to offset calorie expenditures. The elderly must be careful to consume high-quality nutrients, with caloric levels appropriate for their activity and metabolic levels. During pregnancy and lactation, the RDAs for a woman change dramatically to provide for the developing infant. Many doctors prescribe nutrient supplements for pregnant and lactating women.

Promoting Your Health

Determining How Many Grams of Fat You Can Have

Estimate how many calories you consume each day. (For a moderately active, average-size woman, that might be 1500 to 1800; for a similar man, 2000 to 2400.)

fat you can eat daily and still stay at 30 percent

_____ ÷ 9 _____

Number of calories you consume each day

Grams of fat you can eat each day

Multiply by 0.3 to get 30 percent of your maximum amount you should get from fat.

_____ × .3 _____

30 percent of your total daily calories

Divide by 9 (each gram of fat has 9 calories) for the grams of

Recommended Daily Fat Intake			
Daily Calories	Calories from Fat	Fat (grams)	Saturated Fat (grams)
1,000	300	33.3	11
1,200	360	40	13
1,500	450	50	17
1,800	540	60	20
2,000	600	66.6	22
2,500	750	83	28
3,000	900	100	33

Fast Foods: Eating On the Run

For many people, living the "good life" includes the ability to purchase convenient foods whenever time does not allow for shopping and cooking. Although some of these fast foods are inexpensive, "gourmet fast foods" have emerged in supermarkets across the country. Catering to young, upwardly mobile professionals, these microwave dinners are often expensive, high in sodium and preservatives, and lacking in many of the basic nutrients. Meanwhile, McDonald's and Burger King still appeal to millions of Americans. Are all fast foods unhealthy?

The answer to this question is "probably not." Certainly many fast foods are high in fat, proteins, and processed carbohydrates. The majority of them are also high in sodium, catering to our love for "tasty" foods. They usually are high in calories and lack complex carbohydrates. However, many fast-food chains have begun to respond to consumer demands by including salad and fruit bars, hamburgers with tomatoes and lettuce, and

broiled meats. Breadings on fried foods are often "light and crispy" rather than laden with flour and saturated with oils. Leaner cuts of meat are used, and chicken is a staple on many menus. In spite of all of these changes, the burden of responsibility continues to rest with the individual consumer. A person who cares about basic nutrition and is concerned about eating too much fat or protein can choose to purchase healthy foods from fast-food establishments.

Healthy Eating on a Student Budget

For many students, the transition from the home dinner table to the college apartment, student union, or dormitory cafeteria is an unpleasant one. Not only are meals not prepared especially for you, but there also is no one to monitor what you eat, and whether or not you eat. Of equal importance is the fact that grocery money may be limited.

Balancing the need for adequate nutrition with the many other activities that are part of college life often becomes a difficult task. Not surprisingly, for many students, it is often the nutritional part of the total picture that gets slighted. Maintaining a nutritious diet within the confines of student life is extremely difficult. Right? Wrong.

Although students do experience some problems, they can take steps to help ensure a quality diet.

- Buy fruits and vegetables in season whenever possible for lower cost, higher nutrient quality, and greater variety.
- Use coupons and specials whenever possible to get price reductions.
- Shop whenever possible at discount warehouse food chains; capitalize on volume discounts and no-frills products.
- Plan ahead to get the most for your dollar and avoid extra trips to the store; extra trips usually mean extra purchases. Make a list and stick to it.
- Purchase meats and other products in volume, freezing portions for future needs, or purchase small amounts of meats and expensive proteins and combine with beans and plant proteins for lower total cost, lower calories, and lower fat.
- Cook large meals and freeze smaller portions for later use.

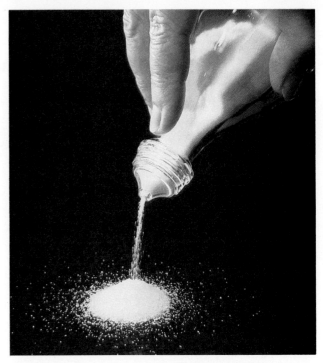

Most Americans consume too much salt, which can contribute to obesity and high blood pressure.

- Drain off extra fat after cooking. Save juices for use in soups and in other dishes.

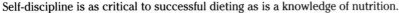

Self-discipline is as critical to successful dieting as is a knowledge of nutrition.

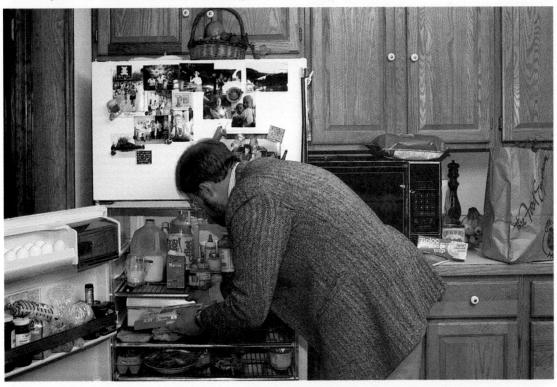

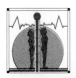

Differences between Old and New FDA Food-Label Requirements

Prompted by consumer groups and major health organizations, the Food and Drug Administration recently passed a set of new requirements for food labeling. These changes should make it simpler for Americans to follow the dietary guidelines—such as cutting down on total fat calories and cholesterol and eating more fiber—that nutritionists and health officials continually emphasize. Here are some of the major differences between the old and new food labels, based on the example of a food label for a single-serving pizza:

NUTRITION INFORMATION	
SERVING SIZE	1/4 PIZZA
SERVINGS PER CONTAINER	4
CALORIES	240
PROTEIN	9 g
CARBOHYDRATE	35 g
FAT	7 g
SODIUM	640 mg

PERCENT OF U.S. RECOMMENDED DAILY ALLOWANCES	
PROTEIN	20
VITAMIN A	15
VITAMIN C	8
THIAMINE	8
RIBOFLAVIN	10
NIACIN	10
CALCIUM	10
IRON	6

THE OLD LABEL

Nutrition labeling was previously required on packaged foods only when a claim was made about nutrient content, or when the product was fortified with vitamins, minerals, or protein. This covered 30 percent of FDA-regulated foods. Another 30 percent of foods displayed nutrition data voluntarily. *That left 40 percent of packaged foods with no nutrition data.*

When a nutrition label was used, it had to include calories, protein, carbohydrates, fat, sodium, iron, vitamins A and C, calcium, thiamine, riboflavin, and niacin. About a dozen other nutrients were listed optionally.

Serving size. Up to the manufacturer. Small sizes were often chosen to make foods seem lower in calories, fat, sodium, etc.

Labels had to list these three B vitamins, even though few Americans are deficient in them.

Ingredients lists. Most foods had to list ingredients. Exceptions were about 300 standardized foods (e.g., mayonnaise, ketchup), which didn't have to list ingredients included in their federal "standard of identity." Ingredients were listed in descending order by weight, without quantities.

Health claims. Starting in the mid-1980s, these proliferated in a legal limbo. About 40 percent of new products now bear health claims. Proposed regulations have stalled. For the most part, the FDA has not fought even the most questionable claims, leaving this to the states.

Labeling terms such as "low-fat," "high-fiber," "light," and "natural" were undefined or poorly defined.

• If you're on a student meal plan, eat at scheduled times so that you won't miss meals and have to buy fast foods at off-hours.

• If you are dissatisfied with cafeteria foods, make your complaints known in writing to the director of student services or the food-service administrator.

Be sure to include recommendations for improvements.

Eating for healthy nutrition need not be difficult. With careful attention to dietary guidelines, a bit of planning, and a lot of common sense, even low-budget, "dine-and-dash" people can promote their own health. Although

NUTRITION INFORMATION	
SERVING SIZE	1/4 PIZZA
SERVINGS PER CONTAINER	4
CALORIES	240
CALORIES FROM FAT	63
PROTEIN	9 g
CARBOHYDRATE	35 g
DIETARY FIBER	2 g
FAT	7g
SATURATED FAT	4 g
CHOLESTEROL	15 mg
SODIUM	640 mg

PERCENT OF U.S. RECOMMENDED DAILY ALLOWANCES

VITAMIN A	15
VITAMIN C	8
CALCIUM	10
IRON	6

THE NEW LABEL

Nutrition labeling is now required on nearly all foods regulated by the FDA (exceptions include spices, foods prepared in retail stores, and restaurant food). Foods regulated by the USDA, including meat and poultry, are *not* covered. Nutritional data for fresh fruits and vegetables will be described on the shelf in booklets.

Serving size. Now requires uniformity of serving size, based on a commonly consumed portion as determined by the FDA.

New data: Amount of saturated fat, fiber, and cholesterol, plus calories from fat (the percentage of calories derived from fat—26 percent for this pizza—will *not* be listed).
Optional: thiamine, riboflavin, and niacin.

Ingredients lists. Nearly all FDA-regulated products, including standardized foods, will list ingredients.

Health claims. These must be supported by "significant agreement" about scientific evidence (this may be tricky to judge). Claims are permitted in these well-established areas: fiber may reduce the risk of colon cancer and heart disease; low fat may reduce the risk of heart disease and cancer; low salt may reduce the risk of high blood pressure; calcium may help prevent osteoporosis. Model messages for claims will be developed by the U.S. Public Health Service.

Formal definitions for such labeling terms as "low-fat" and "high-fiber" will be developed.

SOURCE: *FDA Reports,* November 1991; *University of California at Berkeley Wellness Letter,* July 1990.

being a "junk-food junkie" may not appear to harm you now, your current health and dietary habits will have a major effect on your future health. Research in the field of nutrition increasingly points to the negative effects of a lifetime of poor dietary practices. Your health, now and in the future, depends a great deal on your willing-ness to accept individual responsibility and to take action *now.* Following a diet that uses the information presented in this book in a way that is most appropriate for your lifestyle will have a tremendous impact on how long and how well you live.

- Finding the right nutritional plan can be difficult because of conflicting information from a multitude of sources.

- It is important to recognize the difference between eating because of hunger versus eating due to appetite.

- Nutrition-related problems are major risk factors in a number of major diseases.

- Eating habits are a result of lifelong environmental influences and are difficult to change.

- High-calorie, high-fat, high-protein, high-sodium, high-sugar, and low-complex carbohydrate diets are contributors to many of our current health problems.

- Three major nutrients—fats, carbohydrates, and proteins—are our major sources of energy. The other three nutrients—water, vitamins, and minerals—aid in the body's use of energy.

- Water is an essential element in human survival and maintenance of bodily function.

- Proteins are the major nutrients responsible for the growth and development of tissues.

- Carbohydrates are the major energy suppliers of the body. There are several types of carbohydrates, each consisting of a different chemical makeup.

- Fats perform important functions in the body but must be consumed in moderation.

- Vitamins are either water-soluble or fat-soluble. Water-soluble vitamins (B-complex and C) are not stored by the body and must be consumed daily. Fat-soluble vitamins (A, D, E, and K) are stored and may be toxic if consumed in excess.

- Minerals perform important roles in bodily function, but toxicity may result from megadoses.

- Planning ahead, acting responsibly, and choosing wisely when purchasing and preparing foods will help ensure optimal health results.

7

Managing Your Weight: Consuming and Expending Energy

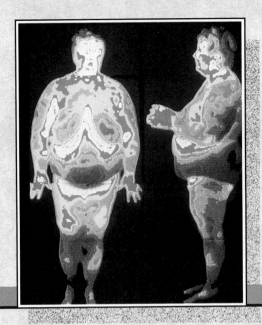

Objectives

- Using the appropriate tables, locate your "ideal" weight based on your height. Explain why this weight may not in fact be your "ideal" weight at all.

- Explain why it is important to know the difference between being overweight and being overfat.

- Describe several techniques for measuring body fat.

- Discuss the possible causes of obesity in terms of why one person may become obese and another may not.

- Explain the factors that must be considered in developing an effective weight-loss program.

Americans are preoccupied with the shapes and contours of their bodies. Television programs, movies, magazines, and the media in general project the image of the "beautiful" person. We are led to believe that if we are thin, with shapely curves or bulging muscles, we will be more desirable or more appealing to others. Spurred by this belief, the majority of Americans spend considerable time and energy battling real or imagined "ugly" bulges or "spare tires." The proliferation of health spas and diet clinics reflects our obsession with thinness.

Seemingly long gone, or at least overshadowed, are the days when dieting meant giving up desserts, eating less, and maintaining secrecy. Now there are liquid-protein diets, freeze-dried diet foods, and diets that can cost up to several thousand dollars, all of which promise fast and effective weight loss. Although many clinics and spas offer safe, scientifically sound methods for weight reduction and body firming, a significant number of weight-loss centers are run by people who lack training in either nutrition or general physiology and merely wish to capitalize on a booming market.

Just how serious is the problem with weight control in the United States today? How many of us are so overweight or underweight that we jeopardize our health?

We do know that the problem of overweight and obese people in contemporary society is extremely complex. Clearly, the ability to lose weight is related to a complex set of factors: genetic predispositions, hormonal imbalances, metabolic functioning, environmental factors, motivations, and beliefs. When hampered by misinformation and influenced by a new wave of quick-weight-loss charlatans, our efforts to lose weight often fail.

Excessive weight is a major contributor to reduced life expectancy, and it has been strongly linked to the development of coronary heart disease, diabetes, gall-bladder disease, hypertension, respiratory ailments, and certain forms of cancer. Excessive weight may also increase the risk of arthritis, low back pain, and numerous other painful conditions. Perhaps just as important are those psychological problems that the extremely overweight person may encounter. Lack of self-esteem and self-assurance are common among obese people, and discrimination against overweight people has been widely documented.

THE HEIGHT-WEIGHT "STANDARD"

The answer to the question of whether you are overweight is somewhat subjective and depends on body structure and how your weight is distributed. Traditionally, people have compared their weight with data from some form of standard height-and-weight chart. These charts usually give the "ideal" weight for a male or female of given height and frame size. If a person's weight is 15 to 20 percent above the ideal weight indicated by the chart, then that person is usually classified as obese.

Height-Weight Tables

Among the most reliable of the height-weight guides is the Metropolitan Life Height and Weight Table, which is reproduced in Table 7.1. Although the table does not indicate a relationship between weight and quality of life, total health, vitality, or appearance, it is still the most commonly used measure of our weight status.

Another formula for people between the ages of 18 and 25 establishes reasonable weights of 110 pounds for a 5-foot-tall man and 100 pounds for a 5-foot-tall woman. For each inch over 5 feet, men and women should add 5 pounds. In addition, a woman should subtract 1 pound for each year under 25.

In recent years, diagnosticians have revised their definition of obesity. Although body weight is certainly an important factor, weight alone does not indicate obesity. The real indicator is how much *fat* your body contains (see Figure 7.1). A male weight lifter may exceed all of the weight charts because of the heaviness and relative density of his muscle tissue. He might be 30 to 40 percent overweight according to the charts and yet still not be obese. Similarly, a 40-year-old woman who prides herself on weighing the same 130 pounds that she did in high school may be shocked to learn that her body now contains over 40 percent fat as compared to 15 percent fat in her high-school days. Weight by itself, although a useful guide, is not a valid indication of obesity.

OVERWEIGHT VERSUS OVERFAT: OBESITY REDEFINED

A more accurate assessment of total body fat requires a different type of measurement. If traditional height-weight charts do not accurately define obesity, what general guidelines should be applied for determining acceptable levels of body fat? **Obesity** is generally defined as an accumulation of fat beyond what is considered normal for a person's age, sex, and body type. The real difficulty lies in defining what is "normal." To date, there are no universally accepted standards for the most "desirable" or "ideal" body weight or *body composition* (ratio of lean body mass to fat body mass). Body composition will be discussed in more detail later in the chapter.

Most researchers agree that men's bodies should contain between 11 and 15 percent total body fat and women should be within the range of 18 to 22 percent

Obesity A weight disorder generally defined as an accumulation of fat beyond that considered desirable for a person's age, sex, and body type.

Table 7.1   Ideal Weights Based on Body Frame

Weights at ages 25 to 29 based on lowest mortality. Weights in pounds according to frame, in indoor clothing weighing 5 pounds for men or 3 pounds for women, shoes with 1-inch heels.

Men					Women				
Height		Small Frame	Medium Frame	Large Frame	Height		Small Frame	Medium Frame	Large Frame
Feet	Inches				Feet	Inches			
5	2	128–134	131–141	138–150	4	10	102–111	109–121	118–131
5	3	130–136	133–143	140–153	4	11	103–113	111–123	120–134
5	4	132–138	135–145	142–156	5	0	104–115	113–126	122–137
5	5	134–140	137–148	144–160	5	1	106–118	115–129	125–140
5	6	136–142	139–151	146–164	5	2	108–121	118–132	128–143
5	7	138–145	142–154	149–168	5	3	111–124	121–135	131–147
5	8	140–148	145–157	152–172	5	4	114–127	124–138	134–151
5	9	142–151	148–160	155–176	5	5	117–130	127–141	137–155
5	10	144–154	151–163	158–180	5	6	120–133	130–144	140–159
5	11	146–157	154–166	161–184	5	7	123–136	133–147	143–163
6	0	149–160	157–170	164–188	5	8	126–139	136–150	146–167
6	1	152–164	160–174	168–192	5	9	129–142	139–153	149–170
6	2	155–168	164–178	172–197	5	10	132–145	142–156	152–173
6	3	158–172	167–182	176–202	5	11	135–148	145–159	155–176
6	4	162–176	171–187	181–207	6	0	138–151	148–162	158–179

Reproduced with permission of Metropolitan Life Insurance Company. Source of basic data: *1983 Build Study,* Society of Actuaries and Association of Life Insurance Medical Directors of America, 1984.

body fat. A man would be considered obese if his body fat exceeded 20 percent of his total body mass. A woman would be considered obese if her body fat exceeded 30 percent of her total body mass. Table 7.2 provides general guidelines for determining how adults aged 18 to 30 compare in terms of overall percentages of body fat. Why the difference between men and women? Much of it may

be attributed to the actual structure of the female body, and to sex hormones. As mentioned earlier, when considering issues of how much or how little fat a person should have, it is important to think of body composition in terms of *lean body mass* and *body fat.* Lean body mass is made up of the structural and functional elements in cells, body water, muscle, bones, and other body organs such as the heart, liver, and kidneys. Body fat is composed of two types: essential fat and storage fat. *Essential fat* is necessary for normal physiological functioning, such as nerve conduction. Essential fat composes ap-

Figure 7.1   Comparisons of an average-weight person and an overweight person. Note the fat deposits under the skin and around the internal organs.

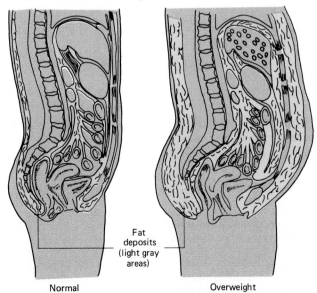

Fat deposits (light gray areas)

Normal   Overweight

Table 7.2   General Ratings of Body Fat Percentages by Age and Gender

Rating	Males (ages 18 to 30) (percent)	Females (ages 18 to 30) (percent)
Athletic*	6–10	10–15
Good	11–14	16–19
Acceptable	15–17	20–24
Overfat	18–19	25–29
Obese	20 or over	30 or over

* The ratings under the athletic category are general guidelines for those athletes, such as gymnasts and long-distance runners, whose need for a "competitive edge" in selected sports may compel them to try to lose as much weight as possible. However, it should be noted that for the average person, such low body-fat levels should be approached with caution.

proximately 3 to 7 percent of total body weight in men and approximately 15 percent of total body weight in women. *Storage fat,* the part that many of us are always trying to shed, makes up the remainder of our fat reserves. It accounts for only a small percentage of total body weight for very lean people and makes up between 5 and 25 percent of the body weight of most American adults. Female bodybuilders, who are often among the leanest of female athletes, may have body-fat percentages ranging from 8 to 13 percent, nearly all of which is essential fat.

Although most of us continually try to reduce body fat, there are levels of body fat below which we dare not go. A minimal amount of body fat is necessary for insulation of the body, for cushioning between parts of the body and vital organs, and for maintaining body functions. In men, this lower limit is approximately 3 to 4 percent. Women should generally not go below 8 percent. Excessively low body fat in females may lead to amenorrhea, a disruption of the normal menstrual cycle. The critical level of body fat necessary to maintain normal menstrual flow is believed to be between 8 and 13 percent, but there are numerous exceptions to this rule and many additional factors that affect the menstrual cycle. Under extreme circumstances, the body often utilizes all available fat reserves and begins to break down muscle tissue as a last-ditch effort to provide nourishment. **Anorexia nervosa, bulimia,** starvation diets, and

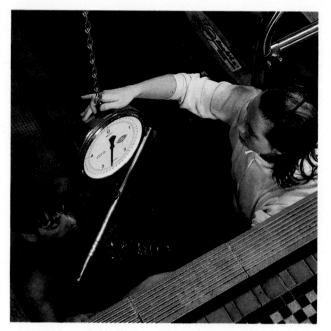

Hydrostatic weighing is the most accurate means of determining percentage of body fat.

certain disease states are some of the conditions that cause the body to behave this way (see the box entitled "Anorexia Nervosa and Bulimia").

Some of us like to say that we are storing up fat to protect ourselves from the great food shortages of the future, but there are certainly limits to the plausibility of this argument! The fact is that too much fat and too little fat are both potentially harmful. The key is for each person to find the right balance. That balance includes achieving a level at which we are comfortable with our appearance and aware of the dangers of excessive fluctuations in our weight (see the box entitled "Weight in Your Mind and Your Body").

TECHNIQUES FOR ASSESSING BODY FAT

Hydrostatic Weighing Techniques

From a clinical perspective, the most accurate method of measuring body fat is through **hydrostatic weighing techniques.** This method measures the amount of water a person displaces when completely submerged. Because fat tissue has a lower density than muscle or bone tissue,

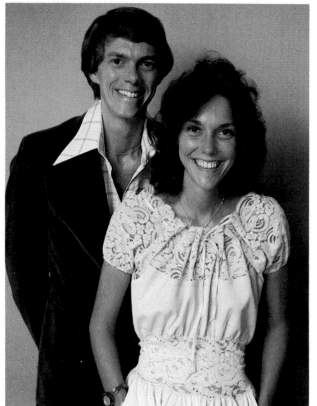

Anorexia nervosa is a psychological disorder related to social pressure to be thin.

Anorexia Nervosa An eating disorder characterized by a severe, self-imposed limitation of food intake.

Bulimia An eating disorder characterized by alternate starvation and binging.

Hydrostatic Weighing Techniques A method of determining body fat by measuring the amount of water displaced when a person is completely submerged.

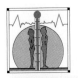

An Obsession with Thinness

Anorexia Nervosa and Bulimia

In recent years, *anorexia nervosa,* an eating disorder characterized by an almost psychotic pursuit of thinness, has emerged as a major health risk for American teenagers. According to recent research, approximately one of every 200 females between the ages of 12 and 18 will become anorexic in any given year. What is anorexia? Who is at risk for this disorder? Can it be prevented? Is treatment available?

A typical anorexic is a young woman raised in a middle-class home where both parents work. Most anorexics suffer from a poor self-image and an overwhelming desire to please others. Many have overprotective mothers, who constantly push them toward perfection, and workaholic fathers, who seldom intervene in family problems. As a result, anorexics often exhibit a compulsive desire for perfection and view their bodies as imperfect, if not grotesque. Although they are already underweight, anorexics are obsessed with losing weight and pursue extreme dietary and exercise habits.

True anorexics resemble skeletons, with few of the curves and soft lines typical of average-weight females. Often, their skin begins to dry and crack, resulting in skin eruptions and infections. In some instances, loss of skin color and hair may cause the victim to look pale. As the condition progresses, there may be a gradual lowering of body temperature, increasing pulse, a bluish tinge around the nails and lips, and eventual cessation of the menstrual cycle (amenorrhea). The final stages of untreated anorexia are not pleasant to witness. The victim may become comatose and assume a fetal position in which muscle twitching and contractions are common. In some cases, the victim's body will attempt to protect itself by growing a furry covering of thick hair to prevent heat loss. Neurological and physiological processes cease. Bowel control, bladder control, and eyesight fail. The final stage is death.

Although anorexia means "lack of appetite," this condition does not develop until late in the starvation process. Victims may be aware of hunger but refuse to eat because of their obsession with fatness. Some take appetite suppressants, laxatives, and diuretics to avoid weight gain. Others exercise to exhaustion and refuse any form of nourishment.

In extreme cases of anorexia, the long-term prognosis for recovery is only approximately 40 percent, even with family and medical assistance. Early diagnosis and strong family support can improve these chances. Many victims experience a cycle of partial recovery followed by reversion to old habits. Untreated anorexics can die of their affliction.

Closely related to anorexia is *bulimia* (often called *bulimia nervosa* or *dietary chaos syndrome*), a disease characterized by uncontrollable cycles of binge eating followed by purging through forced vomiting or the use of laxatives or diuretics. Although bulimia does occur independently of anorexia, between 30 and 50 percent of all anorexics are also bulimic. Bulimics and anorexics come from similar backgrounds and exhibit the same overwhelming need for approval. Unlike anorexia, bulimia is seldom life-threatening, although it is serious enough to merit attention.

Anorexia and bulimia are very difficult to treat. Obviously, anorexics and bulimics need professional help and substantial support from family and friends. Until we come to grips with the societal institutions and patterns of thinking that cause people to become obsessed with the concept of "thinness" in the first place, these disorders will continue to flourish.

---

a relatively accurate indication of actual body fat can be computed by comparing a person's underwater and out-of-water weights. Although this method represents one of the most sophisticated techniques currently available, the equipment is too expensive or inaccessible for most people. In addition, the equipment must be operated by carefully trained technicians to ensure accurate and reliable results.

The Pinch and Skin-Fold Measures

Perhaps the most commonly used method of body fat determination is the **pinch test.** Numerous studies have determined that the triceps area (located in the back of

Pinch Test A method of determining body fat whereby a fold of skin is pinched between the thumb and the index finger to determine the relative amount of fat.

Promoting Your Health

Weight in Your Mind and Your Body

For many people, being overweight can be both emotionally destructive and physiologically damaging. All too often the damage is measured in terms of cardiovascular risk and strain on body parts alone. What is often glossed over is the fact that our perceptions of the world and the people in it may become distorted when viewed through a damaged ego and feelings of guilt and inadequacy.

Although some overweight people manage to adapt very well in a world where a lean body is in vogue, others may have serious problems. Assessing relative psychological comfort and physiological discomfort will give you an idea of how much of a problem your weight is for you and of the importance of prompt action. Take the test below to see how you score.

Psychological Comfort

1. When people look at me, the first thing that they think is that I am overweight.

almost never	*seldom*	*sometimes*	*usually*	*almost always*
4	3	2	1	0

2. I tend to wear large blousy shirts and tops to cover fat rolls.

4	3	2	1	0

3. I find it difficult to find clothes that I like in my size.

4	3	2	1	0

4. I have a hard time finding someone to care about me because all they see is my weight rather than the real me.

4	3	2	1	0

5. I have been passed over for a position I wanted because of my weight.

4	3	2	1	0

6. I tend to use the word *fat* to describe myself.

4	3	2	1	0

7. I worry about getting undressed in front of friends because I don't want them to see how fat I am.

4	3	2	1	0

8. The thing that I am most unhappy about in my life is my weight.

4	3	2	1	0

the upper arm) is one of the most reliable areas of the body for assessing the amount of fat in the *subcutaneous layer* (just under the surface) of the skin. In making this assessment, a person pinches a fold of skin just behind the triceps with the thumb and index finger. It is important to pinch only the fat layer and not the triceps muscle. After selecting a spot for measure, the person assesses the distance between the thumb and index finger. If the size of the pinch appears to be thicker than 1 inch, the person is generally considered overfat.

Another technique, the **skin-fold caliper test**, resembles the pinch test but is much more accurate. In this procedure, the skin between the thumb and index finger is also pinched at various points on the body. However, rather than just making a generalized statement about obesity if the pinch is thicker than 1 inch, this technique uses a specially calibrated instrument called a *skin-fold*

caliper to take a more precise measurement of the fat layer. Besides the triceps area, the points most often used in these measurements are the biceps area (front of the arm), the subscapular area (upper back), and the iliac crest (hip). Once these data points are assessed, special formulas are employed to arrive at a combined prediction of total body fat. In the hands of trained technicians, this procedure can be fairly accurate. However, the heavier a person is, the more prone this technique is to error. For chronically obese people, the difficulties in assessment are magnified because of problems with distinguishing between flaccid muscles and fat. Also, most currently available calipers do not expand far enough to

Skin-Fold Caliper Test A method of determining body fat whereby calipers are used to measure a fold of skin and fat grasped between thumb and index finger.

Promoting Your Health (*Continued*)

Physiological Discomfort

1. I often tire easily after minimal physical exertion.

almost never	*seldom*	*sometimes*	*usually*	*almost always*
4	3	2	1	0

2. I avoid joining many of my friends' activities because I know that I cannot keep up.

4	3	2	1	0

3. My legs, knees, and ankles ache because they have to carry so much weight around.

4	3	2	1	0

4. I am uncomfortable in my clothes because they pinch, rub, and sometimes cause red marks on my body.

4	3	2	1	0

5. Sometimes my heart races so fast after minor exercise that it scares me.

4	3	2	1	0

6. I get winded walking up a flight of stairs.

4	3	2	1	0

7. I avoid exercise because it makes me feel nauseated.

4	3	2	1	0

8. My friends laugh at me behind my back because I am so out of shape.

4	3	2	1	0

Scoring

In scoring the above inventory, you may assess the two categories separately.
Simply add up your total points and rate yourself.
Scoring is as follows for each section:

0–4	Extremely low comfort level. Action is imperative!	13–18	Average comfort level. Look at problem areas.
5–12	Low comfort level. Start analyzing what you need to do to make an impact.	19–24	Above-average comfort level.
		25–32	Excellent comfort level.

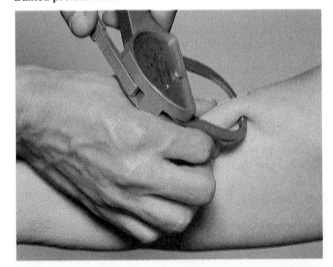

The skin-fold caliper provides one method of assessing percentage of body fat. However, it must be performed by trained professionals.

obtain accurate measurements on the *moderately obese* (20 to 40 percent overweight) or the *morbidly obese* (over 50 percent overweight) person.

The accuracy of the skin-fold caliper test is totally dependent on the skill level of the tester. If the person giving the test is inconsistent in the exact locations of the pinch or if there is difficulty in determining the difference between fat and muscle, the results may be inaccurate.

Another common method of body-fat assessment is the use of **girth and circumference measures**. Diagnosticians use a measuring tape to take girth, or circumference, measurements at various body sites. These measurements are then converted into constants, and a formula is used to determine relative percentages of body fat. Although this technique is inexpensive and easy to

Girth and Circumference Measures A method of assessing body fat that employs a formula based on girth measurements of various body sites.

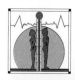

Determining Your Body Mass Index

Is Your Body Mass Putting You at Risk?

Using the BMI Formula

In order to see how you can determine your own Body Mass Index, take as an example a person who weighs 125 pounds and is 64 inches (5 feet, 6 inches) tall.

The BMI formula uses the metric system, so first divide your weight in pounds by 2.2 to convert it to kilograms. For the person in our example, this would work out:

$$125(lb) \div 2.2 = 56.82(kg)$$

Next, convert your height to meters by multiplying your height in inches by 2.54 and dividing the sum by 100. In the example, this would be:

$$64(in) \times 2.54 = 162.56 \div 100 \approx 1.63(m)$$

Then multiply the metric height by itself:

$$1.63 \times 1.63 = 2.66(m)$$

Finally, divide your metric-weight by your metric height in order to determine your BMI. For our example:

$$56.82(kg) \div 2.66(m) = \textbf{21.36 BMI}$$

What the BMI Means

In general, a BMI range of 20 to 25 is considered normal. A suggested desirable range for females is 21.3 to 22.1 and for males, 21.9 to 22.4.* BMI values above 27.8 for men and 27.3 for women have been associated with increased health problems, including high blood pressure and diabetes. The American Dietetic Association, is in its position statement on nutrition and physical fitness, classified people with a BMI greater than 30 as obese and those with a BMI greater than 40 as morbidly obese and in need of prompt medical attention.**

Using the BMI Nomogram

You can also use the nomogram shown here for determining your BMI. To do so, place a ruler between your body weight (left column) and height (right column) and read the number from the middle column—this is your BMI.

* Melvin H. Williams, ed., *Lifetime Fitness and Wellness: A Personal Choice,* 2nd Ed. (Dubuque: Wm. C. Brown, 1990), p. 133.
** American Dietetic Association, "Position of the American Dietetic Association: Nutrition for Physical Fitness and Athletic Performance of Adults," *Journal of the American Dietetic Association,* 87 (1987), 933–39.

---

use, many experts believe that the level of accuracy in prediction is questionable.

Body Mass Index

One of the more widely accepted approaches to weight assessment is a technique developed by the National Center for Health Statistics called the **body mass index (BMI).** Because the BMI is an index of the relationship of weight to height, which is based on a norm of adults between the ages of 20 and 29, it is probably one of the best assessments for most college-aged students. (See the box entitled "Is Your Body Mass Putting You at Risk" for two methods of figuring out your BMI).

Additional Techniques for Assessing Body Fat

Soft-Tissue Roentgenogram A relatively new technique for body-fat determination, the **soft-tissue roentgenogram,** involves injecting a radioactive substance into the body and allowing this substance to penetrate muscle (lean) tissue, enabling distinctions between fat and lean tissue to be made.

Body Mass Index (BMI) A technique of weight assessment based on the relationship of weight to height.
Soft-Tissue Roentgenogram A technique for body-fat assessment in which radioactive substances are used to determine relative fat.

Bioelectrical Impedance Analysis A second method of determining body fat levels, **bioelectrial impedance analysis (BIA),** involves sending a small electric current through the subject's body. The amount of resistance to the current, along with a person's age, sex, and other physical characteristics, is then fed into a computer that uses special formulas to determine the total amount of lean and fat tissue. The water content of the tissue is a key factor in the prediction. One of the newest (and most expensive) body-fat assessment techniques is the **total body electrical conductivity (TOBEC) unit.** Although based on the same principle as impedance, this assessment requires much more elaborate, expensive equipment and is not practical for most people.

Although all of these methods can be useful, they can also be inaccurate and even harmful unless the testers are skillful and well trained. Before agreeing to any such procedure, be sure you are aware of the expenses, risks, and difficulties involved.

Although much of the publicity surrounding obesity focuses on women, large numbers of men have problems with their weight.

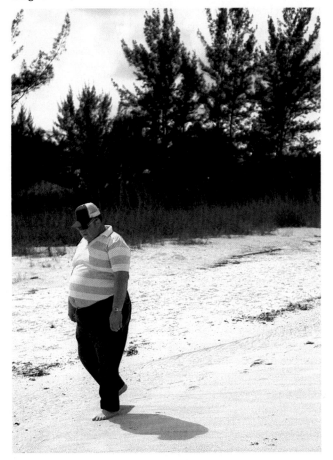

Why Be Concerned about Body Composition?

With all of the techniques available for calculating how fat you really are, how do you decide which is the best for you? Perhaps the best way is to ask yourself how much an exact measure of your body fat means to you. If you are interested in obtaining the most accurate measure before and after a program of diet and exercise, you may find the expense of some of the more sophisticated measures worth the investment. If you simply want a general idea of how much body fat you are carrying around, an inexpensive pinch test, or skin-fold measure, may be all that you need. In contrast, if you know that you are obese based on the bulges around your middle or the size and fit of your jeans, perhaps the exact amount of fat that you have does not matter as much as the fact that you are overweight and need to take action. A quick examination in the mirror may be all you need.

After determining exactly how serious your fat problem is, you must then begin the task of doing something about it. This process involves a careful assessment of the factors that led to your weight problem and the development of a plan of action that will work for you.

ATTACKING THE PROBLEM

Determining the Causes of Obesity

For many researchers, the reason for obesity is quite simple: If you take in more calories that you burn up, you will gain weight. If you do this throughout your lifetime, you will become increasingly obese. If we know what the cause is, we should be able to offer a simple prescription for preventing the problem. Right? Wrong.

Although the calorie explanation of obesity is certainly valid, it offers only one possible reason for a person's weight problem. It does not explain the many additional factors that contribute to the problem and that make the possibility of permanent weight loss very unlikely. It also fails to answer many critical questions. If we know that eating too much will cause us to gain weight, why do we continue to do so? Is there really a metabolic explanation for obesity? Why do fewer than 2 percent of all people who go on a weight-loss program ever demonstrate permanent success? Is pushing yourself away from the table the best method for maintaining weight?

In spite of all the research and all the techniques currently available, controversy still surrounds the reasons that one person becomes obese and another does not. What we do know is that the whole weight-control prob-

Bioelectrical Impedance Analysis (BIA) A technique for body-fat assessment in which electrical currents are passed through fat and lean tissue.

Total Body Electrical Conductivity (TOBEC) Unit Device that uses an electromagnetic force field to assess relative body fat.

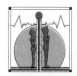

Doomed to Be Fat?

Your Parents and Your Weight

When it comes to gaining weight, the genes you inherited from your ancestors may be more to blame than what you eat or what your parents fed you as a child. Recent studies published in the *New England Journal of Medicine* seem to confirm what many people have long suspected: People can eat identical meals and some will gain more weight than others. In fact, according to a recent study, one person can put on up to 3 times as much weight as another. In addition, if you are overweight, you cannot blame it all on your parents for overfeeding you as a child. According to another study, sets of identical twins who were separated and raised in different families, on widely different diets, still grew up to weigh about the same.

These studies contain the strongest evidence yet that the genes a person inherits are the major factor determining overweight, leanness, or average weight. Although the exact mechanics of the genes remain unknown, it is believed that genes may set metabolic rates, influencing how the body handles calories.

Health professionals are concerned that these studies will paint a "doomed to be fat" picture for many overweight people. However, Albert Stunkard, a psychiatrist at the University of Pennsylvania and author of one of the studies previously mentioned, believes that these conclusions offer hope to those whose extra pounds have been blamed on lack of willpower or hidden psychological needs. In Stunkard's study, the early family environment apparently had no effect at all on adult weight. Based on this finding, Stunkard discounts previous theories that the amount children eat early in life helps determine whether they will be fat as adults. According to Stunkard, it is not the early family environment in which you were raised, but the environment in which you live as an adult that determines whether you will be a fat adult. He points out that diet and exercise will work to modify the genetic effect, but people who are overweight can now be told, "It is very largely due to your genes. You have a specific vulnerability. You are more vulnerable than others; therefore your actions may be even more critical than those of your genetically prone thin friends."

SOURCES: Claude Bouchard et al., "The Response to Long-term Overfeeding in Identical Twins," *New England Journal of Medicine,* 322, no. 21 (1990),:1477–83; and Albert Stunkard et al., "The Body-Mass Index of Twins Who Have Been Raised Apart," *New England Journal of Medicine,* 322, no. 21 (1990), 1483–87.

lem is extremely complex. Many factors appear to influence a person's fat potential.

Heredity   In some animal species, the shape and size of the body are largely determined by the shape and size of the parents. Many scientists have explored the role of heredity in determining human body shapes. Most contend that heredity plays a subtle role in contributing to obesity and argue that obesity has a strong genetic predisposition (tends to run in families). They cite statistics that indicate that 80 percent of children with two obese parents are also obese.* The question of whether these statistics indicate genetic predispositions toward obesity or indicate that children tend to learn eating habits from their environment remains unresolved.

Studies of identical twins who were separated at birth and raised in different environments have provided us with some of our most conclusive evidence that obesity may be an inherited trait. Whether raised in family environments with fat or thin family members, twins with obese natural parents tend to be obese in later life.**

Some scientists believe that heredity is responsible for the "yo-yo" patterns experienced by so many dieters—that is, repeated cycles of weight loss followed by weight gain. These experts theorize that many dieters can lose weight only by becoming far more active and reducing calorie intake to sometimes dangerously low levels.

Hunger, Appetite, and Satiety   Theories abound concerning the mechanisms that regulate food intake. Some sources indicate that the *hypothalamus* (the part of the brain that regulates appetite) closely monitors levels of certain nutrients in the blood. When these levels begin to fall, the brain signals us to eat. In the obese person, it is

---

* Albert Stunkard, *Psychiatric Update: American Psychiatric Association* (New York: Harper & Row, 1985), p. 87.

** G. B. Forbes, "Is Obesity a Genetic Disease?" *Contemporary Nutrition,* June 1981, p. 47.

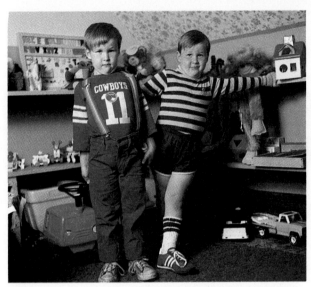
Identical twins, even those separated at birth, often share traits, including obesity.

possible that the monitoring system does not work properly and that the cues to eat are more frequent and intense.

Other sources indicate that thin people may more effectively send messages to the appetite center for regulating metabolic activity. This concept, known as **adaptive thermogenesis,** states that thin people often consume large amounts of food without weight gain because the appetite center of the brain merely speeds up metabolic activity to compensate for the increased consumption. More recent studies have indicated the possibility that specialized types of fat cells, called **brown fat cells,** may send signals to the brain, which controls the thermogenesis response.

The belief that food tastes better to obese people, thus causing them to eat more, has been largely refuted. Scientists do distinguish, however, between **hunger,** an inborn physiological response to nutritional needs, and **appetite,** a learned response to food that is tied to an emotional or psychological craving for food often unrelated to nutritional need. Obese people may be more likely than thin people to satisfy their appetite and eat for reasons other than nutrition.

In some instances, the problem with overconsumption may be more related to **satiety** than to appetite or hunger. People generally feel satiated, or "full," when they have satisfied their nutritional needs and the stomach signals "no more." For undetermined reasons, obese people may not feel "full" until much later than thin people.

Developmental Factors   Some obese people may have excessive numbers of fat cells. This type of obesity, **hyperplasia,** begins to develop in early childhood and perhaps even prior to birth due to the mother's dietary habits. The most critical periods for the development of hyperplasia are the last 2 to 3 months of fetal develop-

ment, the first year of life, and between the ages of 9 and 13. Parents who allow their children to eat without restrictions and become overweight may contribute to a lifelong excess of fat cells in their children's bodies. Central to this theory is the belief that the number of fat cells in a person's body does not increase appreciably during adulthood. However, the ability of each of these cells to swell and shrink, known as **hypertrophy,** does carry over into adulthood. Weight gain may be tied to the number of fat cells in the body and the capacity of each individual cell to enlarge.

An average-weight adult has approximately 25 to 30 billion fat cells, a moderately obese adult about 60 billion to 100 billion, and an extremely obese adult as many as 200 billion.* People who gain large numbers of fat cells in childhood may be able to lose weight by decreasing the size of each cell, but the large numbers of cells appear to remain in waiting, ready for the next calorie binge so that they can fill up and sabotage weight-loss efforts (see Figure 7.2).

Setpoint Theory   In 1982, nutritional researchers William Bennett and Joel Gurin introduced a highly controversial theory concerning the difficulty of losing weight. Their theory, known as the **setpoint theory,** states that a person's body has a setpoint of weight at which it is preprogrammed to be comfortable. If your setpoint is around 160 pounds, you will gain and lose weight fairly easily within a given range of that point.** For example, if you gain 5 to 10 pounds on vacation, it will be fairly easy to lose that weight and remain around the 160-pound mark for a long period of time. Some people have equated this point with the **plateau** that is sometimes reached after a person loses a certain amount of weight. The setpoint theory proposes that after losing a predetermined amount of weight, the body will actually sabotage additional weight loss by slowing down metabolism. In extreme cases, the metabolic rate will decrease to a point where the body will maintain its

---
* Katch and McArdle, *Nutrition*, pp. 138–39.
** William Bennett and Joel Gurin, *The Dieter's Dilemma* (New York: Basic Books, 1982) p. 32.

Adaptive Thermogenesis   Mechanism in which the brain regulates metabolic activity according to caloric intake.

Brown Fat Cells   Specialized type of fat cell that affects the ability to regulate fat metabolism.

Hunger   An inborn physiological response to nutritional needs.

Appetite   A learned response that is tied to an emotional or psychological craving for food, often unrelated to nutritional need.

Satiety   The feeling of fullness or satisfaction at the end of a meal.

Hyperplasia   Condition characterized by excessive numbers of fat cells.

Hypertrophy   The theory that fat cells have the ability to enlarge and shrink.

Setpoint Theory   A theory of obesity causation that suggests that fat storage is determined by a thermostatic mechanism in the body that acts to maintain a specific amount of body fat.

Plateau   A point in a weight-loss program at which a person finds it difficult to lose more weight.

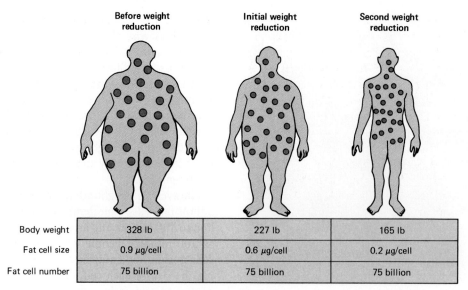

	Before weight reduction	Initial weight reduction	Second weight reduction
Body weight	328 lb	227 lb	165 lb
Fat cell size	0.9 µg/cell	0.6 µg/cell	0.2 µg/cell
Fat cell number	75 billion	75 billion	75 billion

Figure 7.2 One person at various stages of weight loss. Note that, according to theories of hyperplasia, the number of fat cells remains constant but their size decreases.

weight on as little as 1,000 calories per day. Can a person change this predetermined setpoint? Proponents of this theory argue that a person can raise a setpoint over time by continually gaining weight and failing to exercise. Conversely, a person who reduces caloric intake and exercises for a long period of time can slowly decrease the setpoint. Exercise may be the most critical factor in readjustment of the setpoint, although diet may also be important.

Perhaps the greatest impact of this theory was the sense of relief it offered those people who have lost weight, plateaued, and given up, time and time again. Dietary failure may not be due to a lack of willpower alone. Also, nutritional experts have begun to look carefully at popular methods of weight loss. A low-calorie or starvation diet, in addition to being dangerous, may also cause the body to protect the dieter by slowing down metabolism and making weight loss more difficult.

Endocrine Influence Over the years, many people have attributed obesity to problems with their **thyroid gland.** They claimed that an underactive thyroid impeded their ability to burn calories. This belief substituted an "organic" cause for individual responsibility for obesity. How many obesity problems may justifiably be blamed on a poorly functioning thyroid? Most authorities agree that only 3 to 5 percent of the obese population actually have a thyroid problem.

Psychosocial Factors The relationship of weight problems to deeply rooted emotional insecurities, needs, and wants remains uncertain. Because food is often a reward for good behavior from childhood on, people with emotional problems may use food as a reward in otherwise unsatisfying lives. Again, this research is controversial. What is certain is that in the American culture, eating tends to be a focal point of people's lives. Eating is

essentially a social ritual associated with companionship, celebration, and enjoyment. The intimate dinner for two, the office party complete with snacks, and the picnic at the beach all center on eating. Is it any wonder that for many people the social emphasis on the eating experience is a major obstacle to successful dieting? Although some restaurants offer menu items designed to aid dieters, many people have difficulty choosing responsibly when confronted with an entire menu of favorites.

Some theorists have contended that obese people tend to ignore internal cues of hunger and are more likely to use the clock as a guide for "time to eat" than real hunger cues. Other studies refute this hypothesis.

Metabolic Changes Even when at complete rest, the body needs a certain amount of energy. The amount of energy used at complete rest is known as **basal metabolic rate (BMR).** For most adults, BMR is based on approximately 1 calorie per minute. If you were totally immobilized, you would need to burn about 1,400 calories per day to maintain basic metabolism. An extremely sedentary person might require an additional 200 to 300 calories per day, and an extremely active person might require a total of 2,000 to 3,000 calories. For most adults, balancing the amount of calories consumed with a reasonable amount of exercise is often all that is needed to maintain a fairly level weight. Why is it, then, that people who have been able to maintain their weight throughout their adult lives suddenly begin to put on weight in later years? What is responsible for the type of "creeping obesity" that many people experience in middle age and beyond?

Thyroid Gland A two-lobed endocrine gland located in the throat; produces a hormone that regulates metabolism.
Basal Metabolic Rate (BMR) The energy expenditure of the body under resting conditions at normal room temperature.

It is commonly believed that a decline in BMR is a natural part of the aging process. For reasons that are not clearly understood, the body's requirement for energy to maintain basic physiological processes decreases approximately 1 percent per year after 25 years of age. This decline is a major reason that losing weight becomes more of a struggle in later life and gaining weight seems to be as easy as breathing!

Pregnancy The number of overweight women far exceeds the number of overweight men at all ages. Although numerous factors contribute to this situation, one of the most salient appears to be pregnancy. Required to nourish the unborn child and subjected to numerous hormonal fluctuations, the typical pregnant woman struggles between the doctor's scale and her food cravings. The typical woman gains 28 to 30 pounds between conception and the birth of her child. The recommended weight gain is slightly lower, ranging from 20 to 30 pounds. Assuming a baby weighs 8 pounds at birth and allowing for the elimination of fetal supporting tissue, there remains a substantial amount of weight that the new mother must lose. Whereas this excess weight is relatively easy for many women to lose, for others it is the start of a significant weight problem. This is especially true among those women who fail to return to normal weight before becoming pregnant again.

Lack of Physical Activity Of all the factors affecting obesity, perhaps the most critical is the relationship between activity levels and calorie intake. Table 7.3 lists the number of calories expended in a variety of activities. All of us know someone who seems to be able to "eat us under the table" and does not appear to exercise more than we do, yet never seems to gain weight. We often do not understand *how* this person maintains a steady weight. With few exceptions, if we were to follow this person around for a typical day and monitor the level and intensity of activity, we would find the answer to our question. Although the person's schedule may not include running or strenuous exercise, it probably includes a high level of activity. Walking the flight of stairs rather than taking the elevator, speeding up the pace while mowing the lawn, and doing housework burn extra calories. These little extra efforts often go unnoticed and only burn a few calories. Over a period of days, weeks, or months, however, these little extras can make a big difference in weight maintenance.

One pound of body fat contains approximately 3,500 kilocalories (kcal). According to an energy-balance equation, each time you consume an excess of 3,500 kcal, you gain a pound of fat. Conversely, each time your body experiences a deficit of 3,500 kcal, you lose a pound of fat. Clearly, any form of activity that helps your body burn additional calories helps you maintain your weight. In fact, in a study conducted at Stanford University in 1987, a group of men who lost weight through exercise were far more successful at keeping the weight off than were a similar group who lost weight through dieting.

Evidence exists that the majority of overweight people do not eat much more than do thin people. They do, however, move more slowly and less frequently, thus diminishing their chances for weight loss. Because thin people burn more calories, they often feel less sluggish and have more energy than do overweight people.

A major cause of low activity levels is the abundance of labor-saving devices in the modern household. Pushing vacuum cleaners rather than sweeping floors, typing on computer keyboards rather than manual typewriters, and using remote-control buttons on television and stereo equipment cause us to expend fewer calories than did previous generations. The automobile has provided us with a great convenience, but it has not done much to improve our muscle tone or our cardiovascular efficiency.

Recent studies indicate that we may be in a situation of declining health activities, in spite of all of the previous reports of large numbers of people exercising, dieting, and maintaining active involvement in their own health. One of the major aspects of this decline is the increasing number of people with weight problems. Although we have learned a great deal in recent years about the factors that predispose humans to gain or lose weight, a great deal of controversy remains. Perhaps one of the greatest factors that we need to learn about is the most obvious—the individual person.

Individuality Finding specific factors that cause obesity may be impossible. Just as no two people are exactly alike physiologically, no two people are psychologically identical. Each person is a unique result of genetic background, environment, lifestyle, and emotional responses to a lifetime of experiences.

It is highly possible that the causes of obesity are as varied as the people who are obese. Given this complexity, it is obvious that there is no universal cure for weight problems. Instead, we must look for an appropriate mechanism of prevention or intervention for each individual.

SELECTING A WEIGHT-LOSS PLAN

At some point in our lives, almost every one of us will decide to "go on a diet." Whether it be in response to gorging ourselves on the Thanksgiving turkey with all the fixings, noticing the small "spare tire" or "love handles" on our midsections, or for a variety of other reasons, the attempt to lose a few pounds appears to be a common practice in American society. With hundreds of different diets and thousands of different foods to choose from, why do we fail most of the time?

In a 1986 conference on obesity sponsored by the

Table 7.3 Calories Expended in Various Activities*

Activity	Calories per Hour*	Average Calories Used	Activity	Calories per Hour*	Average Calories Used
Sleeping	65	520 (8 hrs.)	Running in place or skipping rope (50–60 steps/min.)	510	255 (1/2 hr.)
Watching TV	80	80 (1 hr.)			
Driving a car	100	50 (1/2 hr.)			
Dishwashing by hand	135	67 (1/2 hr.)	Downhill skiing	595	1,190 (2 hrs. on slope)
Bowling	190	190 (1 hr.)	Swimming, 5.5 min./220 yds.	600	300 (1/2 hr.)
Washing and polishing car	230	230 (1 hr.)	Hill climbing	600	300 (1/2 hr.)
			Touch football	600	300 (1/2 hr. actual play)
Dancing (waltz, rock, fox trot)	250	105 (5 dances, 25 min.)	Soccer	600	600 (1 hr.)
			Snow shoveling, light	610	306 (1/2 hr.)
Walking, 25 min/mi.	255	127 (1/2 hr.)	Jogging, 11 min./mi.	655	327 (1/2 hr.)
Baseball (not pitching or catching)	280	560 (2 hrs.)	Cross-country skiing, 12 min./mi.	700	2,800 (4 hrs.)
Weight training	300	150 (1/2 hr.)	Basketball, full court	750	750 (1 hr.)
Swimming, 11 min/220 yds.	300	150 (1/2 hr.)	Squash, racquetball	775	775 (1 hr.)
			Martial arts (judo, karate)	790	395 (1/2 hr.)
Walking, 15 min./mi.	345	172 (1/2 hr.)	Running, 7.5 min./mi.	800	400 (1/2 hr.)
Volleyball, badminton	350	350 (1 hr.)	Ice hockey, lacrosse	900	900 (1 hr.)
Gardening	390	780 (2 hrs.)			
Calisthenics	415	207 (1/2 hr.)			
Bicycling, 6 min./mi.	415	207 (1/2 hr.)			
Tennis	425	425 (1 hr.)			
Aerobic dancing (med.)	445	222 (1/2 hr.)			

* The bigger and more vigorous you are, the more calories your body uses for a given activity. The calories listed here are for the average 158-pound adult. You will lose 1 pound for every 3,500 calories of exercise, as long as you eat the same amount of food.

SOURCE: C. Kuntzleman, *Diet Free!* (Spring Arbor, Mich.: Arbor Press, 1981).

New York Academy of Science, Dr. William Bennett, a proponent of the setpoint theory, argued that most diet-based approaches to weight loss are a disaster and should be abandoned. According to Bennett, obesity is not a single disease but a group of diseases with different causes and manifestations that require different treatments. He concluded that diets just do not work.* Bennett also claimed that most diet research is inconclusive and does not alert us to the dangers of unsuccessful weight-loss efforts. Since Bennett's early research, many other weight-loss specialists have acquired the "Never Say Diet" mentality. Rather than focusing on dieting to lose weight, these experts promote gradual, "livable" changes and modifications in daily dietary patterns. Cutting down on the number of calories eaten from fats, consuming more fiber and carbohydrates, and eating smaller quantities of favorite, but less nutritious foods, rather than eliminating them completely are cornerstones of this new weight-loss mentality.

Responding to what is perceived as a national frustration with weight-loss efforts, countless bestsellers such as *The Dieter's Dilemma* and *Never Say Diet* reiterate (less scientifically) that losing weight by dieting is often a losing proposition and that dietary modifications are more likely to work overtime.

If all we have to look forward to is the prospect of failure, why should we make the effort? Are all diets equally destined for failure? What has worked? What methods would be best for you? (See the box entitled "Liquid Diets").

Unfortunately, there is no simple answer to these questions. We do know that weight-loss efforts that work for one person do not necessarily work for another. To be successful, weight-loss efforts must consider the unique aspects of the person involved, the underlying causes of the person's weight problem, the conditions that trigger overeating, and, perhaps most important, the factors that motivate the person to follow a reasonable program of diet and exercise.

Nutrition/Exercise Training Clearly, most traditional diets have not been successful. Rather than forcing

---

* William Bennett, *Proceedings: Conference on Human Obesity*, New York Academy of Science, July 1986.

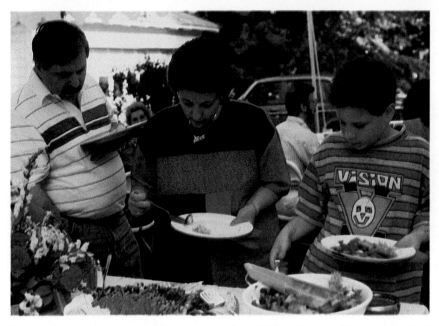

Parents have a significant influence on whether children have problems managing their weight.

a specified "diet" on yourself, perhaps it would be better to think in terms of **nutrition/exercise training.** Teaching yourself to eat and exercise responsibly improves the chances of long-term success. Rather than teaching someone to avoid chocolate cake, truffles, and similar treats, a successful program can teach people that it is okay to indulge sometimes. However, people must then accept responsibility for their actions, practice calorie moderation in other areas, and exercise to burn off the additional calories.

Rather than sticking to the latest fad diet for a few days, growing tired of it, and returning to previous habits (and weight), it is more effective to think in terms of *weekly* rather than daily calorie intake. Thus, if you "blow it" on Saturday, you can make up for it during the next week. The flexibility that this type of program offers often reduces the guilt of failure and enhances the likelihood of future success.

The bottom line of this program is the simple formula explained previously. If you take in more calories than you expend, you will gain weight. If you expend more calories than you take in, you will lose weight. For most people, weight maintenance is a simple balancing formula that should also include exercise designed to keep body parts "firm and functioning."

Regardless of how you approach nutritional and exercise training, you should keep in mind that it is a lifelong process. To be effective, the process should be one that best fits your individual lifestyle and behavior. Although volumes have been written to assist people in choosing a plan, most experts agree on certain criteria, which will be discussed in the next section (see Figure 7.3).

The Role of Exercise in Weight Loss

Approximately 90 percent of the daily calorie expenditures of most people occurs as a result of the **resting metabolic rate (RMR).** The RMR is slightly higher than the BMR and includes the BMR plus any additional energy expended through daily sedentary activities, such as food digesting, sitting, studying, or standing. The **exercise metabolic rate (EMR)** accounts for the remaining 10 percent of all daily calorie expenditures and refers to the energy expenditure that occurs during physical exercise. For most of us, these calories come from light daily activities, such as walking, climbing stairs, and mowing the lawn. If we increase the level and intensity of our physical activity to moderate or heavy, however, the EMR may be 10 to 20 times greater than typical resting metabolic rates and can contribute substantially to weight loss.

Increasing BMR, RMR, or EMR levels will help burn calories. An increase in the intensity, frequency, and duration of your daily exercise levels may have a significant impact on total calorie expenditure. The higher the intensity of the exercise, the more calories you burn. The more often you exercise, the greater the total weekly calorie expenditure. The longer you spend doing

---

Nutrition/Exercise Training   A long-term program of proper eating and exercising.

Resting Metabolic Rate (RMR)   The energy expenditure of the body under BMR conditions plus other daily sedentary activities.

Exercise Metabolic Rate (EMR)   The energy expenditure that occurs during exercise.

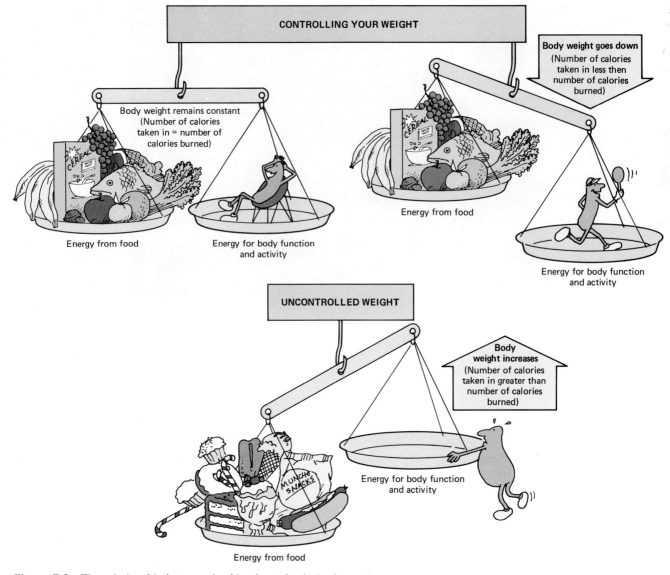

Figure 7.3 The relationship between food intake and calories burned.

a particular exercise, even at a low intensity, the more likely you are to burn additional calories. Thus, walking, even though it may take longer to burn calories than jogging or running, may have a significant effect on your weight if you walk regularly for several weeks.

Strategies to Ensure Success

1. *Design your plan for your needs.* Forget the nutritional gurus who promise quick success. Your plan must fit your personality, your priorities, and your work and recreation schedules. It should allow for sufficient rest and relaxation.

2. *Plan for nutrient-dense foods.* Attempt to get the most from the foods you eat by selecting foods with high nutritional value. Excellent examples of nu-

trient-dense foods include fruits and vegetables, whole-grain breads and cereals, and lean, protein-rich foods such as fish and poultry, low-fat cottage cheese, and skim milk (see Chapter 6).

3. *Balance food intake throughout the day.* Although the evidence is controversial, research indicates that the body may burn calories more efficiently in small amounts than in excessive quantities. Thus, rather than gorging yourself at one main meal, you are probably better off eating several smaller meals interspersed throughout the day.

4. *Plan for plateaus.* As previously indicated, we may have an inner thermostat that attempts to set our weight at a given point. Thus, people who prepare themselves psychologically for plateaus will be less likely to become discouraged. Exercise is probably the critical factor in getting past a plateau.

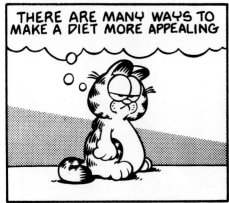
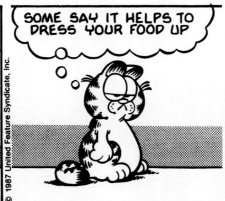
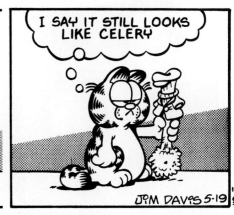

5. *Chart your progress.* For many people, the daily "weigh-in" is a critical factor in maintaining their program. However, particularly for those who have reached a weight plateau, it may be necessary to think in terms of weekly weigh-ins to avoid frustration. After all, it is the longer-range successes that are ultimately the most important.

6. *Chart your setbacks.* Rather than thinking in terms of failure and punishment, it is better to think in terms of temporary setbacks in weight management. By carefully recording emotional states when eating, eating habits, environmental cues, and feelings, dieters may determine why they needed that ice-cream cone or why they chose a pizza instead of a salad. Studies suggest that the "urge" to consume more calories may be greater at certain times of the month, particularly for women during the days immediately before and after menstruation. Thus, successful weight-loss plans might have no accommodate hormonal fluctuations as an influence in dietary habits.

7. *Become aware of your feelings of hunger and fullness.* For many of us, eating becomes time-dependent, and we stop eating only when the food is gone (the old "clean your plate" syndrome). Somewhere during a lifetime of "eating when it is time" instead of eating when it is necessary, we lose the ability to tell when we really are hungry or full. The message that our stomach sends to our brain signaling "full" is not immediate. Sometimes, particularly when we eat too fast, there is a delay between actual fullness and our physical awareness that we have had enough. We continue to eat past the "full" point, causing discomfort and even nausea in some instances. By training ourselves to be more aware of the eating process, learning to recognize true hunger pangs and the first signals that we have eaten enough, we will learn an important lesson in eating patterns.

8. *Accept yourself.* For many people, this aspect of successful weight management is perhaps the most important. Although the rest of the world may appear to be antifat in its thinking, it is probably true that many overweight people are their own worst enemies. It is important to keep your weight in perspective. Unless you feel good about who you are inside, the exterior changes will not help you very much.

9. *Exercise, exercise, exercise.* Although we would all like to wish away our extra pounds, losing weight requires hard work and concentration. Different people benefit from different types of activities. Just because your friends are into jogging or jazzercise does not mean that type of exercise program is best for you. The key is to select an exercise program that is fun and not a daily form of punishment for overeating. Variety may help. Planning a program that includes friends and family may improve the chances of success. It is important to remember that every little effort contributes toward long-term results.

10. *Select a nutritional plan that makes sense.* In today's marketplace of dietary gimmicks and quick-weight-loss schemes, it is important to wade through all the quackery and select an effective and scientifically sound plan. This plan should provide optimum nutrient value per calorie and conform to recommended percentages of fats, proteins, and carbohydrates. The plan should take into consideration your age and total calorie needs. In general, it is best to avoid such products as appetite suppressants, diuretics, and "herbal" or "megavitamin" supplements. A balanced diet consisting of the major food groups is the best rule of thumb.

11. Make exercise a natural part of your day. Instead of setting aside 30 minutes per day to jog, find some form of movement that you really like, and reward yourself with it. Walking, bicycling, swimming, and

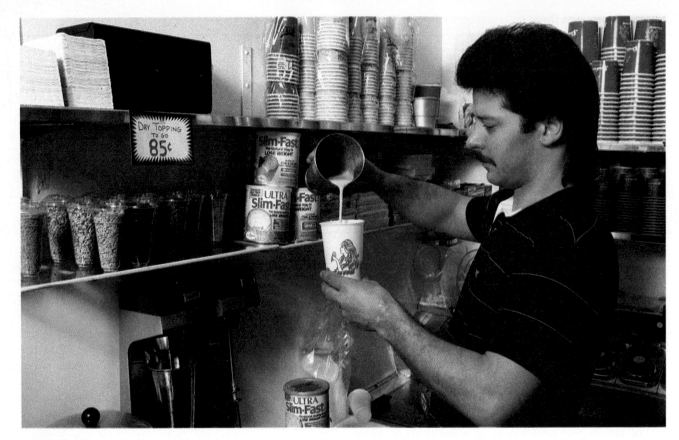

Liquid diets have gained in popularity in recent years even though their use is controversial.

other activities will burn calories, tone muscles, and improve overall health.

Changing Your Eating Behavior

Determining What Triggers Your Eating Behavior Before you can change a given behavior, you must first determine what caused that behavior. Why do you suddenly find yourself at the refrigerator door eating everything in sight? Why do you help yourself to that second and third helping of potatoes or dessert when you know that you should be trying to lose weight?

Many people have found that one of the best ways of assessing their eating behavior is to chart exactly when they feel like eating, where they are when they decide to eat, the amount of time spent eating, other activities engaged in during the meal (watching television or reading), whether they eat alone or with others, what and how much is eaten, and how they felt prior to eating their first bite. A log of those triggers listed in Figure 7.4 should be completed in detail every day for at least a week. Doing so will provide useful clues as to those things in your environment or in your emotional makeup that cause you to want food. Typically, these dietary "triggers" center on problems in everyday living rather than real hunger pangs. By recording this information, your reasons for eating will often become apparent. Many people find that they eat compulsively when stressed or when they have problems in their relationships. For other people, the exact same circumstances diminish their appetite, causing them to lose weight.

Changing Your Triggers Once you recognize the factors that cause you to eat, removing the triggers or substituting other activites for them will help you develop some sensible eating patterns. Some examples of substitute behaviors are listed below:

1. When eating dinner, turn off all distractions, including the television and radio.
2. Replace snack breaks or coffee breaks with exercise breaks.
3. Instead of gulping your food, force yourself to chew each bit several times.
4. Vary the time of day when you eat. Instead of eating by the clock, do not eat until you are truly hungry. Allow yourself only a designated amount of time for eating—but do not rush. Try to get more in touch with real feelings of hunger.

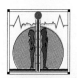

New Miracles or Risky Business?

Liquid Diets

Americans who suffer from obesity have a vast arsenal of seemingly safe, fast, and effortless choices available to help them. The Weight Watchers, Last Chance, Grapefruit, Pritikin, Scarsdale, and Beverly Hills diets are but a few of the hundreds of weight-loss plans that offer solutions to the modern-day dieter. At one time or another, most of the 65 million dieters in the United States have tried one or more of these remedies, usually with very little long-term success.

As people become more frustrated by the high failure rates of these dietary regimens and are spurred on by the dramatic results obtained by television celebrities, they have entered the era of the "liquid diet." Liquid-diet mania typically follows one or two general patterns. In the first category are the liquid "fast" diets such as Optifast and Medifast. In these medically supervised plans, the dieter consumes 5 8-ounce glasses of fortified liquid per day and nothing else. These drinks contain approximately 80 calories each and include about 15 grams of protein, 6 to 10 grams of carbohydrates, less than 1 gram of fat and fiber, and numerous vitamin supplements. The patient undergoes a comprehensive physical examination, and blood and vital signs are closely monitored throughout the process. The second category of liquid diets is over-the-counter products purchased in grocery stores, drugstores, or wherever the product is sold. There is no medical supervision. Typically, these over-the-counter varieties are mixed with low-fat milk, contain approximately 220 calories per 8-ounce serving, and are consumed twice a day, followed by a regular meal.

How popular are these "quick-fix" weight-loss regimens? Are there potential risks associated with these diets? Do they offer long-term results? In 1990, it is estimated that over 20 million Americans will spend nearly $1 billion on medically supervised liquid diets and over-the-counter liquid-diet products. As many as 50 percent of the people who sign up for these medically supervised programs never complete them. More important, people who do lose weight rapidly on such programs are 3 times more likely to regain the weight than are those who lose weight more slowly. Part of the reason for this weight gain is metabolism. When the body is put on what it perceives to be a starvation diet, it tries to protect itself by lowering its energy thermostat and conserving as many calories as possible for essential body processes. A lifetime of semistarvation diets is believed to slow metabolism more and more. In essence, with each diet cycle, the dieter must eat less and less to obtain the desired effect.

Concern over other problems related to liquid diets is rising. Much of this concern relates to the fact that there is very little government regulation of the sale of such products. Potential for fraud and misuse is great. Since 1984, the Food and Drug Administration has required that all very-low-calorie protein diets (providing fewer than 400 calories a day) carry a warning stating that they can cause serious illness and require medical supervision. In spite of such warnings, many people rely on liquid diets alone. They place themselves at risk for blood-pressure fluctuations, cardiac irregularities, loss of excessive amounts of lean muscle, and other serious problems.

Although medical experts seem to believe that such diets play a useful role in rapid weight loss for patients at high risk for heart problems, diabetes, stroke, gallbladder disease, and other medical problems if they do not lose weight rapidly, they strongly question the use of these products for the general public.

5. If you find that you eat all that you can cram on a plate, use smaller plates. Put the old dinner plates away and use the salad plates.

6. If you find that you are continually seeking your favorite foods in the cupboard, do not buy them, or place them in a spot that is not very convenient for you. Having to run upstairs for the sugar bowl will probably force you to think twice before using sugar.

Although the above list could be expanded, it will need to be geared toward your eating behaviors. After

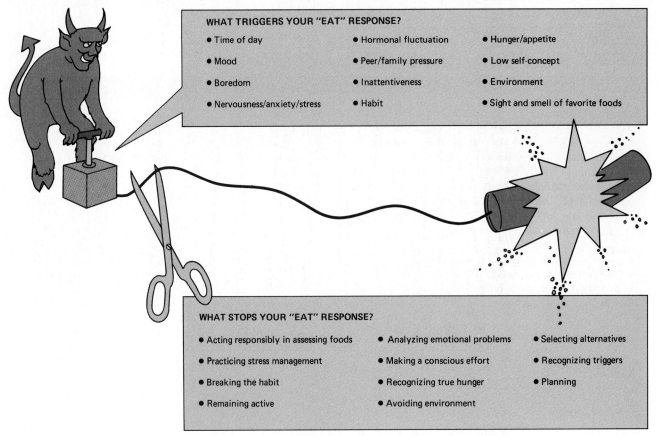

WHAT TRIGGERS YOUR "EAT" RESPONSE?

- Time of day
- Mood
- Boredom
- Nervousness/anxiety/stress

- Hormonal fluctuation
- Peer/family pressure
- Inattentiveness
- Habit

- Hunger/appetite
- Low self-concept
- Environment
- Sight and smell of favorite foods

WHAT STOPS YOUR "EAT" RESPONSE?

- Acting responsibly in assessing foods
- Practicing stress management
- Breaking the habit
- Remaining active

- Analyzing emotional problems
- Making a conscious effort
- Recognizing true hunger
- Avoiding environment

- Selecting alternatives
- Recognizing triggers
- Planning

Figure 7.4 Learn to understand what triggers your "eat" response. Keep a daily log of your responses.

recording your daily intake for a week, devise a list of your own that will allow you to make positive changes.

Selecting a Nutritional Plan That Is Right for You Once you have discovered those factors that tend to sabotage your weight-loss efforts, you will be well on your way to successful weight control. To be successful, you must plan for success. By setting goals that are too far in the future or unrealistic for your current lifestyle, you will doom yourself to failure. Do not worry about losing 40 pounds in 4 months. Worry about losing a healthy 1 to 2 pounds during the first week, and stay with the slow and easy regimen. Reward yourself when you lose those pounds and if you binge and go off your nutrition plan, get right back on it the next day. Remember that you did not gain 40 pounds in 2 weeks and that it is unrealistic for you to punish your body by trying to lose a great deal of weight in a short time.

Seek assistance from reputable sources in selecting a dietary plan that is easy to follow and includes adequate amounts of the basic nutrients. Registered dieticians, some physicians (not all physicians have strong backgrounds in nutrition), health educators and exercise physiologists with nutritional backgrounds, and other health professionals often can provide reliable information. Avoid those quick-weight-loss programs that promise miracle results. The majority of these programs provide fast weight loss at a great expense, and most people regain lost weight after completing their programs. Asking questions about the credentials of the advisor in a weight-loss program, assessing the nutrient value of the prescribed diet, verifying that dietary guidelines are consistent with known factors in dietary research, and analyzing the suitability of the diet to your tastes, budget, and lifestyle are all behaviors that will prevent your being put in a risky, expensive, and unhealthy dietary situation. Any diet that requires radical behavior changes is doomed to failure. Nutritional plans that do not ask you to sacrifice everything you enjoy and allow you to make choices are generally the most successful.

Ultimately, the decision for you to practice responsible weight management is your own. To be successful, you must choose a combination of exercise and eating that fits your needs and lifestyle. Find a workable plan, stick to it, and you will succeed.

SUMMARY

- Excessive body fat is a major problem in American society and contributes to heart disease, diabetes, gallbladder disease, hypertension, respiratory ailments, and certain forms of cancer.

- Between 30 and 50 percent of Americans are overweight. It is important to distinguish between being overweight and being overfat. Overfat is a more accurate indicator of obesity.

- Scales and height–weight tables are not accurate indicators of body fat. Skinfold calipers, hydrostatic weighing techniques, and other techniques are better indicators of fat-to-lean ratios in the body.

- Obesity is generally defined as an accumulation of fat beyond that considered normal for a person's age, sex, and body type.

- Many theories exist to explain the causes of obesity. Heredity; hunger, appetite, and satiety; fat cell theory; setpoint theory; endocrine theory; psychosocial factors; metabolism; pregnancy; and other factors may all be important.

- Body fat is composed of two parts: essential fat and storage fat.

- The most effective weight-loss or fat-loss programs combine exercise, behavior modification, and knowledgeable dietary planning.

- Before planning a weight-loss program, examine the "triggers" that influence you to eat. Changing these triggers may reduce the likelihood of a recurrent obesity problem.

- Because so many people want quick weight loss, quackery is common, and some physicians are willing to surgically remove fat. Both place the consumer at risk and do nothing to change the basic problem.

8

Improving Health Through Aerobic Exercise

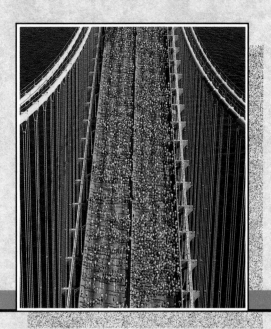

Objectives

- Compare aerobic and anaerobic activity.

- Describe how exercise affects the body.

- Describe the characteristics of CV exercise and explain why some exercises are better for the heart than others.

- Discuss the principles of comfortable exercise and summarize how you can determine exercise intensity and duration.

- Summarize how you can sustain an activity habit.

- List some dangers involved in exercise and describe the steps you can take to safeguard yourself while exercising.

- Describe the various aerobic activities, including their benefits and whatever precautions need to be taken during their performance.

- Describe the benefits of other healthy activities, and discuss an optimal lifestyle strategy.

In recent years Americans have become increasingly interested in improving their overall levels of physical well-being. Jogging, bicycling, swimming, and other forms of physical activity have become an essential part of many individuals typical days. Determining why so many people have donned running shoes or swimming suits or become owners of the latest version of street or mountain bikes has become the subject of a great deal of research. In addition, determining why some individuals put on those shoes, or jump on their bikes and continue in their exercise activities while others quickly head back to their couch and television routines, has become a significant part of behavioral investigations. It is generally assumed that many people start to exercise because of a very real concern for their health and appearance. They want to look and feel better.

Several population studies indicate that virtually any type of activity performed routinely results in **improved health status**. Improved health status means that some aspect of a person's well-being is changed, positively such as higher energy levels, greater resistance to disease, increased bone density and strength, improved emotional health, and overall improved levels of functioning on a daily basis. Increased health status also may indicate protection against premature death and disability. Activity that improves health status can be of very mild intensity, such as gardening, slow walking, housecleaning, and so forth; it can be performed only briefly, but must be performed consistently to obtain a health benefit. When such mild activity includes weight-bearing parts of the body, it is believed to strengthen bone in those areas and prevent future injury.

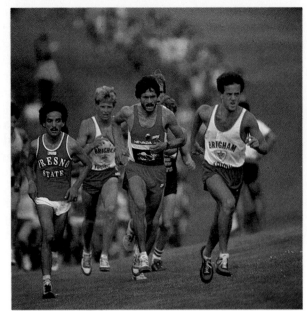

Although some people run competitively, aerobic exercises, such as running, can be practiced by many types of people and can improve cardiovascular health and help the body cope with stress.

Aerobic vs. Anaerobic Activity

Aerobic activity is a different type of activity that is performed at moderate to high intensity and which is believed to be the best type of activity for improving health status while also improving *cardiovascular (cv) fitness*. CV fitness implies improved *aerobic capacity* (VO_2 max), a variable associated with improved functioning of the heart, lungs, blood vessels, and muscles. By their very nature, aerobic activities demand plenty of oxygen and involve large muscle groups. Although rising from the sofa, pushing the vacuum cleaner around the living room, washing dishes, and similar forms of activity may be classified as being physical activity, they are not all aerobic in nature. Thus, while exercise that affects CV fitness also affects health status, it is important to recognize that mild or brief activity, even though it affects health status, generally will not improve CV fitness. Typically, we measure aerobic fitness through a VO_{2max} test performed in a laboratory with a treadmill. The person being tested is asked to walk or run, starting with a relatively low workload which becomes increasingly difficult until he or she reaches maximal exertion. Gener-

ally, the more aerobically fit people are, the more oxygen they can transport efficiently, and the harder and longer period they can exercise. VO_{2max} is expressed in milliliters of oxygen per kilogram of body weight. The higher the value, the higher the level of aerobic fitness, all things being equal. Often, other, less reliable methods of determining VO_{2max} are utilized because of requirements of time, equipment, and skilled personnel. Submaximal bicycle tests, the 1.5 mile walk/run test and 1-minute walking test have been found to be very practical, fairly reliable methods of determining aerobic fitness levels and so are commonly used.

Anaerobics refers to high intensity, short-burst activity in which the muscles rely heavily on the production of energy without adequate oxygen. Sports such as tennis, racketball, handball, squash, sprinting, football, and baseball require all-out efforts for several seconds. To improve your ability to perform these short bursts, you must improve your anaerobic fitness levels. Anaerobic metabolism comes into action at the beginning of any type of exercise as the immediate energy source for all

Improved Health Status A positive change in a person's well being; including higher energy levels, greater resistance to disease, and overall improved levels of daily functioning, which may indicate protection against premature death and disability.

Aerobic Activity A type of activity performed at moderate to high intensity and involving large muscle groups that is considered to be the best type of activity for improving health status through improving cardiovascular (CV) fitness by increasing the efficiency of oxygen intake by the body.

Anaerobics Any high intensity, short-burst activity in which the muscles produce energy without adequate oxygen.

muscle work. This energy source, called **adenosine tri-phosphate (ATP)** is formed in the muscles through the metabolism of carbohydrates and fats. Every muscle needs ATP to perform, and since ATP is metabolized without the need for oxygen, the process is termed anaerobic (without oxygen). In these short bursts of energy, the heart and lungs cannot deliver oxygen to the muscles fast enough; therefore, anaerobic energy sources must take over and provide the fuel for activity. In addition to ATP, other substances, including stored carbohydrates known as **glycogen,** are also used to provide energy during vigorous exercise. The anaerobic use of glycogen produces **lactic acid,** a metabolic end-product that hinders muscle function, particularly when it begins to build up in excessive amounts. Because anaerobic metaboism is very inefficient, high intensity activity can not be sustained for long periods of time.

PHYSIOLOGICAL EFFECTS OF EXERCISE

Exercise causes the physiological systems of the body to respond in a unified way in order to increase the oxygen supply to working muscles. The cardiovascular effects of a single maximal exercise bout are summarized in Table 8.1. Resting values are contrasted with maximal values to illustrate the magnitude of change for each CV variable. *Oxygen consumption* (VO$_2$) is enhanced about 12 to 16 times from rest to maximal exercise. This response is possible due to the large increases in heart rate and stroke volume. Also improved is the tissue uptake of oxygen as indicated by the arterial and venous O$_2$ difference (A-VO$_2$). In addition, elevations in muscle blood flow, blood pressure, and ventilation support the enhanced delivery of oxygen to working tissues.

Adenosine Triphosphate   (ATP) A metabolic by-product and the source of energy for all muscle work.

Glycogen   Stored carbohydrates that provide energy during vigorous exercise.

Lactic Acid   A metabolic end-product hindering muscle functioning, especailly when it builds up excessively.

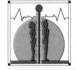

Exercise

What's in It for YOU: Burned Fat? Burned Carbohydrates? Burned Calories?

Muscle glycogen is the primary carbohydrate source of energy during prolonged exercise, but some energy also comes from stored liver glycogen which is transported to the working muscle by the blood as glucose. The primary source of fat for aerobic exercise is triglyceride stored in adipose tissue. This energy is transported to the muscle in the blood and thus, there is a time lag before adipose triglyceride can be used in exercise. Trained individuals rely on triglyceride from muscle more than untrained individuals do.

Although glycogen is a very effective form of stored energy, most energy in the body is stored as fat. The supply of stored carbohydrate (CHO) in the body is relatively limited and can be depleted during prolonged workouts, even though CHO provides more energy per liter than fat. Because of its greater efficiency, CHO is often mistakenly considered the preferred energy source for all types of activity. Muscle glycogen is a very important fuel and is probably used to some

degree in all activities lasting longer than a few seconds. However, the extent that fat or carbohydrate is used as energy depends primarily on the intensity and duration of the exercise bout.

The body's use of fat is slightly higher than the use of CHO at rest, assuming that the use of protein for energy is usually negligible. Protein can provide energy at times when CHO stores are very low, such as after very prolonged exercise or in starvation. When a person exercises mildly, up to moderate intensity (about 50 percent of maximal capacity), the extent of fat used increases, while the use of CHO decreases. At the beginning of light exercise, stored energy sources such as CHO are the most important energy sources, but later in the exercise effort, fat becomes the primary energy source. Fat is indeed the principle energy source, providing up to 75 percent of the total energy requirement after 15-30 minutes of light exercise (50 percent VO$_{2max}$, heart rate about 130 bpm).

Table 8.1 Cardiovascular Response to Acute Maximal Exercise in Healthy Young Adults

CV Parameter	Rest	Maximal Exercise
O_2 Consumption (1/min)	0.25	3.5*
O_2 Consumption (ml/kg/min)	3.5†	50.0*
Heart Rate (bpm)	72	190
Stroke Volume (ml)	70*	120*
Cardiac Output (1/min);	5*	23*
Arterial-Venous O_2 (ml%)	5	15
Blood Pressure (mm Hg)	120/80	180/80
Blood Flow to Working Muscles (1/min)	1	20
Blood Lactic Acid (mg%)	15	100
Respiratory Ventilation 1/min)	6	100*

* Female values are about 10 to 20 percent lower.
† MET.
Unit abbreviations are defined on page ■■.

Repeating exercise bouts over several months or years is called *exercise training,* and it causes changes in the way the cardiovascular system meets the oxygen requirements of the body at rest, during submaximal and maximal exercise. Possibly the most significant alteration in-duced by *aerobic training* is the ability of the heart to pump more blood with each stroke while maintaining a lower heart rate at all levels of work. CV parameters at rest and maximal exercise before and after a training program are contrasted in Table 8.2. At rest, the heart maintains a constant *cardiac output* (~5 1/min) before and after a training program. In the trained state the cardiac output is obtained with a larger stroke volume and lower heart rate than before training partly because of the myocardial *hypertrophy* and improved *contractility* induced by chronic aerobic activity.

After training, the CV adaptation to maximal exercise is characterized by an enhanced stroke volume and slight improvement in A-VO2. Blood flow to working muscles and respiratory ventilation also are increased because of consistent aerobic training. The net result is an increased *maximal oxygen consumption* (VO2max) of about 20 percent compared to before training. The ability of the body to take in and utilize oxygen during maximal work may be the single best measure of overall cardiorespiratory fitness. Numerous tests have been developed to estimate VO2max.

Aerobic exercise may also help relieve tension, promote psychological well-being and self-concept, and improve productivity. Some information from epidemiological research indicates that aerobic exercise training

From moderate to heavy exercise, the use of CHO increases with the exercise intensity, while the use of fat is decreased as the work gets harder. Fat and CHO are used equally for energy at exercise heart rates around 150 bpm. In high intensity exercise, lactic acid from anaerobic CHO metabolism inhibits fat utilization. In maximal exercise CHO provides nearly 100 percent of the required energy if stored ATP and other supplies are depleted.

Another factor that is a critical determinent of energy utilization is exercise duration. Very little fat is used for energy during the initial 15 minutes of exercise. After 20 minutes, fat begins to be burned and contributes an increasingly greater proportion of the energy as exercise is prolonged. Trained individuals use more fat for energy during exercise than untrained individuals do. Individuals who are *endurance* trained, such as marathon runners utilize more fat during prolonged exercise and conserve limited CHO energy. Exercise in hot temperatures stimulates greater use of CHO, while work in the cold causes a greater use of fat than would occur in a temperate environment. Diet also affects the energy type employed during exercise. Increased dietary fat intake enhances the utilization of fat during exercise, while diets high in CHO stimulate the use of CHO. This phenomenon probably relates to the availability of these substrates for muscular use as they are carried in the blood after digestion and absorption.

When exercise ends, the body's increased metabolic rate does not stop immediately, but gradually slows down. This *recovery energy* use can be very small and last only a few minutes or may be large and continue for several hours after exercise. Recovery energy is especially high after prolonged, high intensity exercise. Even following moderate exercise for 45 to 60 minutes, recovery may continue for as long as 12 hours and account for an additional 100 kilocalories of burned energy. In contrast, if you walk at low intensity for 20 minutes, recovery energy may be only 2-3 kilocalories.

Table 8.2 Cardiovascular Adaptations to Aerobic Exercise Training: Maximal Exercise

CV Parameter	Maximal Exercise	
	Before Training	After Training*
O₂ Consumption (1/min)	3.5†	4.4†
O₂ Consumption (ml/kg/min)	50†	60†
Heart Rate (bpm)	190	188
Stroke Volume (ml)	120†	150†
Cardiac Output (1/min)	23†	28†
Arterial-Venous O₂ (ml%)	15	16
Blood Pressure	180/80	190/80
Blood Flow to Working Muscles (1/min)	20†	25†
Blood Lactic Acid (mg%)	100	150
Respiratory Ventilation (1/min)	100†	120†
Heart Size		increased
Myocardial Thickness		increased
Myocardial Contractility		increased
Myocardial Capillary Supply		increased

* Before and after one year of aerobic training.
† Female values are 10 to 20 percent lower.

may improve *longevity*. This hypothesis does, however need further research. It may take several decades, when the participants of the current aerobic fitness boom reach old age, before the effect of chronic activity on longevity can be determined. In the meantime exercisers can take heart (no pun intended) because research evidence suggests that they have healthier, more productive lives than nonexercisers. Chronic exercisers have fewer absences, less time in the hospital, and fewer illnesses than sedentary populations.

EXERCISE AND CARDIOVASCULAR FITNESS

A physically active lifestyle is a key component in CV health. But some types of exercise are better for the heart than others (see Table 8.3). CV activity is aerobic and causes the heart to work moderately for a prolonged period of time. Anaerobic activities are not as effective as aerobic in producing beneficial CV adaptation. Sometimes these short-burst activities can be detrimental to the heart.

Many of the cardiovascular variables such as the lipid profile and body fat require an extended exercise training program (around one year) to be affected. Therefore, rapid reduction in CV disease risk cannot be expected to occur. Instead, exercise should become part of the total long-term lifestyle. The characteristics in Table 8.3 are not meant to be starting points. The CV exercise training program should progress to these goals. Any type of exercise that can meet these criteria is appropriate for CV

fitness. Any low-moderate intensity activity probably will benefit the overall health of an individual even if the activity does not meet all the CV exercise characteristics.

Cardiovascular Detraining

Exercise programs are invariably interrupted because of illness or injury, other job or family priorities, and all too often, insufficient motivation. Withdrawal from training initiates a reversal process in which benefits from exercise begin to decline. Many of the physiological and psychological gains from training recede rapidly. The rate of this decline and the amount of loss due to inactivity may depend on the fitness level of the individual. Persons who have been chronic exercisers for at least one year seem to lose fitness rather slowly. In one research study, habitual exercisers lost only 16 percent of their endurance capacity after three months of detraining. Similarly, heart function, body composition, and blood lipids show little change in exercisers following several weeks of detraining. Even after several months, detrained exercisers have much higher CV fitness levels than untrained people. Many trained individuals notice the psychological detriments of a layoff much more quickly. They recognize that something is missing from their lifestyle and report sluggishness after missing only a few exercise sessions.

On the other hand, individuals without an extensive training base seem to lose CV fitness rapidly. Following short-term training, such as a 12-week aerobic dance class, most of the fitness gains are lost in 4 weeks. This loss can be offset by *maintenance training* in which the aerobic exercise is performed only one or two days per week. This theory suggests that even periodic exercise can be helpful if some exercise sessions are missed. Fitness also may be maintained by reducing exercise duration, for example, from 40 minutes to 20 minutes, while continuing to exercise three to four times per week.

Table 8.3 Characteristics of Cardiovascular Exercise

1. Moderate Intensity: 60% maximal oxygen consumption or 75% maximal heart rate (140–160 beats per min) or 60% heart rate reserve or 12–15 RPE or 7–10 METS
2. Prolonged: At least 30 minutes of continuous activity
3. Continuous: Nonstop activity
4. Frequent: 3–5 times per week, alternate days
5. Calorific: 300–500 kcal/session; 1,200–200 kcal/week
6. Large muscle groups: Total body activity, especially the legs
7. Extended: At least one year program duration

Example activities: jogging, brisk walking, swimming, stepping, level cycling, skilled rope jumping, hiking, rowing, cross-country skiing, some types of aerobic dancing.

However, the intensity of the training must be maintained. That is, if less frequent training is performed, the target heart rate of the initial training program must be maintained in the reduced training workouts.

The key to preventing CV detraining, then, is establishing a long-term (one to two years) fitness base. In addition, maintenance exercise of once or twice per week for 30 to 40 minutes duration *or* three times per week for 15 to 20 minutes duration can prevent the loss of CV fitness. To be successful exercise must be enjoyable and convenient so it can become part of the lifestyle. But even if exercise sessions are missed, it is essential to realize that reduced aerobic exercise can help maintain CV fitness. In addition, activity sessions of even shorter duration or lower intensity may not develop CV fitness but can have other significant health benefits.

STARTING UP AND MAINTAINING ACTIVITY

Getting Ready

One of the problems associated with increasing the activity level is that it is easy to start off too rigorously, to do too much quickly. It may have taken years to get out of shape, so it is helpful to allow plenty of time to get back into shape. Perhaps what needs most to be considered early in an exercise program is personal comfort. You must really enjoy the activity being performed. You say there is no activity you enjoy? Then fitness will be a long uphill battle! Nearly everyone can find some form of movement that is enjoyable and/or relaxing, even if it is a casual walk around the block. Be open to trying new activities, new exercise equipment. You might discover just the right mode for you. But if the activity causes pain or if it is a real chore to perform, it is very likely you will not continue. All the reports about how good an activity is for you do not matter if you will not do it.

Some people find that the best way to begin an exercise program is to take a class or join a gym or health club

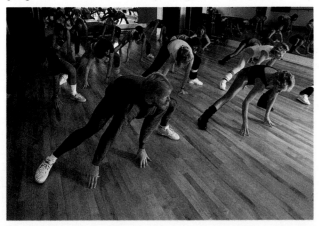

Principles of Comfortable Exercise. A list of some items to consider when exercising is presented in Table 8.4. Initiating the activity may be the hardest part of any conditioning program. If progression is too rapid, aches and pains may arise in previously unheard from places. The key to starting to exercise is to begin at a very low volume and progress slowly. How slow should you progress? Is is impossible to progress too slowly. Add to the exercise load by increasing the intensity or duration, but not both simultaneously. For example, begin with 120 to 130 exercise heart rate one week and add 5 minutes duration at 130 bpm the next week. Progress in this manner until you achieve your prescribed HR goal and target exercise duration (discussed later in this chapter). Many factors are involved in a decision to exercise, but the key is not to overdo early. The exercise must also be convenient; that is, you should feel it does not take too much away from the day's responsibilities. Therefore, exercising at the worksite, at home, or at a conveniently located fitness center usually works best.

The timing of the exercise is an important consideration. It may be uncomfortable for you to exercise in the early morning. Before breakfast, blood glucose levels are low from the long overnight fast. Although the muscles can use more fat in these early morning workouts, the brain needs glucose; this explains why the exerciser may not feel quite right. If early morning time is the most convenient, eating a light carbohydrate breakfast (e.g., one bowl of cereal or one breakfast bar) 60 to 90 minutes prior to exercise may help you feel better during the exercise. On the other hand, exercising just prior to a meal may inhibit caloric intake. *Catecholamines* (adrenalin and noradrenalin) are released during exercise, and these hormones have an inhibitory effect on appetite. They also cause arousal, and so it may be difficult to sleep after exercising.

Table 8.4 Factors for Comfortable Exercise

Factor	Behavior
starting	start at low intensities, short duration
progression	progress slow with intensity *or* duration
convenience	quick to get into and out of, easy to use equipment, showers available
time to exercise	comfortable stomach, before meals, not before sleep
clothing	proper shoes, dress for weather
warm-up	mild intensity at beginning before stretching
stretching	static (not bouncing), before and after exercise
cool-down	progressively decreasing intensity at end
breathing	natural and rhythmic, no breath holding
stitch-in-the-side	empty stomach, stretch torso, warm up

Clothing is another consideration related to comfortable exercise. Obviously, you should dress for the environment. Some general principles, nevertheless, relate to most exercise conditions. For example, proper footwear is critical, especially if the exercise is weight-bearing. Sales personnel at fitness shoe stores usually can provide advice on the shoes best suited for your feet and your activity. Socks with a high sweat-absorbing capacity (cotton blends) and a tight fit are helpful in preventing foot blisters. Cotton and polyester blends in shorts can cause friction on the legs. Loose-fitting nylon shorts are often better for activities such as jogging and walking. A cotton blend T-shirt is recommended for exercise in a temperate climate. Mesh-type shirts offer protection from the sun and allow sweat evaporation in hot weather.

Other factors associated with comfortable exercise relate to the individual exercise bouts. For example, it is important to stretch before and after an exercise session. If the activity is mild enough, for example, slow walking, it is probably advisable to stretch only after the exercise. Some exercise scientists believe it is most beneficial to stretch after the muscle has undergone a *warm-up*. Prior to a hard aerobic exercise session, it may be best to do five minutes of mild aerobic exercise, such as walking, and then stretch. Stretch again after the higher intensity portion of the exercise session.

As with warm-up, physiological systems operate more efficiently with a *cool-down* period. After vigorous exercise, the intensity should be gradually decreased. This strategy allows lactic acid to be removed more rapidly from muscle and blood. More importantly, the continued elevation of cardiac output and blood flow allows the heart to pump more blood out to the recovering muscles and up to the brain. If the exercise is stopped abruptly, blood pools in the active muscles, especially in the legs. Less blood, therefore, is available to get back to the heart and its output is diminished. The lower cardiac output results in a decreased blood flow to the muscles and heart as well as the brain. Dizziness, fainting, or even heart ischemia (lack of blood flow) could result.

Breathing during exercise should be a very natural process. The exerciser should not need to concentrate on the sequence or depth of breathing. A critical guideline related to exercise is never to hold your breath. This advice is especially important when exerting against a load, such as with push-ups, sit-ups, or weight lifting. *Breath holding* increases the pressure in the chest and decreases the amount of blood that can get into the heart, it also makes the heart push harder against this resistance. Air should always be exchanged when performing any type of exercise.

Finally, the *stitch-in-the-side* can be so painful that it causes you to avoid exercise. This pain is thought to be caused by lack of blood flow to the abdominal or respiratory muscles. The ischemia may cause metabolic by-products to accumulate and stimulate pain receptors. By ensuring that no food or stomach gas blocks flow to the

trunk area the stitch can usually be prevented. Therefore, your stomach should be relatively empty during exercise and you should avoid gas-producing meals, even for several hours prior to exercise, if you have predictable pain. In addition, you can stretch the trunk area (e.g., side bends) prior to vigorous exercise to stimulate blood flow to the stomach area. Slow progression of the intensity during the exercise bout also may help prevent the stitch. Once the pain is present, it is difficult to alleviate without completely stopping the exercise. You may even have to stretch the area throughout the day if the pain persists. Fortunately, the stitch-in-the-side represents no real physiological danger.

Determining Exercise Intensity. Monitoring exercise intensity can be valuable regardless of the goals of the exercise program. Even when performing low intensity activity, it is useful to determine the difficulty of the work. When performing moderate intensity aerobic exercise, it is even more critical to monitor the intensity because exercise at the *target heart rate (THR)* will have the most beneficial effect on the CV system. For CV exercise, the THR should be around 75 percent of maximal heart rate (HRmax). For example:

HRmax = 220 − age (yrs)
THR = HRmax × .75

EXAMPLE: HRmax = 220 − 20 yrs = 200 bpm
THR = 200 × .75 = 150 bpm
Use a range of ~5 bpm around the THR, 145–155 bpm.

The THR can also be determined by the *heart rate reserve (HRR)* method, which includes the use of resting heart rate (HRrest):

220 − 20 = 200 bpm
HRrest = 70 bpm
HRR = 200 − 70 = 130 bpm
THR = HRR × 60% + HRrest
THR = 130 × .60 + 78
THR = 148 bpm
Range = 143 − 153 bpm

The use of resting HR should be used with caution, since this variable can be easily affected by such factors as stress, previous exercise, diet, and so on.

The exercise HR should be monitored by counting the pulses at the radial artery (behind the thumb in the wrist) or counting the heartbeats with the hand over the heart. Some researchers have determined that palpating the carotid artery in the neck can slow down the HR and cause an underestimation of the actual HR. If the carotid artery must be used, apply only light fingertip pressure.

Count the beats during exercise or immediately after stopping. Quickly locate the pulse and begin counting with the number 1 and count for 6 seconds. Simply add a zero to this count. The pace can be increased or decreased to achieve the THR.

A variety of electronic HR monitoring devices are available. Most are easy to use and some relatively inexpensive. But many of these devices are movement-sensitive and do not give accurate HR measurements during exercise, especially during bouncing movements used in jogging or stepping. If you desire to obtain an accurate HR measurement *during* exercise, be sure to check whether the instrument is intended for such use.

Some individuals find it too difficult or time consuming to monitor exercise HR, and so other monitoring systems for exercise intensity have been developed. In the *MET (metabolic equivalent)* system, exercise intensity is estimated based on the metabolic cost of an activity as previously tested in a laboratory. For example, jogging at a 10 minutes per mile pace has an energy cost of about 10 mets. Tables of MET values for various activities can be found in a number of exercise science books. MET values around 7 to 10 usually provide an appropriate stimulus to the CV system for young adults.

Another practical method of monitoring exercise intensity is called the *talk test*. This technique is based on the association of lactic acid accumulation to *hyperventilation* (greatly increased breathing). This point of increased breathing is called the *ventilatory threshold*. If you are breathing so hard that talking is difficult, then the intensity is too high. Beginners should control exercise intensity so that very little hard breathing occurs. The exercise should progress just up to the point at which talking is difficult. Periodic "harder breathing" is appropriate after fitness levels are improved.

Although the talk test is a good indicator of ventilatory threshold, for more serious aerobic training, you can more accurately measure or estimate the lactate threshold. In a laboratory setting, this threshold is measured by analyzing blood lactate at several different exercise intensities. Training at the pace that produces slight lactate accumulation in blood may increase the CV and metabolic gains of the exercise. Distance athletes use this pace for their "quality" training sessions. Analysis of blood lactate is not usually possible, so other simpler estimates of this training pace have been developed. One technique uses an all-out 2-mile run. Lactate threshold pace can be estimated from the 2-mile time. Another field test estimate of lactate threshold pace was developed by Conconi in Italy. In this procedure, the athlete increases the pace of running or cycling every 200 yards up to maximal effort, and HR is measured with a watch monitor. The speeds and HRs are plotted on a graph, and the speed at which HR plateaus, or levels off, is close to the lactate threshold pace. Once this training pace is determined, it is used once or twice per week for hard training sessions.

Determining Exercise Duration. Like exercise intensity, the duration of an exercise session should be increased in small increments. To achieve CV fitness, the duration of the exercise eventually should extend from 30 to 45 minutes. The primary reason for this length is to ensure that substantial amounts of stored fat are used during the activity. In addition, prolonged exercise causes additional energy to be burned after the work in recovery. Exercise sessions of shorter durations will benefit health status, especially if the brief exercise is performed each day.

In an unfit individual, the starting duration may be very short and at a low intensity, for example, 5 minutes at a HR of 100 bpm. The intensity and duration should be increased each week, but only one at a time. Once the HR has gradually been increased to near the target zone, the duration should be increased 5 to 10 minutes each week until a duration of 30 to 45 minutes is achieved. It is acceptable to perform exercise of 20 to 30 minutes duration. However, longer exercise sessions are more beneficial and worth the extra time for the additional weight control and physical fitness that are gained.

STAYING POWER

Many of the factors that make starting exercise easier (see Table 8.4) also make it easier to sustain an activity habit. Exercise scientists use the term *adherence* (or compliance) in addressing the problem of dropout. At least half of all people who begin an exercise program stop after a few weeks. No one knows for sure why some people can stick with activity and others cannot. Enjoyment is one factor that seems to be significant. It is critical that individuals choose an activity they like. If you dislike jogging but take it up because it is "good for you," the chances of adhering to the jogging program are

Stairway to aching guards: the Dipnea begins with a 671-step stairway. And then the course gets tough.

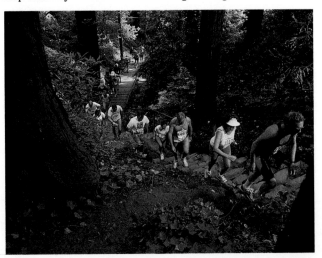

slim. It is also necessary that you feel confident about performing the chosen activity (self-efficacy). If you cannot learn an activity quickly and feel confident in performing it, try a different activity.

It may be wise to find out what you like about the exercise sessions. Is it the social aspects? If so, try to exercise with a partner or group. Is it the setting (environment)? If so, be sure the setting is pleasing to you. Is it the postexercise stretching or relaxation period? If so, be sure to allow enough time for this phase of the session.

Perhaps one of the most discouraging aspects of any exercise program is the slow and subtle payoff. Most people expect too much too quickly. It may take time for exercise to affect your metabolism, your energy level, and your weight. Yet nearly everyone who has maintained a program for at least one year has exhibited desirable effects in any number of body systems. The goal should be a lifetime change, so short-term effects cannot become a major focus. In addition, incorporation of extra activity into your set lifestyle may take time. Be ready to start again after an unexpected layoff or unmotivated time period. Even when you miss "sessions," some of the built-up benefits last a long time and will continue to improve when you get back to the activity.

▌ SPECIAL CONSIDERATIONS

For most individuals any form of movement is better than being sedentary. If a person enjoys an exercise, it may be a valuable activity even if the activity has a dangerous element. But it is helpful to recognize that some activities carry greater risks for injury and illness than others. You may want to avoid these dangers completely or be more cautious when performing a certain activity.

Exercise in Hot Weather

Hot humid weather is one of the most hazardous conditions for exercise. Several strategies can decrease the risk of running in hot weather. If the daytime temperature is higher than 85°F, exercise in the early morning or nighttime is a wise choice. Exercise in the shade will help but sometimes not provide enough protection from the heat. Exercising in an air-conditioned room is the most obvious solution to the heat problem, but this strategy is not always available, and it may increase the inconvenience of the exercise session.

If hot weather exercise is necessary, the most critical strategy is to maintain fluid intake. Large amounts of water loss during exercise in hot weather can lead to *dehydration*. Therefore, fluid replenishment is generally the most important aspect of safe and comfortable exercise in the heat. During brief exercise bouts, cold water is an appropriate replacement fluid because energy replenishment is unnecessary for such brief exercise periods.

As the sessions increase in duration, intensity, or frequency, carbohydrate (CHO) and minerals become more important in the drink. Solutions of 7 to 10 percent CHO (7 to 10 g of CHO per 100 ml of fluid) appear to be optimal for replacing fluid as well as for providing an energy source during exercise. (Most soft drinks are 11 to 12 percent CHO solutions.) As the weather cools down and the duration increases, the concentration of CHO can be increased up to 12 percent. Solutions closer to 7 percent should be used during prolonged exercise in extremely hot weather. Drinks with glucose polymers like polycose may allow greater fluid emptying from the stomach than simple sugars like glucose or sucrose. Most sport drinks now use polycose solutions. Rehydration breaks should occur approximately every 15 minutes when exercising in hot weather. Drink as much as possible during each break, but be careful that you don't drink so much as to cause stomach discomfort during the subsequent exercise.

The use of minerals in exercise drinks has been controversial. Although salt (NaCl) may inhibit water emptying from the stomach, it may stimulate water and CHO absorption from the small intestine to the bloodstream. Thus NaCl should be used in small amounts (0.5 percent solution, not salty tasting) in exercise drinks. Other minerals, such as Mg^+ and K^+, which are often found in sport drinks, also may be advantageous to fluid absorption. It is unnecessary, however, to take mineral supplement tablets except under extreme conditions such as working all day for several days in the heat. Fluid intake should be continued for several hours after exercise in hot weather because the thirst drive lags behind the actual fluid loss. Usually more fluids should be taken in than you feel is necessary; that is, overdrinking is beneficial following exercise in hot weather.

Never wear heavy or insulated clothing during physical activity in hot weather. Dress lightly in a mesh-type shirt to allow air flow next to the skin and to decrease the amount of sun radiation to the skin. A billed or brimmed cap can prevent overexposure of the face and neck to the sun.

Exercise in Cold Weather

Exercise in cold weather usually does not have the degree of danger associated with exercise in hot weather. The increased muscle metabolism keeps the core of the body warm. Heat buildup can be a major danger if heavy insulated clothing is worn. Clothing should be light enough to prevent profuse sweating, which can cause the body to cool too rapidly during recovery in the cold air and cause chills.

Exercise in cold weather has some known metabolic benefits and may be advantageous for conditioned individuals. However, outdoor activity in the cold is generally not recommended for cardiac patients or the elderly. Cold air can cause constriction of blood vessels in the skin that increases the resistance against which the heart must work. Vigorous outdoor activities such as snow shoveling increase the work of the heart. In addition, muscular straining against a heavy load (isometric work) increases the resistance in blood vessels and causes a rapid elevation in blood pressure. The rise in HR and increased vascular resistance in heavy arm exercise adds to the demands on the heart and thus the *myocardial oxygen consumption*. Expiratory strain or breath holding (Valsalva maneuver) causes abrupt increases in heart work. This increased chest pressure is magnified by a full stomach.

Cold air inhalation poses no danger for the healthy lungs and heart. The air passages in the sinuses and chest warm and moisturize the cold air to near-body conditions by the time it reaches the lungs. Any slight burning sensations in the chest are probably caused by the dryness of the cold air. Yet the inhalation of cold air may cause reflex constriction or spasms of the coronary arteries. If a person's coronary circulation is already compromised by atherosclerosis, the combination of the CV effects of the cold can have serious consequences. *Angina pectoris* (chest pain) and irregular heartbeats (arrhythmias) are more common during activity in cold weather than in warm weather.

Exercise in cold weather can be healthy and invigorating. Nevertheless, the increased demands on the CV system mean that an individual should have some degree of CV fitness before performing vigorous activities in this environment. In addition, lifting light loads and breathing throughout the movement are helpful. No muscular straining while breath holding should be performed. Large meals, caffeinated beverages, and cigarette smoking should be avoided prior to activity in cold weather. Individuals with diagnosed heart disease or with any two cardiovascular disease risk factors should avoid heavy, high intensity arm exercise in general, but especially in cold weather.

TYPES OF AEROBIC ACTIVITIES THROUGHOUT LIFE

All aerobic activities basically have two common denominators: They are prolonged and are low to moderate intensity. Characteristics of cardiovascular exercise are presented in Table 8.5. Virtually any activity that can be performed continuously for at least 30 minutes can be called aerobic. The list of potential aerobic activities is very long, but the extent that each exercise is aerobic depends on the manner in which it is performed. All types of aerobic activity are generally beneficial to the heart, but more calories are used during exercise that employs a large proportion of the muscle mass and is weight-bearing, that is, the body weight is supported by the legs, as in jogging.

Jogging/Running

Jogging and running are the most widely used types of aerobic activity. These are activities that nearly everyone can perform, and thus it is natural they initiated the fitness boom. This mode of physical activity requires more energy than most types of aerobics. One reason for the increased *caloric cost* is that a person is likely to "self-select" a relatively vigorous intensity when jogging or running. In other words, it is difficult to exercise at a mild intensity with these activities. Research studies also indicate that jogging stimulates body fat utilization better than many other activities. Jogging or running can be performed in almost any location at any time of day with little or no assistance and very little equipment. The full body weight is supported and lifted during jogging/ running, which increases energy use, but leg injuries are common. Thus it is important that proper precautions be followed. Shoes are the most critical aspect of safe, comfortable jogging. Proper running form, surface considerations, and stretching also are keys to comfortable exercise and injury prevention during jogging.

Aerobic Dance

Aerobic dance is one of the most widely used modes for organized group activity. Some of the national organizations, such as the YMCA, attract over 150,000 participants each year. Aerobic dance videos commonly are found on bestseller lists. A portion of this recent growth

Jogging is one of the most popular forms of aerobic exercise.

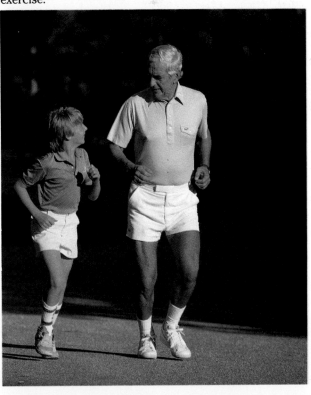

stems from the many modifications available in aerobics-to-music programs, which make such routines attractive to a greater variety of people.

Aerobic dance (or aerobic rhythms) potentially has the same benefits as jogging. It is usually weight-bearing, thereby stimulating increased energy expenditure. Major advantages of aerobic dance also include the variety of exercises performed and the social aspect of exercising with other people. Like jogging, aerobic dance can produce injuries, especially to the legs. But with proper precautions and wise shoe selection, this form of exercise can be highly effective.

The great interest in aerobic dance classes has spurred research into the effects of this activity. Generally moderate intensity classes have produced increases in maximal oxygen consumption, which is the single best measure of aerobic, or CV fitness. The extent of the improvement depends on keeping the HR in the target zone for 30 minutes, the frequency of the program, and the length of time spent in the program. Caloric expenditure and upper body muscle tone can be enhanced with the use of hand weights or wristband weights. However, this practice also can elevate blood pressure and increase the risk of injury. Therefore, limb weights should be handled with caution and probably used only periodically in the aerobic routine and only after some degree of fitness has been attained. (Table 8.5).

Besides the CV and muscular benefits, some research suggests that aerobic dance, like other forms of aerobic activity, can enhance or maintain bone mineral content. In the elderly, who are more susceptible to osteoporosis, this exercise can be especially beneficial.

Because of the great variety of activities and intensities offered with aerobic dance classes, the matching of personal goals with those of the exercise classes must be carefully considered. Some dance activities involve primarily stretching and strengthening exercise. The cardiovascular response to such routines is minor, and thus aerobic dance is not truly an aerobic activity. However, it would be an appropriate choice for individuals with primary goals of improving muscular tone and flexibility. But this routine would be inappropriate for individuals seeking improvement in CV fitness.

On the other hand, some aerobic dance routines can be too strenuous for the heart. Heart rates near maximal frequently have been recorded in aerobic dance classes. Such high intensity may help burn calories but is not beneficial for the heart. In fact, heart rates over 80 percent of maximal can be dangerous to out-of-shape or older individuals. (See guidelines for determining your personal maximal and target heart rates earlier in this chapter.)

One of the newest and most beneficial practices in aerobic dance is individualized pacing to the same music. This personalized intensity has been termed low and high impact. Basically, the intensity is controlled by the height to which the knees are lifted and the extent of the arm movement. By modifying the extent of the leg and arm actions, the target HR can be maintained, regardless of the speed or beat of the music. In addition, individuals of vastly different ages or fitness levels can exercise together to the same music. Injured individuals also may be able to perform low impact exercise without aggravating the injury or necessarily withdrawing from the program. Low impact or low effort movements are appropriate for warm-up and cool-down activities and are ideal for elderly or beginning exercisers. Utilizing the low and high impact method of movement in aerobic dance classes with different levels of participants is helpful.

WALKING

Walking is one of the fastest growing fitness activities in America. Although this is a weight-bearing activity, the impact on the legs is not as great as in jogging or aerobic dance. Still, proper form, shoes, and precautions are necessary. Walking technique should be natural and rhythmic. Very little instruction is necessary. If leg pains result from low intensity walking, the feet and the walking stride should be examined by a *podiatrist*, or foot doctor. This specialist can determine if the anatomy of the foot allows appropriate heel strike and fore-foot takeoff. Slight alterations in the shoe, such as shims and soft orthotics, may result in more comfortable and effective walking.

Walking is an excellent way to incorporate some activity into the regular daily routine. You can walk to and from work or errands, up and down stairs, or around the block with a friend. Healthy walking neither requires a fitness center nor exercise equipment.

Since the body weight is not propelled as vigorously as in jogging, injuries are less prevalent in walkers. This difference, however, also causes walkers to utilize fewer calories. Most individuals can achieve an appropriate target HR by walking. Certainly sedentary, unfit, or elderly populations may find walking to be the ideal exercise. On the other hand, as the fitness level progresses,

Table 8.5   Use of Hand/Arm Weights in Exercise

1. Use only after one month in the exercise program. Never in the beginning unless in good aerobic condition.
2. Use no more than 2-pound weights on each wrist or hand.
3. Do not use weights on upper arms or legs.
4. Use only periodically during the aerobic exercise period.
5. Do not hold weighted hands over the head, as it increases the strain on the heart.
6. Avoid firm grasping of the weight. It is best if the weight can be attached to the limb. Tight grasping is an isometric contraction that can elevate blood pressure.

the target HR is more difficult to achieve by walking. In one study only about half of fit middle-aged males could achieve their target HR, even when they were walking as fast as possible.

Research studies indicate that walking burns as many calories as jogging at speeds above 5 mph. While this speed is not achievable by most walkers, it is possible to increase the caloric cost of walking by speeding up the pace. On the other hand, individuals who use a "self-selected" comfortable walking pace burn only about half the calories as individuals who use a self-selected comfortable jogging pace. But the slower walking pace may have greater relaxation value. At an "easy" pace, a walker uses a little more than half the body weight (in kcal) per mile, while a jogger uses a little less than the total body weight per mile. For example, a 150-pound person uses about 85 kcal per mile when walking and about 140 kcal per mile when jogging. The caloric expenditure of walking increases closer to that of slow jogging if the individual "walks as fast as possible."

Another method of increasing exercise intensity is to use hand, wrist, or ankle weights while walking. In addition, the arm swing can be exaggerated to increase the involvement of the upper body muscles. Adding weights of 3 pounds on each arm and exaggerating the arm swing can nearly double the caloric cost of walking. The added arm involvement also enhances upper body muscle tone. Blood pressure elevation caused by the limb weights is the major disadvantage. (See Table 8.1 for other possible problems.) Therefore, a conservative recommendation is to use 1 to 2 pounds per limb and move the hands no higher than shoulder height. This strategy will increase calorie burning during walking by about 20 percent. In walking, the use of ankle weights causes stride changes that could cause leg muscle soreness or injury. The advantage of burning extra calories when using weights must be weighed against some increased risks.

Stair Climbing/Stepping

Walking or running stairs has been a popular method of training athletes and is frequently used in home exercise programs. Until recently, this mode was limited by access to appropriate stairways. Recently, equipment manufacturers have developed portable in-home stair-climbing devices. The exercise devices are actually stairway treadmills, and the movements involved are a little like going up a down escalator. The foot impact forces are lower than in jogging, but the caloric cost is still high. A handrail can be used, or the caloric use can be increased by swinging the arms during the exercise. This activity is an excellent alternative to jogging to periodically reduce the impact forces on the legs.

Other climbing devices called steppers have a slightly different action than the stairs. Some steppers are more like climbing devices and offer adjustable resistance for both the legs and arms. For those steppers that do not provide resistance for the arms, the upper body can be used by swinging the arms during the stepping activity. Jarring of the legs is minimal with stepping exercise. At high resistance settings, the climbing machine also can be used as a strength exercise for the upper and lower body. At low resistance settings, a beginner can perform this type of exercise. By increasing the resistance and repetition rates on the steppers, the energy expenditure can be very large. Such high intensity exercise should be reserved for fit individuals. This type of equipment can provide excellent diversity and overload for those individuals with training experience. Because of the large muscle mass involvement and the potentially vigorous arm action, it is recommended that HR be monitored on these mechanical stairs and steppers.

Cross-Country Skiing

The cardiovascular and muscular benefits of cross-country skiing have been known for many years. Scandinavian skiers have exhibited some of the highest maximal oxygen consumption values on record. Until recently, snow skiing was reserved for individuals living in cold climates. But now exercise machines are available that simulate cross-country skiing. This type of activity provides excellent total body muscle utilization. Energy expenditure generally is high during skiing exercise because it is weight-bearing and upper and lower body muscles are used. Another caloric advantage of the ski simulator is that individuals self-select a fairly high intensity on the activity. It is difficult to select a mild pace on this total body exercise. In addition, the jarring associated with jogging/running activities is reduced. The adjustable resistances should be kept low for beginners (especially the arm resistance), but they can be increased as fitness level increases. While a person may need patience when learning to use the ski simulator, the results are generally worth the effort. As with all vigorous aerobic exercise, HR should be monitored. Instead of stopping to count pulses, it is more effective as well as safer to use an accurate HR monitor that is not movement-sensitive so that HR can be assessed during the exercise.

Cycling

Like most forms of aerobic activity, cycling with a regular bicycle or stationary cycle is an effective form of CV conditioning. Many people prefer the outdoor scenery associated with bicycling. In addition, this mode of exercise can serve as an inexpensive means of transportation. For some, indoor cycling is more feasible, and the stationary cycle provides an effective mode of aerobic exercise. If the target HR is maintained, then indoor and outdoor cycling will produce similar CV benefits. Since cycling is nonweight-bearing, the caloric expenditure is often less than some other forms of aerobic exercise.

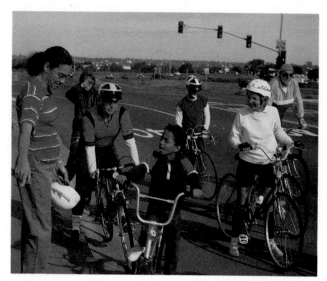
Cycling is a healthful activity for people of all ages.

However, joint and muscle trauma are much less than in typical weight-bearing exercise. Most cycles provide exercise primarily for the legs, but a few of the stationary cycles provide arm exercises as well. Implementing arm exercises with cycling not only enhances energy expenditure, it also increases the effect on upper body muscle tone.

As in all CV exercise, the age-adjusted target HR should be maintained for at least 30 minutes. Most cycles provide easily adjustable leg workloads, permitting control of the HR within a narrow target zone.

Research studies suggest that when you use your arms, upper body exercise should contribute only a small percentage to the total work load. In this way, the larger muscles of the legs do most of the work. Utilizing too much arm musculature in the exercise can increase HR and blood pressure above appropriate aerobic exercise levels. To calculate the exercise work load, you first perform comfortable exercise using only the legs with the exercise HR in the low range of the target zone. Note the work load on the dial, add 10 to 20 percent to the work, and use the arms until this additional work load is achieved. Recheck HR to be sure it is in the target zone. In general, the use of the arms should add no more than 10 to 15 bpm to the legs-only HR.

Rowing

Like cycling, rowing is a nonweight-bearing exercise; therefore it is easier on joints and uses less calories than some other aerobic activities. Rowing stresses the use of the upper torso and arms, although the legs also are utilized. The combination of upper and lower body exercise is a definite advantage. Upper body tone can be an expected benefit. The arm rowing movement primarily involves the biceps, brachioradialis, and brachialis muscles of the upper arm and the trapezius and other muscles of the upper back. On some rowing instruments, the

upper body position can be reversed so that the triceps in back of the arm and pectoral muscles of the chest also can be exercised.

In using the rower, resistance on the arms should be relatively low. Remember that the upper body should contribute only 10 to 20 percent of the total work when both arms and legs are used in exercise. Thus the lower body exercise should be emphasized unless specific goals include more enhanced arm development. Vigorous arm work can be especially unwise in middle-aged individuals just beginning an exercise program. Vigorous upper body exercise is also generally not recommended for individuals with cardiovascular disease.

One disadvantage of most rowers is that the resistance can only be adjusted for the arms; the leg resistance cannot be altered. If the arm resistance is increased very high, then the arms will contribute beyond the acceptable 20 percent of the total work. The NordicRow offers a unique rower with leg as well as arm adjustable resistance. These adjustments allow the work load to be increased at the legs while remaining lower at the arms. Resistance exercises also can be performed separately on arms or legs.

Swimming

Swimming has been called the most complete form of exercise. The diverse movements in the water involve flexibility, strength, and aerobic exercises. Moreover, moving in cool water if often refreshing and relaxing. Swimming is one exercise where fatness can make the exercise easier. Unlike muscle, the fat tissue is less dense than water, and it therefore floats. Since heavier individuals do not have to work as hard to prevent sinking, it is easier to propel the body through the water. This advantage also provides a disadvantage—heavy people use less calories than lean people when swimming.

Since the body is supported by water, the risk of joint

Some people consider swimming to be the most complete form of aerobic exercise.

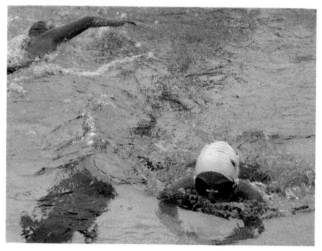

and muscle injury is very low in aerobic swimming. For many years, athletes and racehorses have used water exercises as a means of continuing to exercise when injured. Water activity is also recommended for arthritis and cardiac patients. This mode of exercise may be the least traumatic exercise for joints and muscles of all aerobic activities.

But swimming exercise is not necessarily easy. Swimming can elicit appropriate target HRs and caloric expenditure; however, some research suggests that the exercise target HR should be 10 to 15 beats lower than other aerobic exercise. The horizontal position allows more blood to return to the heart, which increases stroke volume. This increased output with each heartbeat means fewer beats to pump blood out of the heart to the working muscles. The cool water also has a HR lowering effect. One of the ways of judging the potential benefits to the CV system of various exercises is to compare the oxygen pulse (Table 8.6), which is the ratio of total body oxygen consumption (energy used) to HR expressed as milliliters of oxygen per beat. [It is beneficial for total body oxygen consumption to be high while HR is relatively low thus working relatively easy to provide the oxygen to support a relatively high total body work load.] Swimming exercise is associated with a high oxygen pulse because of the relatively high oxygen consumption at a relatively low HR. Swimming, then, is an excellent exercise for improving CV fitness.

Exercise intensity can be varied by stroke and by speed. It is usually best to use both arms and legs together in a swimming workout. Since the resistance of the water on the arms is relatively low, it is unlikely that the arm exercise will be too strenuous for the CV system. The rate of swimming strokes should be varied so that the target HR is maintained for at least 30 minutes. Lap swimming is the easiest way to ensure that swimming is aerobic.

Table 8.6 Oxygen Pulse of Various Activities

Activity	O_2 Pulse (ml/beat)
Swimming	16.0
Jogging	15.0
Walking with Hand Weights	14.5
Walking	14.0
Ski Simulator	14.0
Low-Sit Cycling	13.0
Cycling	12.5
Rowing	12.5
Stepping	12.5
Aerobic Dance	11.5
Circuit Resistance Training	10.5
Racquetball	10.0
Weight Lifting	8.0

NOTE: Values are derived from exercise at the same moderate heart rate (~130 bpm).

Water aerobics offers an excellent alternative to land aerobics. These exercises offer the intensity of land aerobics without the high impact forces on the legs. And, the water offers the potential for greater arm resistance than the air on land, thus providing added upper body benefit.

Circuit Resistance Training

Many different forms of exercise can be performed at moderate intensity and maintained continuously for at least 30 minutes. They can, therefore, be considered aerobic. One mode that is gaining increasing acceptance as an effective fitness activity is *circuit resistance training* (CRT). This type of resistance training is described in

Promoting Your Health

Caloric Cost of Various Aerobic Activities

Activity	Cal/hour*		
Running 6 min/mi	1100	Cycling and arm work	480
Cross-country skiing	725	Cycling 10 mph	400
Jogging 10 min/mi	710	Aerobic dance (low impact)	360
Rope jumping 75 skips/min	650	Walking 17 min/mi	325
Stepping	650		
Rowing	600		
Swimming 40 yds/min	500		
Aerobic dance (moderate)	480		

* Estimates for a 150-pound (68-kilogram) man or woman at a typical pace. Caloric costs are increased or decreased depending on the body weight, terrain, surface, wind, and so on.

Chapter 9. By using relatively light resistance and greater repetitions than traditional weight training, CRT can benefit both the muscular and the CV systems. Another key to the aerobic nature of this activity is the limited rest period (15 to 30 seconds) between exercises. With these limited rest periods and lighter loads, the HR can be maintained within the appropriate CV target zone. CRT is especially useful in maintaining CV fitness and in providing a combination of muscular strength and CV fitness aspects in a program.

While all aerobic activities benefit the CV system, the energy expenditure may be very different for various activities. Therefore, some aerobic exercises will be more effective than others if weight loss is a primary goal. The box entitled "Promoting Your Health" presents a list of caloric costs of various aerobic activities.

▌ OTHER HEALTHY ACTIVITIES

Some activities may be too mild to be classified as effective aerobic or CV exercise. In golf, low intensity walking on the fairways can be beneficial, but this walking is interrupted by the golf swing and the anxious process of searching for a lost ball. Or worse, an electric cart is used, and most of the benefits of this sport are lost. Walking with a push golf cart is the best way to reap the health benefits of this activity. Other games, such as bowling, are so physically mild that they do not tax the CV system enough to improve CV fitness. But they have other healthy effects.

Hunting and fishing are other activities that often are not associated with vigorous effort. The intensity of these activities varies greatly and ranges from the restful watching of the baited fishing line to the maximal effort of dragging decoys and equipment through a muddy marsh. Recent studies on deer hunting in Michigan indicate that the HRs can be very high when stalking and shooting at a deer. In addition, the risk of irregular heartbeats increases due to the excitement of the hunt. Thus hunters should participate in CV fitness exercises prior to the hunting season, and individuals with CV disease should be cautious about the type of hunting and fishing undertaken.

Even though many of these sports and games may not promote large increases in CV fitness, they, along with other activities, can be good for the body. Even routine daily movement can be beneficial to many of the body's systems. Take advantage of opportunities to move around rather than sit. One key to lifelong good health may be your willingness to avoid being sedentary. Mild everyday activities such as housekeeping, walking on errands, and walking stairs may be all the activity necessary to keep you healthy if these tasks are performed frequently.

One strategy for increasing your activity level is to "manufacture activity"; that is, purposefully put yourself in situations that require you to be active. For example, get a pet so that you will be motivated to play with it or walk with it. Maintain a large lawn or mow it more frequently. Plant a flower or vegetable garden to provide motivation to get out and move. Plant trees or bushes and maintain them. Clean the house or the car more often and at a more rapid pace. The list of "work activity" is unending. The motivation for movement may come from active hobbies or from actual work. In either case, this active lifestyle will promote feelings of accomplishment as well as help you improve your health status.

An optimal lifestyle strategy might be to combine healthy activities with fitness activities. It is very beneficial to incorporate some moderate CV exercise in your lifestyle. Thus gardening, cleaning, or golfing can be performed four times per week, and aerobic dance or swimming performed twice per week. It may be necessary to alternate weight-bearing activity with nonweight-bearing activity to decrease the strain on your legs.

Individuals who feel that the intensity and time commitment for any aerobic training are too great can still profit from consistent, low intensity brief activity, especially if it is performed every day. These benefits possibly relate to the relaxing effect of participating in the activity as well as to the physiological adaptations caused by consistently repeating the activity. Therefore, the key criterion for selecting an activity, as indicated, is *enjoyment*. Find something that you like enough to do every day or alternate two enjoyable activities. Exercise has no health value if you dislike it so much that you drop out. Although not all exercise will enhance aerobic capacity, virtually any low intensity, nonstressful activity will enhance health and decrease your risk of disease and death.

9

Muscular Strength: A Key Element of Total Fitness

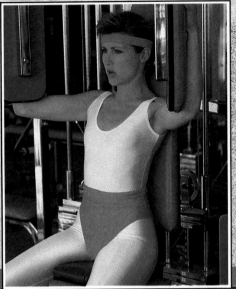

▪ Chapter Outline

- Types of Muscular Contraction
- Methods of Providing Resistance.
- Resistance Training
- Games and Sports

▪ Objectives

- Identify and describe the types of muscular contraction.

- Describe the methods of providing external resistance for muscular exercise.

- Describe the various resistance training programs, including how they work and who should use them.

- Summarize the health and fitness benefits of engaging in sports and games.

The term *total fitness* has a variety of definitions and interpretations. Most people tend to consider muscular strength and tone a part of total fitness. Although exercise scientists agree that aerobic training is the most important component of a fitness program, since the health of the heart, lungs, and blood vessels are so critical to total health, aerobic training alone may not produce adequate muscular function to perform many daily activities efficiently. Movements such as opening a stuck door or lifting a heavy box can cause injury to muscles unused to exerting such force. Although aerobic training improves the function of the muscle groups used in the exercise, it generally does not affect other muscles. Since most aerobic activities rely on the leg muscles, these exercises may not stimulate improvements in upper body strength. Therefore, muscular resistance training must be used to supplement the aerobic program, especially relative to the upper body.

TYPES OF MUSCULAR CONTRACTION

Muscular contractions can be divided into two basic types: (1) **static** or *isometric* in which the internal muscular tension is equal to the external resistance and no movement occurs and (2) **dynamic,** in which muscular tension produces movement. Dynamic contractions in which the internal muscular tension is greater than the external resistance is called *concentric*. In this type of contraction, the muscle shortens and the associated bones move toward each other. In *eccentric* contractions, the internal muscular tension is less than the external resistance, and the bones move apart. The muscle is "stronger" when contracting eccentrically, and it can handle more weight in this "negative" movement than in the "positive" concentric contraction.

The understanding of concentric and eccentric contractions is necessary in exercising properly to strengthen specific muscles. For example, in the sit-up, the same muscle groups are involved in both the up phase and the down phase of the exercise.

Another type of dynamic contraction is *isokinetic,* in which the muscle moves at a specific controlled speed. This type of contraction requires an external device to alter resistance so that the speed of contraction is the same throughout the range of movement. This type of contraction may be important in exercising the muscle at high speeds, which approximate those used during physical activity and sports performance.

Parts of this chapter were adapted from T.R. Thomas, *Muscular Fitness through Resistance Training.* Dubuque:eddie bowers, 1991. Adapted with permission from the publisher.

METHODS OF PROVIDING RESISTANCE

Nearly any type of muscular activity may be beneficial in developing or maintaining the fitness of muscle. Simply raising your arms over the head can have a positive effect on the muscles involved in the movement. In raising the arms over the head, the weight of the hand and arm provide the resistance for the muscles. But improvement in muscular strength and performance, generally requires a method of providing a greater overload resistance to stimulate the muscle to produce greater forces.

Just as there are many kinds of muscular contractions, there are a variety of ways of providing external resistance for muscular exercise. Currently, the study of resistance devices is one of the most dynamic aspects of the fitness boom era. Major equipment manufacturers are spending millions of dollars to develop new resistance machines. The goal of this investment is to make instruments that provide the most appropriate type of resis-

Static Muscular Contractions Muscular contractions in which internal muscular tension equals the external resistance, resulting in no movement.

Dynamic Muscular Contractions Muscular contractions in which muscular tension produces movement.

The use of resistance devices has become an essential feature of the fitness boom.

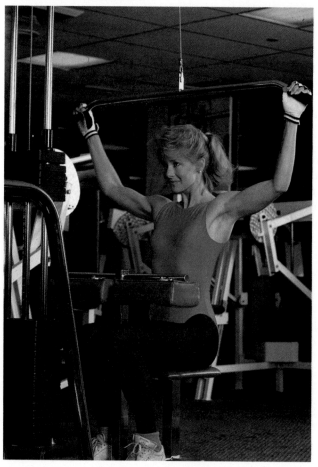

tance for the muscle. Unfortunately, the type of resistance that is actually best for training muscle is unknown. This is an area that is being vigorously researched by exercise physiologists in the United States and other countries.

Static Resistance

When resistance is so strong that your muscles can't move the object, it is termed **static**, or **isometric**. These terms indicate that the load is so heavy, the muscle cannot move it, and thus the muscle length remains the same during the contraction. Because static resistance provides the muscle with stress only at a specific point in the range of motion, strength increases are "angle specific." That is, the strength gained occurs in a very limited area of the working range. If an individual attempted to lift a heavy desk by flexing the biceps muscle, for example, the strength gain would be limited to the arm angle at which the contraction was performed. The elbow angle obviously could be changed several times, which would allow the muscle to be worked through the range. Such changes require a very long workout period for each muscle and generally are not feasible. Regardless, such exercises would have little relevance to the way the muscle is actually used during activity. Few activities employ static muscular contraction.

Another disadvantage of using static resistance is the relatively large increase in blood pressure during the exercise. In addition, the pressure in the chest, called **intrathoracic** pressure, can be elevated. Both of these effects diminish the heart's ability to pump blood to the working muscles and to other organs such as the brain. These effects can be especially dangerous in older individuals. Static or isometric resistance training programs are not recommended for most people. Many better ways exist for providing resistance to the muscle.

Static exercise can be used for brief time periods by young adults when other resistance exercises are unavailable (e.g., when on vacation). In addition, isometric instruments can help test muscular strength. The cable tensiometer, hand grip, and back dynamometers are examples of such testing instruments.

Isotonic Resistance

Isotonic methods are the traditional types of weight lifting. These include the standard free-weight barbell and dumbbell as well as some weight-lifting machines. Isotonic resistance provides a constant load on the muscle throughout the entire range of motion. The muscle must contract with both concentric and eccentric dynamic contractions to raise and lower the weight, respectively. If the isotonic exercise is performed correctly, the muscle is stressed throughout its complete contraction range. *Constant resistance* exercises do not tax each joint angle equally. The skeletal lever system causes the muscle to be stronger at certain angles. Therefore, at points where the muscle is strongest, the weight will tax it less than at points where the muscle is weakest. For example, in the biceps curl, a 100-pound barbell might cause the muscle to develop maximal tension at 180° and 45° joint angles (beginning and end of the lift). But at 100° joint angle (middle of the lift), the muscle is not taxed as much. This constant resistance technique may cause some points in the range of motion to develop greater strength gains than others. Such selective improvement may be beneficial because the weaker points might catch up to the stronger points in the contraction range. On the other hand, constant resistance training may be a disadvantage, since the strongest points in the range may not develop to their full capacity.

Momentum or inertia of the weight also is altered from the start of the lift to the end, which changes the load felt by the muscle through the range of motion. In an attempt to lessen the effect of momentum, free-weight exercise is traditionally performed at slow speeds. Some of the variable resistance and isokinetic machines that do not use weight stacks have eliminated the effect of inertia on the resistance.

Barbell free weights require both the dominant and nondominant limbs to share the load equally. Thus muscular balance between the two sides of the body is better maintained. Moreover, free-weight lifting requires balancing the bar in many directions, not just in the direction of the lift. This versatility may require additional beneficial muscular activity during the exercise.

These potential advantages of free weights are countered by the greater skill required to perform free-weight exercises than machine exercises. Increased danger of losing control and even dropping the weights are risks for the novice. A partner also is required for spotting on some lifts. Because of these potential problems, use of free-weight constant resistance exercises require appropriate training and supervision. Heavy free-weight lifting is recommended only for experienced weight lifters and power athletes whose primary goals consist of maximizing muscular bulk and muscular strength balance.

Variable Resistance

The newest and commercially most competitive area of resistance equipment can be formed in the development of variable resistance machines. With this equipment, resistance is altered throughout the range of motion in an attempt to match the changing capabilities of muscle at different joint angles. Many techniques have been devised to alter resistance during the range of motion. One method uses a pulley cord moving around an irregularly shaped cam; thus the resistance arm distance is altered, and the resistance felt by the muscle is changed

---

Static (isometric) Resistance   Resistance so powerful that muscular force cannot move an object.
Intrathoracic Pressure   The blood pressure in the chest.

throughout its range of motion. Another system mechanically alters the load by physically moving the weights to change the resistance arm length. Such a system causes the resistance to increase continually throughout the concentric phase of the range of motion and decrease during the eccentric phase. These are *linear resistance* changes.

Other examples of innovative mechanisms that produce variable resistance include resistance bands or weight straps. As these straps are stretched through the concentric range of motion, the resistance is increased. In other strength equipment, muscular movement causes an enginelike piston to compress air or fluid in a pneumatic cylinder, thus increasing the resistance through the range of motion.

Additional variable resistance systems are being developed at a rapid pace. Each has a different mechanism that attempts to match resistance with muscular function. The success of these strategies may depend on how well an individual's strength curve of a given muscle matches the specific resistance curve of the machine.

Isokinetic Resistance

Another kind of muscular training that uses a form of variable resistance is isokinetic exercises. In this *same speed* technique, the movement speed is set on a dial. This speed setting is the key distinguishing characteristic of true isokinetic equipment. Speed of the instrument is selected and not the amount of resistance. The machine allows the movement to proceed no faster than the set speed no matter how much tension is produced in the contracting muscle. Thus, an exact resistance can be matched to the force capabilities of the muscle. If a maximal effort is attempted at all joint angles, the machine resistance is maximal at all joint angles. The advantage of such a machine is it can tax the muscle maximally throughout the range of motion. Isokinetic resistance training involves no eccentric contraction, only concentric. This limitation may be an advantage, since eccentric movements have been associated with muscular soreness. Yet the lack of eccentric training also may be a disadvantage because most sports activities require eccentric contractions. For example, the rapid bending of the knees to lower the torso in making a tennis stroke and in gathering for a jump shot or spike require eccentric contractions of the quadriceps muscles.

Isokinetic devices are valuable for muscular function testing. The major advantage of isokinetic testing is it permits the study of muscle function at various angles and in a range of motion as well as high speeds.

Although certain systems of strength equipment seem to have a theoretical advantage, very little research has examined their comparative muscular strength and resistance matchups. Current scientific findings do not support the use of any one type of resistance mechanism. Instead, all systems seem to improve muscular strength. The development of various training devices seems beneficial, since nearly anyone interested in muscular training can find equipment suitable. The selection of one resistance system over another may relate to the specific skill of an individual. For example, machines generally are easier and safer to use than free weights and are more suited to beginning lifters.

Body Weight Exercises

Many techniques can be utilized to develop skeletal muscle fitness without the use of weight equipment. Most of these methods rely on part or all of the body weight to provide the resistance during the exercise. While these techniques may not be as effective as machine training in developing maximal muscular strength and bulk, they are very adequate in improving general muscular fitness.

Many common exercises require the muscles to lift the body weight off the floor. These activities require dynamic muscular contractions, both concentric and eccentric. The sit-up, push-up, and pull-up are examples of these activities. Running or jumping also are body weight-lifting exercises that stress specific muscles and can be used to improve muscular fitness. One limitation to such activities can be the difficulty in exercising opposite muscle groups to maintain muscular balance (e.g., quadriceps and hamstrings).

Body weight activities generally are sufficient to maintain muscular strength and improve muscular tone. With the addition of weights to the body or by increasing the resistance with a partner, substantial strength improvements may be observed.

Sit-ups are a popular body weight exercise.

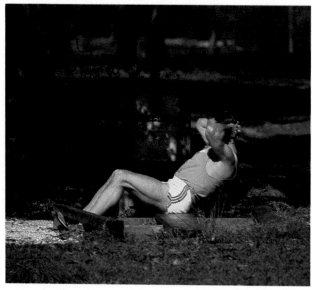

RESISTANCE TRAINING PROGRAMS

Some general principles are important regardless of the goals of the resistance training. Strategies used in the resistance training sessions may, however, vary according to the specific goal of the individual.

Resistance Workout Terms

In traditional weight-training terms, a *repetition (rep)* is moving the resistance through one complete range of motion and returning to the starting position (Table 9.1). The amount of resistance or weight that requires a single maximal contraction is called a one repetition maximum (1 RM). This feat indicates the maximal strength of a specific muscle or group of muscles. The amount of resistance that can be lifted only twice is called a 2 RM, and so on. A training *set* is a single series of multiple repetitions. For example, an individual may perform a 6 RM exercise in each of two sets for a total of 12 repetitions.

Strength Training

Strength is best increased by exerting near maximal forces a few times each workout, that is, high resistance, low repetition exercises. Typically the resistance is 70 to 85 percent of 1 RM, with four to eight repetitions to failure (4 to 8 RM). Early research using untrained men and traditional free-weight training indicated that three sets of six RM on alternative days produced the greatest increments in dynamic strength. Some research evidence suggests that three sets are optimal and five sets produce no greater increase in strength. *Supercompensation*, the

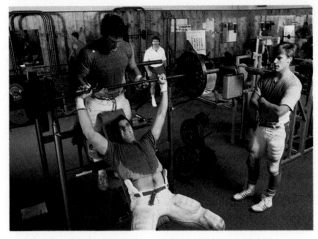

The best strength training program consists of high resistance, low repetition exercises.

muscular rebuilding process, probably requires 24 to 48 hours. This process is longer after more intense, heavy exercise than after light lifting. Supercompensation may take less time in well-trained individuals. The time necessary for muscular rebuilding, therefore, dictates that alternate-day workouts using the same muscle group are probably more effective than working the same muscle group each day. Since most research dealing with dynamic strength training has utilized untrained men, it is unknown if the repetitions, sets, and frequency principles apply to well-trained individuals. Athletes and coaches have sometimes questioned the results of research that used nonathletes. Indeed, strength training research has not always produced results observed by ardent weight lifters. Athletes and other experienced lifters use a variety of heavy resistance programs, apparently with good success. This supports the concept that maximal motor unit recruitment, regardless of the techniques, is a key to muscular strength gains.

Lifting speed does not seem to be a significant factor in the development of muscular strength. When using weights, fast speeds should not be attempted due to the risk of injury and the increased use of momentum in the exercise, which tends to reduce the tension required by the muscle. Similarly, the time between sets does not appear critical to the amount of strength gains. Usually experienced lifters employ trial and error to determine the rest period. Rests of 1 to 3 minutes have been suggested for heavy resistance training.

Heavy resistance training is not inappropriate for most individuals with fitness goals. Adequate strength gains can be achieved with lighter loads and greater repetitions. Even if the goal is to improve performance in recreational sports, a lighter load strength program will be effective. An individual interested in general muscular fitness, sports performance, or muscular tone should employ a "scaled down" strength program of 3 sets of 12 repetitions, using a 15 RM load (about 65 percent of 1 RM) (Table 9.2). In other words, use 12 reps of a

Table 9.1 Resistance Training Workout Terminology

Term	Definition
repetition (rep)	Moving a resistance through one complete range of motion and returning.
one repetition maximum (1 RM)	The amount of resistance that can be moved only one time through the range of motion and returned.
set	A single series of repetitions.
rest period	The time between sets.
work period	The time during which the repetitions are performed.

Table 9.2 Resistance Training Programs

	Resistance Training Goal		
	Strength	Muscular Tone	CV Fitness
Load (% of 1 RM)	65–75	50–60	40–60
Repetitions (number)	10–12	12–20	12–15
Sets (number/exercise)	3	6–10	1–2
Exercises or Stations (number/workout)	10–12	10–12	6–8
Rest Periods (seconds)	120–180	60–90	10–20
Frequency (days/week/ muscle group)	2–3	2–3	3–4

resistance that can be handled for 15 reps. This strategy illustrates a key principle that works for most people: Do not lift to failure. Other principles related to strength resistance training are listed in the box entitled, "Promoting Your Health: Tips for Effective Resistance Training."

Strength Training Phases. In general, heavy loads and few repetitions are utilized to build strength. Also part of this system is *pyramiding,* in which loads are progressively increased during the exercise period. Loads also are pyramided over a given time period in the program. The training regimen uses cycling, or *periodization,* in which the exercise intensity is varied from workout to workout and over set time periods to avoid staleness and training plateaus. Each major muscle group is exercised two times per week, once heavy and once medium. At least two days of rest is taken between sessions using the same muscle groups. The chest and legs are exercised on Monday (heavy) and Thursday (medium), and the back, shoulders, and arms on Tuesday (heavy) and Friday (medium).

A simpler program can be performed by young athletes or adults participating in sports that do not necessarily require maximal strength efforts. In this simpler system three sets of six repetitons (6 RM) are used for each muscle group and all body parts three times per week (alternate days). It is important that the muscles associated with the sport be emphasized and muscular balance maintained. This program is extremely effective in producing strength and hypertrophy gains in previously untrained young adults.

A program similar in intensity to the Epley system can be used for any sport requiring maximal muscular strength and power. Such intense training generally is reserved for high-level competitive athletics and is especially effective in power sports such as football, basketball, volleyball, and track and field. This high intensity program is not necessary or recommended for the recreational athlete.

The cycling "phases" progress from light to maximum intensity:

Promoting Your Health

Tips for Effective Resistance Training

1. Move the resistance through the *full range of motion.*
2. Breathe during each phase of the lift to prevent large increases of intrathoracic pressure.
3. Know the muscle(s) affected by the exercise.
4. Exercise antagonistic muscles to avoid imbalance. For example, quadricep exercises should be accompanied by hamstring exercises and pectoralis exercises accompanied by exercises using the upper back muscles such as the infraspinatus, posterior deltoid, and teres minor.
5. Stretch the active muscle and joints *before and after* exercise to prevent loss of flexibility.
6. Warm up with calisthenics and light lifting before the workout. Cool down with similar light exercises after the workout.
7. Do not exercise just after eating.
8. Do not use the same muscle in sequential exercises. For example, do not perform the shoulder press and bench press in sequence because both use the triceps extensively.
9. Heavy lifting (75 to 100 percent of maximum) is reserved for competitive athletes and weight lifters.
10. After their competitive careers, athletes need to reduce resistance training loads and intensity.

Phase 1
　　10 reps
　　3 sets
　　1st set 65 percent of 1 RM
　　2nd set 70 percent
　　3rd set 75 percent
　　1–2 minutes rest between exercises
　　1–2 week duration

Phase 2
　　8 reps
　　4 sets
　　1st set 65 percent
　　2nd set of 70 percent
　　3rd set 75 percent
　　4th set 75 percent
　　2 minutes rest between exercises
　　1–2 week duration
　　reduce loads by 5 percent on medium days, for
　　example, 1st set = 60 percent of 1 RM

Phase 3
　　6 reps
　　4 sets
　　1st set 65 percent
　　2nd set 75 percent
　　3rd set 75 percent
　　4th set 80 percent
　　2 minutes rest between exercises
　　1 week duration
　　reduce loads by 5% on medium days

Phase 4
　　10, 8, 4, 3 reps
　　4 sets
　　10 reps at 50 percent
　　8 reps at 60 percent
　　4 reps at 80 percent
　　3 reps at 85 percent
　　2 minutes rest between exercises
　　1 week duration
　　reduce loads by 5 percent on medium days

　　Start again at phase 1.

Power training can be incorporated into this strength regimen by using power drills on nonlifting days (Wednesday and weekends) or before the strength routine on leg days (Monday and Thursday). Power drills might include high knee sprinting, stair runs, hopping, jumping, and plyometrics. (An example of plyometrics: Catch a heavy medicine ball with two hands and immediately propel the ball forward.)

Power resistance training also can be performed on a fifth workout day in which lighter loads and faster contractions are used. Loads of about 40 to 60 percent can be used with lifts made as rapidly as possible. Such a program is feasible only when nonweight-resistance equipment is available. Momentum caused by rapidly lifting free weights and weight stacks can reduce the resistance on the muscle and increase the risk of injury.

Some form of power training should be incorporated into the resistance program whether in-season or off-season.

Maintenance. Once strength and power are gained, they are fairly easy to retain. Maintenance training during the season can include using the medium day only, each muscular group used one day per week. As an alternative, one exercise can be performed for each muscle group twice a week (heavy and medium) at intensities equivalent to phase 3 of the cycle.

Muscular Endurance Training

Muscular endurance is best improved by moving a submaximal resistance as many times as possible. That is, low resistance (25 or 50 percent of maximum) is used with many repetitions. The use of traditional resistance training as a means of obtaining endurance is generally not very effective. Not only are such workouts time consuming, but other forms of activity such as distance running, swimming, and cycling produce superior results. Most of the popular endurance programs (e.g., 2 to 3 sets of 12 to 20 RM) are actually providing better muscular strength training than endurance. These programs do increase strength, and when performed in a circuit, can even produce small increases in aerobic capacity. On the other hand, high speed, 30-second isokinetic work bouts may enhance "anaerobic endurance." Such improvement may be valuable in longer anaerobic events such as wrestling and middle distance running.

Muscular Balance

Research studies in sports medicine suggest that muscular balance is very important in preventing muscular injury as well as in enhancing success in certain athletic

Muscular endurance training involves performing more repetitions with less resistance.

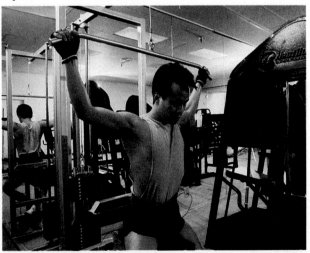

Promoting Your Health

Strength Training Exercises

For the sample exercises listed here, alternatives that affect similar muscular groups can be used. Additional exercises can be selected if the sport demands greater training of specific muscle groups. The sequence of exercises is arranged so that the same muscle group is not used in successive exercises. The complete cycle is performed and then repeated for the second and third sets. If equipment is limited, the second set for a given lift can immediately follow the first set using a 3-minute rest period.

Monday (heavy) and Thursday (medium)
  Chest and Legs

1. Bench press
2. Squat
3. Incline press or chest butterfly
4. Leg curl
5. Heel raise
6. Leg extension or leg press
7. Ankle flexion
8. Hip extension and flexion

Tuesday (heavy) and Friday (medium)
  Arms, Shoulders, Back

1. Arm curl
2. Shoulder press
3. Lat pull
4. Arm extension
5. Upright row
6. Incline shoulder press
7. Bent-over row
8. Shoulder shrug

Monday-Friday (4 times/week)
  Abdominal-Trunk
  One set of 25 each

1. Incline sit-up or Roman-chair sit-up
2. Abdominal curl on machine
3. Knee raise or knee lift

events. Most of the information regarding muscular balance has been obtained by testing the leg muscles. It has been suggested that the hamstrings in the back of the leg should be at least 60 percent as strong as the quadriceps in the front of the same leg when tested at slow speeds, 60° to 120° per second (°/sec).

$$\frac{hamstrings\ strength}{quadriceps\ strength} \times 100 > 60\%$$

When tested at faster speeds of 180°/second or greater, the hamstrings' strength becomes closer in magnitude to the quadriceps and at 300°/second approaches 85 to 90 percent. Thus when the legs are tested at speeds that more closely correspond to sports performance rates, the strength between the two muscle groups approaches equality.

$$\frac{hamstring\ strength}{quadriceps\ strength}\ (at > 180°/sec) \times 100 > 80\%$$

The two hamstring muscles (right and left) should be nearly equal or exhibit no more than 10 percent difference in strength or power at any testing speed. The same is true for the two quadriceps muscle groups.

$$\frac{weak\ hamstrings}{strong\ hamstrings} \times 100 > 90\%$$

$$\frac{weak\ quadriceps}{strong\ quadriceps} \times 100 > 90\%$$

Tests of muscular balance are most accurately performed isokinetically on devices such as the Cybex. If the leg muscles are not in balance, the susceptibility to leg injury is higher. Successful performance is also less likely, especially in competitive sprinting and jumping.

It is unknown whether muscular balances in other parts of the body are as critical as leg balance. An effort nevertheless, should be made to work antagonistic or opposite muscle groups in the training program. For example, triceps exercises should be combined with biceps exercises. Chest exercises should be performed with exercises for the back muscles. It may be tempting to concentrate solely on triceps strength exercises to help improve skills, such as volleyball spike and the basketball shot, since this is the primary arm muscle involved. But complete neglect of the biceps can cause muscular imbalance to develop that may detrimentally affect the skill and increase the risk of injury. Some research indicates that antagonistic muscles are active during movements of the agonist and thus gain some benefit. For example, during the biceps curl, the triceps are active as a stabilizer and therefore benefit from the exercise. These findings imply that it may be unnecessary to spend equal amounts of time on agonist and antagonist muscles. Instead, the primary moves of the activity or sport should be emphasized.

In the general fitness program it is important to lift with opposing muscle groups. Isolating specific muscles may not be as valuable as in athletic weight training. Simply spending equal time using muscles in the front and back of each limb and front and back of the torso should suffice.

Try to make the weaker side work as hard or harder during the exercise as the stronger side. If a double limb machine is used for the training, concentration is necessary to ensure the weak limb is working adequately. Single limb exercises may be necessary to increase the performance of the weaker side or weaker muscle group.

Muscular Tone

The majority of fitness-conscious Americans use muscular training for aesthetic purposes. That is, they want to develop a leaner, stronger appearance. Muscular tone requires two processes: (1) the strengthening and hypertrophying of muscle and (2) the loss of superficial body fat. The use of strength exercises to tone a specific area of the body is called spot reducing. Nearly all types of strength training exercises will strengthen muscle and cause it to increase in size. Moderate changes in strength and lean body weight can occur with resistance as light as 40 to 50 percent of maximum using 10 to 15 repetitions. Although greater hypertrophy occurs with the use of heavier weights, the lighter loads are recommended for muscular toning in the general fitness program (Table 9.2).

Whether resistance exercises will cause the loss of superficial (under the skin) body fat is controversial. Some scientific evidence supports the theory that resistance exercises such as sit-ups and circuit weight training will decrease fat cells in the exercised area and reduce the total body percentage of fat. If fat loss does occur in muscular training, it will be minimal. Greater body fat losses can be expected from vigorous routine aerobic exercises. Weight-bearing activities (walking, jogging, rope jumping) are especially effective. Prolonged aerobic exercise (more than 20 minutes) promotes the mobilization of fat from body depots and the utilization of fat by muscle. Fat is mobilized from at least three areas in order of importance: (1) stomach (abdomen), (2) seat (gluteal), and (3) thigh (femoral). That is, theoretically, it will be most difficult to lose fat from the thigh region and easiest to lose fat from the abdominal region. Regardless, a substantial period of time is required to lose fat in a given area. (See Chapter 7 for more details.)

In summary, a degree of muscular tone can be achieved with resistance exercises. Optimal means of achieving total body tone is the combination of resistance training with aerobic conditioning.

Resistance Training for Cardiovascular Fitness

Depending on resistance training as a means of conditioning the cardiovascular system generally is ineffective. Traditional forms of heavy resistance training produce virtually no improvement in cardiovascular efficiency. In some types of circuit resistance training, small cardiovascular benefits can be obtained. Yet, circuit training itself is not an adequate way to develop optimal cardiorespiratory fitness.

Resistance training causes the heart to work very hard. One reason for this extra strain is the constriction of blood vessels in the muscle caused by the vigorous muscle contraction around the vessels. This narrowing of the vessels increases the resistance to blood flow, and the heart pumps more forcefully in an attempt to push the blood into the muscle.

Another cause for this increased strain on the heart is the pressure in the chest cavity around the heart. One of the most important principles related to safe resistance training is breathing during each phase of the lift. Breathing keeps the air passages open, which prevents the dramatic pressure buildup that can occur in the chest during straining exercise. Closing the air passages during a lift induces a reflex called the Valsalva maneuver, in which the blood flow into the heart is reduced and the heart must pump against a greater resistance, with blood pressure increased. The idea of holding the breath during the lift to maintain torso stability may be correct mechanically, but this practice simply puts too much strain on the heart and vascular system.

Although most scientists agree on the importance of breathing, some controversy exists regarding the timing of exhalation and inhalation. There are two physiological systems to consider: breathing muscles and the heart. Inhalation is an active muscular process requiring more chest muscle activity than exhalation. Since the exercising muscle is strongest in the eccentric (lowering) phase, this easier phase of contraction for the lifting muscles should be associated with the hardest phase of breathing for the respiratory muscles—inhalation. On the other hand, chest (intrathoracic) pressure rises during exhalation, which increases the force of the heart necessary to eject blood. Using this heart physiological process as a guide, the eccentric muscular contraction of the lift should be associated with the hardest phase for the heart—exhalation. Unfortunately, chest muscle and heart activities suggest opposite sequences for breathing. Therefore, physiologically the exhalation-inhalation sequence probably is not critical, and comfort or desires can be used as a guide for breathing. Most experienced heavy lifters inhale during the eccentric phase and exhale during the concentric phase. But more important is simply the act of exchanging air during each phase of the lift. In the general muscular fitness program, coupling the eccentric phase with exhalation and the concentric phase with inhalation is probably better for the heart.

Breathing also must be stressed outside the weight room. Resistance exercises such as sit-ups and push-ups as well as shoveling dirt or chopping wood require the exchange of air during the maneuver. Once again, breath holding should be avoided, which will require some practice at first, since most individuals habitually hold their breath during these types of exercises. Other safety guidelines for heart health are listed in Table 9-3.

Circuit Resistance Training. Resistance training for general fitness is somewhat different in intensity than a program designed to maximize strength and power (see Table 9.2). Cardiovascular fitness is not developed using heavy resistances. Instead, lighter loads are used and the number of repetitions increased. In addition, the time between exercises is reduced to 15 seconds and a sequence of exercises is performed in close succession. The goal of such a routine is to maintain heart rate and oxygen consumption within a target zone necessary to elicit cardiovascular or aerobic training. The exercise intensity should be maintained continuously for 30 to 45 minutes.

A circuit resistance training (CRT) program is the best type of resistance exercise system for producing a desirable aerobic effect. Such a routine will not produce maximal strength and bulk gains. But strength gains can be significant and the continuous moderate exercise promotes beneficial changes in body composition and cardiovascular fitness. Improvements in aerobic capacity also will not be maximal. But adequate gains can be expected and maintenance of aerobic fitness is possible with the CRT routines. Multistation resistance systems are ideal for CRT programs.

This type of program is recommended for individuals interested in aerobic fitness. It is also beneficial for the recreational athlete who seeks general fitness and wishes to improve tennis, racquetball, basketball, or jogging performance. Individuals interested in optimal cardiovascular fitness must use other aerobic activities as the primary exercise. But, CRT can supplement and serve as a short-term substitute for the regular aerobic program. Aerobic exercisers may find the CRT routine a welcome diversion from the normal exercise routine.

Like strength resistance training, CRT can be performed on alternate days. A Monday, Wednesday, Friday program is outlined here, but a better strategy is a two day per week CRT program alternated with a three day per week aerobic program: a total conditioning program of five times per week. For example, jogging or aerobics is performed on Monday, Wednesday, and Friday and the CRT workout on Tuesday and Thursday.

Inserting an aerobic vehicle in the CRT routine can enhance the cardiovascular component of the workout and provide diversity. Aerobic "ergometers" are instruments that provide a means of performing aerobic exercise (see Chapter 8). Some are relatively inexpensive and can provide a warm-up and cool-down exercise as well to be included in the CRT routine. Such exercise should be performed for 3 to 5 minutes at a CRT station to allow the cardiovascular system to adapt to the exercise.

Table 9.3 Guidelines for Resistance Training Based on CV Health

1. Resistance training using loads greater than 50 percent of maximum should not be performed by individuals with known cardiovascular disease or high blood pressure.
2. Resistance training with loads greater than 50 percent of maximum should not be performed without medical clearance by individuals with cardiovascular disease risk factors such as smoking, obesity, or elevated blood fats.
3. Individuals over 45 years of age usually should not perform resistance exercises using loads greater than 60 percent of maximum (~20 RM).
4. Persons interested in general muscular fitness should use loads of 40 to 60 percent of maximum.
5. Persons interested in general muscular fitness should not lift to complete failure.
6. Breathing should be continuous and rhythmic throughout the lifts. The Valsalva maneuver should be avoided.
7. Heavy resistance training using loads greater than 75 percent of maximum should be reserved for competitive athletes.
8. After their competitive playing days, athletes should decrease the loads of resistance training workouts.

CRT Exercises: Generally, free weights are inappropriate for CRT. Machines that allow rapid changes in the loads are best because delays between exercises can lessen the potential cardiovascular effect.

The program we describe is for three times per week and uses lighter weights and more repetitions than the heavy resistance program designed for athletes. For each exercise, 12 to 15 repetitions are performed with loads of 40 to 50 percent of 1 RM. It is neither necessary nor desirable to lift to failure in this type of training. To determine the 40 to 50 percent resistance, simply use a load that causes new fatigue after 18 to 20 repetitions. If no aerobic mode is used, a 15-second rest is taken between each of resistance exercise . After completion of the total sequence (1 to 13), the routine is repeated omitting 1 and 2. After two cycles, the session is ended with cool down (15) and stretching (16). The total routine is designed to be completed in 45 to 50 minutes.
Monday, Wednesday, Friday or
Tuesday, Thursday, Saturday

1. stretching exercises: 6 minutes with no rest period
2. warm-up on cycle: 4 minutes
3. chest press or shoulder press
4. lat pull or pull-up: no rest period
5. ski ergometer: 3 minutes
6. incline sit-ups or abdominal curl
7. leg press or squat: no rest period
8. treadmill walk: 3 minutes
9. trunk extension
10. leg curl
11. knee raise or knee lift
12. heel raise: no rest period
13. rowing ergometer: 3 minutes
14. repeat stations 3 through 13
15. cool-down on cycle: 5 minutes
16. stretching exercises: 6 minutes

Other resistance exercises and other modes of aerobic ergometers can be used in the CRT routine. A single aerobic ergometer can be employed in each three-minute aerobic session during the routine, but a variety may help keep the routine more enjoyable. Try to utilize all muscle groups. More upper body resistance exercises can be substituted for the lower body exercises if jogging, aerobics, skiing, or other leg activities are the primary exercise modes in the aerobic program.

As an alternative to the described CRT program, the ergometers can be employed during the "rest period" itself. Following each resistance exercise, the aerobic ergometer is used for a 30- to 60-second recovery period. In this way, the heart rate remains continuously elevated, and no real rest is taken during the exercise session. This method is often called *supercircuit resistance training*.

▌ GAMES AND SPORTS

Games and sports competition can be excellent motivators for maintaining an active lifestyle. These activities do not produce maximal gains in either CV fitness or muscular strength, but they provide a good combination of health and fitness benefits. Because games and sports contain a social element, they are attractive activities for many adults.

Improving Performance

Usually competitive games are not the best way to begin a fitness program. Vigorous activity should be attempted only after some aerobic fitness base is established. Therefore, perform some moderate aerobic exercise for 3 to 4 weeks prior to playing in vigorous games. Another way to build aerobic fitness is to practice the skill at a low intensity. For example, racketball can be played alone or with a partner at a lower intensity for a few weeks prior to beginning the real competition.

Once the real competition begins, aerobic activity and resistance training can be used to improve performance in the game or sport. Aerobic training makes the game more enjoyable because it helps delay feelings of tiredness. With fatigue delayed, the intensity level can be maintained for the entire contest. Resistance training also can be used to improve sports performance. Overloading the specific muscles used in the sport activity is a key element. Improved muscular strength, power, and control gained from resistance training will benefit performance. In some instances, it may be advantageous to mimic the sport movement with specific resistance exercises. For example, in developing the basketball shot or tennis stroke, an elastic cord or flexible tubing can be used to overload the arm and wrist. Try not to overload the muscle and joints so much that injury results.

Using the same muscle during the game and during the aerobic training and resistance training causes substantial muscle breakdown. The exercised muscles must be allowed to recover. One strategy might be to resistance train after a tennis contest and then allow the arm and leg muscles to recover for 24 to 48 hours before vigorously taxing them again.

Potential Danger

High intensity, vigorous activity can be potentially dangerous. The risk of muscle and joint injury is much greater during these vigorous movements. And these activities place added strain on the heart. Prior aerobic conditioning is one way to ensure that the cardiovascular system is prepared for vigorous anaerobic activity. The box entitled "Playing It Safe: Precautions for High Intensity Activity" lists other precautions related to vigorous activity. One basic precaution is to avoid adding additional load on the heart during the activity. For example, using a plastic sweating suit or heavy hand weights can greatly mutiply the CV strain during high intensity activity.

General Fitness

Games and sports can be an excellent way to increase general fitness and health status. Their primary advantage is that they are enjoyable and thus promote adherence to exercise. If they are not enjoyable or if the individual is always injured, then these vigorous activities will be unlikely to improve fitness.

Heart disease is the number one cause of death among adults in the United States. For most adults, therefore, heart fitness is the primary concern; it is the main goal of the wise exerciser. It may be advantageous to adapt

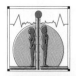

Playing It Safe:

Precautions for High Intensity Activity

1. Establish a solid aerobic fitness base with 4 weeks of aerobic conditioning.

2. Establish a minimal muscle strength base in the primary muscle used during the activity.

3. Do not compound the CV strain by using a rubber suit, hand weights, or exercising in a hot environment.

4. Avoid dehydration by drinking cool fluids at least every 20 minutes of activity (some carbohydrate and mineral preferably).

5. Maintain muscle glycogen stores by eating carbohydrate foods, especially if exercising every day.

6. Do not participate in games that become too competitive and stressful.

games and sports to make the activity more heart healthy. The basic strategy in this plan is to keep the heart rate at a moderate, level pace. To accomplish this task, play the game at a moderate, level pace. For example, in tennis keep moving between points, jog after loose balls, serve rapidly, and so on. In basketball, jog up and down the court, avoid stops in the action, and avoid very short bursts of all-out effort. Some sports such as softball and baseball are not conducive to maintaining a moderate HR. With some creativity and cooperative teammates, most sports activities can be made more heart healthy.

10

Addictions and Addictive Behavior

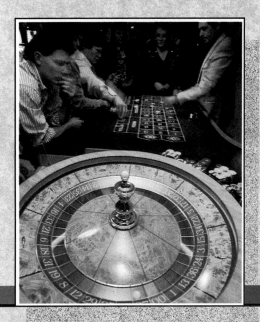

Chapter Outline

- Addiction Defined
- The Scope of Addiction
- Theories of Addiction
- Effects of Addiction on the Family and Society
- Intervention
- Treatment for Addiction

Objectives

- Define addiction and describe the addiction process.

- Name several common addictive behaviors and chemicals

- Name and discuss two categories of disease theories.

- Discuss why the effects of addictive behaviors are not limited to the addict and explain the concepts of codependency and enabling.

- Explain what is meant by intervention and sketch an effective intervention plan.

- Describe the major components of a successful addiction-treatment program.

We have all read and heard about addictive behaviors in the newspapers and on television. The media report crimes and other consequences surrounding the addictive use of substances. We commonly refer to people as "addicts," but what does it really mean to be addicted? The answer to this question was thought to be much simpler when the concept of addiction was limited to drugs. But in recent years, the definition of *addiction* has expanded to include a wide variety of compulsive behaviors. The most commonly recognized addictions today involve the harmful use of alcohol or other drugs, food, sex, relationships, gambling, spending, and work. Many experts now believe that harmful involvement in virtually anything may be classified as an addiction.

▮ ADDICTION DEFINED

Traditionally, diagnosis of an addiction was based on three criteria: (1) the presence of an *abstinence syndrome,* or **withdrawal,** a series of temporary physical and psychological symptoms that occur when the addict stops the addictive behavior; (2) an associated pattern of pathological behavior (deterioration in work performance, relationships, and social interaction); and (3) *relapse,* the tendency to return to the addictive behavior after a period of abstinence. Furthermore, until recently, health professionals were not willing to diagnose an addiction in their patients until medical symptoms appeared. Although withdrawal, pathological behavior, relapse, and medical symptoms are all valid indicators of addiction, they do not explain the apparent addictive behavior of people who do not experience classic withdrawal or who have not developed a medical disease or condition.

Physiological dependence is not the only measure of addiction. Psychological dynamics play an important role, which explains why behaviors not related to the use of chemicals—gambling, for example—may also be addictive. In fact, psychological and physiological dependence are so intertwined that it is not really possible to separate the two. For every psychological state there is a corresponding physiological state. Thus, addictions that have previously been thought to be entirely psychological in nature are now understood to have physiological components.*

The World Health Organization defines **addiction** as "a pathological relationship to any mood-altering experience that has life-damaging consequences."* Initially, addictive behaviors provide a sense of pleasure or stability that is beyond the control of the addict. Eventually,

the addictive behavior is used to provide a sense of normality.

In order to be addictive, a behavior must have the potential to produce a positive mood change, no matter how minor. There is no single chemical or behavior that creates a predictable mood change for everybody. Therefore, people become addicted to a wide variety of chemicals or behaviors. Availability also helps determine whether people choose a specific form of addiction. For example, fewer people become addicted to gambling in states where it is illegal. Because food is readily available in the United States, eating disorders are pervasive in our culture, but they are relatively uncommon in developing countries where food is scarce.

Chemicals produce the most profound addictions, not only because they produce mood change, but also because they cause cellular changes so that the body requires the chemical to function comfortably. However, other behaviors, such as eating, spending, gambling, working, and sex, also create positive mood changes. Moreover, people can (and frequently do) switch from one addiction to another. For example, recovering drug addicts may gradually put on excessive weight through compulsive eating and remain as emotionally isolated as they were when they were taking drugs. For this reason, most treatment programs suggest that recovering substance abusers abstain from all mood-altering chemicals so that they can learn to approach life in a healthy manner.

The Addictive Process

Addiction is a process that begins when a person repeatedly seeks relief from unpleasant feelings or situations, and that evolves over time. Addiction has four major features: (1) *involvement* in the addictive behavior despite negative health, legal, financial, or social consequences; (2) *loss of control,* or the inability to predict what will happen when engaging in the addictive behavior; (3) *denial,* or the inability to perceive that there is a problem; and (4) a strong tendency to *relapse.**

The addictive relationship begins when the person repeatedly seeks the illusion of relief to avoid unpleasant feelings or situations. This pattern is known as *nurturing through avoidance* and is a maladaptive way of taking care of emotional needs.** As addicted people become more and more dependent on the addictive behavior, there is a corresponding decay in relationships with fam-

---

Withdrawal A condition characterized by physical and/or psychological discomforts that result when an addictive behavior is stopped; symptoms may include nausea, vomiting, diarrhea, chills, irritability, or depression.
Addiction Dependence on a substance or behavior to produce a desired mood and manage emotions.

---

* Sidney Cohen, *The Chemical Brain: The Neurochemistry of Addictive Disorders* (Irvine, Cal.: Care Institute, 1988), p. 58.
* John Bradshaw, *Bradshaw On The Family* (Deerfield Beach, Fla.: Health Communications, 1988), p. 5.

* Craig Nakken, *The Addictive Personality* (Center City, Minn.: Hazelden, 1988), p. 23.
** Nakken, *The Addictive Personality,* p. 21.

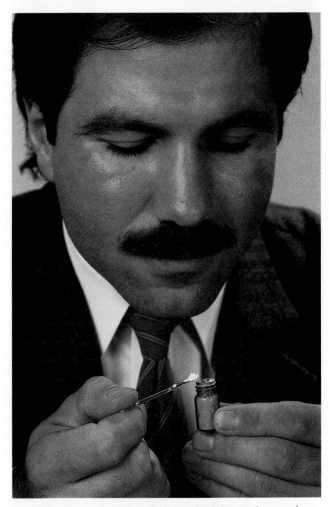

An "addict" is not always what you think he or she may be. In fact, people who are addicted to chemical substances seldom realize or admit that they are addicts.

ily, friends, and coworkers, in performance at work, and in their personal life. Eventually, addicts do not find the addictive behavior pleasurable, but it becomes preferable to the unhappy realities they are seeking to escape (see Figure 10.1).

Figure 10.1 The addictive cycle.

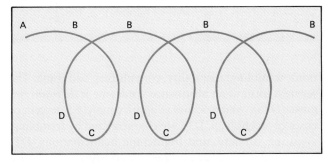

A = pain
B = feel the need to perform the addictive behavior
C = perform the addictive behavior, feel better
D = pain results from performing the addictive behavior

SOURCE: Nakken, *The Addictive Personality*, 1988 p. 24.

People who have destroyed their lives with compulsive behavior are easily identifiable as addicts. People who have had several—or even just a few—episodes of self-destructive behavior, however, are also involved in an addictive process and may also be identified as addicts. For example, virtually all drug addicts who "hit bottom" before beginning recovery can recall potentially dangerous incidents early in their using careers that they ignored. When the people who live around an addict also minimize the importance of a few self-destructive episodes, the stage is set for the addictive cycle to continue.

Addictions are often described in terms of 5 progressive stages: (1) noninvolvement, (2) experimentation, (3) frequent involvement, (4) harmful involvement, and (5) compulsive involvement (see Figure 10.2). Although these stages are useful in describing the extent of one's involvement with an addictive substance or behavior, one should not infer from this model that amount and frequency of involvement are necessarily the most important criteria for diagnosing an addiction. Indeed, *what happens* when the person engages in the addictive behavior may be far more indicative of addiction.

For example, people generally consider it insignificant if a friend uses cocaine only once or twice a year. But if on those occasions the friend experiences illness, blackouts, fights, and personality changes, then the use is a problem. It is very simple: Whatever causes a problem *is* one.

If allowed to continue, addictions progress until the addict is destroyed. Addictions become more resistant to treatment the longer they progress. The current goal is to identify addictions early—before the addict loses everything—and provide appropriate treatment.

In order for a drug or behavior to be addictive, it must have the potential to (1) alter mood, (2) produce tolerance, and (3) create a predictable abstinence syndrome.

Tolerance Tolerance is a phenomenon in which progressively larger doses of a drug are needed to produce the desired effects. Tolerance is the product of the functioning of the liver, which is the main detoxifying organ in the body. The liver becomes increasingly efficient at breaking down the drug and releasing it into the bloodstream for excretion by the kidneys.

Withdrawal Before foreign substances are broken down by the liver, they bind with receptor sites throughout the body, displacing chemicals that are normally present. As a result, the body becomes less efficient at producing these chemicals. If the drug is suddenly withdrawn for any reason, the body will not have the readily available supply of the original chemical needed for reactions at the receptor sites. The startup time for the manufacture of these necessary chemicals is another

Tolerance A condition in which increased amounts of a drug or increased exposure to an addictive behavior are required to produce desired effects.

Living with Addictive Behaviors

Some Facts about the Causes and Consequences of Addiction

- "Compulsive behaviors such as overeating and workaholism are born from feelings of intense cravings for nurturing, affection and personal power . . . . The compulsions become a replacement for nurturing, expression of feelings, self-control, self-worth or security." (Middleton-Moz, *Children of Trauma,* 1989, p. 125)

- One billion packs of cigarettes are sold each year to people under the age of 18 (Office of Inspector General, 1990)

- Drug-using youths who exercise as part of their treatment plan report an 88 percent reduction in multiple drug use and a 44 percent increase in abstinence, according to studies of about 500 teens who participated in the Fitness Intervention Training (FIT) program, Dallas, Texas. (*Journal of Drug Education,* 21, no. 1 [1991], 73–84)

- Passive smoke may cause as many as 53,000 deaths annually among nonsmokers. (Prevention File, 1992)

- Researchers in Berkeley, California, interviewed 468 fifth- and sixth-grade children about the effects of beer advertising on them. The children were likely to have beliefs about beer consumption that were more in line with its advertising image (fun and good times) than the public-health reality (risk). Boys are significantly more likely to believe that beer commercials "tell the truth," while girls were more likely to believe that beer advertising "tried to get kids to drink." (Prevention Pipeline, 1991)

- Of the 1,550 patients admitted by nine New York hospitals during the first quarter of 1990 who screened positive for alcohol problems, 80 percent accepted referral to some type of help. (Prevention Pipeline, 4(4), 1991)

- The U.S. Food and Drug Administration estimates the value of the illegal steroid market at $300–500 million annually. (FDA, 1990)

- Studies show that cigarette consumption has declined over the past decade, but the use of smokeless tobacco (snuff and chewing tobacco) has increased dramatically. (Do-It-Now Publications, 1991)

- Smokeless tobacco products may be more addictive than cigarettes because they contain 3 to 14 times the amount of nicotine as cigarettes. (Do-It-Now Publications, 1991)

- The Metropolitan Life Insurance Company found that in 1990 the average inpatient stay for chemical-dependency treatment cost $7,660. (*Alcoholism and Drug Abuse Weekly,* January 29, 1965)

- When a chemically dependent person receives treatment, insurance claims for health problems of all family members decrease significantly. (*Addictive Behaviors,* 26, no. 2 [1991], 179–87)

- Between 400,000 and 750,000 Americans are addicted to narcotic analgesics. (NIDA, 1989)

- One in 5 Americans (20 percent) is addicted to chemicals, while another 1 in 5 is a steady user. (Harold E. Doweiko, *Concepts of Chemical Dependency,* 1990, p. 3)

- Alcohol and drug addiction are frequently associated with physical abuse. Alcohol alone is estimated to be involved in about 50 percent of cases of spouse abuse and 38 percent of cases of child abuse. (J. D. Beasley, *Wrong Diagnosis, Wrong Treatment: The Plight of the Alcoholic in America* [New York: Creative Informatics, 1987])

24 to 72 hours. Withdrawal symptoms result. Withdrawal symptoms of chemical dependencies are generally the *opposite* of the effects of the drug being withdrawn. For example, a cocaine addict would experience a characteristic "crash" (depression and lethargy), and a barbiturate addict would experience trembling, irritability, and convulsions upon withdrawal. Withdrawal episodes range from mild to severe. Withdrawal symptoms common to many drugs include nausea, vomiting, chills, fever, profuse sweating, headaches, diarrhea, hallucina-

tions, trembling, irritability, convulsions, and coma. The severest form of an abstinence syndrome is *delirium tremens (DTs)*, which occurs in approximately 5 percent of cases of alcoholism. DTs are characterized by trembling, sweating, anxiety, and frightening hallucinations. DTs result in death in 20 to 25 percent of cases.

"Process addictions" such as gambling do not produce tolerance and withdrawal in the classical sense of these terms. However, these addictions produce tolerance in that the addict requires more frequent—or more

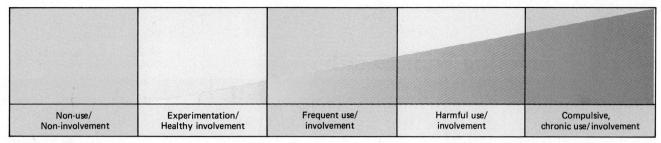

| Non-use/
Non-involvement | Experimentation/
Healthy involvement | Frequent use/
involvement | Harmful use/
involvement | Compulsive,
chronic use/involvement |

Adapted from Doweiko, p. 13.

Figure 10.2 Addiction as a process.

intense—experiences to cause the desired mood changes. And those addicted to these behaviors do, in fact, experience abstinence syndromes which, although they are primarily psychological, (e.g., anxiety) nonetheless constitute a predictable withdrawal phenomenon.

THE SCOPE OF ADDICTION

In comparison to other addictive behaviors, chemical addictions have been well documented over the years, but statistics indicate that a large percentage of the American population suffers from both nonchemical and chemical addictions.

Tobacco

In terms of lost lives, nicotine is by far the most serious addiction. Tobacco use kills over 350,000 Americans each year (see Chapter 11).[*] All forms of tobacco use (cigarettes, pipes, cigars, and smokeless tobacco) are addictive and harmful to health. The American Lung Association estimates that 54 million Americans smoke, and that 90 percent of these smokers would like to quit but feel unable to do so.[**]

Alcohol

Alcohol kills an estimated 100,000 Americans each year, including victims of alcohol-related vehicle accidents and diseases.[‡] The American Psychiatric Association estimates that 10 million adults and 3 million children and adolescents are addicted to alcohol. Another 81 million people are indirectly affected by alcoholism through family and other relationships.[***]

The annual cost of alcoholism to the United States exceeds $116 billion. This figure includes direct costs such as those associated with treatment, crime, and accidents, and indirect costs such as reduced productivity, imprisonment, and premature death (see Chapter 11).[§]

Other Drugs

The incidence of abuse of cocaine and other illegal stimulants (amphetamines and methamphetamines) has been increasing since the mid-1980s. An estimated 4 million to 24 million Americans use cocaine on a regular basis, and between 500,000 and 750,000 Americans are daily users.[*]

Marijuana is used regularly by more than 18 million Americans, 6 million of whom use it on a daily basis (see Chapter 12).[**] These figures are more than 20 times higher than those reported in 1960. This increase is critical in terms of marijuana's reputation as the key gateway drug (see Figure 10.3). A *gateway drug* is one that precedes and leads to the use of other drugs. For a further discussion of gateway drugs, see Chapter 12.

The American Psychiatric Association estimates that no fewer than 7 million Americans are using mood-altering prescription medications without the supervision of a physician.[†] Some physicians continue to prescribe these drugs to their patients who may be addicted, but people who take mood-altering substances without medical supervision run the greatest risk of addiction.

Compulsive Eating

The incidence of compulsive eating is difficult to estimate. However, statistics indicate that obesity, one indicator of compulsive eating, affects approximately 37 million American adults,[*] and 70 percent of compulsive

---

[*] *American Medical Association Encyclopedia of Medicine,* ed. Charles B. Clayman (New York: Random House, 1989), p. 993.

[**] American Cancer Society. *Smokeout Fact Sheet* (1991).

[‡] John R. Seffrin, "Drug and Alcohol Abuse Prevention: A Responsibility, Not a Right," Keynote address at the Drug Prevention Programs in Higher Education Grantee Meeting, Washington, DC (November 17–20, 1989).

[***] Jean Kinney and Gwen Leaton, *Loosening the Grip: A Handbook of Alcohol Information* (St. Louis, Mo.: Mosby–Year Book, Inc., 1991), p. 23.

[§] Ibid., p. 24.

[*] Harold E. Doweiko, *Concepts of Chemical Dependency* (Pacific Grove, Cal.: Brooks/Cole, 1990), p. 58.

[**] Ibid., p. 58.

[†] American Psychiatric Association, "Research on Mental Illness and Addictive Disorders: Progress and Prospects," (1990).

[*] William A. McArdle, Frank I. Katch, and Victor L. Katch, *Exercise Physiology: Energy, Nutrition, and Human Performance,* (Malvern, Pa.: Lea and Febiger, 1991), p. 658.

Promoting Your Health

How to Tell Whether Someone You Know Is Chemically Dependent

For each of the following questions, provide a yes or no answer.

1. Is the person drinking (or using any other drug) more now than he or she did in the past?

2. Are you afraid to be around the person when he or she is drinking or using drugs because of the possibility of verbal or physical abuse?

3. Has the person ever forgotten or denied things that happened during a drinking or using episode?

4. Do you worry about the person's drinking or drug use?

5. Does the person refuse to talk about his or her drinking or drug use—or even to discuss the possibility that he or she might have a problem with it?

6. Has the person broken promises to control or stop his or her drinking or drug use?

7. Has the person ever lied about his or her drinking or using, or tried to hide it from you?

8. Have you ever been embarrassed by the person's drinking or drug use?

9. Have you ever lied to anyone else about the person's drinking or drug use?

10. Have you ever made excuses for the way the person behaved while drinking or using?

11. Are most of the person's friends heavy drinkers or drug users?

12. Does the person make excuses for, or try to justify, his or her drinking or using?

13. Do you feel guilty about the person's drinking or drug use?

14. Are holidays and social functions unpleasant for you because of the person's drinking or drug use?

15. Do you feel anxious or tense around the person because of his or her drinking or drug use?

16. Have you ever helped the person to "cover up" for a drinking or using episode by calling his or her employer or by telling others that he or she is feeling "sick"?

17. Does the person deny that he or she has a drinking problem because he or she only drinks beer (or wine)? Or deny that he or she

---

eaters are obese (20 percent or greater than desired weight).** Obesity is a complex problem, however, that is not always explained by excessive food consumption. Sedentary lifestyle, heredity, and biochemical factors may also play a role (see Chapter 7).

All people are vulnerable to compulsive eating. However, the incidence of eating disorders is higher in women.

Gambling and Spending

Compulsive gambling is a progressive and chronic preoccupation with and urge to gamble. It has been estimated that 1 to 3 percent of American adults are compulsive gamblers. Those most likely to become compulsive gamblers are ages 17 to 34, employed, white, married, pos-

sessing a high-school diploma, and earning between $20,000 and $50,000.***

The widespread use of credit cards in the United States makes compulsive spending very easy. In fact, the very wealthy and those with limited means are equally represented among compulsive spenders. Like other behaviors, spending can be done in either a healthy or an addictive fashion. It is important to distinguish between compulsive shopping and the occasional shopping spree. Compulsive shopping is a chronic pattern of shopping in an attempt to remedy feelings of depression and emptiness. The compulsive shopper often experiences a sense of inner tension that can only be relieved by purchasing something.†

** Donald A. Williamson, *Assessment of Eating Disorders: Obesity, Anorexia and Bulimia Nervosa* (New York: Pergamon Press, 1990), p. 21.

*** Ira Sommers, "Pathological Gambling: Estimating Prevalence and Group Characteristics," *International Journal of the Addictions*, 23, no. 5 (1988), pp. 477–90.

† David W. Krueger, "On Compulsive Shopping and Spending: A Psychodynamic Inquiry," *American Journal of Psychotherapy*, October 1988, pp. 574–83.

Promoting Your Health (*Continued*)

has a drug problem because use is "limited" to marijuana, or diet pills, or some other supposedly harmless substance?

18. Does the person's behavior change noticeably when he or she is drinking or using? (For example, a normally quiet person might become loud and talkative, or a normally mild-mannered person might become quick to anger.)

19. Does the person avoid social functions where alcohol will not be served or where drugs will not be available or permitted?

20. Does the person insist on going only to restaurants that serve alcohol?

21. To your knowledge, has the person ever driven a car while intoxicated or under the influence of drugs?

22. Has the person ever received a summons for driving while intoxicated (DWI) or driving under the influence (DUI)?

23. Are you afraid to ride with the person after he or she has been drinking or using?

24. Has anyone else talked to you about the person's drinking or using behavior?

25. Has the person ever expressed remorse for his or her behavior during a drinking or using episode?

26. If you are married to the person and have children, are the children afraid of the person while he or she is drinking or using?

27. Does the person seem to have a poor self-image?

28. Have you ever found alcohol or drugs that the person has hidden?

29. Is the person having financial difficulties that seem to be related to his or her drinking or drug use?

30. Does the person look forward to times when he or she can drink or use the drugs?

Scoring

If you answered yes to any three of these questions, then there is a good chance that the person you care about has a drinking or drug problem. If you answered yes to any five, then the chance is even greater. And if you answered yes to seven or more, the likelihood is great that the person has a problem with chemical dependency.

Compulsive Work

The central element of workaholism is an irrational commitment to excessive work. Workaholics are unable to take time off or to sustain other interests.‡ Workaholism is considered psychologically harmful because of the lack of balance with nonwork alternatives.

Excessive work that is based on career commitment fosters a great deal of satisfaction and personal fulfillment. However, true workaholics do not work excessively simply because they are committed to their careers. Furthermore, they may not experience significant job satisfaction. The distinction between a workaholic and a person who merely works a great deal is *compulsive* work verses *excessive* work.

The incidence of workaholism is difficult to estimate. People who come from addictive or other kinds of dys-

functional families are more likely than people from healthy families to become workaholics.*** Moreover, work addiction can destroy families just as any other addiction can.

Sex and Relationships

All people need love and intimacy, but the sexual practices of sex addicts involve neither love nor intimacy. In fact, the core issue of sex addiction is the confusion of intensity for intimacy. The sexual behavior of an addict creates an intense feeling, which is then confused with intimacy.§ The sex addict does not nurture or feel nurtured by the person with whom he or she has sex, but by the sexual activity itself. Sex, not the relationship, is the object of the sex addict's affection. It has been estimated

---

‡ Thomas J. Naughton, "A Conceptual View of Workaholism and Implications for Career Counseling and Research," *Career Development Quarterly*, March 1987, pp. 180–87.

*** Bryan E. Robinson, *Work Addiction* (Deerfield Beach, Fla.: Health Communications, 1989), p. 12.

§ Nakken, *The Addictive Personality*, p. 21.

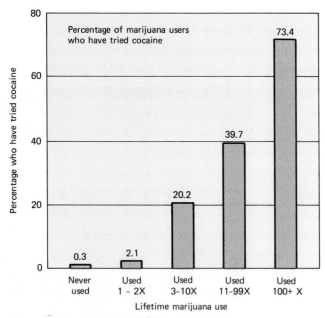

Figure 10.3 Many experts believe that marijuana is a gateway drug. People who use marijuana are more likely to try cocaine and other drugs.

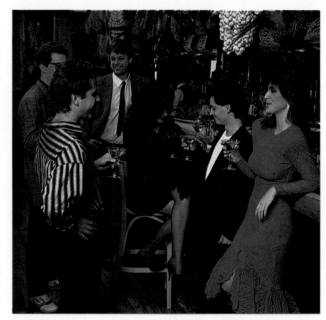

In a culture that glorifies beauty, sex, and Hollywood, it is perhaps no surprise that many people confuse love, intimacy, and sexual intensity. Sex addicts crave sex only, without nurturance or commitment.

that 1 percent of the American population is addicted to sex.*

THEORIES OF ADDICTION

There are many perspectives and theories concerning the cause of addictions. Each theory of addiction focuses on a single causative factor. However, addiction is too complex to be explained by one factor in isolation (see Figure 10.4). The theories discussed here fall into one of two categories: (1) biological, or disease, models, and (2) psychosocial models.

The Disease Model of Addiction

Although the disease concept of addiction has been widely accepted since the mid-1950s, it continues to be a subject of heated debate. Opponents of the disease model suggest that it absolves addicts of responsibility for unacceptable behavior. They also believe that addiction has many causes, not just a single, biological cause.

Proponents of the disease model believe that the model not only allows for acceptance, compassion, and therefore recovery, but also holds addicts fully responsible for seeking treatment for their disease. Proponents of the disease model of addiction also claim that addiction involves a biological component. They apply this theory to the chemical addictions in particular. Studies have

shown that people addicted to mood-altering substances metabolize these substances differently than do nonaddicted people. For example, studies of adult children of alcoholics have shown abnormal concentrations or activity of various neurotransmitters related to mood, specifically norepinephrine, serotonin, endorphine, and enkephalin.** Another study showed greater amounts of norepinephrine in the urine of compulsive gamblers than in the urine of normal subjects† Abnormalities in levels of any of these neurotransmitters may create a biochemically based mood disorder. In order to obtain relief, the person may turn to mood-altering chemicals or behaviors.

Genetic studies also support a disease model of addiction. It has been known for centuries that alcoholism runs in families (see Chapter 11). Studies of family members and twins have repeatedly confirmed the existence of a genetic factor in alcoholism. In the last decade, studies have shown that children of drug-addicted parents are more likely to engage in any of the addictive behaviors than are children of parents who are not addicted. These findings are consistent whether or not children actually live with their addicted parents.‡

Psychosocial Models of Addiction

Psychosocial models of addiction explore the relationship between the addict and social or cultural influences.

---

* Kurt Haas and Adelaide Haas, *Understanding Sexuality,* 2nd ed. (St. Louis: Times Mirror/Hosby, 1990), p. 488.

** Kenneth Blum and James E. Payne, *Alcohol and the Addictive Brain* (New York: The Free Press, 1991), pp. 160–63.

† Doweiko, *Concepts of Chemical Dependency,* p. 147.

‡ Kinney and Leaton, *Loosening the Grip,* p. 76.

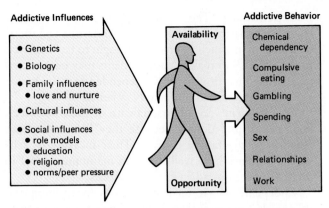

Addictive Influences

- Genetics
- Biology
- Family influences
  - love and nurture
- Cultural influences
- Social influences
  - role models
  - education
  - religion
  - norms/peer pressure

Availability

Opportunity

Addictive Behavior

Chemical dependency

Compulsive eating

Gambling

Spending

Sex

Relationships

Work

Figure 10.4 Addiction is too complex to be explained by a single factor. The Graham model of addiction proposes that addiction is caused by a variety of factors operating together.

Cultural Influences   Cultural expectations and mores help determine whether and how people engage in certain behaviors. For example, although many Italians use alcohol abundantly, there is a low incidence of alcoholism in this culture. Low rates of alcoholism are typically found in those cultures where children are gradually introduced to alcohol in diluted amounts, on special occasions, and within a strong family group. There is strong disapproval of intoxication, which is viewed as not socially acceptable, stylish, nor funny.*** In contrast, such cultural traditions and values are not widespread in the United States, and as a result the incidence of alcoholism and alcohol-related problems is very high.

Societal Influences   Societal attitudes also influence drug abuse and other addictive behaviors. American society's near-worship of youth and beauty plays a significant role in the development of eating disorders in the United States. The attitude that alcohol and other drugs are necessary to have a good time makes it difficult for some people to have fun without using chemicals. The emphasis on materialism and perfectionism has made workaholism not only an accepted practice, but an admirable one.

Role Models   Social learning theory proposes that people learn addictive behaviors by watching parents, caregivers, and significant others. The effects of modeling, imitation, and identification of behavior from early childhood on are well documented. Many studies show that children are more likely to begin smoking if their parents smoke. Compulsive eaters generally have a parent who eats compulsively.

Life Events   Major life events such as marriage, divorce, change in work status, or death of a loved one may trigger addictive behaviors, particularly among women and the elderly. Death of a spouse is the most common event to trigger excessive drinking by an elderly person.

*** Kinney and Leaton, *Loosening the Grip*, p. 86.

Divorce is the most common stimulus of alcoholism and compulsive eating in women. Sexual abuse is another life event that may trigger addictions in women. Substance-abuse treatment programs across the nation report that at least 50 percent of their female patients were sexually abused as children or as adults. Sexual abuse is a common occurrence in addictive families, and the cycle of addiction and sexual abuse is a legacy that sexually abused adults tend to pass on to their own families.**

Personality Influences   Personality may predispose a person to addiction. The question of whether low self-esteem causes addiction or addiction causes low self-esteem has long been argued. Most experts now believe that both relationships exist: A certain degree of low self-esteem predisposes a person to addiction, and addiction further reduces self-esteem. Alcoholics tend to score higher on tests of anxiety, depression, impulsivity, and hostility. People with eating disorders are frequently depressed, have low self-esteem, value perfectionism, and need to be in control. Most addicts seek immediate gratification and need to be in control. In fact, the addictive behavior may give the addict a false sense of control over his or her mood.

Family Influences   Family members whose needs for love, security, and affirmation are not consistently met, who are not allowed to express their feelings, desires, or needs, and who frequently submerge their personalities in order to "keep peace" are prone to addiction. Children whose parents are not consistently available to them or who are victims of sexual abuse, physical abuse, neglect, abandonment, or inconsistent and disparaging messages about their self-worth may experience mental or physical illness, addiction, or even death as a result.

EFFECTS OF ADDICTION ON THE FAMILY AND SOCIETY

During the 1980s, the study of addictions intensified as researchers began to understand and articulate the impact of parental addiction on developing children. Alcoholism served as the model from which the concepts of enabling, codependency, and dysfunctional families emerged. Later, these concepts were applied to families experiencing other addictions and dysfunctions as well.

The effects of any addictive behavior are not limited to the addict. The National Institute of Alcohol Abuse and Alcoholism estimates that 60 to 80 percent of reported violent crimes and crimes against property are attributable to the abuse or sale of alcohol or other

Social Learning Theory   A theory that attributes addictive behavior to identification with or imitation of role models.

** Janet G. Woititz, *Healing Your Sexual Self* (Deerfield Beach, Fla.: Health Communications, 1989), pp. 11–14.

drugs. According to the American College Health Association, 60 percent of sexually transmitted diseases and unwanted pregnancies among college students originate in an unplanned or unprotected sexual encounter between partners under the influence of alcohol or other drugs. Children from families where one or more members were addicts are at high risk for developing their own addictions. Indeed, addictions of all kinds disrupt and destroy families, educations, careers, relationships, and lives.

Dynamics of Family Dysfunction

Adults choose their spouses and can also choose to leave them. Unlike parents, children in dysfunctional families have neither choice nor mobility. The nonaddicted parent may indeed *feel* trapped, but the child *is* trapped. The experience of living in a dysfunctional family is damaging to all members, but children are especially traumatized. Their most basic emotional needs may be rarely or inconsistently met. Many of them face sexual or other forms of abuse.

Children from dysfunctional homes, especially homes where a chemical dependency exists, may suffer to some degree from symptoms of **posttraumatic stress disorder (PTSD)**, a condition first recognized in combat soldiers. PTSD is believed to occur among people with normal defenses who have been subjected to levels of trauma beyond the range that is considered "normal." PTSD is most likely to occur as a result of trauma that is chronic, of human origin, and sustained within a closed social system.*

People who suffer from PTSD experience the following symptoms:

1. *Re-experiencing the trauma.* A sudden reemergence of the feelings, thoughts, and behaviors that were present during the trauma. This experience usually occurs in the presence of a trigger, such as the smell of alcohol, that symbolically represents the original trauma.
2. *Psychic numbing.* The ability to suspend feelings in favor of taking steps to ensure psychological and physical safety.
3. *Hypervigilance.* A "radar" that enables the person to monitor his or her surroundings continuously.
4. *Survivor guilt.* An irrational but painful sense of guilt over having come through a traumatic event more successfully than did others in the same environment.*

Codependency The concept of codependency emerged in the 1980s. **Codependency** refers to a relationship pattern in which a person is thought to be "addicted to the addict." In reality, codependents may be addicted to relationships in general. Codependency is the major outcome of dysfunctional family systems.

Codependents are often unaware of their own feelings, needs, and desires because they live in constant reaction to the family distress. Their measure of self-worth becomes how well they can maintain control in the face of serious adverse consequences.

Codependents assume responsibility for meeting others' needs, to the exclusion of acknowledging or even being aware of their own. This behavior goes far beyond simply performing kind services for another person. Ironically, people who cannot take care of themselves are not really capable of taking care of someone else. This is the paradox of codependency.**

Codependents experience anxiety and weak boundaries in their interpersonal relationships, especially intimate relationships. Because codependents exist solely to take care of others, they lose the sense of their own identity. In interpersonal relationships, the closer the intimacy, the more the codependents sense of self weakens. However, distance between partners elicits a fear of abandonment in the codependent, also weakening the sense of self.†

In an effort to feel connected to others (especially the partner), codependents dismantle their boundaries. As a result, they are unable to tell others what they will and will not tolerate. They allow others to hurt them continually. It is this boundary distortion that allows codependents to be abused, whether physically, psychologically, or sexually.

The environment in which codependents live tends to be chaotic, unpredictable, and highly stressful. As a result, compulsive behaviors, often in the form of addictions, are common among codependents. Addictions enable codependents to medicate the anxiety and depression their circumstances create. Moreover, because they are not able to "fool their bodies" about the pain in their lives, codependents may require a higher than average amount of medical care for stress-related illnesses, such as hypertension, ulcers, headaches, asthma, and rheumatoid arthritis.

It is important to keep in mind that the occasional experience of codependent symptoms discussed here does not make a person codependent. Rather, an intense and rigid *pattern* of codependent behavior identifies a person as codependent.

Post-traumatic Stress Disorder (PTSD) A condition experienced by people who have been subjected to levels of trauma beyond the range that is considered "normal."

Codependency A relationship pattern in which a person takes responsibility for the addict's behavior.

---

* Timmen L. Cermak, *Diagnosing and Treating Codependence* (Minneapolis: Johnson Institute, 1986), p. 55.

* Ibid., pp. 57–58.

** Ibid., p. 11.

† Ibid., p. 19.

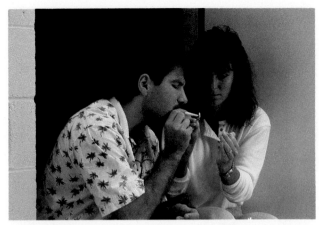

Codependents typically assume responsibility for meeting others' needs, to the exclusion of their own.

quences, people are not made aware of the dangers of their behavior and may therefore continue it. No one but the addict is responsible for his or her behavior. However, anyone who has contact with an addict can be an enabler and may contribute to the addictive behavior.

Enabling is rarely fully conscious and is certainly not intentional, but enablers are generally aware that their behavior allows the addict to continue the addication. Even when this relationship is understood, an enabler may not feel equipped to behave in any other way. Part of ending enabling behaviors involves learning new behaviors.

Whereas some forms of enabling are blatant, other forms are subtle. Consider the brief scenarios in the box on enabling. How obvious is each case? How serious is each one? Can you name other enabling behaviors that are not listed?

Enabling Codependents are the primary enablers of their addicted loved ones. **Enablers** are people who knowingly or unknowingly protect addicts from the natural consequences of their behavior. Without conse-

Enabler   A person who knowingly or unknowingly protects addicts from the natural consequences of their behavior.

Communication

Confronting Addictive Behavior

Most people learn at an early age that it is impolite to confront other people about their behavior, especially if you want to be accepted. Yet the most caring thing you can do for someone who is involved in self-destructive behavior is to get involved. By not confronting the behavior, you subtly show approval.

Confrontation can be frightening. You may hit a wall of denial and hostility. You may even cause a break in the relationship. For these reasons, confrontation should always be done with an attitude of caring and concern.

It may be best to talk to the person in the company of others who are equally concerned and who have had occasion to observe the behavior. This approach reduces the risk associated with talking to the friend alone, and it eliminates some of the potential for denial.

If the person is involved with alcohol or other drugs, wait until he or she is sober so that you can discuss the situation more rationally. The only exception is when someone's safety is at stake. For example, it is appropriate to prevent an intoxicated person from driving.

The goal of the confrontation should be to inform, not to punish. This goal can best be achieved by stating your observations about the person's behavior rather than judging the person for behaving this way.

Do not get sidetracked. Someone who is involved in a harmful behavior will offer numerous explanations as to why your observations are "off-base." An effective denial is to draw attention to someone else to avoid looking bad.

If you believe that your friend has established a pattern of harmful involvement in the behavior, help is needed. It is especially important to make a referral when someone continues the behavior despite promises to stop. Before the confrontation, find out where your friend can receive help. The student health center, the counseling center, a local alcohol and drug treatment program, or a hospital are places to check out.

You can't change someone else by communicating your concern about their behavior. But you can increase the chances that the person will decide to change. People are more likely to change if they can understand the self-destructive nature of their behavior and see that others whom they respect do not approve of it.

▌INTERVENTION

Denial is the hallmark of addiction. Although addicts can become master liars, denial is not the same as a lie. A lie is a deliberate falsification of the truth. **Denial** is the inability to see the truth and is so powerful in addiction that intervention must be designed to break down the addict's denial system.

Intervention is a planned process of confrontation by "significant others"—people who are important to the addict, including spouse, parents, children, boss, and friends. The purpose of intervention is to break down the denial compassionately so that the addict can see the destructive nature of the addiction. It is not enough to get the addict to admit that he or she is addicted. The addict must come to perceive that the addiction is destructive and must be treated.

Individual confrontation is difficult and often futile. However, an addict's defenses generally crumble when significant others collectively share their observations and concerns about the addict's behavior. It is critical that those involved in an intervention communicate how they plan to end their enabling. For example, the spouse should state that he or she will no longer cover bounced checks or make excuses for the addict's antisocial behavior. Significant others must also express support if the addict is willing to begin a recovery program.

Intervention is a serious step toward helping someone who may not want help. Therefore, it should be planned and rehearsed well. Most addiction treatment centers have intervention specialists on staff who can help plan an intervention. In addition, many bookstores carry books on the subject written for families and friends who are concerned about someone who is addicted.

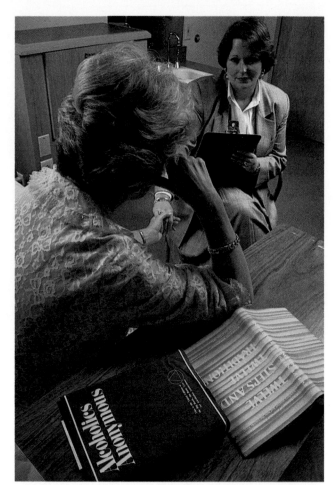

Twelve-step meetings are available in most areas of the United States and in many countries around the world.

Denial The inability to see the truth.

Health in Your Community

The Social Development Strategy

The Social Development Strategy is a drug-abuse prevention approach that reduces risk factors for drug abuse and enhances protective factors.[1] By promoting children's and adolescents' relationships of attachments with non–drug users, by increasing the young people's investment or commitment in the various social units in which

they are involved, and by strengthening their values or beliefs regarding what is healthy and ethical behavior, positive social bonding is enhanced.

1. Oregon Prevention Resource Center and University of Washington School of Social Work, *Oregon TOGETHER! Communities for Drug Free Youth,* 1990.

TREATMENT FOR ADDICTION

Treatment strategies may differ depending on the specific behavior and depth of involvement in the addiction. Today, treatment for most addictions no longer relies solely on individual counseling. Group therapy is more effective in helping addicts to face their denial and find the strength to take responsibility for their behavior. The best treatment programs offer a combination of individual, group, and family therapy and education.

Most states now offer a variety of inpatient and outpatient addiction treatment facilities. Research shows that there is little difference in effectiveness between these two types of facilities. However, inpatient treatment may be most beneficial for people who have relapsed, for those suffering from multiple addictions, and for those who have little support outside of the treatment program.

The most successful treatment programs have the following components: a multidisciplinary staff trained in the understanding and treatment of addictions, individual and group therapy, family education and therapy, and aftercare programs that emphasize involvement in 12-step or other programs of personal growth.

Twelve-step programs are peer support groups patterned after Alcoholics Anonymous. These programs are designed to keep addicts free of their addictions. Twelve-step programs have now been developed for nearly every addiction as well as for families and friends of addicts. They all use a series of 12 steps to guide recovering addicts through a program of personal growth. The groups are available at no cost to anyone with an interest in recovery in practically every community of the nation and in many other countries.

SUMMARY

- In the last decade, the field of addictions was expanded beyond chemical dependency to include a wide variety of compulsive behaviors that are self-destructive.

- In order to become addictive, a behavior must be capable of producing a positive mood change.

- The most commonly recognized addictions include addictions to alcohol and other mood-altering drugs, compulsive eating, sex, relationships, gambling, spending, and work.

- Addictions are characterized by harmful involvement in the behavior despite negative consequences, loss of control, denial, and a tendency to relapse.

- The many perspectives and theories concerning the cause of addictions fall into two categories: (1) biological, or disease, models, and (2) psychosocial models.

- The harmful effects of addiction are not limited to the addict. The family and others close to the addict also suffer.

- Codependency and enabling are overlapping concepts that emerged in the 1980s and that help us to understand the dynamics of addictions in relationships.

- Although the addict alone is responsible for his or her behavior, significant others can increase the chances that the addict will get help by providing an intervention.

- Treatment for addictions may take the form of inpatient or outpatient care, individual and group therapy, and self-help treatments such as the 12-step programs.

11

Alcohol
and Tobacco

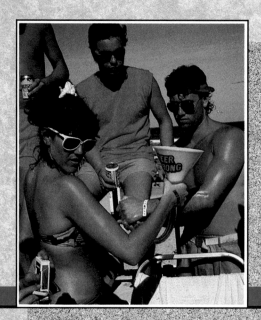

■ Objectives

- Explain why alcohol is a drug and describe its
  chemical composition in terms of how a person gets
  "drunk" on alcohol.
- Discuss the effects alcohol has on human
  metabolism and behavior.
- Describe who uses alcohol and why alcohol use may
  become alcohol abuse (alcoholism).
- Describe the chemical makeup of tobacco and the
  physiological effects of tobacco use.
- Discuss the health risks and hazards of smoking.
- Explain why giving up smoking is so difficult.
- Discuss the social and political issues surrounding
  the advertising, distribution, and sale of tobacco
  products in the United States.

When we hear references to the dangers of drugs, what usually comes to mind? The term "drugs" usually conjures up images of people abusing cocaine, heroin, marijuana, LSD, PCP, and other illegal substances. We conveniently use the word "drugs" to refer to one set of dangerous substances, while we steadfastly refuse to categorize alcohol and tobacco as drugs, primarily because they are socially accepted. Nevertheless, alcohol and nicotine are chemical substances that affect our physical and mental behaviors. The tragedies associated with alcohol addiction and tobacco-related illness receive far less attention than cocaine-related deaths, drug busts, and efforts to eradicate marijuana crops. They are, however, far more common. Alcohol, in particular, may have devastating effects on people of all ages.

The use of alcoholic beverages is interwoven into the fabric and traditions of society. We use alcohol to celebrate everything from christenings to retirements and to help ease the pain experienced in situations involving rejection or loss. We are certainly not unique in this regard; people all over the world and throughout history have used alcohol for everything from social gatherings to religious ceremonies.

An estimated 70 percent of the American population consumes alcoholic beverages regularly. Actual consumption patterns are unevenly distributed throughout the drinking population. Ten percent are heavy drinkers and account for half of all the alcohol consumed. The remaining 90 percent of the drinking population are infrequent, light, or moderate drinkers.

ALCOHOL: AN OVERVIEW

Alcohol is the most widely used (and abused) recreational drug in our society. It is the most popular drug on college campuses, used twice as much as marijuana and five times as much as cocaine.[*] Approximately 85 to 95 percent of college students consume alcoholic beverages. Some 20 to 25 percent abuse alcohol. Indeed, alcohol use has long been a part of the college social scene. Research indicates that students of both sexes increase their alcohol consumption after arriving at college, with the number of female drinkers coming close to or equaling the number of male drinkers.[**] Students may drink for a variety of reasons: to enhance sociability or social interaction, to escape negative emotions, to release otherwise unacceptable emotions, or simply to get drunk.

College is a critical time to become conscious of and responsible about your drinking, if you choose to drink.

Researchers report that the average student spends more money on booze than on books, undoubtably contributing to the fact that alcohol plays a role in 21 percent of all college dropouts. Among those currently in college, between 240,000 and 360,000 eventually will lose their lives because of drinking. Problem alcohol use on our campuses is related to a host of problems, which include injuries, unwanted pregnancies, sexually transmitted diseases, and auto accidents.

A downward trend in per-capita consumption of alcoholic beverages was reported between 1981 and 1989. In 1989, the estimated per-capita consumption was the equivalent of 2.43 gallons of pure alcohol per person.[*] This is the amount of alcohol that a person would obtain by drinking approximately 50 gallons of beer, 20 gallons of wine, or more than 4 gallons of distilled spirits. Wine was the only beverage for which per-capita consumption continued to increase, peaking in 1986 at a level higher than ever previously recorded. This trend may have been a reflection of the availability and marketing of wine coolers, and the increased availability of wine.[**] From 1987 through 1989, wine consumption has decreased, following the trend of other alcohol beverages.[***] In addition, between 1982 and 1987 the proportion of fatally injured drivers who were legally intoxicated dropped from 46 percent to 40 percent.[****]

Most of us recognize the dangers associated with alcohol consumption, yet we deny that such problems could happen to us. We are intellectually aware of the relationship between alcohol and traffic accidents, spouse battering and child abuse, violent crimes, and family disruption, but we tend to believe that these tragedies happen only to other people.

Those who drink often argue that drinking is an inalienable right. Many people do not classify alcohol as a drug simply because they do not wish to see themselves as "drug users." Our society condones and often encourages the use of alcoholic beverages, but does not really teach us about alcohol use. Lip service is often given to "responsible use of alcohol," yet some drug educators would argue that alcohol cannot be used responsibly. In fact, the National Institute on Alcohol Abuse and Alcoholism (NIAAA) has eliminated the phrase "responsible use of alcohol" from its educational materials.

The choice to drink must be made judiciously, with complete information about the risks associated with use. The physiological and psychological reactions of the human organism to alcohol are strong. For this reason, the drug must be approached carefully. To avoid the devastating effects of alcohol abuse, the user must adhere

---

[*] U.S. Department of Health and Human Services, *Alcohol and Health: Special Report to the U.S. Congress* (Washington, D.C.: U.S. Government Printing Office, 1987).

[**] L. D. Johnson, P. M. O'Malley, and J. G. Bachman, *Drug Use among American High School Seniors, College Students and Young Adults, 1975–1990*, Vol. 2 (Rockville, Md.: NIDA, 1991).

---

[*] National Institute on Alcohol Abuse and Alcoholism, "Apparent Per Capita Consumption: National, State, and Regional Trends, 1977–1989," *Surveillance Report*, 22 (1991).

[**] *Alcohol Health and Research World*, 13, no. 4 (1989), 308.

[***] National Institute on Alcohol Abuse and Alcoholism, "Apparent Per Capita Consumption."

[****] U.S. Department of Health and Human Services, *Proceedings of the Surgeon General's Workshop on Drunk Driving, December 14–16, 1988* (1989).

to the same principles of prevention that apply to any potentially harmful substance. Alcohol also interacts adversely with various other drugs (see Table 11.1). The choice to drink must therefore be made in consideration of other substances a person is using.

Alcohol the Chemical

The intoxicating substance found in beer, wine, liquor, and liqueurs is **ethyl alcohol,** or **ethanol.** It is produced during a process called **fermentation,** whereby plant sugars are broken down by yeast organisms, yielding ethanol and carbon dioxide. Fermentation continues until the solution of plant sugars (called mash) reaches a concentration of 14 percent alcohol. At this point, the alcohol kills the yeast and halts the chemical reactions that produce it.

For beers and ales, which are fermented from malt barley, the process stops when the alcohol concentration is 14 percent. After that point, manufacturers add other ingredients that dilute the alcohol content of the beverage. Other alcoholic beverages are produced through further processing called **distillation,** during which alcohol vapors are released from the mash at high temperatures. The vapors are then condensed and mixed with water to make the final product.

The **proof** of an alcoholic drink is a measure of the percentage of alcohol in the beverage. Alcohol percentage is 50 percent of the given proof. Thus, 80-proof whiskey or scotch is 40-percent alcohol by volume, and 100-proof vodka is 50-percent alcohol by volume. The proof of a beverage thus provides an indication of its strength. Lower-proof drinks will produce fewer alcohol effects than the same amounts of higher-proof drinks.

Most wines contain between 12 and 15 percent alcohol. Beers contain between 2 and 6 percent, and ales between 6 and 8 percent (see Table 11.2). The alcoholic content of beers varies according to state laws. Also, since the early 1980s, many breweries and wineries have been marketing "light" (low-calorie) and alcohol-reduced beers and wines.

PHYSIOLOGICAL EFFECTS OF ALCOHOL

Alcohol causes numerous changes in physiological and psychological functioning. The rate of ingestion and the amounts ingested will influence the rate and amount of change.

Metabolism

Unlike molecules found in most other ingestible foods and drugs, alcohol molecules are sufficiently small and fat-soluble to be absorbed throughout the entire length

---

Ethyl alcohol (ethanol) An addictive drug produced by fermentation and found in many beverages.
Fermentation The process whereby yeast organisms break down plant sugars to yield a "mash" that contains ethanol.
Distillation The process whereby mash is subjected to high temperatures to release alcohol vapors.
Proof A measure of the percentage of alcohol in a beverage.

Table 11.1 Drugs and Alcohol: Actions and Interactions

Drug Class/Trade Name(s)	Effects with Alcohol
Anti-alcohol Antabuse	Severe reactions to even small amounts: headache, nausea, blurred vision, convulsions, coma, possible death.
Antibiotics Penicillin, Cyantin	Reduces therapeutic effectiveness.
Antidepressants Elavil, Sinequan, Tofranil, Nardil	Increased central-nervous-system (CNS) depression, blood-pressure changes. Combination use of alcohol with MAO inhibitors, a specific type of antidepressant, can trigger massive increases in blood pressure, even brain hemorrhage and death.
Antihistamines Allerest, Dristan	Drowsiness and CNS depression. Impairs driving ability.
Aspirin Anacin, Excedrin, Bayer	Irritates stomach lining. May cause gastrointestinal pain, bleeding.
Depressants Valium, Ativan, Placidyl	Dangerous CNS depression, loss of coordination, coma. High risk of overdose and death.
Narcotics heroin, codeine, Darvon	Serious CNS depression. Possible respiratory arrest and death.
Stimulants caffeine, cocaine	Masks depressant action of alcohol. May increase blood pressure, physical tension.

SOURCE: *Drugs and Alcohol: Simple Facts about Alcohol and Drug Combinations* (Phoenix: DIN Publications, 1988), no. 121.

Table 11.2 Beverages and Their Alcohol and Calorie Content

Beverage	Alcohol by Volume (approx. %)	Calories (per serving, approx.)
Nonalcoholic beer	0.5	75
Beer, regular	4.5	170
Beer, light	3	70–134
Wine, light beverage	10–14	90 (per 4 fl. oz.)
Sherry and other fortified wines	17–21	140 (per 3.5 fl. oz.)
Champagne	11–12	71 (per 3 fl. oz.)
Sake wine	14–16	39 (per 1 fl. oz.)
Tequila	40	—
Gin	40	120 (per 1.5 fl. oz.)
Brandy	35–40	60 (per 4 fl. oz.)
Vodka	40	95 (per 1.5 fl. oz.)
Rum	40	135 (per 1.5 fl. oz.)
Whiskey	40–54	130 (per 1.5 fl. oz.)

SOURCE: Ken Liska. *Drugs and the Human Body*, 3rd ed. (New York: Macmillan, 1990), p. 186.

of the gastrointestinal system. A negligible amount of alcohol is absorbed through the lining of the mouth. Approximately 20 percent of ingested alcohol is diffused through the stomach lining into the bloodstream. Nearly 80 percent of the liquid passes through the linings of the upper third of the small intestine. Absorption into the bloodstream is rapid and complete.

The concentration of the drink and the amount of food in the stomach at the time of ingestion are two of the major factors affecting the rate of absorption. An alcoholic beverage diluted with fruit juice or other liquid will be absorbed much less rapidly than a drink consisting of straight alcohol. Likewise, if the stomach is full, absorption is slowed because the surface area of the stomach exposed to alcohol is smaller. A full stomach also slows the emptying of the alcohol into the small intestine. Carbonated alcoholic beverages are also more rapidly absorbed than those containing no sparkling additives.

Alcohol is metabolized in the liver, where it is converted by the enzyme *alcohol dehydrogenase* to *acetylaldehyde*. It is then rapidly oxidized to acetate, converted to carbon dioxide and water, and eventually excreted from the body. A very small portion of alcohol is excreted unchanged by the kidneys, lungs, and skin.

Like food, alcohol contains calories. Proteins and carbohydrates (starches and sugars) each contain 4 kilocalories (kcal) per gram. Fat contains 9 kcal per gram. Alcohol, although similar in structure to carbohydrates, contains 7 kcal per gram. The body uses the calories found in alcohol in the same manner it uses carbohydrates. Alcohol calories may be used for immediate energy or may be stored as fat if not immediately needed.

In comparison to the variable breakdown rates of foods and other beverages, the breakdown of alcohol occurs at a fairly constant rate of 0.5 ounces per hour. This amount of alcohol is equivalent to 12 ounces of 5-percent beer, 5 ounces of 12-percent wine, or 1.5 ounces of 40-percent (80-proof) liquor (see Figure 11.1).

Blood alcohol concentration (BAC) is the factor by which the physiological and behavioral effects of alcohol are measured. Legal limits of BAC for operating motor vehicles vary from state to state. Most states set the legal limit at 0.08 to 0.10 percent. Levels of BAC greater than a state's legal limit render the driver legally intoxicated.

A drinker's BAC depends on his or her weight and body fat, the water content in body tissues, the concentration of alcohol in the beverage consumed, the rate of consumption, and the volume of alcohol consumed. Heavier people have larger body surfaces through which to diffuse alcohol; therefore, they will have lower concentrations of alcohol in their blood. Because alcohol does not diffuse as rapidly into body fat as into water, alcohol concentration is higher in a person with more body fat. Because a woman is likely to have more body fat and less water content in her body tissues than does a man of the same weight, she will be more intoxicated than the man after drinking. Table 11.3 compares blood-alcohol levels by sex, weight, and consumption. Although this table can provide an estimate of probable BAC levels, many additional factors may cause considerable variation in these rates. For this reason, you should be cautious when gauging your blood-alcohol levels.

The "breathalyzer" tests used by law-enforcement officers are designed to determine BAC based on the amount of alcohol exhaled in the breath. Likewise, urinalysis can also yield a BAC based on the concentration of unmetabolized alcohol in the urine. Breath analysis and urinalysis can determine whether a driver is legally intoxicated. However, blood tests are the most accurate

---

Blood alcohol concentration (BAC) The amount of alcohol in the blood; the measure against which physiological and behavioral effects of alcohol are compared.

Figure 11.1 Breakdown rate per hour of 3 different alcoholic beverages.

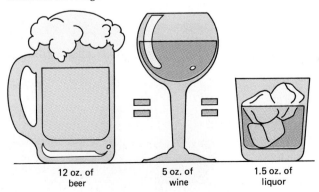

| 12 oz. of beer | 5 oz. of wine | 1.5 oz. of liquor |

Table 11.3   Comparisons of Blood Alcohol Levels by Sex, Weight, and Consumption

Absolute Alcohol (oz.)	Beverage Intake in 1 hr.	Blood-Alcohol Levels (mg/100 ml.)					
		Female (100-lb.)	Male (100-lb.)	Female (150-lb.)	Male (150-lb.)	Female (200-lb.)	Male (200-lb.)
0.5	1 oz. spirits* 1 glass wine 1 can beer	0.045	0.037	0.03	0.025	0.022	0.019
1	2 oz. spirits 2 glasses wine 2 cans beer	0.090	0.075	0.06	0.050	0.045	0.037
2	4 oz. spirits 4 glasses wine 4 cans beer	0.180	0.150	0.12	0.100	0.090	0.070
3	6 oz. spirits 6 glasses wine 6 cans beer	0.270	0.220	0.18	0.150	0.130	0.110
4	8 oz. spirits 8 glasses wine 8 cans beer	0.360	0.300	0.24	0.200	0.180	0.150
5	10 oz. spirits 10 glasses wine 10 cans beer	0.450	0.370	0.30	0.250	0.220	0.180

* 100-proof spirits.

SOURCE: Oakley Ray and Charles Ksir, *Drugs, Society, and Human Behavior,* 5th ed. (St. Louis: Times Mirror/Mosby, 1990), p. 170.

measures of BAC. More and more states are requiring blood tests for people suspected of driving under the influence of alcohol. In some states, refusal to take either the breath or urine tests results in immediate revocation of a person's driver's license.

Behavioral Effects

Behavioral changes caused by alcohol vary with the individual. Generalizations contrasting pre- and postdrinking behaviors are difficult to make. However, alcohol

Law-enforcement officials employ "breathalyzer" tests to determine whether drivers are legally intoxicated.

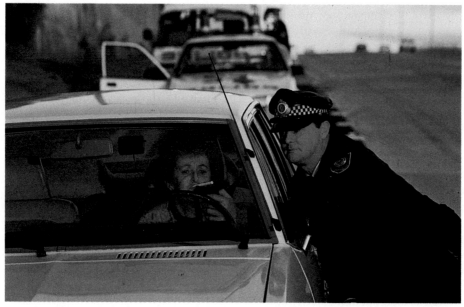

Communication

Communicating Your Concerns When Someone Close to You Drinks Too Much

There may be times when you see someone's drinking getting out of control. You may be affected directly (e.g., if the person says something that embarrasses you) or indirectly (if you see the person act in unusual and embarrassing ways). When you see these kinds of behavior, it may be helpful to talk to the person about your concerns.

Help Is Usually Given in Three Stages:

1. Learn about the illness of alcoholism and various sources of treatment.
2. Guide the person close to you to treatment.
3. Support the person during and after treatment.

Guidelines for Discussing Alcohol Abuse

1. Choose a comfortable time and place when the person is sober.
2. Decide whether the person will respect your feelings or whether there is a more appropriate person (best friend, roommate) to handle the discussion.
3. Find out whether anyone else is affected the same way you are by the person's drinking behaviors.
4. Describe the specific behaviors or remarks that bothered you. Do not be vague about the consequences of the behaviors you describe.
5. Do not criticize, diagnose, or judge your friends' actions. (For example, do not say, "You have a drinking problem.") Explain that you want to share your concerns because you care.
6. After sharing your list of behaviors, let your friend accept or reject what you have said. Do not accept or make excuses; stay on the offensive.

Be aware that your friend may express a range of feelings, from gratitude to anger to indifference. If the person reacts defensively, do not take it personally. You should feel good about doing your friend a service even though it may not be recognized as one at the time. For further information and resources about alcohol, problem drinking, or how to talk to people about their drinking, call Alcoholics Anonymous, Al-Anon, or your local mental-health center, or look for substance-abuse counselors and clinics in the phone book.

SOURCES: Martha Carey, "Lifestyle Workshops," *Human Kinetics.* (Champaign, Ill.: National Institute on Drug Abuse, 1988), p. 310.

---

produces some general behavior effects depending on the BAC. At a BAC of 0.02, the person feels relaxed or euphoric. At 0.05, normal inhibitions are almost eliminated, and some loss of motor impairment and a willingness to talk become apparent. At 0.10, the depressant effects of alcohol become apparent, drowsiness sets in, and motor skills are further impaired, followed by a change in judgment. A driver may not be able to estimate distances or speed. Some drinkers lose their ability to make value-related decisions and may do things they would not do when sober. As the BAC increases, the drinker suffers increased physiological and psychological effects. All these changes are negative. No skills or functions are enhanced because of alcohol ingestion. Rather, physical and mental functions are impaired.

Physical and psychological tolerance to the effects of alcohol can be acquired through regular use. The nervous system adapts over time so that greater amounts of alcohol are required to produce the same physiological and psychological effects. Some people can learn to modify their behavior so that they appear sober even when their BAC is quite high. This behavior is called **learned behavioral tolerance.**

Immediate Effects of Alcohol

The most dramatic effects produced by ethanol are exhibited within the central nervous system, or CNS (see Chapter 2). The primary action of the drug is to reduce the frequency of nerve transmissions and impulses at synaptic junctions within the CNS. This reduction of nerve transmissions results in a significant depression of

---

Learned behavioral tolerance The ability of heavy drinkers to modify their behavior so that they appear to be sober even when they have high BAC levels.

CNS functions, with resulting decreases in respiratory rate, pulse rate, and blood pressure. As CNS depression deepens, vital functions become noticeably depressed. In extreme cases, coma and death can result.

A **hangover** is often experienced the morning after a drinking spree. The causes of hangovers are not well known. Dehydration of cerebral tissues seems to be one cause. Another possible cause is a hypersensitive (allergic) reaction to certain chemicals in alcoholic beverages.

Although home remedies abound, time is really the only effective cure for a hangover. Consuming less than 1 drink per hour, eating before or along with drinking, consuming plenty of nonalcoholic beverages, and getting adequate rest after drinking minimize BAC levels and unpleasant aftereffects.

A **blackout** is a temporary form of amnesia. Blackouts are not necessarily dependent on BAC, although they are usually experienced at higher levels of intoxication and with chronic alcohol intake. Someone who is or has been drinking may appear perfectly normal and may be conscious, talking, walking, and in control. The following day, however, the person has no memory of events that occurred. Blackouts are considered to be one of the first signs of problem drinking or a progression toward alcoholism.

Long-term Effects of Alcohol Abuse

Chronic alcohol consumption over a period of years has a cumulative effect that can be quite serious and may be irreversible. Every system in the body is affected by chronic heavy use of alcohol.

Liver Disease   One of the most common diseases related to abuse of alcohol is **cirrhosis** of the liver, the last stage of liver disease. As a result of heavy drinking, the liver begins to fill with fat. If there is not sufficient time between drinking episodes, the fat cannot be transported away to storage sites, and the fat-filled liver cells stop functioning. Continued drinking can cause a further stage of liver deterioration called *fibrosis*, in which the damaged area of the liver develops fibrous scar tissue. Cell function in the liver can be partially restored at this stage with proper nutrition and abstention from alcohol. If the person continues to drink, cirrhosis results. At this point, the liver cells die, harden, and turn orange, and the damage is permanent.

Effects on the Nervous System   The nervous system is especially sensitive to alcohol. Even people who drink moderately experience shrinkage in brain size and weight and a loss of some degree of intellectual ability. The damage that results from alcohol use is localized primarily in the left side of the brain, which is responsible for written and spoken language, logic, and mathematical skills. The degree of shrinkage appears to be directly related to the amount of alcohol consumed. In terms of

memory loss, the evidence suggests that having 1 drink every day is better than saving up for a binge and consuming 7 or 8 drinks in a night. The amount of alcohol consumed at one time is critical. Alcohol-related brain damage can be partially reversed with good nutrition and abstinence.

Cardiovascular Effects   The cardiovascular system is affected by alcohol in a number of different ways. Evidence suggests that the effect of alcohol on the heart is not all bad. Studies by the National Heart, Lung, and Blood Institute suggest that moderate drinkers suffer fewer heart attacks, have less cholesterol buildup in their arteries, and are less likely to die of heart disease than nondrinkers or heavy drinkers.* However, drinking is not recommended as a preventive measure against heart disease.

There are many more health hazards than benefits relating to alcohol consumption and the cardiovascular system. Alcohol contributes to high blood pressure and slightly increased heart rate and cardiac output. Those who report drinking three to five drinks a day, regardless of race or sex, have higher blood pressure than those who drink less.

The body's red blood cells are also affected by alcohol. Alcohol produces an effect known as *sludging*, in which groups of red blood cells clump together in sticky masses. These clumped red blood cells cannot pass through the tiny capillaries in some parts of the body, leading to oxygen deprivation.

Other Effects   Repeated irritation of the gastrointestinal system by alcohol has been linked to cancers of the esophagus, stomach, mouth, tongue, and liver. Alcohol also affects intestinal function and can cause chronic diarrhea.

Alcohol abuse is a major cause of chronic inflammation of the pancreas, the organ that produces digestive enzymes and insulin. Chronic abuse of alcohol inhibits enzyme production, which further inhibits the absorption of nutrients.

Alcohol and Pregnancy   Alcohol can have harmful effects on fetal development. A disorder called *fetal alcohol syndrome (FAS)* is associated with alcohol consumption throughout pregnancy. FAS is the third most com-

---

Hangover   Unpleasant physical reactions that follow a period of heavy drinking.

Blackout   A temporary form of amnesia, usually occurring at higher levels of intoxication and with chronic alcohol intake.

Cirrhosis   The last stage of liver disease associated with chronic heavy use of alcohol. Liver cells die, and the damage is permanent.

---

* R. D. Moore and T. A. Pearson, "Moderate Alcohol Consumption and Coronary Heart Disease: A Review," *Medicine*, 65, no. 4 (1986), 242–67; Y. Okamoto, Y. Fujimori et al., "Role of Liver in Alcohol-induced Alteration of High-Density Lipoprotein Metabolism," *Journal of Laboratory Clinical Medicine* 111, no. 4 (1988), 484–85.

mon birth defect and second leading cause of mental retardation in the United States. FAS occurs when alcohol ingested by the mother passes through the placenta into the infant's bloodstream. Because the fetus is so small, its BAC will be much higher than that of the mother. Thus, consumption of alcohol during pregnancy can affect the infant far more seriously than it affects the mother. Among the results of FAS are mental retardation, small head, tremors, and abnormalities of the face, limbs, heart, and brain. Infants whose mothers habitually consume more than 3 ounces of alcohol (approximately 6 drinks) in a short time period when pregnant are at a high risk for FAS. Risk levels for babies whose mothers consume smaller amounts are uncertain.

Alcohol can also be passed to a nursing baby through breast milk. For this reason, most doctors advise nursing mothers not to drink for at least 4 hours before nursing their babies, and preferably to abstain altogether.

ALCOHOLISM

How, Why, Who?

Many people do not limit themselves to 1 drink per hour. Their express purpose in consuming alcohol is to become intoxicated. Because this type of drinking can become habitual, it is usually labeled irresponsible use, or **binge drinking**. Problem drinking is more likely to occur among people between the ages of 15 and 24 than in any other age group.* Alcohol use becomes **alcohol abuse** (alcoholism) when it interferes with work, school, or social and family relationships, or when it entails any encounter with the law, including driving while intoxicated (DWI). (See the "Health in Your Community" box for information on avoiding alcohol misuse in social situations.)

The stereotype of the alcoholic as a skid-row bum applies to only 5 percent of the alcoholic population. The remaining 95 percent of alcoholics live in some type of extended family unit. They can be found in all socioeconomic levels, professions, ethnic groups, geographical locations, religions, and races. One in 10 Americans is an alcoholic. Moreover, 25 percent of the American population (50 million people) are affected by the alcoholism of a friend or family member. In all, some 18 million American adults are either alcoholics or have alcohol-abuse problems.**

Women are the fastest-growing component of the population of alcohol abusers. Women tend to become alcoholic at a later age and have fewer years of heavy drinking compared to men. Women at highest risk for alcohol-related problems are those who are unmarried but living with a partner, are in their twenties or early thirties, or have a husband or partner who drinks heavily.

Theories of Alcoholism

How and why alcoholism begins is somewhat of a mystery. It is apparent that alcoholism is a disease with biological, psychological, and social/environmental components. What is not clear, however, is the role that each of these components has in determining whether or not someone will become an alcoholic.

Research into the hereditary and environmental causes of alcoholism has found that high rates of alcoholism exist among family members of alcoholics. Two distinct subtypes of alcoholism have provided important information about the inheritability of alcoholism. *Type 1 alcoholism* is characterized by onset after age 25 in either sex, with mild antisocial behavior or occupational problems. These people avoid harmful situations, are generally not spontaneous, and tend to seek social approval. *Type 2 alcoholics* are typically biological sons of alcoholic fathers and have a history of violence and drug use. They do not seek social approval, lack inhibition, and show a high level of novelty-seeking behavior.*

A 1984 study found a relationship between alcoholism and alcoholic patterns within the family.** Children with one alcoholic parent had a 52-percent chance of becoming alcoholics themselves. With two alcoholic parents, the chances of becoming alcoholic jumped to 71 percent.† The researchers felt that both heredity and environment played parts in the development of alcoholism but were reluctant to say precisely how these factors worked.

Although scientists are hot on the trail of an "alcohol gene," so far they have not managed to find one. In 1990, it appeared the specific gene linked to alcoholism had been discovered. The gene reportedly was a receptor for dopamine, a chemical that plays a crucial role in cell communication and pleasure-seeking behavior. Unfortunately, the gene was not found consistently in every alcoholic studied, and was even found in some individuals who were not alcoholics.* Social and cultural factors may trigger the affliction for many alcoholics who are not genetically predisposed to the disease. Although

Binge Drinking Habitual drinking for the express purpose of becoming intoxicated.

Alcohol Abuse (alcoholism) Excessive use of alcohol that interferes with work, school, or personal relationships or that violates the law.

---

* F. K. Goodwin annd E. M. Gause, "Alcohol, Drug Abuse, and Mental Health Administration," *Prevention Pipeline*, 3, no. 3 (1990), 19.
** S. I. Benowitz, "Studies Help Scientists Home in on Genetics of Alcoholism," *Science News*, September 29, 1984, p. 17.
† John Wells, "Alcohol: The Number One Drug of Abuse in the United States," *Athletic Training*, Fall 1982, p. 172.
* Kenneth Blum, Ernest Noble et al., "Allelic Association of Human Dopamine D_2 Receptor Gene in Alcoholism," *Journal of the American Medical Association*, 262, no. 15 (1990), 2055–59.

---

* National Traffic Safety Association education materials (1987).
** U.S. Department of Health and Human Services, *Proceedings of the Surgeon General's Workshop on Drunk Driving* (1989).

Health in Your Community

Use of Alcohol in Social Situations

Because society has few rules for drinking, we are wise to establish our own rules and limits. These rules should be based on a knowledge of the effects of alcohol and our own common sense.

Many people choose not to drink for religious, health, or personal reasons. No one should have to defend the decision to abstain from the use of alcohol. Social pressure to consume alcoholic beverages is said to be a major influence on the drinking behaviors of people of all ages. Although such pressures may be blatant in our teenage years, they become more subtle as we mature. The first common-sense rule regarding drinking behavior is to honor anyone's decision not to consume alcoholic beverages.

When attending a social gathering at which alcoholic beverages are consumed, the responsible party-goer thinks of drinking in the same way as eating. Very few of us would publicly consume 3 bags of potato chips. (Even binge eaters do their eating in private.) Yet many of us think nothing of guzzling too much alcohol in public. The

responsible drinker sets rules and limits and then abides by them.

Possible rules could include:

1. Know your limits and stay within them. If others are pushing alcohol at you, you can fill your glass with ice or your beer can with water and pretend to continue drinking. You can also simply tell the truth: You prefer not to drink.
2. Stick to the limit of 1 ounce of alcohol in 1 hour. This will not only reduce the possibility of drunkenness but may also leave you in a legal condition to drive home.
3. Wine, beer, and mixed drinks are easier to "nurse" than straight liquor. Stick to these rather than the higher-proof beverages.
4. Eating and drinking at the same time will promote a slower absorption rate of alcohol. Never drink on an empty stomach.
5. Alternate alcoholic beverages with nonalcoholic beverages.

it may be years before a clear genetic link is proven, results from a landmark 600-family study to identify genes that can raise alcoholism risk may be in by 1993.

Although a family history of alcoholism may predispose a person to problems with alcohol, there are numerous other factors that also appear to increase individual risk. Some people begin drinking as a way to dull the senses in order to avoid the pain of an acute loss or some other emotional pain. For example, college students may begin drinking to escape from the stress of college life, disappointment over unfulfilled expectations, difficulties in forming relationships, and loss of the security of home, loved ones, and close friends. Involvement in a painful relationship, death of a family member, and other problems may trigger a search for a way to avoid thinking about problems. Unfortunately, the emotional discomfort that causes many people to turn to alcohol also ultimately causes them to become even more uncomfortable as the depressant effect of the drug begins to take its toll.

Certain social factors have been linked with alcoholism as well. These include urbanization, weakening links to the extended family and general loosening of

kinship ties, increased mobility, and changing religious and philosophical values.

Costs to Society

In a larger sense, the entire society suffers the consequences of alcohol abuse. Half of all traffic fatalities are attributable to alcohol. The annual cost to our society of alcohol-related crimes, medical expenses, accidents, and treatment programs is nearly $117 billion.** Direct health-care costs of alcoholics are estimated to exceed $20 billion yearly. Alcoholism reportedly is directly and indirectly responsible for over 25 percent of the nation's medical expenses and lost earnings. Finally, well over 50 percent of all child-abuse cases are the result of alcohol-related problems. The costs in emotional health are impossible to measure.† Figure 11.2 highlights some of society's alcohol-related problems.

Recognition of an alcohol problem is extremely diffi-

** Ibid.

† U.S. Department of Health and Human Services, *Seventh Special Report to the U.S. Congress on Alcohol and Health*, (1990), p. 22.

Health in Your Community (*Continued*)

6. If you are unfit to drive home, have your host or hostess call a cab or ride with someone who has not been drinking. (Sometimes people go to parties with people who do not drink, secure in the knowledge they will have a safe way to get home.)

7. Understand that being drunk does not excuse your behavior.

8. Remember that it is easy to enjoy yourself without being inebriated. If you like to get drunk just to act silly, try acting silly without the alcohol—it might just be more fun.

For party hosts and hostesses:

1. Be sure there is adequate food and that it is readily available to all guests.

2. Serve beverages that are lighter in alcoholic content than straight liquors.

3. Limit the availability of alcohol to your guests. Do not insist on refilling glasses; wait until asked.

4. Limit the time of drinking.

5. Plan the party to focus on something other than alcohol.

6. Have coffee, tea, or other nonalcoholic beverages readily available throughout the gathering. Put alcoholic beverages away toward the end of the party.

7. If a guest is too drunk to drive home, arrange alternative transportation or allow the guest to stay the night. Never accept a guest's word that he or she is sober enough to drive.

Caution! If a friend passes out from too much to drink, be sure to monitor him or her. Place your friend on his or her side with legs bent, the head turned to the side. Because alcohol is a gastric irritant, vomiting is a possibility. An intoxicated person asleep in a face-down or face-up position could inhale his or her own vomit and suffocate.

Figure 11.2 Alcohol and society.

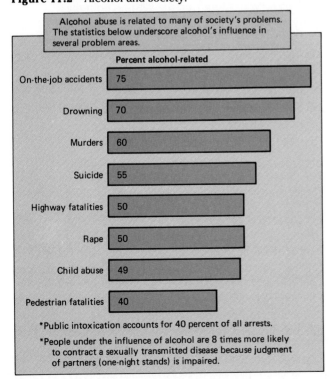

Alcohol abuse is related to many of society's problems. The statistics below underscore alcohol's influence in several problem areas.

Percent alcohol-related

On-the-job accidents	75
Drowning	70
Murders	60
Suicide	55
Highway fatalities	50
Rape	50
Child abuse	49
Pedestrian fatalities	40

*Public intoxication accounts for 40 percent of all arrests.

*People under the influence of alcohol are 8 times more likely to contract a sexually transmitted disease because judgment of partners (one-night stands) is impaired.

cult. The alcoholics themselves deny their problem, often making statements such as "I can stop any time I want to. I just don't want to right now." Family members also deny the existence of a problem, perhaps saying things like, "He really has been under a lot of stress lately. Besides, he only drinks beer." (For a discussion of codependence, see Chapter 10.) The fear of being labeled a "problem drinker" often prevents people from seeking help.

Alcoholics tend to have a number of behaviors in common. Some of the indicators of alcoholism are listed in the accompanying "Promoting Your Health" box. People who recognize one or more of these behaviors in themselves may wish to seek professional help to determine whether alcohol has become a controlling factor in their lives.

Alcoholism and the Family

Only recently have people begun to recognize that it is not only the alcoholic but the alcoholic's entire family that suffers from the disease of alcoholism. Although most research focuses on family effects during the late

Myths and Realities of Alcohol Use

Testing Your Knowledge

Read each of the following sentences carefully and answer true or false.

1. Alcohol is a sexual stimulant.

False. Increasing your alcohol intake decreases your ability to function sexually. Although you may be less inhibited when you are high, you are less likely to be able to follow through.

Alcohol weakens your defenses, lowers your inhibitions, and reduces your ability to make safe, smart decisions about sex partners and activities. As a result, mixing alcohol and sex increases your chances of getting pregnant or getting a sexually transmitted disease, including AIDS. It also can set the stage for date rape.

2. It is okay to mix alcohol with other drugs.

False. Combining alcohol and other drugs is the number-one cause of drug-related death in this country.

Alcohol can cause adverse or potentially fatal reactions in people taking prescription or nonprescription medications. In addition, mixing alcohol and street drugs, such as crack or PCP, is especially risky because the true ingredients and quality of the street drugs are unknown.

3. Drinking only beer or wine does not lead to serious drinking problems.

False. Wine and beer drinkers *can* develop serious drinking problems. A bottle of beer, a wine cooler, a glass of wine, and a shot of hard liquor all have about the same amount of *pure* alcohol—a little more than one-half ounce. Alcohol in wine or beer is absorbed more slowly because it is diluted. Thus, while you probably will not feel the effects of the alcohol as quickly when you drink beer or wine, you are pouring the same amount of alcohol into your system. And you may be developing a serious drinking problem.

4. There is no way to sober up quickly.

True. Time is the only sobering agent. Coffee won't do it. Neither will cold showers, vomiting, or any other remedy you know. To become sober your body must metabolize the alcohol, and this is a slow process. As a rule, it will take 1 hour for a male weighing 150 pounds to metabolize the alcohol in a standard drink (1 glass of wine, shot of liquor, or bottle of beer). Factors such as weight, health, and age will affect how quickly your liver can metabolize the alcohol.

5. Anyone can drink 2 or 3 drinks without their behavior and judgment changing noticeably.

False. Alcohol changes behavior and judgment beginning with the first drink. The change is progressive. The number of drinks it takes for the changes to be noticeable varies for each individual.

The impact of 2, 3, or any number of drinks on your behavior and judgment varies in response to social and physical factors. Social factors include your mood and the setting (both the people and place). Physical factors include your body weight, the amount of food in your stomach, the amount of rest you have had, how quickly the alcohol enters your system, and your health and gender. (Women usually feel the effects of alcohol faster than men even when compared to men of the same weight. Hormonal changes and the use of oral contraceptives also change the impact of alcohol.)

Reprinted with permission from the American College Health Association, "Alcohol: Decisions on Tap," 1988.

stages of alcoholism, the family unit actually begins to react early on as the person begins to show symptoms of the disease. Do certain types of families raise alcoholics? Can actions of family members actually encourage other family members to drink?

An estimated 30 million Americans (1 out of 8) grow up in alcoholic households.* Twenty-two million mem- bers of alcoholic families are 18 or older, and many have carried emotional childhood scars with them into adulthood.** An estimated 7 million children who are 18 or younger live in an atmosphere of anxiety, tension, confusion, and denial. The home is often a battleground filled with stress and embarrassment. The needs of other

* Do It Now Foundation, *Children of Alcoholics*, 1989.

** Office of Substance Abuse Prevention, December, 1991.

Promoting Your Health

Do You Have an Alcohol Problem?

Yes   No

☐ ☐ **1.** Have you ever cut classes in order to drink?

☐ ☐ **2.** Do you drink while studying?

☐ ☐ **3.** Have you ever missed classes because of a hangover?

☐ ☐ **4.** Have you ever done poorly on an exam or assignment because of drinking?

☐ ☐ **5.** Have you ever neglected a school obligation because of drinking?

☐ ☐ **6.** Have friends or family ever told you that you drink too much?

☐ ☐ **7.** Have you ever lost a friend or has a relationship ever suffered from your drinking?

☐ ☐ **8.** Have you ever done or said anything while drinking that you later regretted?

☐ ☐ **9.** Do you urge friends to drink so you won't stand out?

☐ ☐ **10.** Have you begun to associate with a group of friends who drink heavily?

☐ ☐ **11.** Have you ever been injured while drinking?

☐ ☐ **12.** Have you ever awakened after drinking and wondered what happened the night before?

☐ ☐ **13.** Do you ever feel guilty about your drinking?

☐ ☐ **14.** Do you drink to forget your problems?

☐ ☐ **15.** Do you drink to feel more comfortable?

☐ ☐ **16.** Do you ever borrow money or do without other things so you can drink?

☐ ☐ **17.** Have you ever been broke because you spent most of your money on alcohol?

☐ ☐ **18.** Have you ever destroyed or damaged property while you were drinking?

☐ ☐ **19.** Do you ever drive while you are drinking or drunk?

☐ ☐ **20.** Have you been in trouble with police or university authorities because of your drinking or something you did while drinking?

☐ ☐ **21.** Do you ever drink more than you planned?

☐ ☐ **22.** Do you ever have difficulty stopping once you have begun drinking?

☐ ☐ **23.** Do you need a drink to get going in the morning?

☐ ☐ **24.** Do you ever drink alone?

☐ ☐ **25.** Do you ever hide the amount you drink from others?

What Does It Mean?

Answering yes to any of the above questions reveals abusive drinking patterns that merit your attention. The more yes answers, the more urgent your drinking situation and the greater your concern should be. Seek help from your college health center, community mental-health agency, family physician, Alcoholics Anonymous, or other programs available in your community.

Source: Cheryl Graham, *When Is Drinking a Problem?* Oregon State University Student Health Center, 1992.

family members are ignored, and family life centers around the drinking member.

Where to Go for Help

Despite the growing recognition of our national alcohol problem, less than 10 percent of alcoholics in the United States receive any care. Most alcoholics and problem drinkers who seek help have experienced a turning point or dramatic occurrence: A spouse walks out, taking children and possessions; the boss issues an ultimatum to dry out or ship out; the courtroom judge offers the alternatives of prison or a treatment center; a teenage child confesses embarrassment over bringing friends home; a friend or colleague confronts the person about drinking behavior. Regardless of the reasons for seeking help, the alcoholic ready for treatment has, in most cases, reached a low point. Devoid of hope, physically depleted, and spiritually despairing, the alcoholic has finally recognized that alcohol controls his or her life. The first step on the road to recovery is to regain that control and begin to assume responsibility for personal actions.

The Family's Role   Sometimes family members of an alcoholic take action before the alcoholic does. They may go to an organization or a treatment facility to seek help for themselves and their relative. An effective method of helping an alcoholic to confront the disease is through a process called an **intervention**. Essentially, an intervention is a planned confrontation with the alcoholic that involves several family members plus professional counselors. The family members express their love and concern, telling the alcoholic that they will no longer refrain from acknowledging the problem and affirming their support for appropriate treatment. A family intervention is the turning point for a growing number of alcoholics. The alcoholic ready for help has several avenues for treatment: psychologists and psychiatrists specializing in the treatment of alcoholism, private treatment centers, hospitals specifically designed to treat alcoholics, community mental-health facilities, and support groups such as Alcoholics Anonymous.

Treatment Facilities   Private treatment facilities have been making concerted efforts to attract patients through radio and television advertising. Upon admission to a treatment facility, the patient is given a complete physical examination to determine whether underlying medical problems will interfere with treatment. Withdrawal from alcohol can produce serious symptoms, including hyperexcitability, tremors, hallucinations, agitation, irritability, confusion, disorientation, sleep disorders, and convulsions. A severe syndrome known as **delirium tremens (DTs)** is characterized by confusion, vivid hallucinations, and delusions. DTs occur in only a small percentage of patients hospitalized for alcoholism. It most commonly occurs in drinkers suffering from malnutrition, depression, fatigue, or other physical illnesses. For the long-term addict, careful medical supervision is necessary. Withdrawal takes from 7 to 21 days, and most treatment facilities keep their patients from 3 to 6 weeks. Treatment at these centers costs several thousand dollars, but some insurance programs or employers will assume most of this expense.

Through individual and group therapy, the person and family members gradually examine the psychological reasons underlying the addiction. Positive coping skills are also learned and reinforced for use in the situations that would previously have caused the alcoholic to turn to alcohol.

Community mental-health centers and alcohol treatment centers may also be able to help the alcoholic in search of recovery. These centers usually have an attending physician and nurse to help with medical prob-lems, as well as counselors and peer support groups. Fees are generally based on the client's income.

Alcoholics Anonymous (AA) is a private, nonprofit organization founded in 1935. The organization, which relies upon group support to help people stop drinking, currently has over 1 million members and has branches all over the world. People attending their first AA meeting will find that no last names are ever used. No one is forced to speak. Members are taught to believe that their alcoholism is a lifetime problem. They are told that they may *never* use alcohol again. In meetings, they share their struggles with one another. They talk about the devastating effects of their alcoholism on their personal and professional lives. All members are asked to place their faith and control of the habit into the hands of a "higher power." The road to recovery is taken one step at a time.

Drug Therapy   Drug therapy for alcoholism is another treatment option. Disulfiram (trade name, Antabuse) is the drug of choice for treating alcoholics. The drug blocks the enzymes acting in the second stage of alcohol metabolism, causing an accumulation of acetylaldehyde in the body. The effects of accumulated acetylaldehyde are unpleasant: headache, nausea, vomiting, drowsiness, and hangover. These symptoms discourage an alcoholic from drinking. Treatment often fails when the alcoholic decides to stop taking the medication. Antabuse therapy works best in conjunction with some type of counseling.

Can Alcoholics Be Cured?

Success in recovery from alcoholism varies with the individual. A return to alcoholic habits often follows what appears to be a successful recovery. Some alcoholics never recover. Some partially recover and improve other parts of their lives but remain dependent on alcohol. Many alcoholics refer to themselves as "recovering" throughout their lifetime; they never use the word "cured."

A comprehensive treatment approach that includes drug therapy, group support, family therapy, and personal counseling designed to improve living and coping skills is usually the most effective course of treatment for the alcoholic who wishes to break the drinking habit. The alcoholics most likely to recover completely are those who developed their dependencies after the age of 20, those with intact and supportive family units, and those who have reached a high level of personal disgust coupled with strong motivation to recover.

Intervention   A planned confrontation in which family members or friends express their concern about an alcoholic's drinking.

Delirium Tremens (DTs)   A state of confusion brought on by the withdrawal from alcohol. Symptoms include hallucinations, anxiety, and trembling.

Alcoholics Anonymous (AA)   An organization whose goal is to help alcoholics stop drinking; includes auxiliary branches such as Al-Anon and Al-a-teen.

TOBACCO

Each year, smoking claims more lives than alcohol and drug abuse combined. More Americans die each year from tobacco-related health problems than died in World War I, World War II, and the Vietnam War combined. While tobacco companies continue to publish full-page advertisements refuting the dangers of smoking, over 390,000 Americans die each year of tobacco-related diseases.* (See Figure 11.3).

Currently, more than 55 million persons (approximately 26.5 percent of the population aged 17 or older) smoke cigarettes in the United States, consuming more than 533 billion cigarettes a year. This translates to 10,000 cigarettes per smoker. Cigarettes, consumed as intended by the manufacturer, caused over 40,000 premature deaths in this country in 1991.** Despite all of the health risks, there are more smokers today than two decades ago. See Table 11.4 for a profile of who among the American population smokes cigarettes.

---

* American Cancer Society, *Facts on Lung Cancer*, (1991), p. 4.

** U.S. Department of Health and Human Services, *Smoking, Tobacco, and Cancer Program: 1985–1989 Status Report* (September 1990).

Table 11.4   Percentage of Smokers among Select Groups in the United States

Males	Percentage
Overall	31.3
White	30.7
Black	37.2
Hispanic	30.9

Females	Percentage
Overall	25.0
White	25.8
Black	26.0
Hispanic	16.5

Occupation	Percentage
White-collar	25.9
Service workers	30.2
Blue-collar	41.1

SOURCE: "Smoking in the USA," *Health Action Managers* (April 25, 1989), pp. 2–3.

Figure 11.3   Tobacco-Related Deaths Compared to Other Deaths.

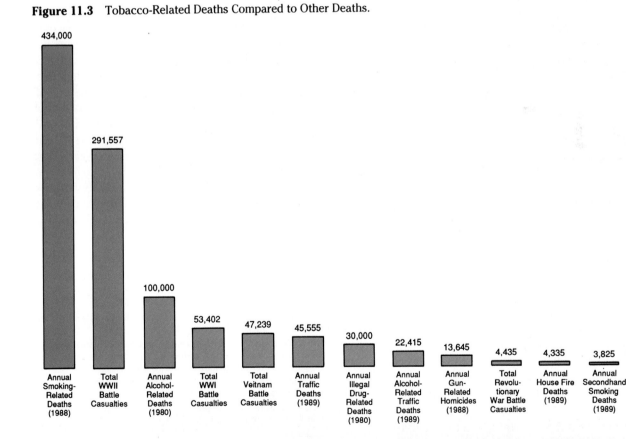

Source: MORBIDITY AND MORTALITY WEEKLY REPORT, Vol 40, No 4, 1991, pp 62-71 U.S. Total Army Personnel Command, Casualty and Mortuary Affairs Division, Washington, DC, R. T. Ravenholt. "ADDICTION MORTALITY IN THE UNITED STATES" 1980. POPULATION AND DEVELOPMENT No 10 Fatal Accident Reporting System 1989, U.S. Department of Transportation, National Highway Safety Administration, National Center for Health Statistics, National Fire Protection Association.

Nicotine and Associated Chemicals

Nicotine Tobacco is available in several forms: cigarettes, cigars, pipe tobacco, snuff, and chewing tobacco (often called "smokeless tobacco"). The chemical stimulant **nicotine** is the major psychoactive substance in all these tobacco products.

In its natural form, nicotine is a colorless liquid that turns brown upon oxidation (exposure to oxygen). When tobacco leaves are burned in a cigarette, pipe, or cigar, nicotine is released and inhaled into the lungs. **Snuff** is a powdered form of tobacco that is inhaled and absorbed through the mucous membranes in the nose. **Chewing tobacco** is taken as a wad, called a "quid," and placed between the gums and teeth. Sucking or chewing the quid releases the nicotine into the saliva, and the nicotine is then absorbed through the mucous membranes in the mouth.

Physiological Effects of Nicotine Nicotine is a powerful central-nervous-system stimulant that produces a variety of physiological effects. Its stimulant action in the cerebral cortex produces an aroused, alert mental state. Nicotine also stimulates the adrenal glands, increasing the production of adrenaline. Physical effects of nicotine stimulation include increased heart and respiratory rate, constriction of blood vessels, and subsequent increased blood pressure because the heart must work harder to pump blood through the narrowed vessels.

Nicotine decreases the stomach contractions that signal hunger. It also decreases blood-sugar levels. These factors, along with decreased sensation in the taste buds, reduce appetite. For this reason, many smokers eat less than do nonsmokers. Smokers weigh an average of 7 pounds less than nonsmokers.

Beginning smokers usually feel the effects of nicotine with their first puff. These symptoms, called **nicotine poisoning,** may include dizziness, lightheadedness, rapid and erratic pulse, clammy skin, nausea, vomiting, and diarrhea.

The effects of nicotine poisoning cease as soon as tolerance to the chemical develops. Medical research indicates that tolerance develops almost immediately in new users, perhaps after the second or third cigarette. In contrast, tolerance to most other drugs, such as alcohol, develops over a period of months or years. (For a further discussion of tobacco addiction, refer to Chapter 10.)

Cigarettes, Cigars, and Pipes Smoking is the most common form of tobacco use. Smoking delivers a strong dose of nicotine to the user, along with an additional 4,000 chemical substances. Among these other substances are various gases and vapors that carry particular matter in concentrations as great as 5 billion particles per cubic millimeter. In contrast, the most air-polluted cities in the world have particulate-matter concentrations of 10,000 particles per cubic millimeter.*

Particulate matter condenses in the lungs to form a thick, brownish sludge called **tar.** Tar contains various carcinogenic (cancer-causing) agents such as benzopyrene and chemical irritants such as phenol. Phenol has the potential to combine with other chemicals and contribute to the development of lung cancer.

In healthy lungs, millions of tiny, hairlike tissues called *cilia* sweep away foreign matter. Once the foreign material is swept up and collected by the cilia, it can be expelled from the lungs through coughing. Nicotine impairs the cleansing function of the cilia by paralyzing them for up to 1 hour following the smoking of a single cigarette. Thus, tars and other solids in tobacco smoke are allowed to accumulate and irritate sensitive lung tissue.

Smokers must remember that tar and nicotine are not the only harmful chemicals in cigarettes. In fact, tars account for only 8 percent of the components of tobacco smoke. The remaining 92 percent is made up of various gases, the most dangerous of which is **carbon monoxide.** In tobacco smoke, the concentration of carbon monoxide is 800 times higher than the level considered safe by the U.S. Environmental Protection Agency (EPA). In the human body, carbon monoxide reduces the oxygen-carrying capacity of the red blood cells by binding at the receptor sites for oxygen. Thus, smoking not only increases heart rate and blood pressure, but it also diminishes the capacity of the circulatory system to carry oxygen, causing oxygen deprivation in many body tissues.

Other gases and dangerous chemicals in tobacco smoke include hydrogen cyanide, vinyl chloride, nitrogen dioxide, formaldehyde, and benzene. Table 11.5 illustrates the concentrations of these gases in one cigarette compared to EPA-recommended safe maximums.

The heat from tobacco smoke can reach 1,616°F and is also harmful to the smoker. Inhaling hot gases and vapors exposes sensitive mucous membranes to irritating chemicals that weaken the tissues and contribute to the development of cancers of the mouth, larynx, and throat.

Filtered cigarettes designed to reduce levels of gases such as hydrogen cyanide and hydrocarbons may actu-

Nicotine The stimulant chemical in cigarettes and smokeless tobacco, a colorless liquid that turns brown upon oxidation.

Snuff A powdered form of tobacco that is sniffed.

Chewing Tobacco A stringy type of tobacco that is placed in the mouth and then sucked or chewed.

Nicotine Poisoning Symptoms often experienced by beginning smokers, including dizziness; diarrhea; lightheadedness; rapid, erratic pulse; clammy skin; nausea; and vomiting.

Tar A thick, brownish substance condensed from particulate matter in cigarette smoke.

Carbon Monoxide A poisonous gas found in cigarette smoke that binds at oxygen receptor sites in the blood.

* Lester Brown, ed., *The State of the World, 1990* (New York: Norton, 1990), pp. 100–101.

Table 11.5 Selected Toxic Substances in 1 Cigarette and EPA-Recommended Safe Maximums

Substance	Hazard	Level in 1 Cigarette	EPA Maximum
Carbon monoxide	Oxygen deprivation	40,000 ppm*	50 ppm
Hydrogen cyanide	Cilia destruction	200 ppm	10 ppm
Nitrogen dioxide	Respiratory irritant	250 ppm	5 ppm
Formaldehyde	Cocarcinogen	90 ppm	2 ppm
Benzene	Carcinogen	67 ppm	0 ppm
Vinyl chloride	Carcinogen	.01 ppm	1 ppm

* parts per million

SOURCES: Gilda Berger, *Smoking Not Allowed* (New York: Franklin Watts, 1987), p. 71; Mike Samuels and Nancy Samuels, *The Well Adult* (New York: Summit, 1988), p. 143.

ally deliver more hazardous carbon monoxide to the user than do nonfiltered brands. Some smokers use low-tar and low-nicotine brands as an excuse to smoke more cigarettes. This practice is self-defeating, as many smokers wind up exposing themselves to more harmful substances than they would if they smoked regular-strength cigarettes.

❚ HEALTH HAZARDS OF SMOKING

There is no doubt that cigarette smoking adversely affects the health of every person who smokes. Each pack of cigarettes has a warning label alerting those who smoke to some of the dangers. Smoking alone has been estimated to be responsible for almost 16 percent of all deaths in the United States each year. Each day cigarettes contribute to deaths or illnesses such as cancer, heart disease, lung diseases, and other causes of mortality.

Cancer The American Cancer Society estimates that tobacco smoking is the cause of 28 percent of all deaths from cancer and more than 90 percent of all cases of lung cancer. Lung cancer, the leading cause of cancer deaths in the United States, kills more than 130,000 Americans a year, 92,000 men and 44,000 women. Less than 10 percent of lung cancers occur among nonsmokers.*

Lung cancer can take from 10 to 30 years to develop, depending on the person. The outlook for victims of this disease is not optimistic. Most lung cancer is not diagnosed until it is relatively widespread in the body. For people with widespread lung cancer, the 5-year survival rate is 13 percent. If a malignancy is diagnosed and

* *Cancer Facts and Figures* (1991) p. 20.

recognized when it is still localized, the 5-year survival rate is 36 percent.

The risk of developing lung cancer is dependent on several factors. First, the number of cigarettes smoked per day is important. A person who smokes 2 packs per day is 15 to 25 times more likely to develop lung cancer than is a nonsmoker (see Table 11.6). People who started smoking in their teens have a greater chance of developing lung cancer than those who started later. Those who inhale deeply when they smoke also increase their chances of developing the disease. Occupational or domestic exposure to other irritants, such as asbestos and radon, also increases the likelihood of developing lung cancer.*

The harmful effects of tobacco are not only linked to lung cancer. Cancers of the lip, tongue, salivary glands, and esophagus are 5 times more likely to occur in smokers than nonsmokers. Smokers are also more likely to develop kidney, bladder, larynx, and pancreatic cancers.

Heart Disease and Circulatory Disorders Half of all tobacco-related deaths occur as a result of some form of heart disease.* Smokers have a 70-percent-higher death rate from heart disease than nonsmokers; heavy smokers have a 200-percent-higher rate than moderate smokers. Smoking cigarettes is as great a risk factor for the development of heart disease as high blood pressure and high cholesterol levels.

Smoking contributes to heart disease by increasing the rate of atherosclerosis, or the buildup of fatty deposits in the heart and major blood vessels. For unknown reasons, smoking decreases blood levels of HDLs (high-density lipoproteins), which help protect against heart attacks. Smoking also contributes to **platelet adhesiveness,** or the sticking together of red blood cells that is associated with blood clots. The oxygen deprivation associated with

Platelet Adhesiveness Stickiness of red blood cells associated with blood clots.

* *Cancer Facts and Figures* (1991), p. 9.
* Mike Samuels and Nancy Samuels, *The Well Adult* (New York: Summit, 1988), p. 140.

Table 11.6 Number of Cigarettes Smoked and Lung Cancer Death Rates—Mortality Ratio per 100,000

Number of Cigarettes Smoked per Day	Mortality Ratio—Men	Mortality Ratio—Women
0	1.0	1.0
1–14	7.8	1.3
15–24	12.7	6.5
25 and above	25.0	30.0

SOURCE: Mike Samuels and Nancy Samuels, *The Well Adult* (New York: Summit, 1988), p. 138.

smoking decreases the oxygen levels supplied to the heart and can weaken tissues. Smoking also contributes to irregular heart rhythms, which can lead to a sudden heart attack. (A more detailed discussion of heart disease is contained in Chapter 13.)

Stroke Smokers are twice as likely to suffer strokes as nonsmokers. A stroke occurs when a small blood vessel in the brain bursts or is blocked by a blood clot, denying oxygen and nourishment to vital portions of the brain. Depending on the area of the brain supplied by the vessel, the stroke can result in paralysis, loss of mental functioning, or death. Smoking contributes to strokes by increasing blood pressure, thereby increasing the stress on vessel walls. Platelet adhesiveness contributes to clotting.

Chronic Obstructive Lung Disorders Chronic obstructive pulmonary disorders (COPD) include bronchitis and emphysema. Smokers' lungs are chronically inflamed because of the constant introduction of vapors, gases, and foreign materials into the lungs. The cilia and mucus-producing cells are forced to work overtime.

Chronic bronchitis may develop because the inflamed lungs develop more mucus and constantly try to rid themselves of the mucus and foreign particles. This results in the "smoker's hack" experienced by most smokers. Smokers are more prone to respiratory ailments such as influenza, pneumonia, and colds than are nonsmokers. (See Figure 11.4)

Emphysema is a chronic disease in which the alveoli are destroyed, making breathing difficult. Whereas healthy people expend only about 5 percent of their energy breathing, people with advanced emphysema expend nearly 80 percent of their energy breathing. Simple movements such as standing up from a seated position may be painful and difficult for the emphysema patient. Approximately 80 percent of all cases of emphysema are related to cigarette smoking.

Women and Smoking A study released in 1989 indicated that female smokers have a higher risk of developing cervical cancer than do female nonsmokers.

Emphysema A chronic lung disease in which tiny air sacs in the lungs are destroyed, making breathing difficult.

Figure 11.4 How cigarette smoking damages the lungs.

Smoking is a sure way to damage your health; it contributes to about one death in seven in the U.S. The main harmful effects come from nicotine, carbon monoxide, and tar. The first two contribute to heart disease, whereas tar causes lung disease and cancer.

Nonsmoker
Cilia
Cells lining airways

Smoker
Smoke particles
Extra mucus produced

Nonsmoker
Bronchiole
Blood capillaries
Alveoli

Smoker
Coalesced alveoli

How smoking damages the lungs
Smoke particles irritate the lung airways, causing excess mucus production (top right). They also indirectly destroy the walls of the lungs' alveoli, which coalesce (above left and right). Both factors reduce lung efficiency. In addition, tar in tobacco smoke has a direct cancer-causing action.

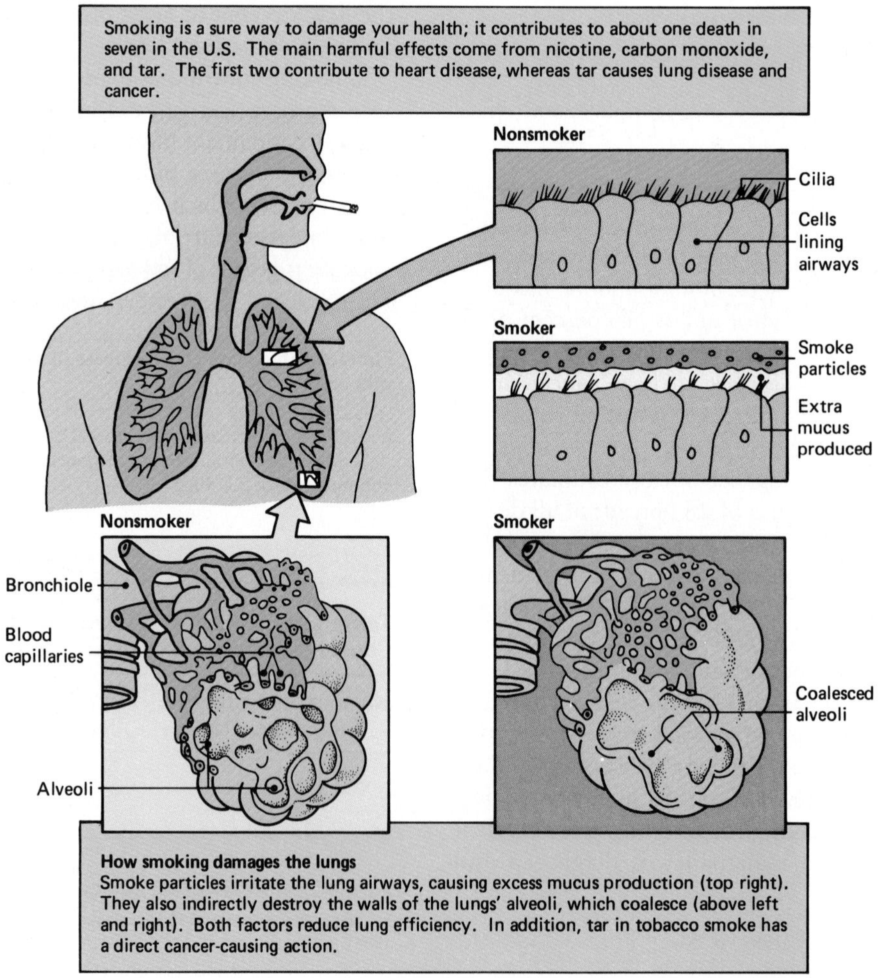

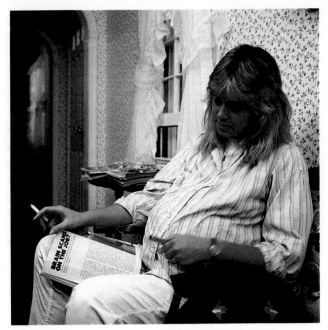
Smoking during pregnancy may endanger fetuses and newborn infants.

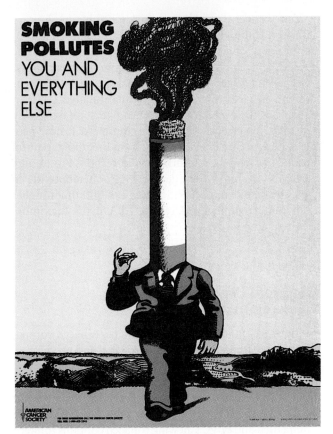
Environmental tobacco smoke contributes to health problems of nonsmokers as well as smokers.

The risk seemed to be higher for women under the age of 30.**

Although cigarette smoking is dangerous for all women, it presents special risks for fetuses and pregnant women. Each year in the United States, approximately 50,000 miscarriages are attributed to smoking during pregnancy. On average, babies born to mothers who smoke weigh less than those born to nonsmokers. Infant mortality rates are higher among babies born to smokers. Research also indicates that babies born to women who smoked during pregnancy are more likely to die of **sudden infant death syndrome (SIDS)** than are babies born to mothers who did not smoke. SIDS, or "crib death," occurs when an infant, usually under 1 year of age, dies during its sleep for no apparent reason (see Chapter 14).

Women who smoke and use oral contraceptives run a high risk of stroke and heart attack. These women run a 20-times-greater chance of stroke than nonsmokers and a 30-times-greater chance of having a heart attack than female nonsmokers. Smoking in women also contributes to osteoporosis, a condition involving bone loss.

Environmental Tobacco Smoke

As the population of nonsmokers rises, so does the demand for the right to breathe clean air. Although only 30 percent of Americans are smokers, air pollution from smoking in public places continues to be a problem.

Environmental tobacco smoke is sometimes called **secondhand smoke.** People who breathe smoke from someone else's smoking product (sidestream smoke) or smoke exhaled by a smoker (exhaled mainstream smoke) are said to be *involuntary,* or *passive, smokers.* Approximately 30 percent of the American population is exposed to secondhand smoke on a regular basis.*

Although involuntary smokers breathe less tobacco smoke than do active smokers, they still face risks from exposure to tobacco smoke. A National Academy of Sciences report on involuntary smoking stated that approximately 2,400, or 2 percent, of all lung cancer deaths are attributable to passive smoking.** An American Cancer Society study found that nonsmokers exposed to 20 or more cigarettes a day at home were twice as likely to develop lung cancer as those exposed to 19 or fewer cigarettes.†

Sudden Infant Death Syndrome (SIDS) Death that occurs without apparent cause in babies under 2 years of age, some cases may be associated with tobacco use by the mother during pregnancy.

Secondhand Smoke The cigarette, pipe, or cigar smoke breathed by nonsmokers; also called "sidestream smoke."

* Robert D. Tollison, *Clearing the Air: Perspectives on Environmental Tobacco Smoke* (Lexington, Mass.: Lexington Books, 1988), p. 7.
** *Cancer Facts and Figures*, p. 21.
† *Facts on Lung Cancer*, p. 5.

** "Cigarettes and Cervical Cancer," *Health Action Managers* (April 25, 1989), p. 3.

Lung cancer is not the only risk faced by involuntary smokers. Children of smokers have a greater chance of developing colds, bronchitis, pneumonia, chronic coughs, and ear infections than children of nonsmokers.

Cigarette, cigar, and pipe smoke in enclosed areas presents hazards to nonsmokers. An estimated 10 to 15 percent of the population of nonsmokers are extremely sensitive (hypersensitive) to cigarette smoke. These people experience itchy eyes, difficulty in breathing, painful headaches, nausea, and dizziness in response to minute amounts of smoke. The level of carbon monoxide in cigarette smoke in enclosed places is 4,000 times higher than that recommended by the EPA in its maximum clean-air standards.

Cigarette Use Declines, Chewing Increases

In the wake of antismoking campaigns, tobacco companies have increased their advertising for, and production of, chewing-tobacco products. Chewing tobacco and snuff (smokeless tobacco) are used by approximately 12 million Americans, 3 million of whom are under the age of 21. Most users of smokeless tobacco products are young men and boys. Chewing tobacco contains tobacco leaves treated with molasses and other flavorings. As previously mentioned, the user places a quid of tobacco between the teeth and gums, and the quid is sucked or chewed to release the nicotine. Once the quid becomes ineffective, the user spits it out and inserts another.

Dipping is another method of using chewing tobacco. The dipper takes a small amount of tobacco and places it between the lower lip and teeth to stimulate the flow of saliva and release the nicotine. Dippers usually swallow the product rather than spit it out. Dipping rapidly releases the nicotine into the bloodstream. The negative effects of dipping usually occur more quickly than those associated with chewing.

Chewers and dippers do not face the specific hazards associated with heat and smoke, but they do run other tobacco-related risks. All forms of tobacco contain nicotine, and its stimulant effects may create the same circulatory and respiratory problems for chewers as for smokers.

Additional risks of chewing tobacco include **leukoplakia,** a condition characterized by leathery white patches inside the mouth produced by contact with the irritants in tobacco juice. Between 3 and 17 percent of diagnosed leukoplakia cases develop into oral cancer. Users of smokeless tobacco are 50 times more likely to develop oral cancer than are nonusers.‡

---

‡ National Cancer Institute, *Chew or Snuff Is Real Bad Stuff* (1988).

QUITTING

Simply put, quitting smoking is difficult. The chemical effects of nicotine are strong enough to hook many smokers with the first puff. There are four progressive symptoms associated with nicotine addiction. First, the addicted user has usually made several serious but unsuccessful attempts to stop using tobacco. Second, the user's attempts to quit have led to withdrawal symptoms. Symptoms of **nicotine withdrawal** include irritability, restlessness, nausea, vomiting, and intense cravings for tobacco. Third, the user continues to use tobacco even in the face of serious health problems that are exacerbated by tobacco use. Finally, the chemical produces *tolerance,* whereby increased dosage is required to achieve the same effects.

The person who wishes to quit smoking has several options. Some people quit "cold turkey"—they merely decide not to smoke again. Others rely on organizations, such as the American Cancer Society, that offer short-term quitting programs based on behavior modification and a system of self-rewards. Still others turn to treatment centers. Such centers may be part of large franchises, or they may be part of a local medical clinic's community outreach plan. Some people work privately with their physicians to reach their goals.

Nicotine-replacement products have helped some people quit tobacco use. Patients use a prescription chewing gum called Nicorette to help them reduce their nicotine consumption over a period of time. Under the guidance of a physician, the user chews between 12 and 24 pieces of gum per day for up to 6 months. The user experiences no withdrawal symptoms and fewer cravings for nicotine in the beginning, and the dosage is reduced as time passes until the user is completely weaned.

Prospective quitters must decide which method or combination of methods will work best for them. Financial considerations, personality characteristics, and level of addiction should all be analyzed when choosing a plan for quitting.

TOBACCO AND SOCIAL ISSUES

The production and distribution of tobacco products in the United States and abroad involves many political and economic issues. During the 1980s, tobacco products were one of the United States' top five exports. Tobacco-growing states derive substantial income from tobacco

---

Leukoplakia A condition characterized by leathery white patches produced by contact with the irritants in tobacco juice.

Nicotine Withdrawal A series of conditions, including nausea, headaches, and irritability, suffered by smokers who cease using tobacco.

production, and federal, state, and local governments benefit enormously from cigarette taxes.

More recently, nationwide health awareness has led to a decrease in the use of tobacco products among U.S. adults.

Advertising

Tobacco companies spend hundreds of millions of dollars advertising their products. Advertising of tobacco products is the most pervasive evidence of company efforts to keep their products in the public eye. With the number of U.S. smokers declining by about one million each year, the industry must actively recruit new smokers. Campaigns are directed toward all ages and social and ethnic groups. Since children and teenagers constitute 90 percent of all new smokers, much of the advertising has been directed toward young people.*

Tobacco companies have aimed campaigns at young people telling them that smoking is a mature, elegant, sophisticated activity. Cartoon characters such as Camel's Old Joe have been used in advertising campaigns on campuses, in magazines, and even promoting a line of clothing. A recent study indicated that over 95 percent of school-age children can identify this character.** As a result of such campaigns, millions of young people try to convey their sophistication by lighting up.

* Joseph R. DiFranza, M.D., and John Richards, Jr., M.D., "RJR Nabisco's Cartoon Camel Promotes Camel Cigarettes to Children," *Journal of the American Medical Association*, 266 (1991), 3149–53.
    ** Ibid.

Seventy-five percent of all smokers begin smoking before their twenty-first birthday.

Gender-based Advertising Advertisements in "women's" magazines imply that cigarette smoking is a "liberated" thing to do. These ads have apparently been working. From 1975 through 1988, cigarette sales to women increased dramatically. In 1987, statistics indicated that cigarette-induced lung cancer had surpassed breast cancer as the leading form of cancer death among women.*

Women are not the only targets of cigarette advertisements. Men, of course, figure prominently. They may be depicted changing clothes in a locker room, charging over rugged terrain in off-road vehicles, or riding bay stallions into the sunset. Such advertisements are blatant appeals to a need to feel and appear masculine.

Conclusion

Tobacco products are directly responsible for the deaths of 350,000 Americans each year, or more than 1,000 people per day. If this same number of people were killed daily in plane crashes, we would be outraged at the airline industry. Tobacco companies continue to argue that there is no conclusive evidence linking smoking to serious diseases and that tobacco use is a choice each of us has a right to make. However, medical evidence has shown nicotine to be a highly addictive substance, and many people are beginning to wonder just how much choice is involved in the use of tobacco

* *Cancer Facts and Figures*, p. 9.

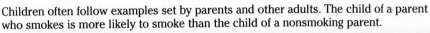

Children often follow examples set by parents and other adults. The child of a parent who smokes is more likely to smoke than the child of a nonsmoking parent.

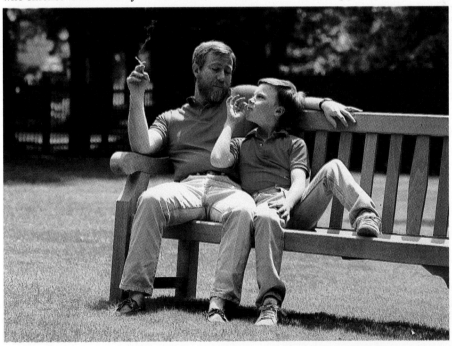

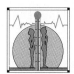

The First Link in the Chain of Abuse

Tobacco: The Gateway Drug

A causal relationship has been found to exist between cigarette smoking and use of other substances. Recent research has revealed distinctive age-related patterns of drug use that begin in the preteens and teens with the consumption of beer and wine, then cigarettes, and finally marijuana, psychedelics, and other illicit substances in the late teens and early twenties. Those who have not experimented with any of these substances by age 21 are unlikely ever to do so.

Surveys conducted throughout the years concerning the gateway effect of tobacco products have revealed the following statistics.

• Current smokers aged 12 to 17 were 10 times more likely to be actively using marijuana than were nonsmokers (49 percent versus 5 percent) and were 14 times more likely to be actively using cocaine, hallucinogens, or heroin (14 percent versus 1 percent).

• Two-thirds of high-school seniors who smoked a pack of cigarettes a day were actively using illicit drugs, versus 10 percent among those who never smoked. Daily marijuana use was 20 times higher among smokers than nonsmokers.

• Over 90 percent of all alcoholics are heavy cigarette smokers, and smoking is nearly universal among heroin addicts and patients on methadone maintenance.

There are various reasons for the causal connection. The discovery that cigarette smoking or alcohol can change a person's mood and emotional state may lead to the desire to explore other mind-altering substances. Furthermore, the act of smoking cigarettes conditions the person to inhale a foreign substance, which may lead to smoking marijuana or crack, a derivative of cocaine that is usually smoked in a pipe.

The gateway effect of tobacco is an important association. Most recovered alcoholics and drug addicts released from treatment centers continue to smoke cigarettes. The gateway effect may explain the high relapse rates among alcoholics and abusers of illicit drugs, because these people have never learned to overcome the first link in the chain of abuse.

Source: K. H. Ginzel, "Tobacco as a 'Gateway' Drug," *Tobacco and Youth Reporter* (Autumn 1989), p. 9.

products. Once people begin smoking or chewing tobacco, their chances of quitting are slim (less than 15 percent).

Education seems to be part of the answer. People with college educations are less likely to smoke than are those with an eighth-grade or high-school education. Another solution to the problem may be additional government measures to restrict the sale of tobacco products to young people. To meet the surgeon general's goal of a smoke-free society before the year 2000, we must take drastic steps to keep people from starting a habit that is a virtual death sentence.

▌SUMMARY

▪ Alcohol is a central-nervous-system depressant used by 70 percent of all Americans. Effects of this drug include impaired judgment and coordination and changes in emotional and intellectual functioning.

▪ Alcoholism is caused by a combination of biological, psychological, and environmental components.

▪ Alcohol is a causative factor in traffic accidents, child and spouse abuse, violent crimes, and family breakdown.

■ Every system in the body is affected by heavy use of alcohol. Chronic alcohol consumption can cause cirrhosis of the liver, high blood pressure, and increased risk of cancer of the esophagus, stomach, and liver.

■ Approximately 26.5 percent of Americans aged 17 or older smoke. There are more smokers today than two decades ago.

■ Smoking tobacco products have been linked directly to lung cancer, heart and circulatory disease, emphysema, and mouth and throat cancers.

■ The active drug in tobacco products is nicotine, an extremely addictive substance that has been recognized to be as addictive as heroin and cocaine.

12

Prescription, Over-the-Counter, and Illegal Drugs

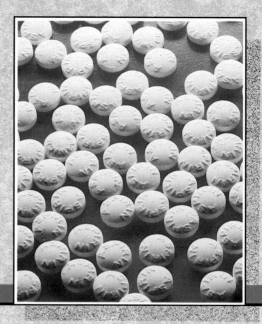

■ Objectives

- Explain why drugs work in the body and name the six categories of drugs.
- Discuss the differences between drug use and drug abuse and explain how hazardous drug interactions occur.
- List some of the ways that drugs may be taken into the body.
- Discuss the classifications of prescription and OTC drugs.
- State why caffeine may be considered addictive and define caffeinism.
- Describe what is meant by "illicit drugs" and discuss why people use them.
- For each of the five categories of illicit drugs, list specific drugs and some of their effects on the body.
- Discuss drug use and abuse in the United States, stating some specific problems and costs of drug abuse and outlining some possible solutions.

A **drug** is a chemical substance with the potential to alter the structure and functions of a living organism. Tens of thousands of these chemicals are available to us. Many of us take drugs, whether by our own choice or when prescribed by a physician. But how often do we take drugs without clearly understanding what chemicals we are putting into our bodies? This chapter will discuss the use of drugs in general, including prescription drugs, over-the-counter (OTC) preparations, and illicit drugs. The use of any chemical substance involves risks. These risks can be minimized through careful study and decision making regarding those chemicals that we choose to take and those that we take because of social pressure.

DRUG DYNAMICS AND DRUG CATEGORIES

How Drugs Work

Drugs work because they physically resemble the chemicals produced naturally within the body (see Figure 12.1). For example, painkillers resemble the endor-

phins ("morphine within") that are manufactured in the body (see Chapter 3). Most bodily processes result from chemical reactions or changes in electrical charge. Because drugs possess an electrical charge and a chemical structure similar to those chemicals that occur naturally in the body, they can affect physical functions in many different ways.

A current explanation of drug actions is the **receptor site** theory, which states that drugs attach themselves to specific receptor sites. These sites are specialized cells to which a drug can attach because of its size, shape, electrical charge, and chemical properties. Most drugs can attach at multiple receptor sites located throughout the body in such places as the heart and blood system, the lungs, liver, kidney, brain, and gonads (testicles or ovaries). The physiology of drug activity and its effect on human behavior is very complex.

Drug A chemical substance with the potential to alter the structure and functions of a living organism.

Receptor Sites Places in the body where drugs can attach themselves.

Figure 12.1 How drugs work.

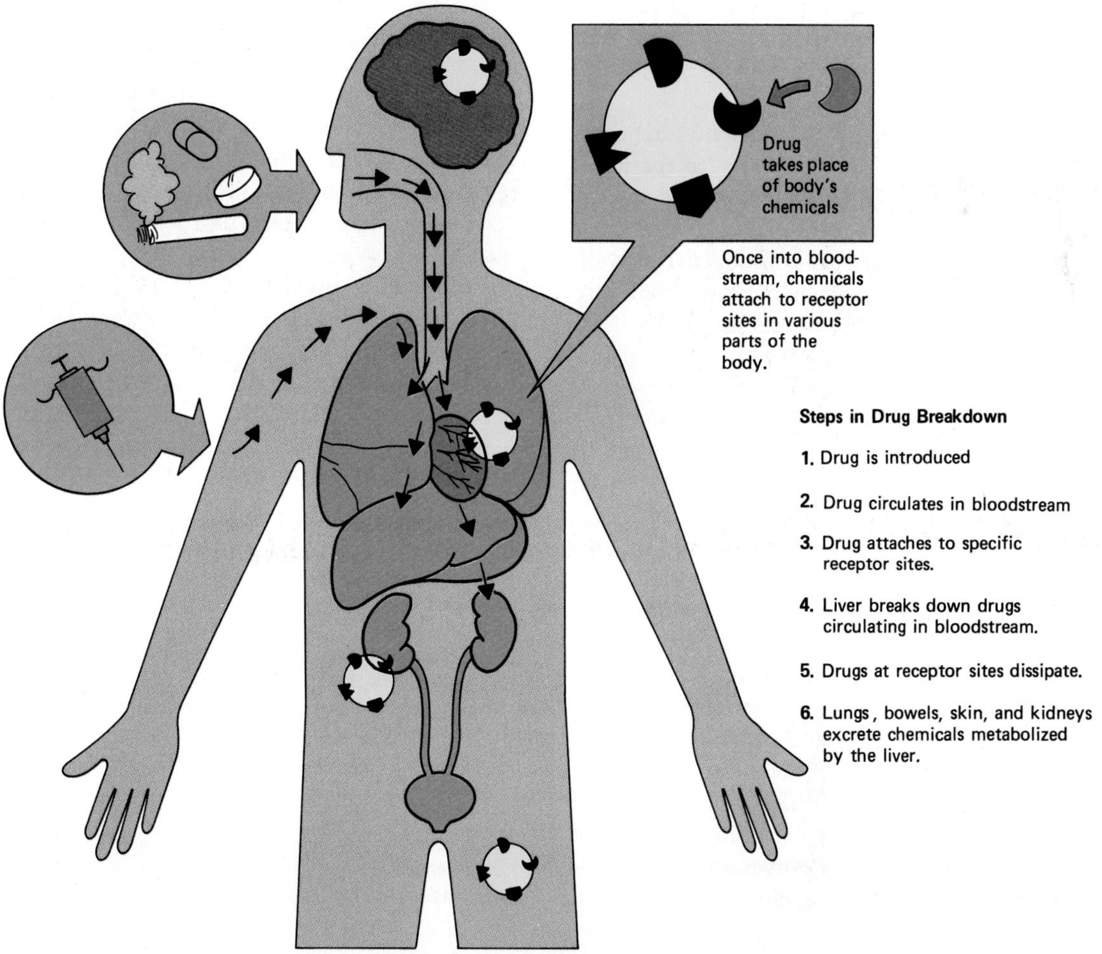

Drug takes place of body's chemicals

Once into bloodstream, chemicals attach to receptor sites in various parts of the body.

Steps in Drug Breakdown

1. Drug is introduced

2. Drug circulates in bloodstream

3. Drug attaches to specific receptor sites.

4. Liver breaks down drugs circulating in bloodstream.

5. Drugs at receptor sites dissipate.

6. Lungs, bowels, skin, and kidneys excrete chemicals metabolized by the liver.

Drug Categories

Drugs can be divided into six categories: prescription drugs, OTC preparations, recreational substances, herbal preparations, illegal drugs, and commercial drugs. Illicit and recreational drug use will be discussed later in this chapter. Each category includes drugs that stimulate the body, some that depress body functions, and others that produce sensory hallucinations. The categories also include drugs that have the potential to alter a person's mood or behavior. Such drugs are called **psychoactive drugs**.

Prescription drugs are those substances that must be obtained through the written prescription of a licensed physician. More than 40,000 types of prescription drugs are currently available, and these drugs should be used only under the care of a licensed medical practitioner. The physician determines the dosage for the individual patient at the time the prescription is written. Taking someone else's prescription can be dangerous, and deliberately sharing a prescription with another person is illegal.

Over-the-counter drugs can be purchased in pharmacies, supermarkets, and discount stores. These preparations do not require a physician's prescription because they are considered safe to use when the manufacturer's instructions are followed correctly. Common examples include analgesics (pain relievers), cold- and flu-symptom relievers, some appetite suppressants, laxatives, sleeping aids, sunscreens, and various ointments. More than 300,000 of these products are available in stores and pharmacies.

Recreational drugs belong to a somewhat vague category, depending upon the definition of "recreation." Generally, this category contains chemicals used to help people relax or socialize. Most of the drugs in this category are legally sanctioned and are psychoactive as well. Alcohol, tobacco, coffee, tea, and chocolate products are usually included in this category (see Chapter 11).

Illicit drugs, or **illegal drugs**, are the most notorious substances. Although laws governing their use, possession, cultivation, manufacture, and sale differ from state to state, the illicit drugs are generally recognized as harmful. Some groups consider all illicit drugs to be harmful, whereas other groups consider certain illegal drugs, such as marijuana, to be safe. Illegal drugs include heroin and other opium derivatives, cocaine, LSD, mescaline, PCP ("angel dust"), amphetamines, and marijuana. All of these substances are psychoactive.

Herbal preparations constitute another vague category. Included among these 750 substances are herbal teas and other products of botanical origin.

Commercial preparations are the most universally used yet least recognized chemical substances. More than 1,000 of these substances exist, including such seemingly benign items as food additives, perfumes, cosmetics, household cleansers, paints, glues, inks and dyes, gardening chemicals, pesticides, and industrial by-products.

In this chapter, we will concentrate on the first four categories: prescription, over-the-counter, recreational, and illegal drugs.

DRUG USE, ABUSE, AND INTERACTION

The sheer number of legal and illegal drugs available to people today is overwhelming. Many people fail to take time to ensure their personal safety when considering the use of a drug. Adopting an attitude that "the doctor knows best," or "Cindy down the hall uses it, and she's fine," or even "I can handle myself" is an evasion of personal responsibility.

Using, Misusing, and Abusing Drugs

Although drug abuse is frequently referred to in the context of illicit and recreational psychoactive drugs, many people abuse and misuse prescription and over-the-counter medications. **Drug misuse** is generally considered to be the use of a drug for a purpose for which it was not intended. For example, using a friend's high-powered prescription painkiller for your headache is a misuse of that drug. However, this is not too far removed from **drug abuse**, which is the excessive use of any drug. Also, as we saw in Chapter 10, the misuse and abuse of drugs may lead to *addiction*, the habitual reliance on a substance (or behavior) to produce a desired mood, regardless of psychological dependence.

Clearly there are risks and benefits associated with the use of any type of chemical substance. Intelligent decision-making involves clearheaded evaluation of the risks and benefits. If, after considering all the facts, you feel that the benefits outweigh the risks, you may decide to use a particular drug. Sometimes, however, un-

---

Psychoactive Drugs Drugs that have the potential to alter mood or behavior.

Prescription Drugs Medications that must be obtained through the written prescription of a licensed physician.

Over-the-counter (OTC) Drugs Medications that can be purchased without a physician's prescription in pharmacies or supermarkets.

Recreational Drugs Chemicals used to help people relax or socialize. Often legally sanctioned.

Illicit (illegal) Drugs Substances generally considered to be harmful and whose use is prohibited by law.

Herbal Preparations Substances that are of plant origin.

Commercial Preparations Substances that include cosmetics, household cleaning products, and industrial waste.

Drug Misuse The use of a drug for a purpose for which it was not intended.

Drug Abuse The excessive use of a drug.

The Risks and Benefits of Drug Use

Preparing a Drug Profile

In order to compare drug risks and benefits, you might want to make a profile for each drug. A *drug profile* consists of a set of questions to be answered about a particular drug. Potential users who do not compile a complete profile may subject themselves to greater risk than those who do.

Following are the key drug-profile questions that should be asked before you decide to use a given drug.

QUESTION 1   What is the chemical in the drug?

At first glance, this question may seem simplistic. In the case of an OTC preparation, the consumer may be allergic to a particular chemical in a product. Intelligent consumers read labels to determine whether the product contains substances to which they might be allergic.

QUESTION 2   Where within the body are the receptor sites?

Drugs are transported by the blood to areas where they are able to interact with other chemicals and influence many different bodily processes. The areas that drugs target are called *receptor sites.* If we know where the receptor sites are located, then we can choose an appropriate drug to affect that area.

QUESTION 3   What are the main effects of the drug?

This question relates to the major effects the consumer can expect from a drug.

QUESTION 4   What are the usual side effects of the drug?

This question is crucial. Because there are multiple receptor sites, all drugs produce side effects. The main effect of anticancer drugs is to kill cancer cells; the side effects are the destruction of intestinal and hair-follicle cells, resulting in nausea and hair loss.

QUESTION 5   What are the possible adverse reactions to the drug?

In addition to main effects and side effects, drugs have the potential to create adverse reactions. Most adverse reactions are allergic reactions. These unpleasant reactions occur when the body's immune system identifies a chemical as a foreign invader and seeks to destroy it. Something goes wrong in the recognition process, however, causing damage to healthy tissue.

Hypersensitivity reactions may consist of skin rashes, itching, swelling, watery eyes, runny nose, skin discoloration, and hives. More serious reactions include *anaphylactic shock,* which involves respiratory failure and cardiac arrest.

Physicians are frequently able to find alternative medicines for patients allergic to particular prescription drugs. If a drug has a high potential for causing allergic reaction (as with penicillin), most physicians monitor the patient carefully.

---

foreseeable reactions or problems arise, even after the most careful deliberation.

In order to compare drug risks to benefits, you might want to create a profile for each drug. A *drug profile* consists of a set of answers to specific questions about each drug. The box titled "The Risks and Benefits of Drug Use" provides you with the kinds of questions you may use to prepare a drug profile.

Individual Response to Psychoactive Drugs: Set and Setting   Individuals differ in the way in which they respond to psychoactive drugs. Two external factors that affect both main effects and side effects of psychoactive drugs are *set* and *setting*. **Set** is the total internal environment of a person at the time a drug is taken. Physical,

emotional, and social factors work together or against one another to influence a drug's effect on a particular person. Expectations of what the drug will or will not do are also part of the set. For example, the person who reads two pages of reported side effects for a particular drug may experience more side effects than a person who is not exposed to this information.

In other cases, set may be related to the user's mood. A depressed person using marijuana for a lift may find that the drug actually deepens the depression. Likewise, a person who is already giddy may become even sillier after using the drug.

Set   The internal environment of a person at the time a drug is taken.

If set refers to the internal environment, **setting** is the user's total external environment. It encompasses both the physical and social aspects of that environment at the time the psychoactive drug is taken. Wild colors, heavy-metal rock music, and a noisy crowd of people will generally have the opposite effect of a quiet place with soft music and relaxed company.

Drug Interactions

People who share medications, use outdated prescriptions, or use medications as a substitute for dealing with personal problems may face serious health consequences. However, people engaged in **polydrug use**—the use of several medications or illegal drugs at once—face the very dangerous problems associated with drug interactions. The msot hazardous interactions are synergism, antagonism, inhibition, and intolerance.

Synergism is also known as *potentiation*. Mathematically, synergism could be expressed as $2 + 2 = 10$. When drugs have a synergistic interaction, the effects of the individual drugs are multiplied beyond what would normally be expected.

A synergistic interaction is most likely to occur when two or more **central-nervous-system depressants**—any drugs that cause a decrease in heart rate, breathing, nerve reflexes, or blood pressure— are used concurrently (that is, at the same time). Although there are many drugs that have the potential for synergistic interactions, one of the worst combinations is alcohol and barbiturates (sleeping preparations such as Seconal and phenobarbital). The combination of these depressants leads to a slowdown of the brain centers that control respiration, heart rate, and blood pressure, leading to coma and possibly death. Many prescription and OTC drugs carry special labels warning the user not to combine the drug with certain other drugs or with alcohol.

Antagonism, although not usually as serious as synergism, can produce unwanted and unpleasant effects. In an antagonistic reaction, the drugs in question work at the same receptor site so that one drug *blocks* the action of the other. The blocking drug occupies the receptor site so the other drug cannot attach, creating alterations in absorption and action.

Setting   The external environment of a person at the time a drug is taken.

Polydrug Use   The use of multiple medications or illicit drugs simultaneously.

Synergism (potentiation)   An interaction of two or more drugs that produces more profound effects than would be expected if any of the drugs were taken separately.

Central-nervous-system Depressant   Any drug that causes a decrease in heart rate, breathing, nerve reflexes, or blood pressure.

Antagonism   A type of interaction in which two or more drugs work at the same receptor site.

Promoting Your Health

Alternatives to Drug Use

People use drugs for a variety of reasons—to achieve altered states of consciousness, for example, or to cope with the stress of everyday life. Fortunately, many nondrug alternatives are available that can accomplish the same results. Below is a checklist of positive, nondrug behaviors. Label each behavior *true* or *false* depending on whether it applies to you.

_____ I engage in regular exercise several times a week.

_____ When I feel a need for excitement or risk taking, I engage in some sort of activity, such as hiking, biking, or outdoor adventure.

_____ I find challenge and satisfaction in my work.

_____ I participate in political or social activities that add meaning and a sense of accomplishment to my life.

_____ Religion or spirituality plays an important role in my life.

_____ I practice meditation or biofeedback to help myself relax.

It is not necessary to answer *true* to *all* of these statements. In fact, many people probably lead a very healthy lifestyle without engaging in many of these activities. In most cases, however, the fewer *true* responses you indicated, the greater the risk that you will use drugs as a coping mechanism. If you answered *false* to most or all of these statements, you might want to consider whether changes in your lifestyle would be desirable. How could you go about changing these aspects of your life?

Source: Adapted from Richard G. Schlaadt and Peter T. Shannon, *Drugs,* 3rd ed. (Englewood Cliffs, NJ: Prentice Hall, 1990).

Inhibition is a type of interaction in which the effects of one drug are eliminated or reduced by the presence of another drug at the receptor site. One common inhibitory reaction occurs between antacid tablets and aspirin. The antacid inhibits the absorption of aspirin, making it less effective as a pain reliever.

Intolerance occurs when drugs combine in the body to produce extremely uncomfortable reactions. One such reaction occurs when the drug Antabuse is used to help alcoholics give up alcohol. The Antabuse binds liver enzymes (the chemicals the liver produces to break down alcohol), making it impossible for the body to metabolize alcohol. The interaction of Antabuse with alcohol results in nausea, vomiting, and occasionally fever.

Cross-tolerance occurs when a person develops a physiological tolerance to one drug and shows a similar tolerance to certain other drugs as a result. Taking one drug may actually *increase* the body's tolerance for another drug. For example, cross-tolerance can develop between alcohol and barbiturates, two depressant drugs.

USING DRUGS: ROUTES OF ADMINISTRATION

Route of administration refers to the way in which a given drug is taken into the body. Common routes include oral ingestion, injection, inhalation, inunction, and suppository.

Oral ingestion is the most frequently used method of administration. Orally ingested drugs include tablets, capsules, and liquids. Oral ingestion generally results in a relatively slow absorption because the drug must pass through the stomach, be subjected to digestive juices, and move on to the small intestine before entering the bloodstream.

Depending on the drug and the amount of food in the stomach, effects of ingested drugs are manifested within 20 minutes to 1 hour after ingestion. The only exception to this is alcohol, part of which is absorbed directly into the bloodstream from the stomach.

Injection is another common form of administration. Injection involves the use of a hypodermic syringe to introduce the drug into the body. This method can result in rapid absorption, depending on the type of injection. **Intravenous injection** puts the chemical in its most con-

---

Inhibition   A type of interaction in which the effects of one drug are eliminated or reduced by the presence of another drug at the receptor site.

Intolerance   A type of interaction in which two or more drugs produce extremely uncomfortable symptoms.

Cross-tolerance   The development of a tolerance to one drug that reduces the effects of another, similar drug.

Route of Administration   The manner in which a drug is taken into the body.

Oral Ingestion   Intake of drugs through the mouth.

Injection   The introduction of drugs into the body via a hypodermic syringe.

Intravenous Injection   The introduction of drugs directly into the bloodstream.

Promoting Your Health

Medical Terms and What They Mean

• What do the initial PDR stand for?

Physicians Desk Reference. Members of the American Medical Association (AMA) receive an update each year. Written in medical terminology, the book lists drugs by chemical (generic) name, manufacturer, and common trade name. Each description includes a synopsis of rules for use and all potential side effects.

• What is "overmedicating"?

When a physician relies excessively on prescribing drugs to treat medical problems, rather than selecting alternative forms of healing.

• How does "multiprescribing" differ from overmedicating?

Multiprescribing involves the use of several different drugs at the same time for different conditions, whereas overmedicating may refer to the use of a single drug.

• What do the initials GRAS stand for?

Generally Recognized as Safe. Drugs on the GRAS list have a low incidence of adverse reactions or undesirable side effects.

• What do the initials GRAE stand for?

Generally Recognized as Effective. Drugs on the GRAE list, when taken properly, work for their intended purpose.

• What is an "iatrogenic disease"?

A medical problem that results from some form of treatment by a health-care professional.

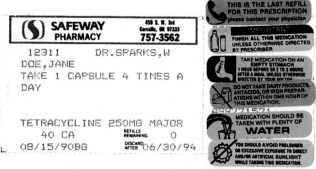

Prescription drug labels must contain pharmacy name, pharmacist's initials, prescription number, patient's name, physician's name, directions for use, side effects, and warning labels if they apply.

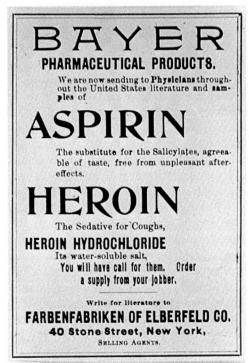

Drug advertising has been used for years. This ad from the early twentieth century promoted one product that we still use today (aspirin) and another drug that is now illegal (heroin).

centrated form directly into the bloodstream. Effects will be felt within 3 minutes, making this route extremely effective, particularly in medical emergencies. However, injection of unknown substances into the bloodstream may cause serious and even fatal reactions. In addition, some serious diseases are also transferred in this way. For this reason, intravenous injection can also be one of the most dangerous routes of administration.

Intramuscular injection results in much slower absorption than intravenous injection. This type of injection places the hypodermic syringe into muscular tissue, usually in the buttocks or the back of the upper arm. Normally used to administer antibiotics and vaccinations, this route of administration ensures a slow and consistent dispersion of the drug into the body tissues.

Subcutaneous injection puts the drug into the layer of fat directly beneath the skin. Street drug users often call this route "skin popping." Common medical use is for administration of local anesthetics. A drug administered in this manner will circulate even more slowly than an intramuscularly injected drug because it takes longer to be absorbed into the bloodstream.

Inhalation refers to administration through the nostrils. This method of administration transfers the drug rapidly into the bloodstream through the alveoli (air sacs) in the lungs. Effects are frequently noticed immediately after inhalation, but they do not last as long as with the slower methods. Only small amounts of a drug can be absorbed and metabolized in the lungs.

Inunction occurs when a chemical enters the body through the skin. One common example is the small adhesive patches that are used to alleviate motion sickness. These patches, which contain a prescription medicine, are applied to the skin behind the ear, where they slowly release their chemicals to provide relief for nauseated travelers.

Suppositories are drugs that are mixed with a waxy medium designed to melt at body temperature. A suppository is inserted into the anus until it is past the rectal sphincter muscles, which will hold it in place. (Some types of suppositories are for use in the vagina.) As the

wax melts, the drug is released and absorbed through the rectal walls into the bloodstream. This area of the anatomy is well vascularized (contains many blood vessels), and effects are usually felt within 15 minutes. Some OTC laxatives and hemorrhoid treatments are administered by suppository. In hospital settings, anal suppositories may be the chosen route of administration of painkillers for patients unable to tolerate ingestion or injection.

PRESCRIPTION AND OVER-THE-COUNTER (OTC) DRUGS

Even though prescription drugs are administered under medical supervision and over-the-counter (OTC) drugs are carefully regulated by the FDA, the wise consumer still takes precautions. Hazards and complications arising from the use of prescription and OTC drugs are

---

Intramuscular Injection The introduction of drugs into the large muscles of the buttocks or upper arms.

Subcutaneous Injection The introduction of drugs into the fatty tissue under the skin.

Inhalation Breathing a drug into the nostrils.

Inunction The introduction of drugs into the body by rubbing them onto the skin.

Suppositories Medications placed in a waxy medium designed to melt at body temperature; inserted into the anus.

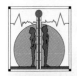
Your Drug IQ

common. Responsible decision making about drug use requires the consumer to acquire basic drug knowledge.

Classifying Prescription Drugs

Prescription drugs can be divided into dozens of categories. Those of most interest to college students are discussed below. Others are explored in the chapters on fertility management, infectious and noninfectious diseases, cancer, and heart disease.

Antibiotics are drugs used to fight bacterial infection. They may be dispensed by intramuscular injection or in tablet or capsule form. Some, called *broad-spectrum antibiotics,* are designed to control disease caused by a number of bacterial species. These medications may also kill off "helpful" bacteria in the body, thus triggering secondary infections.

Analgesics are pain relievers. The earliest pain relievers were made of derivatives of the opium poppy. Most pain relievers work at receptor sites, interrupting pain signals. Some analgesics are available as OTC drugs.

Other analgesics are called **prostaglandin inhibitors.** Prostaglandins are chemicals that resemble hormones and are released by the body in response to pain. When a painful stimulus such as a cut or scrape occurs, prostaglandins are released by the nerve cells near the site of the pain. (Scientists believe that the additional pain caused by the release of prostaglandins signals the body to begin the healing process.) Prostaglandin inhibitors restrain the release of prostaglandins, thereby reducing the pain. The most commonly used of the prostaglandin inhibitors are ibuprofen (Motrin) and sodium naprosyn (Anaprox). Both are prescribed to relieve arthritis pain or menstrual cramps.

Most analgesics have side effects, the most common of which is drowsiness due to the depression of the central nervous system. Some labels caution specifically against driving or operating heavy machinery when using the drug, and most state that analgesics must not be taken with alcohol.

Sedatives are central-nervous-system depressants that induce sleep and relieve anxiety. Used heavily in the 1950s and 1960s in the form of Quaaludes, phenobarbital, or Seconal, they have gradually fallen out of favor because of the risks of addiction and detoxification problems.

Tranquilizers are another category in the long list of central-nervous-system depressants. They are classified as "major" tranquilizers and "minor" tranquilizers.

The most powerful tranquilizers are used in the treatment of major psychiatric illnesses. When used appro-

---

Antibiotics Prescription drugs designed to fight bacterial infection.
Analgesics Pain relievers.
Prostaglandin Inhibitors Drugs that inhibit the production and release of prostaglandin hormones associated with arthritis or menstrual pain.
Sedatives Central-nervous-system depressants that induce sleep.
Tranquilizers Central-nervous-system depressants that relax the body and calm anxiety.

priately, they are strong sedatives capable of reducing violent aggressiveness and self-destructive impulses.

The so-called minor tranquilizers enjoyed much notoriety in the late 1960s and early 1970s. Known by the trade names Valium, Librium, and Miltown, these central-nervous-system depressants were commonly prescribed to women who suffered from anxiety. Because these drugs have high potential for addiction, many people became physically and psychologically dependent on them. Today, physicians are more likely to suggest psychotherapy or counseling for their patients.

Antidepressants are powerful substances used to treat clinically diagnosed cases of depression. These drugs act to inhibit the release of neurotransmitters in the brain, thereby elevating the user's mood. They are not, as their name implies, chemicals to produce happiness.

Amphetamines are stimulants that are prescribed less commonly now than in the past. Like many drugs, they are purchased both legally and illegally. These powerful stimulants suppress appetite and elevate respiration, blood pressure, and pulse rate. Tolerance to these stimulants develops rapidly, and the user trying to cut down or quit may experience unpleasant **rebound effects**, severe withdrawal symptoms peculiar to stimulants, which include depression, irritability, violent headaches, nausea, and deep fatigue.

Generic Drugs

Generic drugs have gained popularity in the past few years and are available as alternatives to more expensive brand-name drugs. **Generic drugs** are medications sold under their chemical name. They are also manufactured by reputable pharmaceutical companies. Although they contain the same active ingredient as their brand-name counterparts, controversy exists as to the effectiveness of some generic drugs.

There may be disadvantages in using generic drugs if basic ingredients are substituted for other substances similar in chemical makeup. Substituting even a minor ingredient could affect the way the drug is absorbed, causing discomfort or even an allergic reaction in some patients. Therefore, patients must be aware of any reactions to medications taken in the past.

Generic drugs can help to reduce health-care costs. Often, their price is less than one-half the price of the brand-name drug. However, not all drugs are available as generics. Many pharmacists offer the patient the option of using a generic if the doctor approves. In some instances, generic equivalents are not recommended.

Classifying Over-the-Counter Drugs

Over-the-counter drugs are those nonprescription drugs we use in the course of self-diagnosis and self-medication. Many of us, in our eagerness to save the money ordinarily spent on an office visit to a physician,

diagnose our own illness and go to the nearest discount pharmacy to stock up on the latest and best-advertised cure for what ails us.

In an effort to cure ourselves, American consumers spend an excess of $10 billion yearly on OTC preparations for relief of everything from runny noses to ingrown toenails. There are over 40,000 OTC drugs available to us, but there are more than 300,000 brand names. Most of these drugs are manufactured from a basic group of 1,000 chemicals. Combining as few as 2 and as many as 10 substances creates the many different OTC drugs available to us.

Despite a common belief that OTC products are both safe and effective, indiscriminate use and abuse can occur with these drugs just as with all others. In fact, many OTC drugs have the potential to produce dependency, tolerance, and addiction as well as adverse toxic reactions. Table 12.1 lists some of the possible side effects of OTC drugs.

The FDA has categorized 26 types of OTC preparations. Those most commonly used are analgesics, cold/cough/allergy preparations, asthma relievers, stimulants, sleeping aids, appetite suppressants, laxatives, and diuretics.

Analgesics   Analgesics, or pain relievers, come in several forms. Aspirin and acetaminophen are the two most commonly used ingredients in OTC pain relievers. The active chemical in aspirin relieves pain, brings down fever, and reduces the inflammation and swelling associated with arthritis. However, aspirin can be a gastric irritant, causing internal bleeding from small vessels in the stomach walls. Combining aspirin with alcohol can compound this problem.

Research has linked aspirin to a potentially fatal condition called Reye's syndrome. Children, teenagers, and young adults (up to age 25) who are treated with aspirin while recovering from the flu or chicken pox are at risk for developing the syndrome. Aspirin substitutes are recommended for all children regardless of the illness they may be experiencing.

Acetaminophen is an aspirin substitute found in Tylenol and related medications. Like aspirin, acetaminophen is an effective analgesic and antipyretic (fever-reducing drug). It does not, however, provide relief from inflamed or swollen joints. Side effects with acetaminophen are minimal. Overdose can occur, however, and may cause liver damage.

In 1985, certain drugs containing ibuprofen (prostaglandin inhibitors) were released for OTC purchase.

Antidepressants   Prescription drugs used to treat clinically diagnosed depression.

Amphetamines   Prescription stimulants not commonly used today because of the dangers associated with them.

Rebound effects   Severe withdrawal effects experienced by users of stimulants, including depression, nausea, and violent headaches.

Generic drugs   Drugs marketed by their chemical rather than a brand name.

Table 12.1 Some Side Effects of OTC Drugs

Drug	Possible Hazards
Acetaminophen	• Bloody urine, painful urination, skin rash, bleeding and bruising, yellowing of the eyes or skin (even for normal doses) • Difficulty in diagnosing overdose because reaction may be delayed up to a week • Severe liver damage and death (for dose of about 50 tablets) • Liver damage from chronic low-level use
Antacids	• Reduced mineral absorption from food • Possible concealment of ulcer • Reduction of effectiveness for anticlotting medications • Prevention of certain antibiotics' functioning (for antacids that contain aluminum) • Worsening of high blood pressure (for antacids that contain sodium) • Aggravation of kidney problems
Aspirin	• Stomach upset and vomiting, stomach bleeding, worsening of ulcers • Enhancement of the action of anticlotting medications • Potentiation of hearing damage from loud noise • Severe allergic reaction • Association with Reye's syndrome in children and teenagers • Prolonged bleeding time (when combined with alcohol)
Cold medications	• Loss of consciousness (if taken with prescription tranquilizers)
Diet pills, caffeine, decongestants	• Organ damage or death from cerebral hemorrhage
Ibuprofen	• Allergic reaction in some people with aspirin allergy • Fluid retention or edema • Liver damage similar to that from acetaminophen • Enhancement of action of anticlotting medications • Digestive disturbances (half as often as with aspirin)
Laxatives	• Reduced absorption of minerals from food • Creation of dependency
Toothache medications	• Destruction of the still-healthy part of a damaged tooth (for medications that contain clove oil)

Generally marketed as arthritis or menstrual-cramp relievers, these drugs are milder versions of the prescription varieties. Examples include Nuprin and Advil. Research is being conducted to assess reports of gastrointestinal bleeding caused by ibuprofen products.

Cold, Cough, Allergy, and Asthma Relievers   These substances are popular OTC remedies for the symptoms that affect millions of sufferers. The operative word in their titles is *reliever*. Most of these medications are designed to alleviate some or all of the discomforting

Over-the-counter labels must include product name and ingredients, manufacturer's and packer's name and address, directions for use, dosages, warnings, and conditions for which the product is intended.

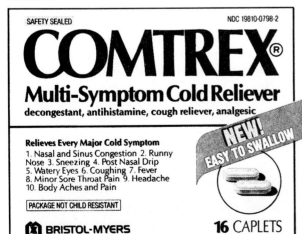

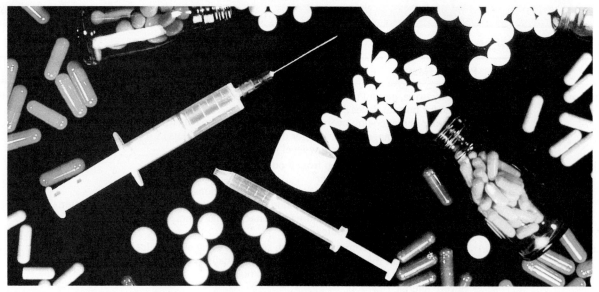
Because Americans have such a great variety of drugs available to them, they must research these substances carefully.

symptoms associated with these upper-respiratory maladies. Unfortunately, these drugs only relieve symptoms temporarily. They do not cure the disease.

Expectorants are formulated to loosen phlegm, allowing the user to cough it up and clear congested respiratory passages. *Antitussives* are used to calm or curtail the cough reflex. These are most effective when the cough is dry or does not produce phlegm. *Antihistamines* are central-nervous-system depressants that dry runny noses, clear postnasal drip, clear sinus congestion, and reduce tears. *Decongestants* are designed to reduce nasal stuffiness due to colds. Finally, *anticholinergics* are substances that are often added to cold preparations to suppress nasal secretions and tears. Some cold compounds contain alcohol in concentrations that may exceed 40 percent.

OTC Stimulants   Nonprescription stimulants are sometimes used by college students who leave assignments and other obligations until the last minute. The active ingredient in OTC stimulants is caffeine. It acts to heighten wakefulness, increase alertness, and relieve fatigue.

Sleeping Aids and Relaxants   These drugs are often used to induce the drowsiness that precedes sleep. The principal ingredient in OTC sleeping aids is an antihistamine called *pyrilamine maleate*. Chronic reliance on sleeping aids may lead to addiction; people accustomed to using these products may find it impossible to sleep without them.

Dieting Aids   Drugs to help us lose weight are available over the counter. Some of them are advertised as "appetite suppressants." The active chemical is phenylpropanolamine. Its stimulant effects can cause danger-

ous reactions in people suffering from diabetes or heart or thyroid ailments.

Some people rely on a **laxative** or **diuretic** ("water pill") to aid in weight reduction. Frequent use of laxatives for weight loss disrupts the body's natural elimination patterns and may cause constipation or even obstipation (inability to have a bowel movement). The use of laxatives to produce weight loss has generally unspectacular results and can rob the body of needed fluids, salts, and minerals.

Use of diuretics as part of a weight-loss plan is also dangerous. Not only will the user gain the weight back upon drinking fluids, but diuretic use may contribute to dangerous chemical imbalances. The potassium and sodium eliminated by diuretics play important roles in maintaining electrolyte balance. Depletion of these vital minerals may cause weakness, dizziness, fatigue, and sometimes death.

CAFFEINE AND CAFFEINISM

Caffeine is a drug derived from the chemical family called **xanthines**. Two related chemicals, *theophylline* and *theobromine*, are found in tea and chocolate, respectively.

The xanthines are mild central-nervous-system stimulants. They enhance mental alertness and reduce feelings of fatigue. Other stimulant effects include increases in heart-muscle contractions, oxygen consumption, metab-

---

Laxative   A medication used to soften stool and relieve constipation.
Diuretic   A drug that increases the excretion of urine.
Caffeine   A stimulant found in coffee and cola drinks.
Xanthines   The family of stimulants to which caffeine belongs.

Table 12.2 Caffeine Content of Various Products

Product	Caffeine Content (average mgs per serving)
Coffee (5-oz. cup)	
Regular brewed	65–115
Decaffeinated brewed	3
Decaffeinated instant	2
Tea (6-oz. cup)	
Hot steeped	36
Iced	31
Soft Drinks (12-oz. servings)	
Dr. Pepper	61
Mountain Dew	54
Coca-Cola	46
Pepsi-Cola	36–38
Chocolate	
1 oz. baking chocolate	25
1 oz. chocolate candy bar	15
1/2 cup chocolate pudding	4–12
Over-the-Counter Drugs	
NoDoz (2 tablets)	200
Excedrin (2 tablets)	130
Midol (2 tablets)	65
Anacin (2 tablets)	64

olism, and urinary output. These effects are felt within 15 to 45 minutes of ingesting a caffeine-containing product.

Until the mid-1970s, caffeine was not medically recognized as addictive. The effects of chronic caffeine use were called "coffee nerves." This syndrome is now recognized as *caffeine intoxication,* or **caffeinism.** Symptoms of caffeinism include chronic insomnia, jitters, irritability, nervousness, anxiety, and involuntary muscle twitches. Withdrawing the caffeine may compound the effects and produce severe headaches. (Some physicians ask their patients to take a simple test for caffeine addiction: If you get a severe headache after abstaining from anything containing caffeine for 4 hours, you are addicted.)

Different products contain different concentrations of caffeine. An 8-ounce cup of coffee contains between 100 and 150 milligrams of caffeine; caffeine concentrations vary with the brand and the strength of the brew. Small chocolate bars contain up to 15 milligrams of caffeine and theobromine. A comparison of various caffeine-containing products can be found in Table 12.2.

▌ THE LURE OF ILLICIT DRUGS

Whether we choose to use licit or illicit drugs, are forced to watch someone we love experience problems with drugs, become the victim of a drug-related crime, or are forced to pay increasing taxes for law enforcement, drug treatment, or other social services, drugs touch all of us on a daily basis. **Illicit drugs** are those drugs that are illegal to possess, produce, and sell. A 1988 survey conducted by the National Institute on Drug Abuse (NIDA) indicates that over 38 percent of the American population over the age of 12 have used some type of illicit drug at least once.[*]

Patterns of drug use vary considerably by age group and type of drug used. For example, in 1988 over 56 percent of college students had used marijuana and nearly 20 percent had used cocaine at least once in their lives. In contrast, 30 percent of adults 25 and over had used marijuana, and only about 4 percent had ever used cocaine (see Table 12.3).

The use of illicit drugs by Americans has declined significantly in recent years. In one study, the number of persons who used marijuana, cocaine, or any other illicit drug within the 30 days prior to the survey had dropped from 23 million in 1985 to 14.5 million in 1988. However, the survey found continued intense use of cocaine within the cocaine-using population.[*]

Why People Use Illicit Drugs

Human beings appear to have a need to alter their **consciousness,** or mental state of being. We like to feel good. Sometimes we like to change our awareness of things and feel different. Consciousness can be altered in many ways. Children spinning until they become dizzy and adults enjoying thrilling high-speed activities are altering their consciousness. Many of us listen to music, skydive, ski, skate, read, daydream, meditate, pray, or have sexual relations to change our awareness or to alter our consciousness.

For many people, drugs offer an easy way to alter consciousness. For example, smoking a marijuana cigarette requires less time and effort than climbing a mountain. The "high" achieved is not necessarily the same, but both actions produce altered awareness.

Illicit drugs in particular produce altered awareness. The laws against their use recognize the potential dangers associated with these substances. These same laws contribute to the mystique and risk surrounding illicit drug use.

The reasons for using drugs may vary from one situation to another and from person to person. A person's

---

Caffeinism Symptoms brought on by excessive caffeine use, which include chronic insomnia, irritability, anxiety, muscle twitches, and headaches.

Illicit drugs Drugs that are illegal to possess, produce, and sell.

Consciousness The mental state of being; awareness.

---

[*] National Institute on Drug Abuse, *NIDA Capsules* (Rockville, Md.: NIDA, U.S. Department of Health and Human Services, August 1991).

[*] "Household Survey Shows Declining Drug Use Nationwide," *Alcohol and Drug Review,* 10, no. 1 (1990), p. 11.

Table 12.3 Drug Use by Type of Drug and Age Group: 1972, 1974, and 1988

Type of Drug	Percent of Youths (12–17)				Percent of Young Adults (18–25)				Percent of Older Adults (25+)			
	Ever Used		Used in Past Month		Ever Used		Used in Past Month		Ever Used		Used in Past Month	
	1972	1988	1974	1988	1972	1988	1974	1988	1972	1988	1974	1988
Marijuana and hashish	14.0	17.4	12.0	6.4	47.9	56.4	25.2	15.5	7.4	30.7	2.0	3.9
Inhalants	6.4	9.2	0.7	2.0	9.2	12.6	—	1.7	—	3.9	—	0.2
Hallucinogens	4.8	3.5	1.4	0.8	16.6	13.8	2.5	1.9	1.3	6.6	—	—
Cocaine	1.5	3.4	1.0	1.1	9.1	19.7	3.1	4.5	1.6	9.9	—	0.9
Heroin	0.8	0.8	—	—	4.6	0.4	—	—	0.5	1.1	—	—
Psychotherapeutics												
Stimulants	4.0	4.2	1.0	1.2	12.0	11.3	3.7	2.4	3.0	6.6	—	0.6
Sedatives	3.0	2.4	1.0	0.8	10.0	5.6	1.6	0.9	2.0	3.3	—	0.3
Tranquilizers	3.0	2.0	1.0	0.2	7.0	7.8	1.2	1.0	5.0	4.6	—	0.6
Analgesics	—	5.8	—	0.9	—	9.4	—	1.5	—	4.5	—	0.4
Cigarettes	52.0	42.3	25.0	11.8	68.8	75.0	48.8	36.2	65.4	79.8	39.1	29.8
Smokeless tobacco	—	—	—	4.0	—	—	89.3	85.3			54.5	54.8
Alcohol	54.0	50.2	34.0	25.2	81.6	90.3	—	6.0	73.2	88.6	—	3.0

Approximate wtd. N = 8,800
— = no data available

SOURCE: National Institute on Drug Abuse, *National Household Survey on Drug Abuse* (Rockville, Md.: NIDA, U.S. Dept. of Health and Human Services, August 1989).

Activities like this can produce a "high" without drugs.

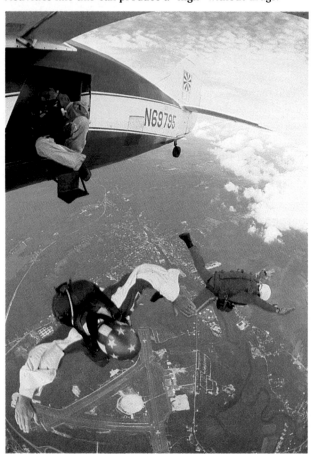

age, gender, genetic background, physiology, personality, experiences, and expectations are all factors.

The use of illicit drugs has physical, emotional, social, and legal consequences. Social and cultural determinants of drug use should not be overlooked when examining the issue of illicit drugs. People who develop drug problems generally begin with the belief that they will receive benefits from, and can control, their drug use. Initially, they often view drug taking as a fun and controllable pastime. The majority of illegal drugs produce physical and psychological dependence, and the belief that these substances can be used regularly without developing addiction is foolish.

ILLICIT DRUGS: WHAT THEY ARE AND WHAT THEY DO

Illicit drugs may be grouped into five categories: *stimulants*, like cocaine; *marijuana* and its derivatives; *depressants*, such as the opiates; *psychedelics and deliriants*; and *"designer drugs."* In addition, inhalants and solvents, though they may be purchased legally, represent a dangerous alternative for people who cannot afford to buy illicit substances.

Stimulants

Cocaine The rise of **cocaine,** or "coke," as the drug of choice among upper- and middle-class Americans has been chronicled in the media since the early 1980s. Approximately 5 million Americans from all socioeconomic groups use cocaine regularly; almost 3 million may be addicted. As many as 10 percent of college students reported using cocaine during the past year (see Table 12.3).* Cocaine is thought to be the second most popular drug among college students, after marijuana. While the number of people using cocaine occasionally has dropped, the number who use cocaine more than once a week has grown.** Professional athletes have been banned from competition for cocaine use. National toll-free cocaine hotlines have been established. The country has become more aware of cocaine abuse since the use of the relatively inexpensive cocaine derivative called *crack* became a national epidemic in the mid-1980s.

NIDA describes cocaine as "the most powerful naturally occurring stimulant."*** Despite a few chemical similarities to less potent stimulants such as caffeine, cocaine is very dangerous and should not be compared with these substances. In appearance, cocaine is a crystalline white alkaloid powder derived from the leaves of the South American coca shrub (not realted to cocoa plants). Coca grows only in the Andes at elevations between 1,500 and 5,000 feet. Coca leaves have been chewed for their stimulant effects for thousands of years by the Inca Indians and their descendants.

PHYSICAL EFFECTS OF COCAINE Cocaine can be administered in several ways. The powdered form of the drug is "snorted" through the nose. Smoking and intravenous injections are two more dangerous means of ingesting cocaine.

Cocaine is both an anesthetic and a central-nervous-system stimulant. In tiny doses, however, it can slow heart rate. Larger doses increase heart rate. Other effects of cocaine include temporary relief of depression, euphoria (an intense feeling of well-being), talkativeness, restlessness, and heightened self-confidence. Cocaine also acts as an appetite suppressant.

The effects of cocaine are felt rapidly. Snorted cocaine enters the bloodstream through the lungs in less than 1 minute and reaches the brain in less than 3 minutes.

The cocaine "high" lasts from 5 to 20 minutes. When it abates, the desire for the pleasurable feelings is difficult to control and the user wants more. Spending over $1,000 a day is not unusual for a crack addict. Studies with primates showed that these animals preferred co-caine to life itself; they repeatedly took the drug given them until they died.

Freebase Cocaine Freebase is a form of cocaine that is more powerful and costly than chips or powder. Street cocaine (cocaine hydrochloride) is converted to pure base by removing the hydrochloride salt and many of the "cutting agents." The end product is not water-soluble and is ingested by smoking the drug through a water pipe.

Because freebase cocaine reaches the brain within seconds, it is more dangerous than cocaine that is snorted. It produces a quick, intense high that disappears quickly, leaving an intense craving for more. Freebasers typically increase the amount and frequency of the dose. Often they become severely addicted and experience serious health problems and financial ruin.*

Crack Crack is the street name given to freebase cocaine that has been processed from cocaine hydrochloride using ammonia or sodium bicarbonate (baking soda) and water and heating the substance to remove the hydrochloride. Crack can also be processed with ether, but this is much riskier because ether is a flammable solvent. The term *crack* refers to the crackling sound that is heard when the mixture is smoked (heated), presumably due to the chemical reaction of the sodium-bicarbonate residue.

Crack is typically sold in small vials, folding papers, or heavy tinfoil and is often smoked in a pipe. The drug resembles the hard shavings of slivers of soap.

Crack is sometimes called "rock," an alias that should not be confused with *rock cocaine.* Rock cocaine is a form of cocaine hydrochloride that is primarily sold in California. White in color, it is about the shape of a pencil eraser.

There is no definitive way of estimating the extent of crack use in the United States, but according to NIDA estimates, there are 4 to 5 million people who use crack at least once a month.** Crack houses, crack-addicted babies, crack-related crimes, and other problems focused on by the media have drawn national attention to the enormity of the crack problem since the drug first gained notice around 1986.

Cocaine Addiction and Society Cocaine addicts often suffer both physiological damage and serious disruptions of their lifestyle, including loss of jobs and self-esteem. It is estimated that the costs of cocaine addiction in the United States may exceed $100 million. However,

---

Cocaine A powerful stimulant drug made from the leaves of the South American coca shrub.

Freebase The most powerful distillate of cocaine.
Crack A distillate of powdered cocaine that comes in small, hard chips.

---

* *Drug Abuse Update,* September 1990.
** Centers for Disease Control, April 1990.
*** National Institute on Drug Abuse, Statistical Series, *Annual Data Report,* 1989.

* National Institute or Drug Abuse, *NIDA Capsules* (April 1989), pp. 18–19.
** Ibid.

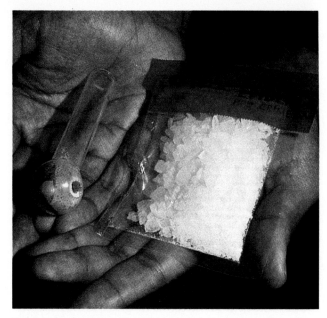
Ice is an inexpensive illicit drug with long-lasting effects. It is typically smoked through a pipe.

Occasionally, the drug may be cut with arsenic or other cocainelike powders.

Medicinal Uses of Cocaine   Turn-of-the-century medical professionals saw great hope for the use of cocaine as an anesthetic but changed their opinions when they saw their patients developing dependency. Although synthetic drugs are now usually preferred, cocaine was and still is used in some eye, ear, nose, and throat surgeries.

Crank and Ice   Newer illicit stimulants such as *crank* and *ice* have created further concerns because their effects last considerably longer than those produced by crack and cocaine. The elevated mood and excitability caused by **crank,** an amphetaminelike stimulant, last from 2 to 4 hours. For this reason, crank is becoming more and more popular among people whose occupations require long periods of wakefulness, such as truck drivers.

Ice is an even more potent stimulant that has begun to gain popularity in the United States, particularly in

Crank   An amphetaminelike stimulant with effects that last longer than those of crack or cocaine.
Ice   A potent stimulant that has long-lasting effects and is inexpensive.

there is no way to measure the costs of wasted lives. In the early 1980s, 1 person in 7 in the $50,000 income bracket was a regular user of crack or cocaine.* Today, even more people from all income levels are using these drugs. The average cost of crack is reported to range from $5 to $15 per small piece, or "quarter rock"; however, costs vary considerably in various regions of the country. Five thousand new users try cocaine or crack each day. Federal agencies estimate that 5 to 6 million people use the drug at least once a month.**

Crack-addicted babies are costing hospitals $500 million a year. Cocaine use can cause premature birth, low birthweight, birth defects, and respiratory and neurological problems. Many crack babies' hospital bills go unpaid.***

The DEA has found no successful method to fight the growing cocaine and crack epidemic in the United States. Cocaine has been called unpredictable by drug experts, deadly by coroners, dangerous by former users, and disastrous by the media. Unfortunately, the risks associated with the use of the drug apparently do not override the attraction of the high that users feel they receive.

Because cocaine is illegal, a complex network has developed to manufacture and sell the drug. Buyers may not always get the product they think they are purchasing. Cocaine marketed for snorting may be only 60 percent pure and is usually mixed, or "cut," with other white powdery substances such as mannitol or sugar.

The number of babies born addicted to drugs has been increasing at an alarming rate.

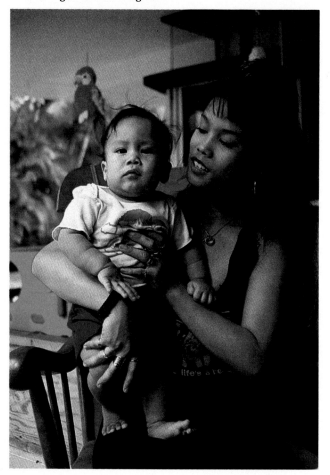

* Mark S. Gold, *800-Cocaine* (Toronto: Bantam Books, 1984), pp. 1–3.
** National Institute on Drug Abuse, Statistical Series, *Annual Data Report, 1989.*
*** American Public Health Association, *The Nation's Health* (April 1990), p. 5.

Hawaii, where it has reportedly surpassed marijuana and cocaine as the leading problem drug.

Ice is so named because it is the crystallized, colorless, odorless form of methamphetamine. (It is also called "crystal meth."). Called *shabu* by the Japanese and *hiroppon* by the Koreans, ice can be manufactured in the laboratory using easily obtained chemicals. Purer and more crystalline than the crank manufactured in many large U.S. cities, most ice comes from Asia, particularly South Korea and Taiwan.

Typically, ice quickly becomes addictive. Some users have reported severe cravings after using the drug only once. The effects of ice are long-lasting. They include wakefulness, mood elevation, and excitability, all of which appeal to work-addicted young adults, particularly those who must work long hours in high-stress jobs. Because the drug is also very inexpensive, it has become popular among young people looking for a quick high. A penny-sized plastic bag, called a "paper," may cost $50 and when smoked can keep a person high for a few days or up to a week. In contrast, an ounce of cocaine causes a high that lasts only 5 to 20 minutes.

Addicts call the sensation from smoking ice "amping," for the amplified euphoria it gives them. However, as is true of other *methamphetamines* (sympathetic-nervous-system stimulants), the "down side" of this drug can be devastating. Prolonged use can cause fatal lung and kidney damage as well as long-lasting psychological damage. In some instances, major psychological dysfunction has lasted as long as 2½ years after use. Aggres-sive behavior is also associated with the drug's use, as evidenced by the dramatic increase in the number of ice-related violent crimes.[*] The number of babies born severely addicted to the drug is also increasing at an alarming rate.

Marijuana

Although archaeological evidence documents **marijuana** use as far back as 6,000 years ago, the drug did not become popular in the United States until the 1960s. Marijuana use receives less media attention today than it did in the 1960s, but it is still widespread, with an estimated 29 million regular users. Among college students, marijuana is the most popular illegal drug (see Table 12.4).[**] Despite the decrease in media attention, damaging effects associated with the use of marijuana are still being discovered.

Marijuana The plant material derived from the *cannabis indica* or *cannabis sativa* plant (hemp); a psychoactive stimulant that intensifies reactions to environmental stimuli.

---

[*] Michael A. Lerner, "The Fire of Ice," *Newsweek*, November 27, 1989, pp. 37–38.

[**] Ken Liska, *Drugs and the Human Body*, 3rd ed. (New York: Macmillan, 1990), p. 243; and Richard G. Schlaadt and Peter Shannon, *Drugs*, 3rd ed. (Englewood Cliffs, N.J.: Prentice Hall, 1990), p. 251.

Table 12.4   Trends in Use of Drugs among College Students 1 to 4 Years beyond High School

	\multicolumn{9}{c}{Percent Who Used in Last Twelve Months}	1987–1988 Change
	1980	1981	1982	1983	1984	1985	1986	1987	1988	
Approx. Wtd. N =	(1,040)	(1,130)	(1,150)	(1,170)	(1,110)	(1,080)	(1,190)	(1,220)	(1,310)	
Marijuana	51.2	51.3	44.7	45.2	40.7	41.7	40.9	37.0	34.6	−2.4
Inhalants	3.0	2.5	2.5	2.8	2.4	3.1	3.9	3.7	4.1	+0.4
Hallucinogens	8.5	7.0	8.7	6.5	6.2	5.0	6.0	5.9	5.3	−0.6
LSD	6.0	4.6	6.3	4.3	3.7	2.2	3.9	4.0	3.6	−0.4
Cocaine	16.8	16.0	17.2	17.3	16.3	17.3	17.1	13.7	10.0	−3.7
Crack	—	—	—	—	—	—	1.3	2.0	1.4	−0.6
Heroin	0.4	0.2	0.1	0.0	0.1	0.2	0.1	0.2	0.2	0.0
Other Opiates	5.1	4.3	3.8	3.8	3.8	2.4	4.0	3.1	3.1	0.0
Stimulants	22.4	22.2	—	—	—	—	—	—	—	—
Stimulants, Adjusted	—	—	21.1	17.3	15.7	11.9	10.3	7.2	6.2	−1.0
Sedatives	8.3	8.0	8.0	4.5	3.5	2.5	2.6	1.7	1.5	−0.2
Barbiturates	2.9	2.8	3.2	2.2	1.9	1.3	2.0	1.2	1.1	−0.1
Methaqualone	7.2	6.5	6.6	3.1	2.5	1.4	1.2	0.8	0.5	−0.3
Tranquilizers	6.9	4.8	4.7	4.6	3.5	3.6	4.4	3.8	3.1	−0.7
Alcohol	90.5	92.5	92.2	91.6	90.0	92.0	91.5	90.9	89.6	−1.3
Cigarettes	36.2	37.6	34.3	36.1	33.2	35.0	35.3	38.0	36.6	−1.4

— = no data available

SOURCE: National Institute on Drug Abuse (Rockville, Md.: NIDA, U.S. Dept. of Health and Human Services, 1989).

PHYSICAL EFFECTS OF MARIJUANA The active chemical in marijuana is **tetrahydrocannabinol (THC)**. Marijuana itself is any plant material derived from either the *cannabis sativa* or *cannabis indica* (hemp) plants. The total plant mixture (stems, leaves, and seeds) contains between 0.5 percent and 3.0 percent THC. The average percentage of THC for marijuana sold in the United States is 1.0. As growers have improved the quality of their crops, this percentage has been increasing.

THC is found in several other forms. **Ghanja** consists of the top leaves and flowers of the plant and may contain up to 5 percent THC. **Hashish** is the sticky resin of the plant and contains about 10 percent THC. *Hash oil* is a substance produced by percolating a solvent such as ether through dried marijuana to extract the THC. Hash oil is a tarry liquid that may contain up to 63 percent THC. It may also contain potentially hazardous solvent residue.

Marijuana can be brewed and drunk in tea. It may also be baked into breads or brownies. THC concentrations in such products are impossible to estimate. Most of the time, however, marijuana is rolled into cigarettes (joints) or packed firmly into a pipe. Some people smoke marijuana through water pipes called "bongs." Effects are generally felt within 10 to 30 minutes and usually wear off within 3 hours.

The most noticeable effect of THC is the dilation of the blood vessels in the eyes, which produces the characteristic bloodshot eyes. Smokers of the drug also exhibit coughing, dry mouth and throat ("cotton mouth"), increased thirst and appetite, lowered blood pressure, and mild muscular weakness, primarily exhibited in drooping eyelids.

EFFECTS OF CHRONIC MARIJUANA USE Because the use of marijuana is illegal in most parts of the United States, and because the drug has only been widely used since the 1960s, long-term studies of its effects have been difficult to conduct. Also, studies conducted in the 1960s involved marijuana with THC levels that were only a fraction of the levels found in plants today. Thus, the results of these studies may not be relevant to the more toxic forms of the drug presently in use. Most of the current information gathered about chronic marijuana use has been obtained from countries such as Jamaica and Costa Rica, where the drug is not illegal. These studies of chronic users (10 or more years) indicate that long-term use of marijuana causes lung damage comparable to that caused by tobacco smoking. The chemicals do not damage the heart, but the effects of inhaling burning material do. Inhalation of marijuana transfers carbon monoxide into the bloodstream. Because the blood has a greater affinity for carbon monoxide than it does for oxygen, the oxygen-carrying carrying capacity of the blood is diminished. The heart must then work harder to pump the vital element to oxygen-starved tissues.

Debates concerning the effects of marijuana on the reproductive system have yet to be resolved. Studies conducted in the mid-1970s suggested that marijuana inhibited testosterone (and thus sperm) production in males and caused chromosomal breakage in ova and sperm. Subsequent research in these areas is inconclusive. The question of whether the high-level THC plants currently available will promote increased risk is, as yet, unanswered. Likewise, the issue of the effects of marijuana on the immune system remains in question.

Marijuana and Medicine Although recognized by the U.S. government as a dangerous drug, marijuana has at least two medicinal uses. It has been used to help control the side effects, such as nausea, produced by chemotherapy, the chemical treatments for cancer, though it is not used as a treatment for the disease itself. Some reports claim that marijuana also reduces the pressure in the eyeball caused by *glaucoma* (a progressive disease characterized by increased fluid pressure in the eyeball). There may be adverse effects in both of these medicinal uses, and legal drugs that work as well as marijuana are available in both cases.*

Depressants

The Opiates

HISTORY OF OPIATE USE The *opiates* are among the oldest analgesics known to humans. These drugs, also called **narcotics**, are derived from the parent drug **opium**, a dark, resinous substance made from the milky juice of the opium poppy. Other opiates include *morphine, codeine, heroin,* and *black tar heroin.*

The word *narcotic* comes from the Greek word for *stupor* and is generally used to describe sleep-inducing substances. For many years, opium was widely used by the medical community to relieve pain, induce sleep, curb nausea and vomiting, stop diarrhea, and sedate psychiatric patients. During the late nineteenth and early twentieth centuries, many patent medicines contained opium. Suppliers advertised these concoctions as cures for everything from menstrual cramps to teething pains.

Some opiates are still used today for medical purposes. **Morphine**, a derivative of opium, is sometimes

---

Tetrahydrocannabinol (THC) The chemical name for the active ingredient in marijuana.

Ghanja The top leaves of the cannabis plant.

Hashish The sticky resin of the cannabis plant.

Narcotics Drugs that induce sleep and relieve pain; primarily refers to the opiates.

Opium The parent drug of the opiates—that is, drugs that are made from the seedpod resin of the opium poppy.

Morphine A derivative of opium; sometimes used by medical practitioners to relieve pain.

---

* "U.S. Rescinds Approval of Marijuana as Therapy," *New York Times*, March 11, 1992, p. A21.

Marijuana Update

Effects of the Most Common Illegal Drug

Marijuana is by far the most extensively used illicit drug. According to a 1988 survey, nearly 62 million Americans have tried marijuana at least once, and 29 million had used the drug in the past year. Although marijuana use has declined since 1982, 16 percent of all 20-to-40-year-olds surveyed in 1988 reported using marijuana at least once in the last month.

Findings from several studies sponsored by NIDA indicate the following effects of marijuana:

Effects on the Brain

Several animal studies appear to indicate that THC affects the *hippocampus,* the major component of the brain's limbic system responsible for learning, memory, and sensory integration. Pathological changes in the brain may resemble the mild losses associated with normal aging. However, whether such chemical changes may place long-term marijuana users at risk for serious or premature memory disorders remains in question.

Effects on Reproduction

A great deal of research has focused on the effects of THC on male reproduction. More recently, research has focused on the effects of THC on female reproduction as well. Recent studies suggest that pregnant women who smoke marijuana are at higher risk of suffering stillbirth or miscarriage and of delivering low-birthweight babies and babies with abnormalities, especially of the nervous system. Babies born to women who use marijuana during pregnancy are five times more likely to have features exhibited by children with fetal alcohol syndrome. In addition, THC passes through the placenta to the baby; therefore, the baby of the mother who recently smoked marijuana may be born "high." All of these risks are greatest toward the end of a pregnancy but may occur at any time.

Effects on Heart Rate

Recent studies indicate that the combination of marijuana and cocaine can cause a greater increase in heart rate and blood pressure than does either drug used alone. The following results were obtained by testing the heart rate while subjects sat quietly. The implications for drug use while engaging in physically stressful activity may be serious.

- Marijuana alone—average increase of 29 beats per minute
- Cocaine alone—average increase of 32 beats per minute
- Marijuana and cocaine combined—average increase of 49 beats per minute over longer time.

Effects on Accidents

Research revealed that one-third of the most seriously injured accident victims admitted to a trauma unit in a Maryland hospital had detectable levels of marijuana in their blood, indicating use within 2 to 4 hours prior to admission. The study also found that 4 out of every 10 people under the age of 30 were under the influence of marijuana at the time of their accidents.

Effects on Self-Awareness

Many marijuana users believe that the drug makes them function better and improves self-awareness. In reality, the drug may serve only to buffer or mask problems. Studies have found that use of marijuana actually impairs self-awareness.

Adapted from National Institute on Drug Abuse, *NIDA Capsules: Marijuana Update* (May 1989), pp. 12–14.

---

used in hospitals and prescribed by doctors for relief of severe pain. **Codeine,** a drug derived from morphine, is found in prescription cough syrups and in other painkillers. Several prescription drugs, including Percodan, Demerol, and Dilaudid, contain synthetic opiates. All opiate use is strictly regulated.

Physical Effects of the Opiates Opiates are powerful central-nervous-system depressants. In addition to relieving pain, these drugs lower heart rate, respiration,

---

Codeine A drug derived from morphine; used in cough syrups and certain painkillers.

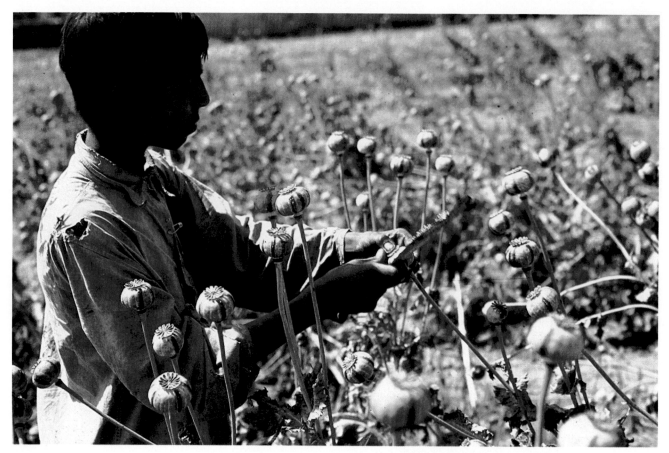

Cultivation of the opium poppy, from which the opiates—opium, morphine, codeine, and heroin—are produced.

and blood pressure. Side effects include weakness, dizziness, nausea, vomiting, euphoria, decreased sex drive, visual disturbances, and lack of coordination. Of all the opiates, heroin is the most notorious. Because all opiate addiction follows a similar progression, heroin will be used as a model for narcotic abuse.

HEROIN ADDICTION **Heroin** and **black-tar heroin** are illegal opiates. Heroin is a white powder derived from morphine. Black-tar heroin is a sticky, blackish, foul-smelling substance that is 60 to 70 percent pure. Once considered a cure for morphine dependency, heroin was later discovered to be more addictive and more potent than morphine. Today, heroin has no medical use.

In addition to its depressant effects, heroin causes drastic mood swings in some users, with euphoric highs followed by depressive lows. Symptoms of tolerance and withdrawal can appear within 3 weeks of the first use of the drug. The most common route of administration is intravenous injection of powdered heroin mixed in a solution. Many users describe the "rush" they feel when injecting themselves as intensely pleasurable, whereas others report unpredictable and unpleasant side effects. The effects of heroin are of relatively short duration and begin to wear off within an hour. The temporary nature

of the effect contributes to the drug's high potential for addiction.

The physiology of the human body contributes greatly to opiate addiction. Opiatelike substances called *endorphins* have multiple receptor sites within the body, particularly in the central nervous system. Endorphins attach themselves at these points, creating feelings of painless well-being (see Chapter 8). Medical researchers have referred to endorphins as the body's own opiates. When endorphin levels are high, people feel euphoric. The same euphoria occurs when opiates or related chemicals are active at the endorphin receptor sites.

TREATMENT FOR ADDICTION Programs to help heroin addicts kick their habits are not very successful, and the rate of recidivism (tendency to return to previous behaviors) is high. Some addicts resume their drug use even after months or years of drug-free living. The craving and desire for the injection rush is very strong. The discipline needed to seek alternative nondrug highs has

Heroin An illegally manufactured derivative of morphine, usually injected into the bloodstream.
Black-tar heroin A dark-brown, sticky substance made from morphine, a derivative of opium poppies that is more potent than heroin.

in many cases proven inadequate in helping an addict stay clean.

Methadone maintenance is one type of treatment available for people addicted to heroin or other opiates. Methadone is a synthetic narcotic that blocks the effects of opiate withdrawal. In most cases, withdrawal symptoms begin within 6 hours of the last dose of the opiate. Within 24 to 72 hours, the addict experiences severe symptoms. Methadone is similar enough to the opiates to control the tremors, chills, vomiting, diarrhea, and severe abdominal pains of withdrawal. Methadone dosage is decreased over a period of time until the addict is weaned off the drug, although the potential for addiction to methadone exists.

Methadone maintenance is controversial. Critics contend that the program merely substitutes one addiction for another. Proponents argue that people on methadone maintenance are less likely to engage in criminal activities to support their habits. In fact, many methadone-maintenance programs are state- or federally financed and are available to clients free of charge or at reduced costs.

Addiction to heroin and other opiates has become less common since the late 1970s. One recent contributing factor to this decline is believed to be the increase in the incidence of AIDS, a deadly virus transmitted through the use of contaminated syringes (see Chapter 18). Drug abusers are now opting for other drugs, like cocaine, that are not administered via needles. Nevertheless, nearly half a million people in the United States are addicted to the opiates.

Psychedelics and Deliriants

Psychedelics The term **psychedelic** was adapted from a Greek phrase meaning "mind manifesting." Drugs classified as psychedelics supposedly expand consciousness by enabling the user to experience parts of the mind that are not normally accessible. The major receptor sites for most of these drugs are in the part of the brain that is responsible for interpreting outside stimuli before allowing these signals to travel to other parts of the brain. This area is called the **reticular formation** and is located in the brainstem at the upper end of the spinal cord. When a psychedelic drug is present at a reticular-formation receptor site, messages become scrambled, and the user may see wavy walls instead of straight ones, or may smell colors or hear tastes. This mixing of sensory messages is known as **synesthesia**.

In addition to synesthetic effects, users may also recall events that have been hidden in the subconscious mind, or they can become less inhibited than they are in a nondrug state. These experiences do not have to be drug-induced but can be self-induced by people who are willing to work to achieve them.

Some psychedelic drugs are erroneously labeled "hallucinogens." Hallucinogens are substances that are capable of creating auditory or visual **hallucinations**, images that are perceived but are not real. Not all of the psychedelic drugs are capable of producing hallucinations. The most widely recognized psychedelics are LSD, mescaline, psilocybin, and psilocin. All are illegal and carry severe penalties for their manufacture, possession, transportation, and sale.

LSD Of all the psychedelics, **lysergic acid diethylamide (LSD)** has achieved the most notoriety. This chemical was first synthesized in the 1930s by two researchers in Switzerland. Because LSD seemed capable of unlocking the secrets of the mind, psychiatrists initially felt it could be beneficial to patients unable to remember and recognize suppressed traumas. From 1950 through 1968, the drug was used for such purposes.

An odorless, tasteless, white crystalline powder, LSD is today most frequently dissolved in water to make a solution that can then be used to manufacture the street forms of the drug, which include sugar cubes, tablets, blotter acid, and windowpane. *Sugar cubes* are made by putting a droplet of LSD onto a commercially prepared sugar cube. *Tablets* are the most commonly sold form of LSD. *Blotter acid* is made by placing a droplet of LSD on a piece of blotter paper, which is then chewed or swallowed by the user. A blotter "page" is 11-by-14 inches and contains 1,000 tabs or "hits." *Windowpane* (sometimes called "clear light") consists of small squares of clear gelatin that contain LSD. Users place the gelatin in their mouths or eyes, where it easily dissolves into the bloodstream. Crystal LSD looks a bit like rock candy. One gram provides 10,000 hits. Effects usually last from 10 to 12 hours.

Despite its reputation for being primarily a psychedelic drug, LSD produces a large number of physical effects, including slightly increased heart rate, elevated blood pressure and temperature, gooseflesh (roughened skin), increased reflex speeds, muscle tremors and twitches, perspiration, increased salivation, and mild nausea. The drug also stimulates uterine muscle contractions and should not be used by pregnant women because it can induce premature labor and miscarriage.

Research into the effects of long-term LSD use has been inconclusive. As with any illegally purchased drug, users run the risk of purchasing an impure product.

Methadone maintenance A treatment for people addicted to opiates that substitutes methadone, a synthetic opiate, for the opiate of addiction.

Psychedelics Drugs that distort the processing of sensory information in the brain.

Reticular formation An area in the brainstem that is responsible for relaying messages to other areas in the brain.

Synesthesia A drug-created effect in which sensory messages are incorrectly assigned—for example, hearing a taste or smelling a sound.

Hallucinations Images (auditory or visual) that are perceived but are not real.

Lysergic acid diethylamide (LSD) Psychedelic drug causing sensory disruptions; also called "acid."

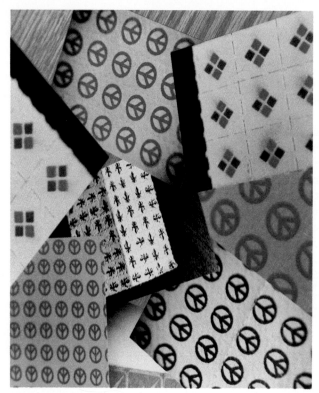

Pages of blotters containing LSD show the distinctive symbols popular with students, who eat the tabs. Police and school officials say the psychedelic drug is enjoying a comeback among teenagers.

The psychological effects of LSD vary from person to person. Set and setting are the most important factors influencing the effects of the drug. A person may experience *euphoria,* a common psychological state produced by the drug, but *dysphoria* (a sense of evil and foreboding) may also be experienced. The drug also shortens attention span, causing the mind to wander. Thoughts may be interposed and juxtaposed as well; thus, the user may be able to imagine several different thoughts simultaneously. Users become introspective, and suppressed memories may surface, often taking on bizarre symbolism.

"Bad trips" are the most publicized risk of LSD. These negative experiences are commonly related to set or setting. In the 1960s and 70s such bad trips eventually led to a decline in LSD use. However, during the late 1980s and early 1990s, LSD has experienced an upsurge in popularity.

Many LSD users become depressed for 1 or 2 days following a trip and turn to the drug again to relieve this depression. The result is a cycle of LSD use to relieve post-LSD depression, which often leads to psychological addiction.

MESCALINE **Mescaline** is one of the hundreds of chemicals derived from the **peyote** cactus. The small, buttonlike cactus grows in the southwestern United States and parts of Latin America. Natives of these regions have long used the dried peyote buttons during religious ceremonies. In fact, members of the Native American Church (a religion practiced by thousands of North American Indians) have been granted special permission to use the drug during religious ceremonies.

Users normally swallow 10 to 12 dried peyote buttons. These buttons taste bitter and usually induce immediate nausea or vomiting. Longtime users claim that the nausea becomes less noticeable with frequent use.

Those who are able to keep the drug down begin to feel the effects within 60 to 90 minutes. Unlike LSD, mescaline is a powerful hallucinogen. It is also a central-nervous-system stimulant.

Products sold on the street as mescaline are likely to be synthetic chemical relatives of the true drug. Street names of these products include DOM, STP, TMA, and MMDA. Any of these can be toxic in small quantities.

PSILOCYBIN **Psilocybin** and *psilocin* are the active chemicals in a group of mushrooms sometimes called "magic mushrooms." Psilocybe mushrooms, which grow throughout the world, can be cultivated from spores or harvested wild. Because many mushrooms resemble the psilocybe variety, people who use wild mushrooms for any purpose should be certain of what they are doing. Mushroom varieties can easily be misidentified, and mistakes can be fatal.

Psilocybin is similar to LSD in physical effects. These effects generally wear off within 4 to 6 hours.

The Deliriants **Delirium** is an agitated mental state characterized by confusion and disorientation. Almost all of the psychoactive drugs will produce delirium at high doses, but the **deliriants** produce this condition at relatively low (subtoxic) levels.

PCP **Phencyclidine,** or **PCP,** is the best-known deliriant. Phencyclidine is a synthetic substance that has been used as a tranquilizer for large animals. It became a black-market drug in the early 1970s. A white, crystalline powder that users often sprinkle onto marijuana cigarettes. PCP is dangerous and unpredictable regardless of the method of administration. Common street names for the drug include "angel dust" for the crystalline powdered form and *PeaCe Pill* for the relatively unpopular tablet form of the drug.

The effects of PCP depend on the dosage. A dose as small as 5 mg will produce effects similar to those of

---

Mescaline A hallucinogenic drug derived from the peyote cactus.
Peyote A cactus with small buttons that when ingested, produce hallucinogenic effects.
Psilocybin The active, hallucinogenic chemical found in psilocyte mushrooms.
Delirium An agitated mental state characterized by confusion and disorientation that can be produced by psychoactive drugs.
Deliriant A substance that produces delirium, including PCP and some herbal substances.
Phencyclidine (PCP) Commonly called "angel dust," a deliriant formerly used as an animal tranquilizer.

strong central-nervous-system depressants. These effects include slurred speech, impaired coordination, reduced sensitivity to pain, and reduced heart and respiratory rate. Doses between 5 and 10 mg cause fever, salivation, nausea, vomiting, and total loss of sensitivity to pain. Doses greater than 10 mg result in a drastic drop in blood pressure, coma, muscular rigidity, violent outbursts, and possible convulsions and death.

Psychologically, PCP may produce euphoria or dysphoria. It is also known to produce hallucinations as well as delusions and overall delirium. Some users experience a prolonged state of "nothingness."

Longterm effects of PCP use are unknown. The original manufacturer applied for a permit to market the drug as a tranquilizer for humans in the late 1960s but withdrew the application upon discovering the unpredictable and traumatic effects upon test subjects.

Designer Drugs

Designer drugs are structural analogues (drugs that produce similar effects) of drugs already included under the Controlled Substances Act. They are manufactured by underground chemists to mimic the psychoactive effects of controlled drugs. At present, there are three types of synthetic drugs available through the illegal drug market: analogues of *phencyclidine* (PCP), analogues of *fentanyl* and *meperidine* (both synthetic narcotic analgesics), and analogues of *amphetamine* and *methamphetamine*, which have hallucinogenic and stimulant properties.*

Amphetamine and methamphetamine analogues are the most common forms of designer drugs on college campuses today. These analogues often cause hallucinations and euphoria. *Ecstasy*, which was dubbed the "LSD of the eighties," is one such analogue that has become popular on many college campuses. It is actually a chemical called methylenedioxymethylamphetamine, or MDMA, and it is similar to the hallucinogen MMDA.

Users claim that the drug provides the rush of cocaine combined with the mind-expanding characteristics of the hallucinogens. Psychological effects of MDMA include confusion, depression, anxiety, and paranoia. Physical symptoms may include muscle tension, nausea, blurred vision, faintness, chills, or sweating. MDMA also increases heart rate and blood pressure and may destroy neurons that regulate aggression, mood, sexual activity, and sensitivity to pain.†

A number of deaths were initially attributed to MDMA, but subsequent research indicated that these deaths were actually related to other factors. Researchers are continuing to explore the effects of this and other designer drugs.

Inhalants and Solvents

Inhalants and solvents are not commonly recognized as drugs. They are legal to purchase and universally available but are potentially dangerous. These drugs are generally used by young people who lack the financial resources to purchase illicit substances.

Some of these agents are organic solvents representing the chemical byproducts of the distillation of petroleum products. Rubber cement, model glue, paint thinner, lighter fluid, varnish, wax, spot removers, and gasoline belong to this group. Most of these substances are sniffed by users in search of a quick, cheap high.

Because they are inhaled, the volatile chemicals in the products reach the bloodstream within seconds. An inhaled substance is not diluted or buffered by stomach acids or other body fluids and is thus more potent and more dangerous than it would be if swallowed. This characteristic makes inhalants particularly dangerous, as does the fact that dosage is extremely difficult to control because each of us has unique lung and breathing capacities.

Effects of inhalants usually last for less than 15 minutes. Users may experience dizziness, disorientation, impaired coordination, reduced judgment, and slowed reaction times. The effects of inhalants and solvents are very similar to those of central-nervous-system depressants. Combining inhalants with alcohol produces a synergistic effect. In addition, these substances can cause severe liver damage, possibly leading to death.

An overdose of fumes from inhalants can cause unconsciousness. If the user's oxygen intake is reduced during the inhaling process, death can result within 5 minutes. Solvent fumes irritate the mucous membranes that line the nose, mouth, and throat. Accidental ingestion of any of these products can cause serious illness and death.

AMYL NITRITE Sometimes called "poppers" or "rush," amyl nitrite is often prescribed to alleviate chest pain in heart patients. It is packaged in small, cloth-covered glass capsules that can be crushed to release the active chemical. The drug relieves chest pains because it causes rapid dilation of the small blood vessels and reduces blood pressure. It also produces fainting, dizziness, warmth, and skin flushing.

ILLEGAL DRUG USE IN THE UNITED STATES

Stories of people who have tried illegal drugs, enjoyed them, and suffered no consequences may tempt us to try them. We may tell ourselves it's "just this once," convincing ourselves that one-time use will be harmless.

---

* National Institute on Drug Abuse, *NIDA Capsules: Designer Drugs*, August 1989, pp. 17–21.

† Ibid.

Amyl nitrite A drug that dilates blood vessels and is often used to relieve chest pains.

Table 12.5 Differences among Drug Users, Abusers, and Nonusers

Drug users, abusers, and nonusers differ significantly in their behaviors. Results of a survey designed to measure the differences are summarized here.

Abusers (%)	Attitudes/Behaviors	Users (%)	Nonusers (%)
47	Are unable to finish projects	26	26
48	See things as hopeless	17	19
47	Feel something or someone stops any progressive move forward	21	18
42	Feel angry or frustrated most of the time	24	20
36	Often find it difficult to get through the day	19	18
34	Have never found a group they felt they belonged to	8	8
66	Have run away from home	37	—
36	Have failed classes	16	16
70	Have been expelled from school	41	—
62	Have purposely damaged property	43	—
89	Keep drugs on hand	41	—
51	Sell drugs for profit	14	—

SOURCE: Richard G. Schlaadt and Peter T. Shannon, *Drugs of Choice,* 2nd ed. (Englewood Cliffs, N.J.: Prentice Hall, 1986), p. 33.

Given the dangers surrounding these substances, however, potential users should carefully consider non-drug alternatives. Many such alternatives, although often time-consuming, are more rewarding and usually contribute more to personal growth than do chemically induced experiences.

The differences in attitudes and behaviors of both drug users and drug abusers are outlined in Table 12.5. Whereas both users and abusers choose to take drugs, users tend to understand better how drugs fit into their lives. An attempt to comprehend the risks and benefits distinguishes users from abusers and may convince some people that nonuse is the best choice.

Risks associated with drug use extend beyond the personal level. The decision to use any illicit substance encourages illicit drug manufacture and transportation and contributes to the growing national drug problem.

How Great Is the National Drug Problem?

Illegal drugs affect every sector of private and public life in the United States. The DEA estimates that illegal drug sales in the United States in 1980 totaled $79 billion, an amount that exceeded the annual sales volume of all but the largest U.S. corporations. Retail sales of heroin alone surpassed $8 billion. Viewed from a different perspec-

tive, in 1984 the U.S. marijuana crop was estimated by the House Select Committee on Narcotics Abuse to range between $10 billion and $50 billion. By comparison, according to U.S. Department of Agriculture statistics, the nation's corn crop that year totaled $19.5 billion, the hay crop $11.5 billion, and the soybean crop $11.3 billion. Thus, illegal drugs are not only "big business," but they are believed to be one of the largest businesses in the United States.*

The financial burden of illegal drug use on the U.S. economy is staggering. Health-care costs attributable to illicit drug abuse total $60 billion annually. Crime-related costs are approximately $176 billion annually. The value of illicit drugs crossing the U.S. borders is between $27 billion and $110 billion annually.

In comparison to these costs, government funds to prevent such abuse are small. The amount allocated for prevention and treatment of drug abuse in 1985 was $230 million. Drug enforcement costs taxpayers $1.8 billion annually.** Critics of national policy on drug control and prevention claim that more dollars are needed to fight what they term a problem of "epidemic proportion."

Solutions to the Illicit-Drug Problem

Americans are alarmed about the increasing use of illegal drugs, particularly crack and other forms of cocaine. We have been warned through the media about the "chemical menace" to our society.

Past antidrug strategies included total prohibition and "scare-tactic" methods. Both approaches proved to be ineffective. Prohibition of alcohol during the 1920s created more problems than it solved, as did prohibition of opiates in 1914. Likewise, prohibition of other illicit drugs has neither eliminated them nor curtailed trafficking of illegal substances across U.S. borders.

Drug Education   In general, researchers in the field of drug education agree that a multimodal approach to drug education is needed. Students should be taught the difference between drug use and abuse. Factual information that is free from scare tactics must also be presented; moralizing about drug use and abuse does not work. Programs that teach people to control drugs rather than allowing drugs to control them are needed, as are programs that teach about the influences of set and setting. Reinforcement of positive self-esteem is mandatory for all levels of students. It is not adequate to "just say no," especially when no alternatives to drugs exist. At-risk groups must be targeted for study so that we can begin to better understand the unique circumstances that make

---

* Liska, *Drugs and the Human Body,* 1991, 3rd ed., p. 243; and Schlaadt and Shannon, *Drugs of Choice,* 2nd ed., p. 216.

** Tom Morganthau, with Nikki Finke Greenberg, Andrew Murr, Mark Miller, and George Raine, "Crack and Crime," *Newsweek,* June 16, 1986, pp. 16–22.

Recognizing Drug-Abuse Tendencies

If you knew you were severely allergic to a particular food, you would probably avoid eating it. Our unique physiology makes even one-time use of illicit drugs dangerous. What is it that makes people use drugs the first time? We know that people with addictive personalities (Chapter 8) run the risk of drug addiction. Other characteristics or desires, though, influence that first step. Look at the questions below. A "yes" answer to any of these means you might be induced to try an illegal drug. As you examine the list, think of nondrug alternatives.

1. Do you frequently wish you could ignore your problems and become indifferent to them?

2. Do you feel "down" for long periods of time? Do you wish for a "high"?

3. Do you like to take physical risks (race-car driving, skydiving, daredevil stunts)?

4. Do you like to be a nonconformist?

5. Are you susceptible to peer pressure?

6. Are you frequently plagued with vague anxieties or feelings of unworthiness?

7. Do you long for knowledge of your subconscious?

8. Do you ever wish to be oblivious to everything?

9. Do you like to be silly and have a good time?

Most of us experience some of these feelings at some time in our lives. These common human feelings are what make drugs seductive. For the abuser, drugs offer instant gratification. We have a choice when we experience these feelings: find an equally satisfying nondrug alternative or give in to what could be a fatal urge.

Drugs obtained from a cocaine bust.

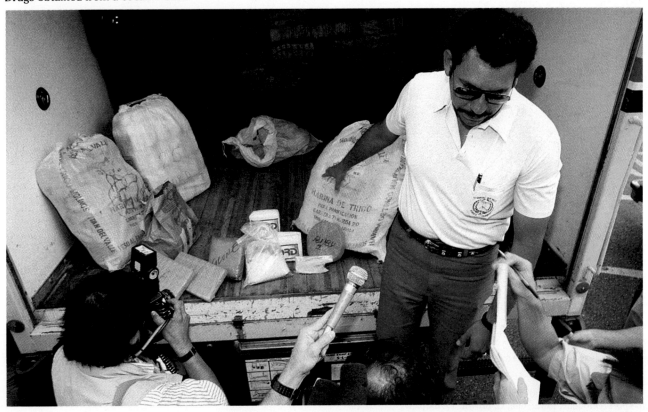

each group more or less prone to drug use. Time, money, and effort from educators, parents, and policy makers are needed to ensure that today's youth are given the love and security necessary for building productive and meaningful lives.*

Other Possible Solutions Various strategies for combating drug abuse have been suggested, including stricter border surveillance to reduce drug trafficking, longer prison sentences for drug pushers, increased gov-ernment spending for drug prevention and enforcement of antidrug laws, and greater cooperation between gov-ernment agencies and private groups and individuals. All of these approaches will probably help up to a point, but none offers a total solution to the problem. Drug abuse has been a part of human behavior for thousands of years and is not likely to disappear in the near future. For this reason it is especially important that we educate ourselves and develop the self-discipline necessary to avoid dangerous drug dependencies.

▌ SUMMARY

▪ The six categories of drugs are prescription medica-tions, OTC medications, recreational substances, illicit substances, commercial preparations, and herbal sub-stances.

▪ Over-the-counter drug categories include analgesics, cold/cough/asthma relievers, stimulants, sleeping aids, sedatives, dieting aids, laxatives, and diuretics.

▪ People use illicit drugs for many reasons, including personal exploration, religious ceremonies, creative in-spiration, and rebellion.

▪ Illicit drugs fall into five categories: stimulants, such as cocaine; marijuana and its derivatives; depressants, such as the opiates; psychedelics and deliriants; and de-signer drugs.

▪ Crack is purer than cocaine and is thus more danger-ous. Highly addictive, crack can lead to death as a result of heart failure.

▪ Marijuana appears to have gained a permanent place in American society. One in 6 Americans is a regular user.

▪ The opiates are a type of narcotic used for pain relief.

▪ Ice and crank are part of a newer and more potent group of illicit drugs, and their widespread use is a fur-ther reminder of the ingenuity of drug users.

---

* Raymond Tricker and David L. Cook, *Athletes at Risk: Drugs and Sport* (Dubuque, Iowa: Wm. C. Brown, 1990), p. 47.

13
Cardiovascular Disease and Cancer: Understanding Your Risks

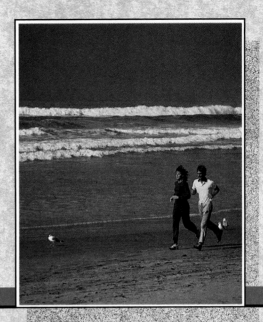

▪ Objectives

- Describe each part of the cardiovascular system, including its function(s) and how it works. Then list your alterable and unalterable risk factors for cardiovascular disease, describe its symptoms, explain how it can damage your heart, and what if anything you can do to treat or prevent it.

- Describe the six most common types of heart disease, including causes, symptoms, and treatment.

- Summarize the advances in diagnosis and treatment of heart disease, including their advantages and disadvantages compared to other methods.

- Present a profile of cancer, including the two major theories about why cells become malignant. Then describe symptoms and methods for diagnosis.

- Discuss each of the most widely suspected causes of cancer and what can be done if possible to prevent cancer or reduce the risk of it.

- List the four classifications of cancer and identify who is most at risk. Then identify which factors influence incidence and mortality, summarizing the types of cancer.

- Summarize the most effective cancer prevention and treatment strategies. Then discuss why the cancer experience is now less disruptive for many patients.

The old adage used by economists, "There's no such thing as a free lunch," applies well—though perhaps unappetizingly—to the history of diseases in our society. Medical technologies have succeeded in reducing the incidence and severity of infectious and noninfectious diseases, such as polio and smallpox, that previously maimed and killed many people. However, other technologies, such as the automobile and the television set, have provided us with convenient and sedentary lifestyles that help keep the incidence of cardiovascular disease and cancer high. In this chapter we discuss the causes of cardiovascular disease and cancer, with a special emphasis on how you can reduce your risk of developing them.

CARDIOVASCULAR DISEASE AND THE CARDIOVASCULAR SYSTEM

During the last century, the American way of life became synonymous with the "good life," a life filled with abundant food, the best in medical treatment, and technological gadgetry. Slowly but surely we began to consume more than our share of protein-rich, high-fat, high-sugar, high-sodium, and high-calorie foods, to the point where over 30 percent of all American adults have become obese. To compound this problem, we have shunned exercise and have opted for riding escalators and elevators rather than taking stairs. Millions of us continue to consume cigarettes and alcohol. Is it any wonder that **cardiovascular diseases** are the leading cause of death in the United States today, accounting for more than 50 percent of all deaths, nearly 3 times the number caused by the second leading killer, cancer, and more than all other diseases combined?

Although it is difficult to place a dollar value on the cost of human life, the economic burden of cardiovascular disease in our society is overwhelming (see Figure 13.1). Estimates of lost wages, lost productivity, and medical expenses exceed $94.5 billion every year. The 1991 edition of *Heart and Stroke Facts,* published by the American Heart Association, indicates that 5,000,000 people alive today have a history of heart attack, angina pectoris (chest pain), or both. In 1991, over 1.5 million Americans were stricken with heart attacks, and more than 500,000 died. The majority of these, 300,000, will die during the 2 to 3 hours they wait before seeking medical assistance.*

We can prevent or reduce the risks for CVD by taking steps to change certain behaviors. For example, controlling high blood pressure and reducing our intake of saturated fats and cholesterol are two things we can do to reduce the risk for heart attacks. By maintaining our

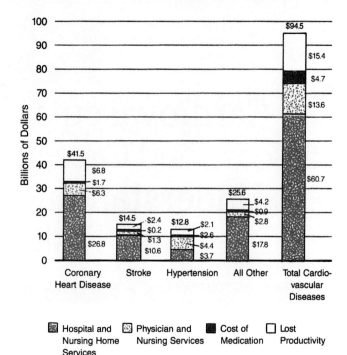

*Individual components may not add to the total given due to rounding.

Figure 13.1 Estimated cost of major cardiovascular diseases in the United States in billions of dollars (1990).

weight, lowering our intake of sodium, and changing our lifestyles to reduce stress, we can lower blood pressure. We can also monitor the levels of fat and cholesterol in our blood and adjust our diets to prevent clogging of arteries.

The Cardiovascular System

The **cardiovascular system,** which is made up of the heart and blood vessels, is extremely complex. In order to understand the implications of cardiovascular disease, we must first understand the underlying mechanisms of the heart and the circulatory system.

The heart is a four-chambered pump, roughly the size of a man's fist. It is a highly efficient, highly complex, and extremely flexible organ.

Under normal circumstances, the human body contains approximately 6 quarts of blood. This blood transports nutrients, oxygen, waste products, hormones, and enzymes throughout the body. It also regulates body temperature, cellular water levels, and acidity levels of body components. The blood also aids bodily defenses by protecting us against toxins and other microorganisms. An adequate blood supply is essential to our health and well-being.

Cardiovascular Diseases Diseases of the heart and circulatory system.
Cardiovascular System The heart and blood vessels, which transport blood throughout the body.

---

* American Heart Association, 1991, *Heart and Stroke Facts,* pp. 3–4.

How does the heart ensure that blood is transferred "on demand" to necessary body parts? How does this small organ manage to contract 100,000 times each day, pumping the equivalent of 4,300 gallons of blood to all areas of the body?

The four chambers of the heart work together to achieve the necessary results (Figure 13.2). The two upper chambers of the heart, called **atria** or *auricles,* are large collecting chambers that receive blood. The two lower chambers are known as **ventricles,** or *pumping chambers.* Small valves regulate the steady, rhythmic flow of blood between chambers and prevent the backwash of blood between chambers at inappropriate times.

Although heart activity actually depends on a complex interaction of biochemical, physical, and neurological signals, the following is a simplified version of the steps involved in heart function:

1. Deoxygenated blood enters the right atrium from the body after having been circulated.
2. From the right atrium, blood moves to the right ventricle and is pumped through the pulmonary artery to the lungs, where it receives oxygen.
3. Oxygenated blood from the lungs then returns to the heart, entering the left atrium.
4. Blood from the left atrium is forced into the left ventricle.

5. The left ventricle pumps blood through the aorta to all body parts.

Many blood vessels are involved in this process. **Arteries** take blood away from the heart, except for pulmonary arteries, which carry deoxygenated blood to the lungs, arterioles (small blood vessels), and capillaries. **Capillaries** are minute blood vessels with thin walls that permit the exchange of oxygen, carbon dioxide, nutrients, and waste products with body cells. Carbon dioxide and waste products are returned to the lungs and kidneys through **veins** and *venules* (small veins).

The average adult heart at rest beats 70 to 80 times per minute. Well-conditioned hearts may beat 50 to 60 times per minute to achieve the same results. When overly stressed, a heart may beat over 200 times per minute. A healthy heart functions more efficiently and is less likely to suffer damage from overwork than an unhealthy one.

Atria   The two upper chambers of the heart that receive blood.
Ventricles   The two lower chambers that pump blood through the blood vessels.
Arteries   Vessels that carry blood away from the heart to other regions of the body.
Capillaries   Minute blood vessels that allow for the exchange of oxygen, carbon dioxide, nutrients, and waste products with body cells.
Veins   Vessels that carry blood to the heart.

Figure 13.2   Anatomy of the heart.

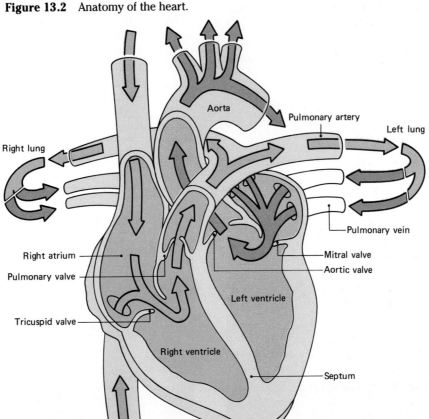

Risk Factors for Cardiovascular Disease

Under ideal circumstances, a person will live a long and healthy life, despite the possibility of developing cardiovascular disease. A knowledge of these factors that contribute to cardiovascular disease can lead to health-promoting lifestyle changes. Different risks can have a compounded effect when combined. For example, if you have high blood pressure, smoke cigarettes, have a high cholesterol level, and have a family history of heart disease, you run a much greater risk of having a heart attack than someone with only one of these risks.

Alterable Risk Factors: What You Can Do Factors that increase the risk for cardiovascular disease fall into two categories: those that can be controlled and those that cannot. The following risk factors can be controlled. As you read about each factor, ask yourself whether it applies to you. Remember that for each factor there are several steps you can take to improve your cardiovascular health and reduce your risks for cardiovascular disease.

CIGARETTE SMOKING The risk for cardiovascular disease (CVD) is 70 percent greater for smokers than for nonsmokers. When the ill effects of smoking are combined with other risk factors, the danger increases by more than the net effects of just adding the risks together.

Although we do not fully understand how cigarette smoking damages the heart, several possible explanations are offered. Nicotine increases heart rate, heart output, blood pressure, and oxygen use by heart muscles. Because the carbon monoxide in cigarette smoke displaces oxygen in the tissue, the heart is forced to work harder to obtain sufficient oxygen. Another theory states that chemicals in smoke may damage the lining of the coronary arteries, allowing cholesterol and plaque to accumulate more easily. This additional buildup constricts the vessels, thus increasing blood pressure and causing the heart to work harder.

BLOOD FAT AND CHOLESTEROL LEVELS Excess fats in the body can contribute to CVD. Especially dangerous is atherosclerosis, or cholesterol buildup along the walls of blood vessels. In past years, cholesterol levels of between 200 and 250 milligrams per 100 milliliters of blood (mg/dL) were considered normal. Recent research indicates that levels between 180 and 200 mg/dL are more desirable in reducing the risk of CVD. It is also important to monitor the levels of lipoproteins in the blood. For more information on cholesterol and lipoproteins, see the box entitled "Monitoring Cholesterol Levels: What the Numbers Mean to You."

Triglycerides are among the most prevalent forms of fat in the American diet. They are also manufactured by the body. Although some CVD patients have elevated triglycerides, a causal link between elevated triglycerides and CVD has yet to be established.

HYPERTENSION **Hypertension** refers to persistent, sustained high blood pressure. If it cannot be attributed to any specific cause, it is known as *essential hypertension.* Approximately 90 percent of all cases of hypertension fit this category. *Secondary hypertension* refers to hypertension caused by specific factors, such as kidney disease, obesity, or tumors of the adrenal glands. In general, the higher your blood pressure, the greater your risk of CVD. Although hypertension affects nearly 61 million Americans, as many as half of them may be unaware of their condition. Known as the "silent killer," hypertension usually has no symptoms, making it one of our more dangerous health threats. Common forms of treatment include dietary changes (reducing salt and calories), weight loss (when necessary), the use of diuretics and other medications (only when prescribed by a physician), regular exercise, and the practice of relaxation techniques and effective coping and communication skills.

Hypertension   Sustained, elevated blood pressure; can be essential or secondary.

A normal artery (left) and an atherosclerotic artery (right). As cholesterol builds up along the walls of arteries, the risk of heart attacks increases.

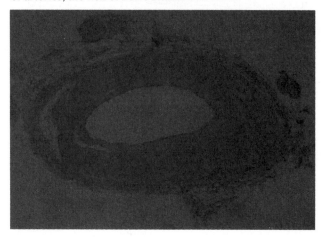
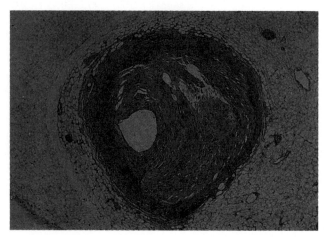

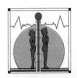

Monitoring Cholesterol Levels

What the Numbers Mean to You

If a blood test reveals that you have a high level of total cholesterol (more than 240 mg/dL), the first thing you should do is have the test retaken to make sure that the reading is accurate. (Remember that prior to having your blood drawn, you must not eat or drink anything for 12 hours.) If your total cholesterol is still high, you should request that a lipoprotein analysis be done to determine the level of low-density and high-density lipoprotein (LDL and HDL) in your blood.

Lipoprotein analysis, which also requires that you fast for 12 hours, measures the level of 3 substances: total cholesterol, HDL, and triglycerides. The level of LDL is derived using a standard formula:

$$LDL = \text{Total cholesterol} - HDL - (\text{Triglycerides} \div 5)$$

For example, if the level of total cholesterol is 200, the level of HDL is 45, and the level of triglycerides is 150, the LDL level would be 125 (200 − 45 − 30).

In general, LDL, often referred to as "bad cholesterol," is more closely associated with cardiovascular risks than is total cholesterol. However, most authorities agree that by looking only at LDL, we ignore the positive effects of HDL ("good cholesterol"). Perhaps the best method of evaluating risk is to examine the percentage of HDL in total cholesterol. If the percentage of HDL is less than 35, the risk increases dramatically.

The ratio of HDL to total cholesterol can be controlled by lowering LDL levels or raising HDL levels. The best way to lower LDL levels is to reduce your dietary intake of the major sources of saturated fat. (For more information on nutrition and cholesterol, see Chapter 13.) However, medications can also be used. You can raise your HDL levels by performing aerobic exercise at least 3 or 4 days per week for 20 minutes or more each time. For significant improvement, however, you must exercise for 2 to 5 hours over a 5- to 7-day period. Also, cigarette smokers can raise their HDL levels simply by quitting smoking. Although some researchers have also found that consuming one or two alcoholic drinks per week can raise HDL levels, this finding remains controversial. Overall, it is easier to lower levels of LDL than it is to raise levels of HDL.

Adapted from *Harvard Medical School Health Letter,* 14, no. 5 (1989), p. 5.

Blood pressure is measured in two parts and is expressed as a fraction—for example, 110/80, or 110 over 80. Both values are measured in millimeters of mercury (mm Hg). The first number refers to **systolic pressure,** or the pressure being applied to the walls of the arteries when the heart contracts, pumping blood to the rest of the body. The second value is **diastolic pressure,** or the pressure applied to the walls of the arteries during the heart's relaxation phase. During this phase, blood is reentering the chambers of the heart, preparing for the next heartbeat.

Normal blood pressure varies for different people depending on weight and physical condition, and varies for different groups, such as women and minority groups. For the average person, 110 over 80 is a normal blood pressure level. If your blood pressure exceeds 140 over 90, you probably need to take steps to lower it.

EXERCISE, DIET, AND OBESITY   Although the role of exercise in preventing CVD was discussed in Chapter 9, it is important to reiterate that a sedentary lifestyle increases individual risk for heart-related disorders. Moreover, physically inactive people also tend to be overweight and are more likely to smoke and to pay less attention to overall health behaviors than active people. Like exercise, diet and obesity are believed to play a role in CVD. Researchers are not certain whether dietary intake (high-fat, high-sugar, high-calorie diets) contributes to CVD or whether the heart of an obese person is strained to excess by having to push blood through the many miles of capillaries that supply each pound of fat. A heart that continuously has to move blood through an overabundance of vessels will probably be unduly strained and may become damaged.

DIABETES   Diabetics, particularly those who have taken insulin for a number of years, appear to run an increased risk for the development of CVD. In fact, CVD

Systolic Pressure   Upper number in fraction; pressure on walls of arteries when the heart contracts.
Diastolic Pressure   Lower number in fraction; pressure on walls of arteries during relaxation phase of heart activity.

is the leading cause of death among diabetic patients. Because overweight people run an increased risk of diabetes, distinguishing between the effects of the two conditions is difficult. Diabetics also tend to have elevated blood fat levels, increased atherosclerosis, and a tendency toward deterioration of small blood vessels, particularly in the eyes and extremities. Through prescribed regimens involving dietary control, exercise, and medication, much of the increased risk for CVD may be controlled.

EMOTIONAL STRESS   During the 1960s and 1970s, stress was considered a leading cause of CVD. More recent studies have challenged this apparent link between emotional stress and heart disease.

Unalterable Risk Factors   There are, unfortunately, some risk factors for CVD that we cannot prevent or control. The most important are listed here.

- *Heredity:* Having a family history of heart disease appears to increase risks significantly. The question of whether this is because of genetics or environment remains unresolved.
- *Age:* Seventy-five percent of all heart attacks occur in people over age 65. Risk of CVD increases with age for both sexes.
- *Sex:* Men are at much greater risk for CVD. Women under 35 are of very low risk except where high blood pressure, kidney problems, or diabetes are present. Women who take oral contraceptives and smoke have a greater risk. Hormonal factors and lifestyle of women appear to reduce risk.
- *Race:* Blacks have 45 percent greater risk of hypertension and, thus, a greater incidence of CVD than do whites.

HEART DISEASE

Although most of us associate heart disease with heart attacks, there are actually a number of different types of heart disease. Current efforts are aimed at treating and preventing the most common forms of heart disease:

- Heart attack (myocardial infarction)
- Irregular heartbeat (arrhythmia)
- Chest pain (angina pectoris)
- Congestive heart failure
- Congenital and rheumatic heart disease
- Stroke (cerebrovascular accident)

Prevention and treatment of these diseases vary from changes in diet and lifestyle to use of medications and surgery.

Heart Attack

Most of us who were raised on a weekly dose of doctor programs on television will recognize the "Code Blue" *myocardial infarction* (M.I.), or similar terminology often used to describe a **heart attack.** Although we have heard the term frequently enough, many people do not know exactly what a heart attack is.

A heart attack involves a blockage of normal blood supply to an area of the heart. This condition is often brought on by a **coronary thrombosis,** or blood clot, in the coronary artery. When blood does not flow readily, there is a corresponding decrease in oxygen flow with resultant tissue necrosis (death).

If the heart blockage is extremely minor, the otherwise healthy heart will adapt remarkably well, often developing new, small blood vessels that reroute needed blood through other areas. This system, known as *collateral circulation,* is a form of self-preservation that allows a damaged heart muscle to heal.

In situations where heart blockage is more severe, the body is unable to respond, and additional lifesaving support is critical. The hour following a heart attack is the most vital, because over 40 percent of heart attack victims die within this time. For information on how to assist a heart-attack victim, see the box entitled "What to Do in the Event of a Heart Attack."

The victim of a heart attack today has a variety of options that previous victims did not. Medications designed to strengthen heartbeat, control irregularities in rhythm, and relieve pain are widely prescribed. Triple and quadruple bypasses and angioplasty have become relatively commonplace procedures in hospitals throughout the nation.

Heart Attack   Damage to the heart resulting from a blockage of the normal blood supply to the heart.
Coronary Thrombosis   A blood clot occurring in the coronary artery.

Because 40 percent of heart-attack victims die within the first hour, immediate action is vital to a patient's survival.

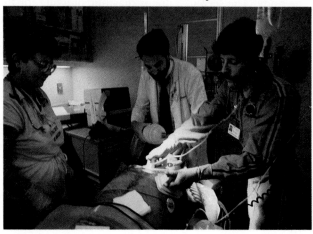

Hot Reactors: High Risks for Heart Attack?

Although such factors as smoking, high-fat diet, and sedentary lifestyle have been conclusively linked to increased risk for cardiovascular disease, there is still a great deal of controversy surrounding the role of other variables in contributing to CVD. Although it was widely assumed that the Type A personality who suffered from high stress levels was a "time bomb" moving toward a heart attack, this theory has not been proven clinically.

Researcher-physician Robert S. Eliot has demonstrated that approximately 1 out of 5 people has an extreme cardiovascular reaction to stressful stimulations. These people experience alarm and resistance so strongly that when under stress their bodies produce large amounts of stress chemicals, which in turn cause tremendous changes in the cardiovascular system, including remarkable increases in blood pressure. These people are the *hot reactors*. Although their blood pressure may be normal when they are not under stress—for example in a doctor's office—their blood pressure may increase dramatically in response to even small amounts of everyday stress.

Are Hot Reactors Always Type A's?

According to Eliot, sometimes hot reactors are Type A's, but usually they are not. In fact, he believes that these are actually two very different conditions. Whereas hot reactors respond with an extreme cardiovascular response to mildly challenging mental and physical tasks, Type A behavior is often demonstrated by overt verbal or external physical reactions. People at highest risk for CVD are those whose blood vessels constrict in response to stress over a period of years, which severely weakens the heart.

Cold reactors are those people who are able to experience stress in their lives (even live as Type A's) but are able to avoid harmful cardiovascular responses to stressful events. Cold reactors internalize stress, but their "self-talk" and perceptions about the stressful events lead them to a nonresponse state. Their cardiovascular system remains virtually unresponsive.

Preventing Hot Reactor Response

Although Eliot believes that Type A behavior is not as important as being a "hot reactor" in assessing CVD risk, he advocates many of the same types of prevention techniques:

- *Changing your self-talk.* It is your *perceptions* of events that often make you ill, rather than the actual events. Rationally thinking a problem through is important.

- *Learning appropriate relaxation techniques.* Although relaxation and mediation are often used only as "quick fixes" for hot-reactor responses, these techniques should be used as a part of a comprehensive relaxation program.

- *Improving fitness levels.* Regardless of your reaction to stress, a well-tuned body has a much better chance of avoiding CVD.

- *Managing alcohol, cigarettes, caffeine, and pills.* Each of these factors increase CVD risk. In a hot reactor, the combined effects can be deadly.

- *Eating right.* Following sensible dietary guidelines with respect to fat, sodium, and high-calorie foods is essential.

- *Making the most of your support and leisure.* The role of a strong network of friends and family is critical to reduced CVD risk. Numerous studies have shown that people who feel "connected" and who have a sense of belonging tend to be better able to keep life events in perspective, control the hot-reactor response, and reduce their risk of CVD.

SOURCE: Robert S. Eliot, "Changing Behavior: A New Comprehensive and Quantitative Approach," Keynote Address, Fourth Annual Meeting of American College of Cardiology on Stress and the Heart, July 3–5, 1987, Jackson Hole, Wyo.

Arrhythmias

An **arrhythmia,** or an irregularity in heartbeat, may be suspected when a person complains of a racing heart in absence of exercise or anxiety. *Tachycardia* is a term used to describe this abnormally fast heartbeat. On the other end of the continuum is *bradycardia*, a condition where heartbeat is abnormally slow. When a heart goes into *fibrillation*, it exhibits a totally sporadic pattern of

---

Arrhythmia An irregularity in heartbeat.

beating with extreme inefficiency in moving blood through the system. If untreated, this condition may be fatal.

In many instances, excessive caffeine or nicotine consumption can trigger an arrhythmia episode. For the most part, in the absence of other symptoms, arrhythmias are not serious. However, severe cases may require drug therapy or external electrical stimulus to prevent serious complications.

Angina Pectoris

As a result of atherosclerosis and other circulatory impairments that reduce the heart's oxygen supply, heart-disease patients often suffer from varying degrees of **angina pectoris,** or chest pains. Many people suffer from short episodes of angina whenever they exert themselves physically. Symptoms may range from slight feelings of indigestion to a feeling that the heart is being crushed. Generally, the more serious the oxygen deprivation, the more severe the pain. Although angina pectoris is not a heart attack, it does indicate underlying heart disease.

Congestive Heart Failure

When the heart is damaged and begins to fill with blood, its chambers are often taxed to the limit. Patients who are afflicted with rheumatic fever, pneumonia, or other cardiovascular problems often have weakened heart muscles. These weakened muscles respond poorly when stressed, and blood begins to pool in the heart. This

Angina Pectoris Severe chest pain occurring as a result of reduced oxygen flow to the heart.

Promoting Your Health

What to Do in the Event of a Heart Attack

Because heart attacks are serious and frightening, we would prefer not to think about them. However, knowing how to act in an emergency could save your life or that of somebody else. This box contains advice on how to manage such a situation.

Know the Warning Signals of a Heart Attack

- Uncomfortable pressure, fullness, squeezing, or pain in the center of your chest lasting 2 minutes or longer.
- Pain spreading to your shoulders, neck, or arms.
- Severe pain, dizziness, fainting, sweating, nausea, or shortness of breath.

Not all these warning signs occur in every heart attack. If some of these symptoms do start to occur, however, don't wait. Get help immediately!

Know What to Do in an Emergency

- Find out which hospitals in your area have 24-hour emergency cardiac care.
- Determine (in advance) the hospital or medical facility that's nearest your home and office, and tell your family and friends to call this facility in an emergency.

- Keep a list of emergency-rescue-service numbers next to your telephone and in your pocket, wallet, or purse.
- If you have chest discomfort that lasts for 2 minutes or more, call the emergency rescue service.
- If you can get to a hospital faster by going yourself and not waiting for an ambulance, have someone drive you there.

Be a Heart Saver

- If you're with someone who is showing the signs of a heart attack, and the warning signs last for 2 minutes or longer, act immediately.
- Expect a denial. It's normal for a person with chest discomfort to deny the possibility of anything as serious as a heart attack. Don't take no for an answer, however. Insist on taking prompt action.
- Call the emergency rescue service, or
- Get to the nearest hospital emergency room that offers 24-hour emergency cardiac care.
- Give CPR (mouth-to-mouth breathing and chest compression) if it's necessary and if you're properly trained.

Source: American Heart Association, *1991 Heart and Stroke Facts,* p. 18.

pooling causes enlargement of the heart and decreases the amount of blood that can be circulated. Blood begins to accumulate in other body areas, such as the vessels in the legs and ankles. If untreated, congestive heart failure will result in death. Most cases respond well to treatment that includes diuretics (water pills) for relief of fluid accumulation, modified diet, reduced intake of salt, and restricted activities.

Congenital and Rheumatic Heart Disease

Approximately 1 out of every 125 children is born with some form of **congenital heart disease** (present at birth). These may range from a slight **murmur** caused by valve irregularities, which some children outgrow, to serious complications in heart function that can be corrected only with surgery. Underlying causes are unknown but are believed to be related to hereditary factors, maternal diseases such as German measles during fetal development, or chemical intake by the mother during pregnancy. Because of advances in the area of pediatric cardiology, the prognosis for children with congenital heart defects is better than ever before.

   Rheumatic heart disease can cause similar heart problems in children. It is attributed to rheumatic fever, which often results from an unresolved streptococcal infection of the throat (strep throat). In a small number of cases, this infection can lead to an immune response in which antibodies as well as the bacteria attack the heart.

Stroke: Reducing Your Risk

In 1991, approximately 400,000 people in the United States suffered from a **stroke.** Of these, 150,000 died and the rest were left with varying degrees of disability ranging from slight to severe incapacitation. What is a stroke? Essentially, it is an injury to the brain caused by basic problems with blood vessels supplying the brain (see Figure 13.3). There are two main types of such problems:

1. Blocked arteries reducing the supply of fresh blood to the brain, and
2. Ruptured blood vessels causing bleeding in or around the brain.

   Depending on the part of the brain affected and the size of the blockage or rupture, the stroke damage may be minor or major. Some people experience a **transient ischemic attack (TIA)** or minor, temporary strokes that may be precursors of more serious, impending strokes.

   Strokes may be caused by several factors. The most common cause is the buildup of fatty substances inside of the artery wall, known as **atherosclerosis.** This buildup can become so severe that the blood flow to the brain is blocked. A diet that is high in saturated fat and cholesterol, high blood pressure, diabetes, and smoking all contribute.

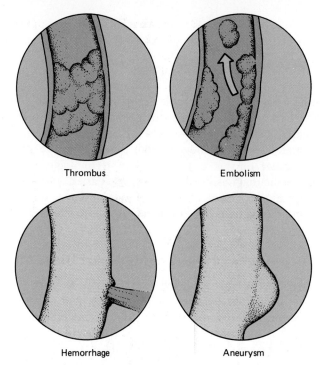

Figure 13.3   This figure illustrates some of the most common blood-vessel disorders.

   Blocked arteries can also occur as a result of a dislodged blood clot, or **embolus,** that is thrown from the heart, inflammation of the walls of the blood vessels, excessive blood clotting, or effects of birth-control pills. Actual bleeding in the brain can be caused by such things as high blood pressure, leukemia, aneurysms, tumors, or anticoagulant medications such as Coumadin.

   Although not all strokes can be prevented, there are several things that you can do to reduce your risk.

- Control high blood pressure
- Reduce intake of fat and cholesterol
- Manage your diabetes
- Avoid smoking and excessive alcohol
- Ask your doctor about taking aspirin to reduce clotting at the early stages
- Pay careful attention to heart-disease risks
- See your doctor regularly
- Avoid unnecessary stress, control stress more effectively

Congenital Heart Disease   Heart disease that is present at birth.

Murmur   Heart sounds made as a result of blood pressing through irregular valve closures.

Rheumatic Heart Disease   A heart disease caused by untreated streptococcal infection of the throat.

Stroke   A condition occurring when the brain is damaged by disrupted blood supply.

Transient Ischemic Attacks   (TIA) Minor or temporary strokes that may be precursors of more severe strokes.

Atherosclerosis   A buildup of fatty substances inside an artery wall, and the most common cause of strokes.

Embolus   Blood clot that is forced through the circulatory system.

NEW WEAPONS IN DIAGNOSIS AND TREATMENT OF HEART DISEASE

There has been considerable debate in recent years over the best treatment choices for people suffering from a heart blockage (*cardiovascular occlusion*). Several advances have come about in both the diagnosis and the treatment of this condition. New technologies have made the diagnosis of these problems easier. Also, new surgical procedures, new medications, and new ways of using medications have made therapy more effective.

Techniques of Diagnosing Heart Disease

Several techniques are being used to diagnose heart disease, including stress tests, angiography, and positron emission tomography scans. An **electrocardiogram** (**ECG**) is a record of the electrical activity of the heart taken during a stress test. During stress tests, patients walk or run on a treadmill while the heart is monitored. A more accurate method of testing for heart disease is **angiography,** in which a needle-thin tube called a catheter is threaded through blocked heart arteries, a dye is injected, and an X-ray is taken showing the blocked areas. A more recent and more effective method of measuring heart activity is **positron emission tomography,** also called a **PET** scan, which produces three-dimensional images of the blood as it flows through the heart. During a PET scan, a patient receives an intravenous injection of a radioactive tracer. As the tracer decays, it emits positrons that are picked up by the scanner and transformed by a computer into color images of the heart.

Angioplasty Versus Bypass Surgery

During the 1980s, **coronary bypass surgery** appeared to be the ultimate technique for treating patients who had coronary blockages or had suffered a heart attack. In bypass surgery, a blood vessel taken from another site in the patient's body (usually a leg vein) is implanted to transport blood by bypassing blocked arteries. But experts have begun to question the effectiveness of bypass operations. Are they necessary? Are there alternatives that may offer equally effective results without the risks of surgery?

Bypass patients typically spend 10 days or more in the hospital to recuperate from the surgery. The average cost of the procedure is $25,000. The death rate is generally 2 percent at medical centers where surgical teams do large numbers of these operations. At hospitals where the procedure is performed infrequently, the death rate can be much higher. A new procedure called **angioplasty** (sometimes called *balloon angioplasty*) is associated with fewer risks and is believed by many experts to be more

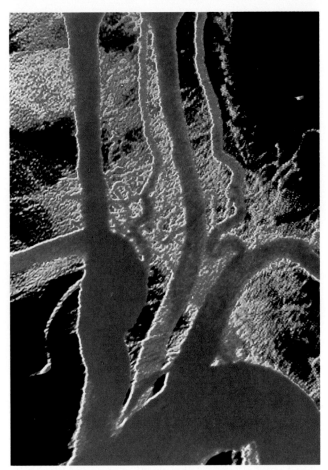

This angiograph shows an X-ray image of arteries arising from the aortic arch.

effective in selected cardiovascular cases. This procedure is similar to angiography. As in angiography, a needle-thin catheter is threaded through the blocked heart arteries. In angioplasty, however, the catheter has a balloon at the tip, which is inflated to flatten fatty deposits against the artery walls, allowing blood to flow more freely.

Angioplasty patients are generally awake but sedated during the procedure and spend only 1 or 2 days in the hospital after treatment. Most people can return to work within 5 days. Only about 1 percent of all angioplasty patients die during or soon after the procedure. Compared to bypass operations, angioplasty is far less expen-

Electrocardiogram (ECG)   A record of the electrical activity of the heart taken during a stress test.

Angiography   Technique for examining blockages in heart arteries in which a catheter is inserted, a dye injected, and an X-ray taken.

Positron Emission Tomography (PET)   Method for measuring heart activity by injecting a patient with a radioactive tracer which is scanned electronically to produce a three-dimensional image of the heart and arteries.

Coronary Bypass Surgery   A surgical technique whereby a blood vessel is implanted to bypass a clogged coronary artery.

Angioplasty   A technique in which a catheter with a balloon at the tip is inserted in a clogged artery; the balloon is inflated to flatten fatty deposits against artery walls.

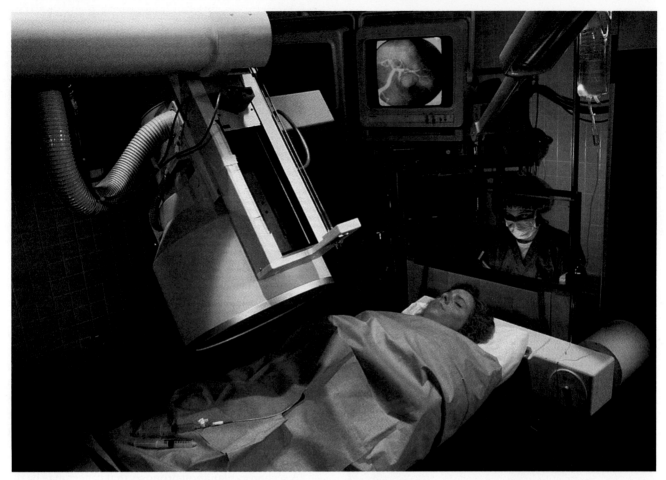

Angiography is a common technique used to detect blocked blood vessels.

sive, costing about $10,000. However, there are some hidden hazards to angioplasty. In 3 to 7 percent of cases, the blood vessel that is stretched open by the balloon collapses spontaneously, and a bypass has to be done anyway. In addition, in about 30 percent of all angioplasty patients, the treated arteries become clogged again within 6 months. Some patients may undergo the procedure as many as 3 times within a 5-year period. Some surgeons argue that with such a high rate of recurrence, a bypass might be a more effective method of treatment.

CANCER: THE SILENT ENEMY

Although overshadowed by the grim specter of the AIDS epidemic, cancer continues to be one of the most dreaded diseases of the century.* **Epidemiologists** estimate that over 76 million Americans now living—about 30 percent of our population—will eventually develop cancer. Over the years, cancer will strike approximately 3 out of 4 families.

Cancer can strike at any age, although it occurs more

frequently among older people. Overall, cancer is the second leading killer in the United States, surpassed only by heart disease. Statistics indicate that over 514,000 people will die of cancer in the United States in 1991 (about 1400 per day) and another 1,000,000 new cases of cancer will be diagnosed. These numbers do not include incidence rates for some of the minor, easily treatable forms of cancer, such as early-stage, nonmelanoma skin cancers. In these instances, removal of the affected patch of skin is often the only treatment necessary. In 1991, American Cancer Society reports indicated that our most common form of cancer, nonmelanoma skin cancer, appeared to affect over 620,000 new victims annually.

Profile of a Deadly Killer

Cancer is a large group of diseases characterized by uncontrolled growth and spread of abnormal cells. Understanding the underlying process by which normal healthy cells become malignant may seem difficult.

Epidemiologists Professionals who study the causes, incidence, and distribution of diseases in a population.

Cancer A large group of diseases characterized by uncontrolled growth and spread of abnormal cells.

---

* Cancer statistics in this chapter are from the American Cancer Society, *Cancer Facts and Figures, 1991.*

However, if a cell is thought of as a small computer, programmed to operate in a particular fashion, the process becomes clearer. Under normal conditions, the healthy cell is protected by a powerful overseer, the immune system. These healthy cells perform their daily functions of growing, replicating, and repairing body organs. When something interrupts the normal cell programming, however, uncontrolled growth and abnormal cellular development, or **neoplasms**, result. This neoplasmic mass often forms a clumping of cells known as a **tumor.**

Not all tumors are **malignant** (cancerous); in fact, most tumors are **benign** (noncancerous). Benign tumors are generally harmless unless they grow in such a fashion as to obstruct or crowd out normal tissues or organs. A benign tumor of the brain could be life-threatening were it to grow in a manner that caused blood restriction and resulted in a stroke.

The only way to determine whether a given tumor or mass is benign or malignant is through **biopsy,** or microscopic examination of cell development.

Benign and malignant tumors differ in several important ways. Benign tumors generally are composed of ordinary-looking cells enclosed in a fibrous shell or cap-

A cancer cell surrounded by killer T cells. Unregulated cells that avoid detection by T cells cause cancer.

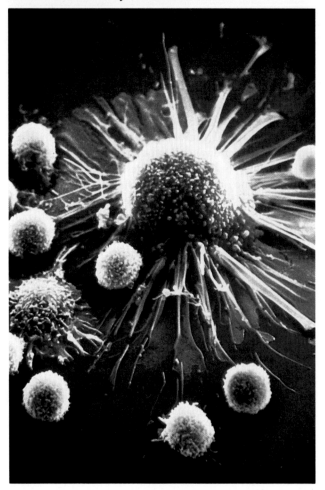

sule that prevents their spreading to other body areas. Malignant tumors are usually not enclosed in a protective capsule and therefore can spread to other organs. This process, known as **metastasis,** makes some forms of cancer particularly **virulent.** By the time they are diagnosed, malignant tumors frequently have spread throughout the body, making treatment extremely difficult. Unlike benign tumors that expand to take over a given space, malignant cells actually invade surrounding tissue, emitting clawlike protrusions that disrupt the chemical processes within the healthy cells. More specifically, the malignant cells disturb the *ribonucleic acid (RNA)* and *deoxyribonucleic acid (DNA)* within the normal cells. Tampering with these substances, which control cellular metabolism and reproduction, produces **mutant cells** that differ in form, quality, and function from normal cells.

Although we can describe the process by which malignant cells spread throughout the body, we are not certain as to why this process occurs. We also do not know why some people harbor malignant cells but never develop cancer. Scientists have proposed two major theories for the changes that occur in cells.

One theory proposes that cancer may result from some spontaneous error that occurs during cell reproduction. Perhaps those cells that are overworked or show signs of age are more likely to break down, causing errors in the genetic makeup of cells and producing mutant cells.

A second explanation proposes that cancer may be the result of some form of external agent or agents that enter a normal cell and cause the cancerous process to begin. Numerous environmental **carcinogens** (cancer-causing agents) such as radiation, chemicals, hormonal drugs, immunosuppressant drugs (drugs that suppress the normal activity of the immune system), and other toxic substances are considered possible disease agents. Perhaps the most common and most dangerous carcinogenic agent is the tar found in cigarettes. This theory of environmental carcinogens clearly has profound implications for our industrialized society. As in most disease-related situations, the greater the dose or the exposure to environmental hazards, the greater the risk of disease.

Neoplasm   A cancerous tumor.

Tumor   An abnormal mass of tissue that grows more rapidly than surrounding tissues.

Malignant   Very dangerous or harmful—likely to cause death, as in a cancerous tumor.

Benign   Harmless; refers to a noncancerous tumor.

Biopsy   Microscopic examination of tissue to determine if cancer is present.

Metastasis   Process by which cancer spreads from a localized area to different areas of the body.

Virulent   Level of high infectiousness and resultant seriousness of a disease.

Mutant Cells   Cells that differ in form, quality, or function from normal cells.

Carcinogens   Cancer-producing agents.

Similarly, those occupations that involve high exposures to environmental carcinogens or that otherwise stress the body's immune system have high risks for cancer.

Although numerous factors may increase individual risk for cancer development, it is important to discuss those that have received most recognition by researchers in recent years.

PROBABLE CAUSES OF CANCER

Although the underlying mechanisms behind the development of cancer cells have been outlined, much research needs to be conducted before the exact mechanisms can be understood. Scientists have classified many substances as possible carcinogens, but we cannot state with certainty that these substances produce cancer in human beings. Some of the most widely suspected causes of cancer are discussed in the following section.

Oncogenes

Research on certain viruses that are believed to cause tumors in animals led to the discovery of **oncogenes**, cancer-causing genes that are present on chromosomes. Although oncogenes are typically inactive or in a type of dormant state, scientists theorize that certain conditions such as age, exposure to carcinogens, stress, viruses, and radiation may activate these oncogenes. Once activated, they begin to grow and reproduce in an out-of-control manner.

Many **oncologists** (physicians who specialize in the treatment of malignancies) believe that the oncogene theory may be an important link in understanding how individual cells function. Through better understanding of normal cell functioning, researchers may be closer to developing an effective treatment for cancerous cells.

Biological Factors

Some theorists believe that we may actually inherit a genetic predisposition toward certain forms of cancer.[*] Much of the research in this area, however, remains inconclusive. Although a rare form of eye cancer appears to be passed from mother to child by means of a direct genetic link, most cancers have not been proven to be genetically linked. Whether we can inherit a tendency toward a cancer-prone, weak immune system remains controversial. Future research may reveal that we inherit a particular disease-fighting potential as a genetic trait. However, the complex interaction of hereditary predisposition, lifestyle, and environment on the develop-

ment of cancer makes the likelihood of determining a single cause fairly remote.

Although an actual link between heredity and cancer has not been found, cancers of the breast, stomach, colon, prostate, uterus, ovaries, and lungs appear to run in families. Hodgkin's disease and certain leukemias show similar *familial* patterns. Whether these familial patterns are attributable to actual genetic susceptibility or to the fact that people in the same families experience similar environmental risks remains uncertain.

Occupational Factors

As previously mentioned, the nature of a person's occupation may contribute to the development of various forms of cancer. In 1991, the American Cancer Society estimated that about 5 percent of all cancer deaths result from occupational risks. Other estimates place this number even higher. Risks vary according to the amount of exposure and the length of exposure time.

One of the most common occupational carcinogens is asbestos, a fibrous substance widely used in the construction, insulation, and automobile industries. Also, people who routinely work with certain dyes and radioactive substances may have increased risks for cancer. Working with coal tars, as in the mining professions, or working near possible inhalants, as in the auto-painting business, is also hazardous. Herbicides, especially pesticides, are potential carcinogens that are found in excessive amounts in many water supplies.

Social and Psychological Factors

Many researchers claim that social and psychological states may play a major role in determining whether a person gets sick. A number of therapists have even begun preventive-treatment centers where the primary focus is placed on "being happy" and "thinking positive thoughts." Is it possible to laugh away cancer?

Although orthodox medical personnel are skeptical of preventive-treatment centers, it is difficult to rule out the possibility that negative emotional states contribute to disease development. People who are lonely or depressed and lack social support have been shown to be more susceptible to cancer than their mentally healthy counterparts. Similarly, people who experience chronic stress and have poor nutritional or sleeping habits develop cancer at a slightly higher rate than the general population. Experts believe that severe depression may actually reduce the activity of the body's immune system, thereby wearing down bodily resistance.

Although psychological factors play a major role in

---

* T. G. Krontirus, "The Emerging Genetics of Human Cancer," *New England Journal of Medicine*, 309 (1983), 404; A. G. Knudson, "Genetics of Human Cancer," *Annual Review of Genetics*, 20 (1986), 23.

Oncogenes   Suspected cancer-causing genes present on chromosomes.

Oncologists   Physicians who specialize in the treatment of malignancies.

cancer development, exposure to substances such as tobacco and alcohol may account for the largest numbers of cancer deaths. Cigarette smoking or exposure to cigarette smoke is believed to account for about 83 percent of all lung cancer cases and about 30 percent of all lung cancer deaths. Heavy consumption of alcohol has been related to oral cancer and cancer of the larynx, throat, esophagus, liver, and colon.*

Cancer and Diet

Can our diets affect our chances of developing cancer? In a 1982 report, the National Academy of Sciences indicated that diet may be a factor in as many as 60 percent of cancers in women and 40 percent in men.

Chemicals in Foods   Although certain chemical additives and preservatives have been linked to some forms of cancer, the majority of these substances play useful roles in food preservation. One such preservative, *sodium nitrate* (a chemical used to preserve and give color to red meat) is one of the most highly publicized carcinogens. Research indicates that the actual carcinogen is not sodium nitrate but the *nitrosamines*, substances formed when the body digests the sodium nitrates. Despite this evidence, sodium nitrate was never banned, primarily because it prevents the formation of poisonous botulism in meats. (It should be noted that the bacteria found in the intestinal tract may contain more nitrates than a person could ever take in from cured meats or other food products.) One possible benefit of this concern was the introduction of meats that were nitrate-free or contained reduced levels of the substance.

The FDA has developed a list of chemicals suspected of causing cancer. Recent sources indicate that this list may contain as many as 14,000 substances.

Nutrition and Cancer   Rather than concerning itself with the ill effects of possible chemicals and carcinogens, current research has focused on the nutrient components of the modern diet. The American Cancer Society, after years of extensive study, has come up with the following nutritional guidelines for cancer prevention:

1. *Avoid obesity.* Sensible eating habits and regular exercise will help you avoid excessive weight gain. If you are 40 percent overweight, your risk increases for colon, breast, gallbladder, prostate, ovarian, and uterine cancers.

2. *Cut down on total fat intake.* A diet high in fat may be a factor in the development of certain cancers,

such as breast, colon, and prostate cancer. Eating fewer fatty foods will enable you to control your body weight more easily.

3. *Eat more high-fiber foods.* Regular consumption of cereals, fresh fruits, and vegetables is recommended. Studies suggest that diets high in fiber may help to reduce the risk of colon cancer.

4. *Include foods rich in vitamins A and C in your daily diet.* Choose dark green and deep yellow fresh vegetables and fruits as sources of vitamin A, such as carrots, spinach, sweet potatoes, peaches, and apricots; and oranges, grapefruit, strawberries, and green and red peppers for vitamin C. These foods may help lower risk for lung cancer and cancers of the larynx and esophagus.

5. *Include cruciferous vegetables in your diet.* Certain vegetables in this family—cabbage, broccoli, Brussels sprouts, kohlrabi, and cauliflower—may help prevent certain cancers from developing. Research is currently in progress to determine which are the substances in these foods that may protect us against cancer.

6. *Eat moderately of salt-cured, smoked, and nitrate-cured foods.* In areas of the world where salt-cured and smoked foods are eaten frequently, there is a higher incidence of cancer of the esophagus and stomach.

7. *Keep alcohol consumption moderate, if you do drink.* The heavy use of alcohol, especially when accompanied by cigarette smoking or chewing tobacco, increases risk of cancers of the mouth, larynx, throat, esophagus, and liver.*

Possible Viral Causes

The belief that it is possible to "catch" cancer has not been eliminated from modern thinking. Evidence that the herpes-related viruses may be involved in the development of some forms of leukemia, Hodgkin's disease, cervical cancer, and Burkitt's lymphoma has surfaced in recent years. Although the research is inconclusive, many scientists believe that the virus may play a role in providing an opportunistic environment for subsequent cancer development. It is likely that a combination of other risk factors and immunological bombardment by viral or chemical invaders may substantially increase the risk of cancer.

Radiation

Although radiation used in medical diagnosis and therapy has been linked to increased risk for cancer, the naturally occurring radiation from the sun is perhaps one

* J. E. Fielding, "Smoking: Health Effects and Controls (Part I)," *New England Journal of Medicine*, 313, 8 (1985), 491–497; *Reducing the Health Consequences of Smoking: 25 Years of Progress*, A Report of the Surgeon General, Executive Summary (U.S. Department of Health and Human Services, DHHS Publication No. [CDC] 89–8411, 1989, pp. 3–32).

* *The Surgeon General's Report on Nutrition and Health* (U.S. Dept. of Health and Human Services, Public Health Service DHHS Pub. No. 88-50210, 1988).

of the greatest risk factors. Farmers, lifeguards, and construction workers, whose occupations force them to be in the sun for prolonged periods, run an increased risk for the most common form of cancer—cancer of the skin. Most skin cancers are easily treatable on an outpatient basis. However, **malignant melanoma,** a virulent cancer of the *melanin* (pigment-producing) portion of the skin, can be fatal. Any chronic irritations of the skin or changes in a wart or mole should be watched closely for possible cancer development. Avoiding excessive exposure to the sun and applying high-numbered sun-protection-factor (SPF) lotion are the best forms of protection.

Combined Risks

Currently, many factors are believed to contribute to cancer development. How large a role each risk factor plays is unknown. Experts believe, however, that combining risk factors can dramatically increase a person's risk for cancer. For example, a person who smokes heavily and works as an auto-body painter runs a much greater risk for developing lung cancer than a person who has only one of these risks.

CANCER: AN IDENTIFIABLE ENEMY

Cancer Classifications

The term "cancer" refers not to a single disease but to hundreds of different diseases. Each cancer has a unique set of characteristics and is named according to the type of tissue from which it arises. The typical classification of cancers follows:

Carcinomas: Epithelial tissues (tissues covering body surfaces and lining most body cavities) are the most common sites for cancers. Carcinoma of the breast, lung, intestines, skin, and mouth are examples. These cancers affect the outer layer of the skin and mouth, as well as the mucous membranes. They metastasize through the circulatory or lymphatic system initially and form solid tumors.

Sarcomas: Sarcomas occur in the mesodermal or middle layers of tissue, such as in bones, muscles, or general connective tissue. They metastasize primarily through the blood in the early stages of the disease. These cancers are generally less common but more virulent than carcinomas, and they also form solid tumors.

Lymphomas: Lymphomas develop in the lymphatic system, the infection-fighting regions of the body. They metastasize through the lymph system. Hodgkin's disease is an example of one type of lymphoma. Lymphomas also form solid tumors.

Leukemia: Cancer of the blood-forming parts of the body, particularly the bone marrow and spleen, is called leukemia. A nonsolid tumor, leukemia is characterized by an abnormal increase in the number of white blood cells.

Although these classifications indicate the general types of cancer, virulence and general prognosis are determined through careful diagnosis by trained oncologists. Once laboratory results and clinical observations have been made, cancers are rated by level and stage of development. Those diagnosed as *carcinoma in situ* are localized and are often curable. Cancers that are given higher level or stage ratings have spread further and are less likely to be cured.

Approximately 514,000 people died from cancer in 1991, which amounted to 1,400 cancer deaths each day, or one every 62 seconds. Of every 5 deaths in the United States, 1 is from cancer. Figure 13.4 indicates the most common sites for cancer occurrence and the death rates for each type of cancer.

Who Gets Cancer?

Cancer is mainly a disease of middle and old age, although it can strike at any time. In fact, cancer kills more children between the ages of 1 and 14 than any other disease. More than half of all cases of cancer are diagnosed after age 65. Up to age 50, the incidence of cancer is higher in women; after age 60, there is a dramatic increase in cancer among men.*

Not everyone is equally at risk for all types of cancers. Cancer incidence and mortality vary greatly by age, sex, race, and socioeconomic status. The National Cancer Institute (NCI) estimates that blacks have greater incidence and mortality rates than do whites for most of the primary cancer sites. In addition, blacks have a lower 5-year survival rate than whites—38 percent versus 50 percent. Researchers at the NCI believe that these differences may be due more to socioeconomic status and to limited access to health care than to racial characteristics.**

Types of Cancer

Lung Cancer Although lung cancer rates have dropped among white males during the last decade, the incidence among white females (particularly young

---

Malignant Melanoma A virulent cancer of the melanin (pigment-producing portion) of the skin.

---

* National Cancer Institute, *Cancer Rates and Risks* (U.S. Dept. of Health and Human Services, NIH Publication No. 85–691, Bethesda, Md., April 1985).

** National Cancer Institute, *Cancer Control Objectives for the Nation: 1985–2000* (Division of Cancer Prevention and Control, U.S. Dept. of Health and Human Services, Final Draft, Bethesda, Md., February, 1989).

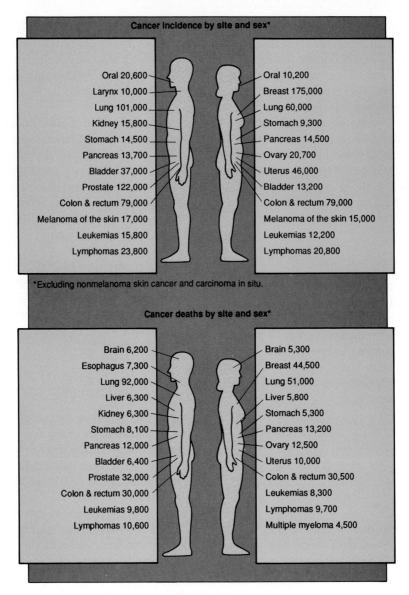

Cancer incidence by site and sex*

Oral 20,600
Larynx 10,000
Lung 101,000
Kidney 15,800
Stomach 14,500
Pancreas 13,700
Bladder 37,000
Prostate 122,000
Colon & rectum 79,000
Melanoma of the skin 17,000
Leukemias 15,800
Lymphomas 23,800

Oral 10,200
Breast 175,000
Lung 60,000
Stomach 9,300
Pancreas 14,500
Ovary 20,700
Uterus 46,000
Bladder 13,200
Colon & rectum 79,000
Melanoma of the skin 15,000
Leukemias 12,200
Lymphomas 20,800

*Excluding nonmelanoma skin cancer and carcinoma in situ.

Cancer deaths by site and sex*

Brain 6,200
Esophagus 7,300
Lung 92,000
Liver 6,300
Kidney 6,300
Stomach 8,100
Pancreas 12,000
Bladder 6,400
Prostate 32,000
Colon & rectum 30,000
Leukemias 9,800
Lymphomas 10,600

Brain 5,300
Breast 44,500
Lung 51,000
Liver 5,800
Stomach 5,300
Pancreas 13,200
Ovary 12,500
Uterus 10,000
Colon & rectum 30,500
Leukemias 8,300
Lymphomas 9,700
Multiple myeloma 4,500

SOURCE: American Cancer Society, *Cancer Facts and Figures, 1991.*

Figure 13.4 Cancer incidence and deaths by site and sex—1991 estimates.

teens) and black males and females continues to rise and caused 143,000 deaths in 1991. In 1987, lung cancer surpassed breast cancer as the leading cause of cancer death among women.

Symptoms of lung cancer include a persistent cough, blood-streaked sputum, chest pain, and recurring attacks of pneumonia or bronchitis. For smokers, especially those who have smoked for over 20 years, and those who have been exposed to asbestos or radiation, the risk is multiplied. Some researchers have theorized that as many as three-fourths of all lung cancer cases could be avoided if people did not smoke. Substantial improvements in the overall prognosis have been noted in smokers who quit at the first signs of precancerous cellular changes and allowed their bronchial linings to return to normal.

Treatment for lung cancer depends on the type and stage of cancer. Surgery, radiation therapy, and che-motherapy are all options. Unfortunately, despite advances in medical technology, survival rates for lung cancer have improved only slightly during the last 10 years. Only 13 percent of lung cancer patients live 5 or more years after diagnosis. These rates improve slightly with early detection.

Breast Cancer Based on current rates, over 45,000 people (4,700 females and more than 300 males) will die of breast cancer in 1991, making it the leading cause of death for women 35–50 years of age in the United States. It is also the most common type of cancer to affect women after skin cancer. Overall, an American woman has a 1 in 9 chance of developing breast cancer over the course of her lifetime, and of those who get cancer, 1 out of 4 will die.* The number of cases continues to soar,

---

* American Cancer Society, *Cancer Facts and Figures, 1991.*

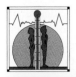

Mammograms

Un Underused Weapon in the Cancer War

Mammograms have proven their effectiveness many times over in recent years. A 1987 study found that women whose tumors were discovered early by mammogram had a much greater chance of a *lumpectomy* (surgery that spares the breast and removes only the tumor) and a 5-year survival rate that was nearly 23 percent better than those who had not had mammograms.

In spite of these facts, fewer than one-third of women over 40 have mammograms every 1 or 2 years as experts recommend. What is the reason for this poor showing at the doctor's office? Several factors may contribute to this underuse:

- *Fear of radiation* Although this is often a reason given for not getting a mammogram, mammograms give off less than one-tenth of the radiation they did 20 years ago, less than the cosmic rays you'd experience on an airplane flight.
- *Failure to recommend* Many doctors continue to feel that mammograms aren't necessary for women not in high-risk categories. Yet 3 out of 4 breast-cancer victims have no known risk! No woman over 40 should consider herself safe.
- *Cost* Costs may range from $50 to $200 and are often not covered by insurance. Medicare just

began paying for this in 1991. Many women postpone these visits because food, shelter, and clothing are higher priorities.

- *Conflicting views on scheduled tests* The American Cancer Society urges a mammogram every 1–2 years for women between 40 and 49, and annually thereafter. The American College of Physicians disagrees, claiming that a mammogram is *not* cost-effective for women under 50, since only 20 percent of the malignancies are in this group. This sort of controversy is all that many women need to justify not seeking medical help earlier.

- *Controversy over quality and accuracy* The proliferation of machines has led to use by unskilled technicians and numerous inaccuracies in diagnosis. Patients should select a high-volume, accredited facility. According to some experts, the "touch factor" is important: If you're not uncomfortable as the machine compresses your breast, you're probably not getting a good scan. Knowing when to seek help and checking for the most reputable facility are key factors in accurate diagnosis.

Source: *Time,* Special Report on Breast Cancer, January 14, 1991, p. 52.

Regular mammography is an essential part of regular physical examination.

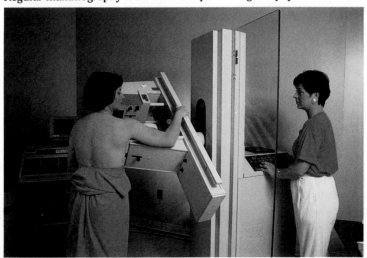

with an increased incidence of over 30 percent between 1982 and 1989.**

Although these figures appear bleak, it is important to note that 5-year survival rates for diagnosed cases have increased from 68 percent in 1970 to nearly 77 percent in 1991. Of these 77 percent, nearly 63 percent are alive 10 or more years later.***

Warning signals for breast cancer include: persistent breast changes, such as a lump, thickening, swelling, irritation, discharge, pain, or tenderness, or any unusual "feelings" or discomfort in the breast. A key factor in survival rests with individual recognition of early symptoms. Figure 13.5 provides a brief overview of one of the best early-detection methods, breast self-examination (BSE).

Fortunately, women with breast cancer have several treatment options, ranging from the simple *lumpectomy* surgery to *radical mastectomy* to various combinations of radiation or chemotherapy (as illustrated in Figure 13.6). To ensure the best treatment possible, the breast-cancer patient should seek more than one opinion before making a decision.

Colon and Rectal Cancers   Although colon and rectal cancers are the second leading cause of cancer deaths, many people are unaware of their potential risk. Bleeding from the rectum, blood in the stool, and changes in bowel habits are the major warning signals. People who are over the age of 40, who have a family history of colon and rectal cancer, have a personal or family history of *polyps* (benign growths) in the colon or rectum, or have inflammatory bowel problems such as *colitis* run an increased risk. Diets high in fats or low in fiber may also increase risks.

Because colorectal cancer tends to spread slowly, the prognosis is quite good if it is caught in the early stages. Treatment often consists of radiation or surgery. Chemotherapy, although not used extensively in the past, is being examined as a possibility. A permanent *colostomy*, the creation of an abdominal opening for the elimination of body wastes, is seldom required for patients of colon cancer and even less frequently for rectal cancer.

Prostate Cancer   Cancer of the prostate is the third leading cause of cancer death in males, killing an estimated 30,000 men in 1991. Most signs and symptoms of prostate cancer are nonspecific, acting much like an infection or enlarged prostate. Symptoms include pain or difficulty in urinating, blood in the urine, and pain in the low back, pelvis, or upper thighs. Risk factors include a high-fat diet and a tendency toward prostate cancer in the immediate family.

Fortunately, even with so many generalized symptoms, most prostate cancers are detected while they are still localized. These patients have an average 5-year

survival rate of 84 percent. Because the incidence of prostate cancer increases with age (80 percent of all cases are diagnosed in men over 65), every man over the age of 40 should have an annual prostate examination.

Skin Cancer   Although discussed previously, the importance of skin cancer should not be underestimated. Whereas most people do not die of the highly curable basal or squamous cells cancers, malignant melanoma is increasing at the rate of 4 percent per year. Any unusual skin condition, especially a change in the size or color of a mole or other darkly pigmented growth or spot, should be suspect. Scaliness, oozing, bleeding or the appearance of a bump or nodule, the spread of pigment beyond the border, or change in sensation, itchiness, tenderness, or pain are all warning signs of melanoma.

Treatment of skin cancer depends on the seriousness of the condition. Surgery is used in 90 percent of all cases. Radiation therapy, *electrodesiccation* (tissue destruction by heat), and *cryosurgery* (tissue destruction by freezing) are also common forms of treatment. For melanoma, surgery may involve removal of the regional lymph nodes, radiation, or chemotherapy.

Testicular Cancer   Testicular cancer is currently one of the most common types of solid tumors found in males entering early adulthood. Males between the ages of 15 and 34 are at greatest risk. There has been a steady increase in tumor frequency over the past several years among this age group.

Although the exact cause of testicular cancer is unknown, several possible risk factors have been identified. Males with undescended testicles appear to be at greatest risk for the disease. In addition, some studies indicate that there may be a genetic influence on individual risk.*

In general, testicular tumors are first noticed as a painless enlargement of the testis or as an apparent thickening in testicular tissue. Because this enlargement is often painless, it is extremely important that all young males practice regular testicular self-examination (see Figure 13.7). If a suspicious lump or thickening is found, medical follow-up should be sought.

Ovarian Cancer   Ovarian cancer is often silent, showing no obvious signs or symptoms until late in its development. The most common sign is enlargement of the abdomen (or a feeling of bloating) in women over the age of 40. Other symptoms include vague digestive disturbances, such as gas and stomach aches that persist and cannot be explained.

The risk for ovarian cancer increases with age, with the highest rates among women in their sixties. Women who have never had children are twice as likely to develop ovarian cancer as those who have. In addition, having one or more primary relatives (mother, sisters,

** Ibid.
*** Ibid.

* Stanley Robbins and Vinay Kumar, *Basic Pathology* (Philadelphia: Saunders, 1987), p. 617.

Do you know that 95% of all breast cancers are discovered first by women themselves? And that the earlier breast cancer is detected, the better the chance of complete cure?

Of course, most lumps or changes are not cancer. But you can help safeguard your health by making a habit of examining your breasts once a month – a day or two after your period or, if you're no longer menstruating, on any given day. And if you notice anything changed or unusual – a lump, thickening or discharge – contact your doctor right away.

how to examine your breasts

how to look for changes

Step 2
Raise your arms above your head and repeat the examination in step 1.

Step 1
Sit or stand in front of a mirror with your arms at your sides. Turning slowly from side to side, check your breasts for:
• changes in size or shape
• puckering or dimpling of the skin
• changes in size or position of one nipple compared to the other

Step 3
Gently press each nipple with your fingertips to see if there is any discharge.

how to feel for changes

Step 2
Imagine that your breast is divided into four quarters.

Step 4
Now do the same for the lower, inner portion of your breast. You may feel a ridge of firm tissue under your breasts, if your breasts are larger than average. Or, if you are thin, you may feel a rib through your breasts. This is perfectly normal.

Step 6
With your arm still down, feel the upper, outer part of your breast, starting with your nipple and working outwards.

Step 1
Lie down and put a pillow or folded bath towel underneath your left shoulder. Then place your left hand under your head. (From now on you will be feeling for a lump or thickening in your breasts.)

Step 3
With the fingers of your right hand held together, press firmly but gently, using small circular motions to feel the inner, upper quarter of your left breast, starting at your breastbone and working toward the nipple. Also examine the area around the nipple.

Step 5
Next, bring your arm down to your side and feel under your left armpit for swellings.

Step 7
Finally, with your arm still down, examine the lower, outer quarter in the same manner.

Step 8
Now place the pillow under your right shoulder and repeat steps 1-7, this time using your left hand to examine your right breast.

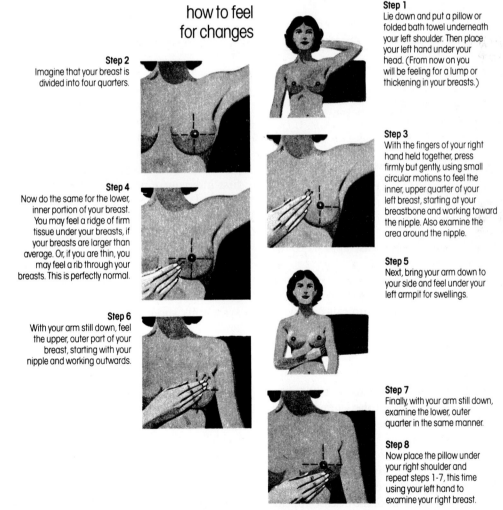

Figure 13.5 Breast self-examination: the 10-minute habit that could save your life.

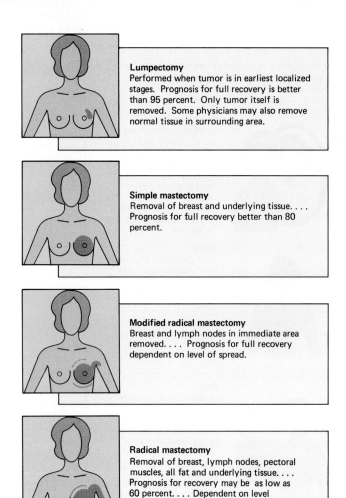

Lumpectomy
Performed when tumor is in earliest localized stages. Prognosis for full recovery is better than 95 percent. Only tumor itself is removed. Some physicians may also remove normal tissue in surrounding area.

Simple mastectomy
Removal of breast and underlying tissue.... Prognosis for full recovery better than 80 percent.

Modified radical mastectomy
Breast and lymph nodes in immediate area removed.... Prognosis for full recovery dependent on level of spread.

Radical mastectomy
Removal of breast, lymph nodes, pectoral muscles, all fat and underlying tissue.... Prognosis for recovery may be as low as 60 percent.... Dependent on level of spread.

Figure 13.6 Selected surgical procedures for diagnosed breast cancer. These surgeries typically include the use of radiation and/or chemotherapy in treatment.

What can I do?
Cancer of the testes—the male reproductive glands— is one of the most common cancers in men 15 to 34 years of age. It accounts for 12 percent of all cancer deaths in this group.

Your best hope for early detection of testicular cancer is a simple three-minute monthly self-examination. The best time is after a warm bath or shower, when the scrotal skin is most relaxed.

Roll each testicle gently between the thumb and fingers of both hands. If you find any hard lumps or nodules, you should see your doctor promptly. They may not be malignant, but only your doctor can make the diagnosis.

Following a thorough physical examination, your doctor may perform certain X-ray studies to make the most accurate diagnosis possible.

Vas deferens
Epididymis
Nodule

Figure 13.7 Key points in testicular self-examination.

grandmothers) who have had the disease appears to increase individual risks.

To protect yourself, annual thorough pelvic examinations are important. Pap tests, although useful in detecting cervical cancer, do not reveal ovarian cancer. If you have any of the above symptoms and they persist, see your doctor. If they continue to persist, get a second opinion.

Uterine Cancer In 1991, an estimated 47,000 new cases of uterine cancer developed in the United States. Most of these cases developed in the body of the uterus, usually in the *endometrium* (lining). The rest developed in the *cervix,* located at the base of the uterus. Overall incidence of early-stage cervical cancer has increased slightly in recent years in women under the age of 50. In contrast, invasive, later-stage forms of the disease appear to be decreasing. Much of this apparent trend may be due to more effective regular screenings of younger women using the *Pap test,* a procedure in which cells taken from the cervical region are examined for ab-

normal cellular activity. Although these tests are very effective in detecting early-stage cervical cancer, they are less effective in detecting cancers of the uterine lining and are not effective in detecting cancers of the fallopian tubes or ovaries.

Risk factors for cervical cancer include early age of first intercourse, multiple sex partners, cigarette smoking, and certain sexually transmitted diseases. For endometrial cancer, a history of infertility, failure to ovulate, obesity, and prolonged estrogen therapy appear to be major risk factors.

Early warning signs of uterine cancer include bleeding outside of the normal menstrual period or after menopause or persistent unusual vaginal discharge. These symptoms should be checked by a physician immediately.

Leukemia Leukemia is a cancer of the bloodforming tissues, which leads to proliferation of millions of immature white blood cells. These abnormal cells crowd out normal white blood cells (which fight infection), platelets (which control hemorrhaging), and red blood cells (which prevent anemia). As a result, symptoms such as fatigue, paleness, weight loss, easy bruising, repeated infections, nosebleeds, and other forms of hemorrhaging occur. In children, these symptoms can appear suddenly. Chronic leukemia can develop over several months and have few symptoms.

Leukemia can be acute or chronic in nature and can strike both sexes and all age groups. Although many people believe that leukemia is a childhood disease, leu-

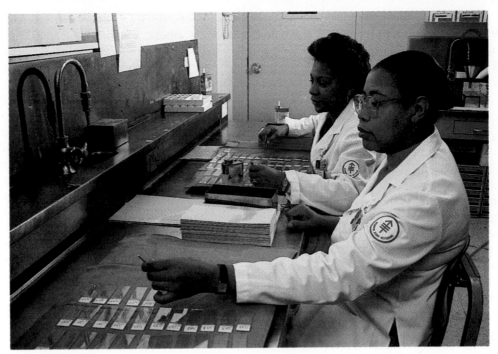

Pap smear results are reviewed by trained professionals to determine if cancer cells are present.

The occurrence of cancer in children often causes great pain and emotional suffering for parents.

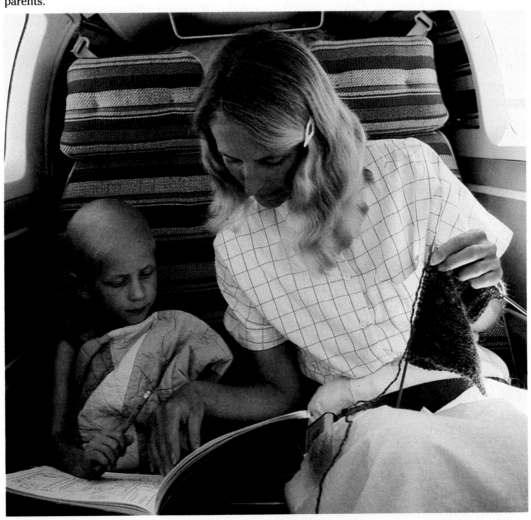

kemia struck many more adults (25,500) than children (2,500) in 1991. Although the prognosis for leukemia patients is much better today than it was in the 1960s, leukemia still poses a significant threat to those people who contract it.

CAN WE AVOID CANCER?

Although we seem to live in a world filled with carcinogens, nevertheless there are things we can do to protect ourselves from cancer. Perhaps the most basic preventive measure is to avoid known carcinogenic substances whenever possible and to reduce the level and duration of exposure when they cannot be avoided. Although cancer affects nearly every family in America, current research indicates that we may be gaining ground on this age-old enemy.

Preventing Cancer

Recent studies have indicated that lifestyle and environment play major roles in cancer development and that cancer mortality can be significantly reduced through specific lifestyle changes and preventive actions.

We should be aware of American Cancer Society (ACS) guidelines regarding an anticancer diet as well as the minimal ACS recommendations regarding the early detection and diagnosis of cancer. It is not enough to rely on the medical community for these services. Everyone should know the seven warning signals of cancer, which can be remembered as the word "CAUTION":

*C*hange in the size or color of a wart or mole

A sore that does not heal or that heals slowly

*U*nusual or unexplained bleeding from the bowel, nipples, or vagina, or the presence of blood in the urine

*T*hickening or lump in the breast or on the lip or tongue

*I*ndigestion that persists or loss of appetite

*O*bvious change in bowel or bladder habits

*N*agging or persistent cough or hoarseness and difficulty swallowing

Although none of these symptoms definitely means that you have cancer, they should not be ignored, particularly if they persist for several weeks. Because many people deny the possibility of illnesses, especially those they fear, they frequently ignore many warning signs.

Detecting Cancer The earlier a person is diagnosed as having cancer, the better the prospect for survival. We must all accept responsibility for personal cancer detection. Responsibility entails making sure that appropriate

diagnostic tests are completed whenever any warning signals appear. Various high-tech diagnostic techniques exist to detect cancer. **Magnetic resonance imagery (MRI)** involves the use of magnetic fields, radio waves, and computers instead of radiation to generate an image of internal tissue of the body. Another diagnostic tool, **computerized axial tomography (CAT scan)**, is a machine that uses radiation to view internal organs not normally visible by X-rays. **Xeroradiograms** are three-dimensional X-ray mammograms used to detect breast cancer. These medical techniques, along with regular self-examinations and check-ups, play an important role in the early detection and prevention of cancer.

Each person must also make a realistic assessment of individual risk factors and try to reduce personal risk. Even if you have a history of cancer in your immediate family, you can reduce your risk for cancer by changing your dietary patterns and avoiding known carcinogens and other environmental hazards. In addition, paying careful attention to those factors listed in the "Promoting Your Health" box entitled "Prevention of Cancer" may significantly decrease your chances of getting cancer.

Cancer Treatments

Although cancer treatments have changed dramatically over the last 20 years, *surgery,* in which the tumor and surrounding tissue are removed, is still common. Today's surgeons tend to remove less surrounding tissue than previously and to combine surgery with either **radiotherapy,** the use of radiation, or **chemotherapy,** the use of any of over 50 drugs, to kill cancerous cells.

Radiation works by destroying malignant cells or stopping cell growth. Fortunately, radiation is more effective in destroying malignant cells than in destroying healthy cells, although some healthy cells are inadvertently destroyed in the process. Radiation is most effective in treating localized cancer masses. In recent years, many scientists have questioned whether radiotherapy increases the risks for other types of cancer. Despite these questions, radiation continues to be one of the most common forms of treatment.

When cancer has spread throughout the body, it is necessary to use some form of chemotherapy. Currently, over 50 different anticancer drugs are in use, some of which have excellent records of success. A chemotherapeutic regimen including four anticancer drugs in combination with radiation therapy has resulted in remark-

Magnetic Resonance Imagery (MRI) A device that uses magnetic fields, radio waves, and computers to generate an image of internal tissues of the body for diagnostic purposes without the use of radiation.

Computerized Axial Tomography (CAT scan) A machine that uses radiation to view internal organs not normally visible by X-rays.

Xeroradiograms Three-dimensional X-ray mammograms.

Radiotherapy The use of radiation to kill cancer cells.

Chemotherapy The use of drugs to kill cancerous cells.

Promoting Your Health

Prevention of Cancer

Primary prevention refers to steps that might be taken to avoid those factors that might lead to the development of cancer.

Smoking	Cigarette smoking is responsible for 85 percent of lung-cancer cases among men and 75 percent among women—about 83 percent overall. Smoking accounts for about 30 percent of all cancer deaths. Those who smoke two or more packs of cigarettes a day have lung-cancer mortality rates 15 to 25 times greater than non-smokers.
Sunlight	Almost all of the more than 600,000 cases of nonmelanoma skin cancer diagnosed each year in the United States are considered to be sun-related. Recent epidemiologic evidence shows that sun exposure is a major factor in the development of melanoma and that the incidence increases for those living near the equator
Alcohol	Oral cancer and cancers of the larynx, throat, esophagus, and liver occur more frequently among heavy drinkers of alcohol.
Smokeless tobacco	Use of chewing tobacco or snuff increases risk of cancer of the mouth, larynx, throat, and esophagus and is highly habit-forming.
Estrogen	For mature women, estrogen treatment to control menopausal symptoms increases risk of endometrial cancer. Use of estrogen by menopausal women needs careful discussion between the woman and her physician.
Radiation	Excessive exposure to ionizing radiation can increase cancer risk. Most medical and dental X-rays are adjusted to deliver the lowest dose possible without sacrificing image quality. Excessive radon exposure in homes may increase risk of lung cancer, especially in cigarette smokers. If levels are found to be too high, remedial actions should be taken.
Occupational hazards	Exposure to several different industrial agents (nickel, chromate, asbestos, vinyl chloride, etc.) increases risk of various cancers. Risk from asbestos is greatly increased when combined with cigarette smoking.
Nutrition	Risk for colon, breast, and uterine cancers increases in obese people. High-fat diets may contribute to the development of cancers of the breast, colon, and prostate. High-fiber foods may help reduce risk of colon cancer. A varied diet containing plenty of vegetables and fruits rich in vitamins A and C may reduce risk for a wide range of cancers. Salt-cured, smoked, and nitrite-cured foods have been linked to esophageal and stomach cancer. The heavy use of alcohol, especially when accompanied by cigarette smoking or chewing tobacco, increases risk of cancers of the mouth, larynx, throat, esophagus, and liver.

SOURCE: *Cancer Facts and Figures, 1991*, p. 17.

able survival rates for some cancers, including Hodgkin's disease.

Whether used alone or in combination, each type of treatment has possible side effects, including excessive nausea, nutritional deficiencies, hair loss, and general fatigue. The newest technique in cancer therapy involves **immunotherapy,** a process that stimulates the body's own immune system to help combat the cancer cells.

Interferon, a protein produced by the body upon viral invasion, is believed to provide a protective mechanism for otherwise healthy cells, thus making it more difficult for cancer to gain a foothold.

Immunotherapy A process in which the body's own immune system helps to combat cancer cells.

Life after Cancer: Patient Concerns

Heightened public awareness and an improved prognosis for cancer victims have made the cancer experience less disruptive for many patients. Unfortunately, many recovering cancer patients experience problems with job discrimination and are unable to obtain health or life insurance. Although several states have enacted legislation assisting people who have become victims of insurance cancellations and other problems, much remains to be done.

On the personal side, assistance for the cancer patient is more readily available than ever before. Cancer support groups, cancer-information workshops, and low-cost medical consultation for those who cannot afford to pay are just some of the more positive aspects of the cancer situation. Increasing efforts in the area of cancer research, improved diagnostic equipment, and more advanced treatments provide some hope for the future.

SUMMARY

- Cardiovascular diseases are the leading cause of death in the United States today, responsible for more than 50 percent of all deaths, nearly 3 times the number caused by cancer and more than all other diseases combined.

- Risk factors for cardiovascular disease include cigarette smoking, blood-fat and cholesterol levels, hypertension, exercise, diet and obesity, and emotional stress. Many of these factors have a compounded effect when combined.

- Dietary changes, exercise, weight reduction, and attention to lifestyle risks can reduce CVD susceptibility.

- The major treatable heart diseases in the United States include heart attacks, arrhythmia, angina, congestive heart failure, congenital heart defects, rheumatic heart disease, and strokes.

- New methods developed for treating heart blockages include coronary bypass surgery and angioplasty. Also, beta blockers and calcium channel blockers are being used to reduce high blood pressure and to treat other symptoms, and anticoagulants (such as aspirin) are being used to prevent blood clotting, which can cause heart attacks.

- There are currently over 5 million Americans with a history of cancer, most of whom have a much better prognosis for 5-year survival than people in previous decades.

- Cancer is the second leading killer in the United States, behind heart disease. Cancer occurs more frequently among older people but also kills more children between the ages of 3 and 14 than any other disease.

- Major types of cancer include carcinomas, sarcomas, lymphomas, and leukemia.

- Possible causes of cancer include biological factors, occupational factors, social and psychological factors, dietary factors, viral factors, oncogenes, medical causes, radiation, and combinations of these factors.

14

Infectious and Noninfectious Diseases

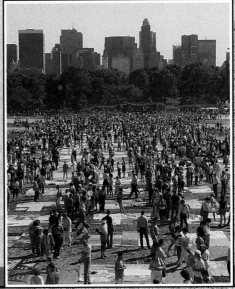

Objectives

- Identify and describe each of the most common risk factors that cause disease.

- Identify the six most common pathogens. Then give an example of a disease caused by each, describing its symptoms and treatment.

- Discuss how the body defends itself against pathogens.

- Describe the mode of transmission for STD's, their common and unique characteristics, methods of diagnosis, and treatment as well as damage caused if untreated.

- Discuss the origins of AIDS and how it is transmitted. Then summarize the symptoms of AIDS, how it is diagnosed, prevention strategies, where to seek help, and chances for a cure.

- Describe the common characteristics of noncommunicable and chronic diseases.

- Identify each respiratory disorder, including its causes, symptoms, and, when indicated, prevention and treatment strategies.

- Identify the most common neurological disorders, and summarize their causes, symptoms, and treatment.

- Identify the most common female disorders, and summarize their causes, symptoms, and treatment.

- Identify the most common disorders related to digestion, and summarize their causes, symptoms, and treatment.

- Identify the most common diseases of the bones and

joints, and summarize their causes, symptoms, and treatment.

- Identify other modern diseases and summarize their causes, symptoms, and treatment.

G reek mythology tells of a Golden Age when people lived completely free of illness until Pandora opened the "Box of Evils" and inflicted disease upon humanity. Many other cultures have embraced myths of an idyllic "Garden of Eden" that was violated, turning disease and pestilence loose upon civilization.

Scientific evidence, however, indicates that disease has always been a part of our existence. Fossils provide evidence that infections, arthritis, cancer, heart disease, and similar ailments have afflicted humans and animals since prehistoric times. Preserved mummies discovered in ancient burial places indicate the presence of disease as well as surprisingly sophisticated methods of treatment.

Throughout most of history, people believed that illness was caused by "single agents." Early treatment of disease was often based on what physicians and others could hear, see, smell, taste, or feel. For example, tasting urine to detect the sweetness indicative of diabetes was a common practice.

It was not until the nineteenth century that the relationship between microscopic germs and disease was established. The **germ theory** became widely accepted through the efforts of three men: Louis Pasteur, Joseph Lister, and Robert Koch. Louis Pasteur, a French chemist, was interested in why foods such as meat and wine often spoiled. He began looking at decaying meats through primitive microscopes and determined that living organisms caused this problem. Through a process of trial and error, he determined that heating fluids such as wine to a temperature just below the boiling point destroyed many of these germs. This process, later called **pasteurization,** has contributed greatly to reducing the bacterial contamination of certain foods.

Joseph Lister, an English surgeon, was concerned with the reasons for the 45-percent mortality rate among surgical patients. Recognizing the relationship between the infection of wounds and bacterial growth, Lister proposed the sterilization of surgical instruments and disinfection of surgical sites. These procedures greatly enhanced the chances of survival among patients suffering from a variety of ailments.

Finally, in the late nineteenth century, the German scientist Robert Koch clearly established the bacterial causes of many infections and the methodology involved in culturing and reproducing bacteria in laboratory settings. For his efforts, Koch received the Nobel Prize in 1905.

The work of these and other scientists had a tremendous impact on the treatment of diseases in the United States. Today, the presence of a multitude of microscopic organisms is an accepted fact. We know that the air we breathe, the food we eat, and our own body cavities are breeding grounds for a host of potential enemies, most of which are much too small to be seen.

Certain organisms, called *endogenous* microorganisms, normally live within the human host. For example, endogenous bacteria within the intestines aid in the digestion of nutrients and serve a variety of necessary functions. If you are in good health and your immune system is functioning properly, endogenous organisms are generally harmless. However, in sick people these organisms can overrun the body and cause serious health risks.

Exogenous microorganisms are those organisms that do not normally inhabit the body. When these microorganisms invade the body, infection and illness can result. Exogenous microorganisms are responsible for pneumonia, strep throat, sexually transmitted diseases, and other illnesses. How serious these afflictions become or whether a person actually "gets" a given disease depends on a variety of factors.

FACTORS CONTRIBUTING TO THE DISEASE PROCESS

The discovery of microscopic causes of diseases initially reinforced the single-cause theory of specific diseases. However, over the years it became obvious that there were other reasons to explain why one person became ill and even died while another remained unaffected. (See Figure 14.1.)

Today, there is a much greater appreciation for the role of multiple factors in the disease process. Before a disease can occur, the *host* must be susceptible, meaning

Germ Theory   A scientific theory that demonstrated the relationship between germs and disease development.

Pasteurization   Process in which foods are heated to near boiling point for approximately 30 minutes to kill bacteria.

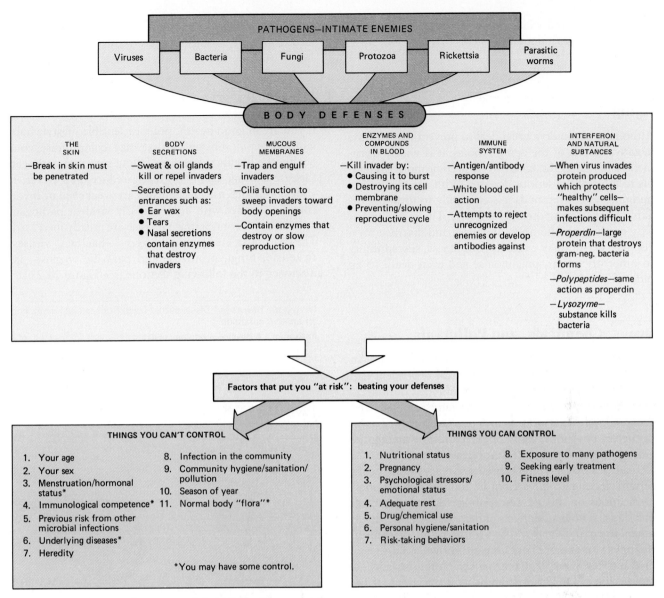

Figure 14.1 Factors that put you "at risk": beating your defenses.

that *resistance* levels must be suppressed, an *agent* capable of transmitting a disease must be present, and the *environment* must be hospitable to the organism. We talk about people having a number of *risk factors* that may make them more susceptible to a given ailment. People who are overweight or in poor physical condition, who smoke, or who experience a great deal of stress in their lives may have increased risks of succumbing to a variety of illnesses. Some of the most common risk factors are discussed above.

Heredity

In recent years, scientists studying the factors that contribute to longevity have theorized that the single greatest determinant of individual life expectancy is your par-

ents' life expectancy. Being born into a family with a history of atherosclerosis, breast cancer, or other heredity-related disorders may decrease your own life expectancy. Some people from families with a high incidence of diabetes mellitus may contract the disease even though they take precautions to avoid it. Still other diseases are caused by direct chromosomal inheritance. **Sickle-cell anemia**, a disease that primarily affects black people, is carried in the genes themselves. If both parents carry the trait, the likelihood of their child contracting the disease is even greater.

Scientific research has also focused on the possible inherited capacity of immune systems. It is believed that certain people may actually inherit immune systems that

Sickle-cell Anemia   Genetic disease commonly found among black people resulting in organ damage and premature death.

are susceptible to a wide variety of invasive organisms, while others inherit immune systems that are more resistant to disease.

Aging

Although we can do a great deal to prevent many of the negative effects of the aging process, it is widely documented that after the age of 40 we become more vulnerable to most of the serious diseases. With age, the body's immune system responds less efficiently to invading organisms, increasing the risk of illness. The same flu that may produce an afternoon of nausea and diarrhea for a younger person may cause days of illness, susceptibility to other organisms, pneumonia, and even death to an older person.

Drugs, Chemicals, and Pollutants

It is easy to document the negative effects of alcoholism and other forms of drug and chemical dependency in modern society. However, the costs of direct or indirect illnesses brought on by weakened immune responses and general bodily deterioration may pose even greater risks. Recurrent infections, colds, and hepatitis are among the more common drug-related problems.

One area that has largely been ignored is the impact of certain legitimate prescription and over-the-counter medications on disease susceptibility. Many medicines may cause serious side effects or increase susceptibility to other diseases. Diseases that are the result of medical treatment for another condition are known as **iatrogenic diseases.** For example, women given antibiotics such as tetracycline for relief of streptococcal infections of the throat often develop vaginal "yeast" infections as the tetracycline begins to work in other areas of the body. By increasing the acidity of the vaginal area, this antibiotic actually creates ideal conditions for bacterial yeasts to develop.

Environmental pollutants such as chemicals, particles, radioactive substances, or infectious pathogens may contaminate the air, water, soil, or food supply and make people who are exposed to them extremely ill (see Chapter 16).

Lifestyle

It is difficult to assess the impact of heredity, aging, drugs, and chemicals on individual disease susceptibility. The effects of these factors will vary according to a person's lifestyle. People who subject themselves to overwork, excessive stress, lack of sleep, inadequate exercise, poor nutrition, substance abuse, and other health risks significantly increase their chances for illness. Lifestyle is one of the greatest contributors to disease, and the rela-

tionship of lifestyle to total health will be covered throughout the various sections of this text.

▌ PATHOGENS

If you are in good health, practice sensible lifestyle habits, and avoid substances that may compromise your health, the likelihood of your falling prey to a **pathogen** (disease-causing agent) is greatly reduced. However, if your bodily-defense mechanisms are weakened or if you come in contact with a particularly virulent pathogen, your risks for contracting a disease are greatly increased. The six most common pathogens—bacteria, viruses, rickettsia, fungi, protozoa, and parasitic worms—are discussed in the following sections (see Figure 14.2).

Iatrogenic Diseases   Diseases that result from medical treatment for another condition.
Pathogen   A disease-producing organism.

Figure 14.2   This figure shows examples of the 6 major pathogens known to cause diseases in humans.

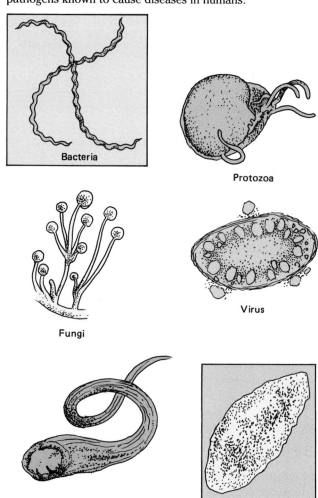

Bacteria

Bacteria are single-celled organisms that are plantlike in nature but lack *chlorophyll* (green coloring material). There are three major types of bacteria: cocci, bacilli, and spirilla. Bacteria may be viewed under a standard light microscope.

Although there are several thousand species of bacteria, only approximately 100 of these cause diseases in humans. Many bacteria cause disease by secreting poisonous substances called **toxins**. These toxins can be extremely powerful.

Bacterial infections can take many forms. The following are among the most common.

Staphylococcal Infections Perhaps one of the most common forms of bacterial infection is the staph infection. **Staphylococci** are normally present on our skin at all times and usually cause few problems. When there is a cut or break in the **epidermis**, or outer layer of the skin, the staphylococci may enter and cause a localized infection. If you have ever suffered from acne, boils, styes (infections of the eyelids), or infected wounds, you have had a staph infection.

At least one staph-caused disorder, **toxic shock syndrome**, can be fatal. Although most cases of toxic shock syndrome have occurred in menstruating women, the disease was first reported in 1978 in a group of children and continues to be reported in men, children, and non-menstruating women. Most cases that are not related to menstruation occur in patients recovering from wounds, surgery, and similar incidents. Although tampons are strongly implicated, the actual mechanisms that produce this disease remain uncertain.

To reduce the likelihood of contracting toxic shock syndrome, take the following precautions: (1) Avoid superabsorbent tampons except during the heaviest menstrual flow, (2) change tampons at least every 4 hours, and (3) use napkins at night instead of tampons. Call your doctor immediately if you have any of the following symptoms during menstruation: high fever, headache, vomiting, diarrhea, chills, stomach pains, or shocklike symptoms such as faintness, rapid pulse, or pallor (which can be caused by a drop in blood pressure), or a sunburnlike rash, particularly on fingers and toes.

Streptococcal Infections Another common form of bacterial infection is caused by microorganisms called **streptococci**. A "strep throat" (severe sore throat characterized by white or yellow pustules at the back of the throat) is the typical streptococcal problem. However, *scarlet fever* (an acute fever, sore throat, and rash) and *rheumatic fever* (said to "lick the joints and bite the heart") are also serious streptococal infections.

Pneumonia In the late nineteenth and early twentieth century, **pneumonia**, along with influenza, was the leading cause of death in the United States (see Chapter 1).

This disease is characterized by chronic cough, chest pain, chills, high fever, fluid accumulation, and eventual respiratory failure. One of the most common forms of pneumonia is caused by bacterial infections and responds readily to antibiotic treatment. However, pneumonia may also be caused by the presence of viruses, chemicals, or other substances in the lungs. In these cases, treatment may be more difficult. Although medical advances have reduced the incidence and severity of pneumonia, it remains the fifth leading cause of death in the United States.

Legionnaire's Disease. This bacterial disorder gained widespread publicity in 1976 at the American Legion convention in Philadelphia when several Legionnaires contracted the disease and died before the invading organism was isolated. Symptoms are similar to pneumonia, but identification is often difficult. Thus, among those people whose resistance may be lowered, particularly the elderly, this disorder often poses serious consequences if adequate treatment is not given. **Penicillin**, an antibiotic used to fight various bacterially caused ailments, was found to be ineffective as a treatment; erythromycin (Ilotycin) later proved effective.

Tuberculosis One of the leading killers in the early 1900s, **tuberculosis** (T.B.) was largely controlled in the United States until recently. Caused by bacterial infiltration of the respiratory system, this disease continues to be a serious problem in many regions of the world. Most school systems in the United States require potential staff to undergo tuberculosis screening. Universities typically require all students be screened for tuberculosis prior to enrollment. Unfortunately, in spite of all of our technological advances and screening procedures, T.B. threatens to become an epidemic disease once again unless drastic prevention methods are initiated. Poverty, overcrowding, poor sanitation and ventilation, ignorance, apathy, and a variety of other factors have contributed to an epidemic spread of T.B. In addition, persons suffering from immunological deficiencies, such as those caused by HIV diseases, appear to be particularly vulnerable. Public health professionals believe that without major changes in education and our social service system, tuberculosis will once again be a leading killer in the U.S.

Bacteria Single-celled organisms that may be disease-causing.

Toxins Poisonous substances produced by certain microorganisms and causing various diseases.

Staphylococci Round, gram-positive bacteria, usually found in clusters.

Epidermis The outermost layer of the skin.

Toxic Shock Syndrome A potentially life-threatening bacterial infection of the vagina.

Streptococci Round bacteria, usually found in chain formation.

Pneumonia Bacterially caused disease of the lungs.

Penicillin Antibiotic used to treat a variety of bacterially caused ailments.

Tuberculosis A bacterial disease caused by the infiltration of the respiratory system.

Periodontal Diseases Diseases of the teeth and gums, called **periodontal diseases,** affect 3 out of 4 adults after the age of 35. Improper tooth care, including lack of flossing, poor brushing, and absence of dental care, lead to increased bacterial growth, caries (decay), and gum infections. If left untreated, serious consequences, such as permanent tooth loss, can result.

Bacterial Contamination of Foods One of the common ailments associated with summer cookouts is **salmonellosis** (often called "food poisoning"). The typical victim is someone who has been munching on food left on picnic tables long after the meal has ended, especially on a hot summer day. This food has usually warmed to air temperature and is an ideal place for bacterial growth and toxin production. During the 6 to 8 hours after the food is consumed bacteria and resultant toxins multiply, causing severe nausea, stomach cramps, diarrhea, and fever. Mayonnaise, eggs, insufficiently cooked poultry, and certain forms of prepared meats and sausages are likely to harbor salmonella bacteria.

An even more lethal form of bacterial infection is caused by the **botulism** organism. These **anaerobic** organisms grow in air-free environments, particularly in improperly canned foods. Symptoms include nausea, dizziness, and weakness in the early stages, followed by central-nervous-system problems. Paralysis of the respiratory system often leads to death within 36 to 48 hours after ingestion of the botulism bacteria. How much botulism ingestion is too much? Because of the extremely virulent nature of this organism, just the mere act of sticking a finger in a can and licking it to see if it's "any good" may be enough to kill you. One pint of botulism toxin would theoretically be enough to kill everyone on earth! Although the toxin itself is broken down by boiling the canned food for a minimum of 10 minutes, there remains a potential risk for infection in spite of these precautions.

Even though we have made considerable progress in our war against bacterial infections, the battle is far from over. Bacterial strains have become increasingly resistant to antibiotics that were powerful weapons in past decades. Penicillin, the miracle drug of the 1940s, is often worthless against many of today's bacterial strains. Even more serious is the threat of the "new breed" of bacterially caused sexually transmitted diseases that appear to be resistant to modern drugs.

Viruses

Viruses are the smallest of the pathogens, being approximately 1/500th the size of bacteria. Because of their small size, they are visible only under an electron microscope and were identified in humans only in this century. Not until the 1960s were viruses effectively grown outside the body in tissue cultures.

At the present time over 150 viruses are known to cause diseases in humans. The role of viruses in the development of various cancers and chronic disease is still unclear. In fact, viruses themselves are perhaps the most unusual of the microorganisms that infect humans.

Essentially, a virus consists of a protein structure that contains the nucleic acids ribonucleic acid (RNA) or deoxyribonucleic acid (DNA). They have no capacity for carrying out the normal cell functions of respiration and metabolism. Some scientists even question whether or not viruses should be considered living organisms. Viruses cannot be grown and cannot reproduce on their own; rather, they must exist in a parasitic relationship with the cells they invade.

Once viruses attach themselves to host cells, they inject their own RNA and DNA, causing the host cells to begin reproducing new viruses. Once they take control of the cell, these new viruses overrun it until it fills to capacity and bursts, putting thousands of new viruses into circulation to begin the process all over again. This whole reproduction process may take as little as 20 seconds!

Because viruses cannot reproduce outside of living cells, they are particularly difficult to culture in a laboratory, making detection and study of the organism extremely time-consuming. Treatment is also difficult because many viruses withstand heat, formaldehyde, and large doses of radiation with little effect on their structure. In addition, some viruses may have an **incubation period** (the length of time required before symptoms of illness appear) measured in *years* rather than hours or days. Termed **slow viral infections,** these viruses in their semidormant state cause slowly developing illnesses. AIDS is the most recent deadly example of a slow-acting virus.

Drug treatment for viral infections is limited. Drugs that are powerful enough to kill viruses also kill the host cells. However, some drugs are available that block stages in viral reproduction and do not damage the host cells.

Another form of virus protection exists within our own bodies. When exposed to certain viruses, the body begins to produce a protein substance known as **interferon.** Although interferon does not destroy the invading microorganisms themselves, it sets up a protective mechanism to aid healthy cells in their struggle against the

---

Periodontal Diseases Disease of the tissue around the teeth.

Salmonellosis Form of bacterially caused food poisoning with symptoms of nausea, vomiting, and diarrhea.

Botulism An extremely virulent form of food poisoning caused by botulism bacteria or their toxins.

Anaerobic Able to live in the absence of free oxygen.

Viruses Minute parasite microbes that live inside another cell.

Incubation Period The time between exposure to a disease and the appearance of the symptoms.

Slow Viral Infections Viruses with long incubation periods and slowly progressive symptoms.

Interferon A protein substance produced by the body; aids the immune system by protecting healthy cells.

invaders. Although interferon offers a promising new area of antiviral activity, it should be noted that not all viruses stimulate interferon production.

Some of the most common viral infections are described in the following pages.

The Common Cold On an everyday basis, perhaps no ailment is as bothersome as the runny nose, itchy eyes, and generally uncomfortable feeling associated with the common cold. Cold-related symptoms are responsible for more days lost from work and more uncomfortable days spent at work than any other ailment.

Caused by any number of viruses (some experts claim there may be over 100 different viruses responsible for the common cold itself), colds are *endemic* (present to some degree) among people throughout the world. Current research indicates that otherwise healthy people carry cold viruses in their noses and throats most of the time. These viruses are held in check until a person's resistance is lowered. Thus, in the true sense of the word, it is possible to "catch" a cold from the airborne droplets of another person's sneeze or from skin-to-skin or mucous-membrane contact. In fact, recent studies indicate that the *hands* may be the greatest avenue of cold and other viral transmission. It should be obvious that covering your mouth with a tissue or handkerchief when sneezing is better than covering it with your bare hand, particularly if you next use your hand to touch food in a restaurant, shake your friend's hand, or open the door.

Although numerous theories exist as to how to "cure" the cold, including taking megadoses of vitamin C, there is little hard evidence to support any of them. The best rule of thumb is to keep your resistance level high. Also, avoiding people with newly developed colds (colds appear to be most contagious during the first 24 hours of onset) appears to be advisable. Once you contract a cold, bed rest, plenty of fluids, and aspirin for relief of pain and discomfort are the most "tried and true" remedies. Depending on the nature of the symptoms, several over-the-counter preparations have proven effective on a short-term basis.

Influenza Among otherwise healthy people, **influenza,** or "flu," is usually not serious. Its symptoms, including aches and pains, nausea, diarrhea, fever, and coldlike ailments, generally pass very quickly. However, in combination with other disorders, or among the elderly (people over the age of 65), those with respiratory or heart disease, and the very young (children under the age of 5), the flu can be very serious.

To date, three major varieties of flu virus have been isolated, with many different strains within each variety. The "A" form of the virus is generally the most virulent, followed by the "B" and "C" varieties. Although you may contract one form of the disease and develop immunity to it, this will not necessarily give you immunity to other forms of the disease. There is little that can be done to treat the flu once it has infected someone. Some vac-cines have proven effective against certain strains of flu virus, but they are totally ineffective against others. In spite of minor risks, it is recommended that people over the age of 65, pregnant women, people with heart disease, and those with other illnesses be vaccinated.

Infectious Mononucleosis An affliction particularly of college-aged students, **mononucleosis,** or "mono," is often jokingly referred to as the "kissing disease." The initial symptoms of this disorder include sore throat, fever, headache, nausea, chills, and a pervasive sense of weakness or tiredness. As the disease progresses, lymph nodes may become increasingly enlarged, and jaundice, spleen enlargement, aching joints, and body rashes may occur.

Theories on the causes and treatment of mononucleosis are highly controversial. Caused by the *Epstein-Barr virus,* mononucleosis is readily detected through a *monospot test,* a blood test that measures the percentage of specific forms of white blood cells. Because many viruses are caused by transmission of body fluids, many people once believed that young people passed the disease on by kissing. Although this is a possible cause, mononucleosis is not believed to be highly contagious. It does not appear to be easily contracted through normal everyday personal contact. Multiple cases among family members are rare, as are cases between intimate partners.

Treatment of mononucleosis is often a lengthy process that involves bed rest, balanced nutrition, and medications to control the symptoms of the disease. Gradually, the body develops a form of immunity to the disease and the person returns to normal activity levels. The danger of relapse from returning prematurely to classes, work, and other activities is very real. Also, medical authorities disagree over whether you can "catch" mononucleosis more than once. Recently, a growing number of health authorities have theorized that in some instances we may never actually get rid of the disease completely. Although symptoms may disappear, the disease itself may lie dormant until a person's resistance is down, at which time it may reappear.

Hepatitis One of the most highly publicized viral diseases is **hepatitis.** In some regions of the country and among certain segments of the populace, hepatitis has reached epidemic proportions. Massive educational programs aimed at prevention of this disease have been initiated in the hopes of preventing new outbreaks.

Hepatitis is generally defined as a virally caused inflammation of the liver, characterized by symptoms that include fever, headache, nausea, loss of appetite, skin rashes, pain in the upper right abdomen, dark-yellow

---

Influenza A common viral disorder of the respiratory tract.

Hepatitis One of four major virally caused diseases (types A, B, C, D) in which the liver becomes inflamed, producing symptoms including fever, headache, and jaundice.

Prevention and Treatment

Lyme Disease

Lyme disease is a bacterial tissue transmitted through the bite of a poppy-seed-sized tick. Like AIDS, it has spread rapidly in recent years, infecting large numbers of people. The disease was first identified in Lyme, Connecticut, in 1975 by the rheumatologist Dr. Allen Steere when he noticed unusual patterns of arthritis cases in the town. After ruling out possible environmental causes for the disease, researchers eventually identified the corkscrew-shaped organism called a *spirochete* (named *borrelia burgdorferi*) that was the cause of this disease. During the complex 2-year growth cycle of the disease, the spirochete infects the tick and resides on the tick's salivary glands. During this period, the tick lives on rodents such as the white-footed mouse and on deer. Once the tick attaches itself to a human, it generally takes 24 hours before the spirochete is transmitted through tick saliva. People infected with Lyme disease typically go through 3 distinct stages.

In stage 1, the spirochete spreads under the skin at the site of the bite. Between 2 and 30 days after the bite, 30 to 80 percent of those bitten display a characteristic "bull's-eye" rash near the area of the bite. Other symptoms vary dramatically and may include fever, flulike symptoms, and swelling of lymph nodes. If the rash remains untreated, it will eventually disappear, but the infection will remain, at which time the victim will enter stage 2 of the disease. In this phase, the spirochete may spread throughout the patient's blood or lymph fluids to various sites of the body, where small rashlike sores may develop. Severe headaches, mild neck

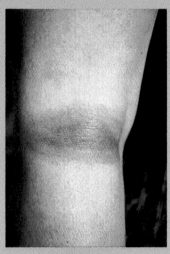

The "bull's-eye" rash characteristic of Lyme disease appears between 2 and 30 days after the tick bite.

stiffness, extreme fatigue, and possible neurological and cardiac abnormalities may occur. In addition, victims may experience brief attacks of arthritic pain in the knees and other joints. In the third and final stage, arthritic and neurological symptoms may become much more severe. Although fatalities from the disease are rare, the risks are increased for people with cardiovascular abnormalities, particularly for already ill patients.

The wide range of symptoms of Lyme disease makes diagnosis in the early stages difficult. In these early stages, antibiotics such as tetracycline and doxycycline are the common modes of treatment and are extremely effective in halting the

---

(with a brownish tinge) urine, and the possibility of *jaundice* ("the disease your friends diagnose" because of the yellowing of the whites of the eyes and the skin).

At the present time, four distinct forms of hepatitis have been isolated: *hepatitis A,* known as infectious hepatitis; *hepatitis B, non-A, non-B hepatitis;* and a newly discovered form of the disease called *hepatitis D.* Two additional forms of hepatitis are also under investigation.

Hepatitis A
Hepatitis A is the viral disease traditionally passed on throughout the world through the fecal-oral route. Historically labeled as "infectious" hepatitis, this form of the disease is the one that has become a

major sexually transmissible disorder because of exchanges of body fluids between infected persons. Any time there is poor sanitation, particularly with water contamination, this disease tends to surface. Day-care centers are possible high-risk areas because of poor hygiene of workers when changing infants, failure to wash hands, and other poor sanitary practices. The incubation period for this disease is 3 to 4 weeks, and its eventual symptoms include fever, malaise, nausea, abdominal discomfort, and eventual jaundice. Gammaglobulin injections given during the first 7 to 10 days after exposure may protect the victim. The problem with this disease is that it is often cyclical, and relapses are fairly common.

Prevention and Treatment (*Continued*)

disease. In later stages, treatment becomes more difficult, involving such methods as intravenous antibiotics for the bacteria and steroids for relief of inflammatory symptoms.

Despite an arsenal of effective treatments, the disease continues to escalate. Although it has primarily been concentrated in nine states (Minnesota, Wisconsin, Massachusetts, New Jersey, New York, Rhode Island, Pennsylvania, Connecticut, and California), cases have been reported in over 45 states.* The disease has also spread through parts of Europe since the early 1900s. Each summer, an increasing number of people and animals are infected by the disease.

Prevention of the problem appears to be the best method of control; however, many past efforts have been unsuccessful. Attempts to wipe out deer populations in high-infestation areas have resulted in the ticks' migrating to other mammal hosts. Attempts to reduce the mouse population, which is critical to the life cycle of the organism, have proven ineffective and possibly counterproductive. As the mouse population declined in treated areas, the ticks tended to migrate to the remaining mice (a single mouse may carry more than 40 ticks), resulting in a higher transmission rate of the disease.

The most plausible means of prevention appears to rest with individuals. If you are in a tick-infested area, observing the following list of preventive actions may significantly reduce your risk.

1. Provide your dogs and cats with tick collars. Routine checking of pets for ticks and prompt removal of ticks are essential. Also, keeping your pets out of your bed and off the furniture during tick season may help.

2. Teach small children to stay out of tall brush and grasses. They should also learn to check for "moving freckles." If a tick is found, remove it with tweezers by pulling straight back (not twisting). Never use matches or nail polish, which may cause the tick to "throw up" as it dies, increasing the risk of an infected wound.

3. If you must work outdoors, wear long pants and tuck the legs into high-top shoes or socks. Wear white or light colors and tightly woven fabrics that reduce your risk of exposure to ticks. Check often for ticks, particularly in good hiding places such as your genital area or scalp.

4. If you can't wear heavy clothes spray insect repellent on your skin or clothing. If you do cover up, spray permethrin (sold as Permanone) on your clothes, particularly on pants and socks.

5. If you do find a tick that is firmly lodged in your skin, seek medical help. Ask about what signs and symptoms to look for, and promptly start antibiotic therapy if symptoms begin.

* Oregon State Health Division, "Lyme Disease Update," *Communicable Disease Summary,* 42, no. 21 (July 15, 1990).

Hepatitis B

Another virally transmitted form of hepatitis is hepatitis B, or *serum hepatitis*. Traditionally, the hepatitis-B virus was passed on through blood transfusions or sharing of contaminated needles among addicts, with an incubation period averaging 60 to 90 days. Massive screening of blood for the hepatitis antibodies has virtually eliminated this form of transmission. However, isolated problems in hospitals still occur through inadvertent pricking of fingers by hospital staff. The hepatitis-B antigen has been found in nearly all body secretions, with blood, saliva, and semen being high risks for possible infection. Symptoms of hepatitis B are similar to, but more severe than, those associated with hepatitis A,

with potential high risk for liver damage. Treatment is also more difficult, with a more serious prognosis and increased potential for remission and relapse.

Non-A, non-B Hepatitis

This form of hepatitis, also called hepatitis C, has received considerable attention in recent years. Although the antigens found in this disease resemble the hepatitis-A and -B forms, they cannot be classified as either one. Symptoms are similar to the other forms of the disease, and treatment follows similar patterns. To date, this unidentified agent is believed to be responsible for more transmission of post-transfusion hepatitis than either the hepatitis-A or -B forms (accounting for over 90 percent of the cases).

There is growing concern over possible sexual transmission.

Hepatitis D

The newest form of this disease, hepatitis D, may have more serious health consequences than any other strain. Also known as *delta hepatitis,* this form can only infect people who have hepatitis B. It is most often spread through intimate contact with intravenous drug users, and symptoms indicate more severe reactions than with the other forms of the disease. Treatment of any of the forms of viral hepatitis is somewhat limited. A proper diet, bed rest, and antibiotics to resist bacterial invaders that might cause additional problems with resistance are recommended.

Vaccines for hepatitis are available, although they are very expensive and are not widely used. People at high risk for hepatitis B, including people who use injected drugs or who require regular blood transfusions, are most frequently recommended for vaccination. None of the vaccines appears to be effective against hepatitis D.

Mumps Prior to 1968, **mumps** was a common viral disorder among children. That year, scientists discovered an effective vaccine. The disease appeared to be largely under control, with reported cases declining from 80 per 100,000 people in 1968 to less than 2 reported cases per 100,000 people in 1984.* Failure to vaccinate has been responsible for increasing numbers of mumps cases in recent years, however.

Approximately one half of all mumps infections are inapparent, with only minor symptoms. Typically, there is an incubation period of 16 to 18 days, followed by symptoms of the virus lodging in the glands of the neck. The most common symptom is the swelling of the parotid (salivary) glands. One of the greatest dangers associated with mumps is the potential for sterility in men who contract the disease in young adulthood. Some victims may also suffer hearing loss.

Chicken Pox Caused by the *herpes zoster varicella* virus, **chicken pox** displays the characteristic symptoms of fever and tiredness, commonly 13 to 17 days after exposure, followed by skin eruptions that itch, blister, and produce a clear fluid. The virus is present in these blisters for approximately 1 week. Symptoms are generally mild, and immunity to subsequent infection appears to be lifelong. Because no vaccine is available, most children contract the disease. However, scientists believe that after the initial infection, the virus goes into permanent hybernation and, for most people, there are no further complications. For a small segment of the population, however, the zoster virus may become reactivated. Blisters will develop, usually on only one side of

the body, and usually stop abruptly at the midline. Cases in which the disease covers both sides of the body are far more serious. This disease, known as *shingles,* affects over 5 percent of the population each year. More than one half of those infected are over 50 years of age.

Measles Measles is a viral disorder that often affects young children. Symptoms, appearing about 10 days after exposure, include an itchy rash and a high fever. **German measles,** or *rubella,* is a milder viral infection that is believed to be transmitted by inhalation, after which it multiplies in the upper respiratory tract and passes into the bloodstream. It causes a rash, especially on the upper extremities, but is not a serious health threat and usually runs its course within 3 to 4 days. The major exceptions are among newborns and pregnant women. Rubella can damage the fetus, particularly during the first trimester, creating a condition known as *congenital rubella* in which the infant may be born blind, deaf, retarded, or with heart defects. Immunization has reduced the incidence of both measles and German measles. However, measles epidemics are occurring with increasing frequency in recent years. Infections in children not immunized against measles can lead to fever-induced problems such as rheumatic heart disease, kidney damage, and neurological disorders.

Rabies The **rabies** virus infects many warm-blooded animals. Bats are believed to be **asymptomatic** (symptomless) carriers. Their urine, which they spray when flying, contains the virus, and the air of densely populated bat caves may be dangerous to breathe. In most other hosts, the disease is extremely virulent and usually fatal. A characteristic behavior of rabid animals is the frenzied biting of other animals and people. Not only does this cause injury but it also spreads the virus through the infected animal's saliva. The most obvious symptoms of the disease are extreme cerebral excitement and rage, spasms in the pharynx (throat) muscles, especially at the sight of water, and the inability to drink water.

The incubation period for rabies is usually 1 to 3 months, yet documented cases range from 1 week to 1 year. The disease is almost always fatal if not treated immediately with the rabies vaccination.

Mumps A common viral disorder, most usually among children.

Chicken Pox A viral disease that infects most children, causing itchy skin and blistery skin eruptions.

Measles A viral disease that produces symptoms including an itchy rash and a high fever.

German Measles Termed "rubella"; a milder form of measles that causes a rash and mild fever in children and may cause damage to a fetus or a newborn baby.

Rabies A viral disease of the central nervous system often transmitted through animal bites.

Asymptomatic Without symptoms or symptom free.

---

* Centers for Disease Control, *Morbidity and Mortality Weekly,* April 30, 1990.

Rickettsia

Rickettsia were once believed to be closely related to viruses but are now considered to be a small form of bacteria. They produce toxins and multiply within small blood vessels, causing vascular blockage and tissue death. Rickettsia require an insect *vector* (carrier) for transmission to humans. Two common forms of human rickettsial disease include *Rocky Mountain spotted fever,* carried by the tick, and *typhus,* carried by the louse, flea, or tick. Both diseases can be life-threatening. They produce similar symptoms, including high fever, weakness, rash, and coma. A person does not actually have to be bitten by a vector to contract these diseases. Because the vectors themselves harbor the developing rickettsia in their intestinal tracts, insect excrement deposited on the skin which enters the body through abrasions and scratches may be a common source of infection.

Fungi

Hundreds of species of **fungi** inhabit our environment and serve useful functions. Moldy breads, cheeses, and mushrooms used for domestic purposes pose no harm to humans. However, some species of fungi can produce infections. *Candidiasis* (a vaginal yeast infection), athlete's foot, ringworm, and jock itch are examples of fungal diseases. Keeping the affected area clean and dry and treating it with appropriate medications will generally bring prompt relief from the majority of these infections.

Protozoa

Protozoa are microscopic, single-celled organisms that are generally associated with tropical diseases such as *African sleeping sickness* and *malaria.* Although these pathogens are prevalent in the developing countries of the world, they are largely controlled in the United States. The most common protozoal diseases in the United States are *trichomoniasis,* an infection discussed further in the sexually-transmitted-diseases section of this chapter, and *giardiasis,* a common parasite found in mountain streams in some regions of the United States.

Giardiasis is a protozoal infection caused by the organism *giardia enteritis,* which affects the small intestine. This disease is gaining worldwide attention as a major cause of diarrheal diseases. It is prevalent in some areas of the United States, particularly in mountain streams and polluted water supplies that are contaminated by either animal or human feces. The giardia enteritis cysts are ingested and hatch internally. Although the symptoms, including acute diarrhea, stomach cramps, fatigue, and weight loss, are not life-threatening, they are serious. Not everyone shows all of the symptoms. Victims of giardiasis can transmit the disease through their feces. Day-care centers that do not emphasize sanitation often harbor the disease. Prevention includes proper sanitation and hand-washing procedures. Drinking water can be kept free of these microorganisms through boiling, adding iodine tablets, or using a sophisticated water-purification system. Some people add a few drops of household bleach to their water about 20 minutes before drinking it, but this procedure must be carefully regulated. For people who have contracted giardiasis, prescription drugs are needed to rid the body of the protozoan.

Parasitic Worms

Parasitic worms are the largest of the pathogens. Ranging in size from the relatively small *pinworms,* typically found in children, to the relatively large *tapeworms,* found in all forms of warm-blooded animals, most parasitic worms are more of a nuisance than an actual threat. Of special note here are the new forms of worm infestations commonly associated with eating raw fish in Japanese sushi restaurants.

▌BODY DEFENSE MECHANISMS

Although all of the pathogens described in the preceding sections pose potential threats if they gain entry to the body (Figure 14.3 summarizes the stages of the course of a disease and recovery), the chances of this occurring are actually quite small. They must first overcome a number of effective barriers, many of which were established in the body prior to birth.

The Skin and Body Linings

The first of these barriers is the skin itself. In order to penetrate through the outer layer of skin, the pathogen must first survive the acidity of the skin, which normally destroys most forms of bacteria. Tears, saliva, and perspiration contain chemicals that kill bacteria. Even if the organism survives this initial line of defense, it must then find a route of entry through hair follicles, breaks in the skin due to injury, sweat glands, or normal body openings. Having gained initial entry, the pathogen must then escape the internal mucosa of the body linings. This mucosa is a constantly moving, sticky mass that traps organisms, much like flypaper. *Cilia,* tiny hairlike projections that move in a sweeping action toward body cavities, attempt to sweep offending microorganisms toward areas where they can be eliminated. Pathogens that survive these initial barriers reach the stomach,

---

Rickettsia Bacterialike organisms that live inside other living cells.

Fungi A group of plants that lack chlorophyll and do not produce flowers or seeds; several microscopic varieties are pathogenic.

Protozoa Microscopic single-celled organisms.

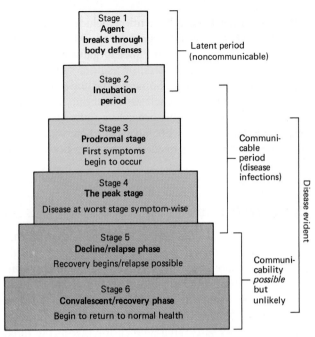

Figure 14.3 Stages of the course of a disease and recovery. Stages include the break in body defenses, incubation period, prodromal stage, peak stage, decline/relapse, and convalescent/recovery stages. Periods of likely communicability are indicated.

intestines, or other internal areas (depending on where they gained initial entry) and usually are destroyed. Those that are not destroyed by the body's first line of defense must then deal with an even more powerful additional line of defense.

Body Fluids/Cells

Whether threatened by an invading organism, a physical object (such as a sliver), or a chemical irritant, the body reacts in a similar way to defend itself. The blood supply to the area increases, bringing more oxygen-carrying red blood cells known as *erythrocytes* to the area. Specialized white blood cells known as *leukocytes* rush to the site of infection to fight the invading organism. Another type of white blood cell that is particularly effective in protecting the body, especially against bacterial infections, is the *phagocyte* ("cell that eats"). Phagocytes rush to an infected area, engulf the invaders, and digest them. This white-blood-cell activity is often signaled by pyogenic (pus-forming) buildup at the site of infection. In addition to cell activity, various enzymes and compounds in the blood itself can kill an infectious organism by causing it to break open, destroying its cell wall, or preventing it from multiplying.

Fever

If the infection is localized, pus formation, redness, swelling, and irritation often occur. These symptoms indicate that the invading organisms are being fought

systematically. Another indication is the development of a fever. (Normal body temperature is 98.6° F.) Fever is often caused by toxins secreted by the pathogens that interfere with the control of body temperature. Although this elevated temperature is often harmful to the body, it is also believed to act as a form of protection. Elevations of body temperature by even 1 or 2 degrees provide an environment that destroys some types of disease-causing organisms. Also, as body temperature rises, the body is stimulated to produce more white blood cells, which destroy more invaders.

Pain

Although often not considered an actual body defense mechanism, the role of pain in the body's response to invasion cannot be ignored. In a general sense, pain is a response to injury. Although pain may be caused by the direct stimulation of nerve endings in an affected area, it may also be *referred pain,* meaning that the pain can be present in a given place although the source may be elsewhere. An example of this is someone having a heart attack who experiences referred pain in the arm or jaw. Regardless of the cause of pain, most pain responses are accompanied by inflammation. Whatever its origin, pain is often the earliest sign that an injury has occurred. Usually, the pain response causes the person to slow down or stop the activity that was aggravating the injury, thereby protecting against further damage. Because it is often one of the first warnings that some form of disease is present, persistent pain should not be overlooked or masked with short-term pain relievers.

The Immune System

If all these systems are breached, the body turns to its most powerful line of defense, the immune system. **Immunity** is the state of being resistant to injury, particularly by toxic chemicals, foreign substances, or parasites. When the body is invaded by one of these agents, it responds by forming substances that harm or destroy the invaders. Substances that invade and cause an immune response are called **antigens**. The body recognizes both the size and the shape of an invading antigen and produces specific **antibodies** that work to destroy or lessen the effects of the antigen. Antibodies work only on the specific antigens that activate them. Flu antibodies work on flu antigens, measles antibodies work on measles antigens, and so on.

Regardless of the bodily reaction, the immune system generally is a powerful and effective ally in the effort to prevent disease. In each of the above instances, it is the

Immunity   State of being protected from infectious disease.

Antigens   Substances that invade and cause an immune response.

Antibodies   Substances produced by the body to lessen the effects of the antigen.

white blood cells that are the operative protecting agents. The **lymphocytes** are white blood cells found in the circulating blood, lymph nodes, bone marrow, and certain glands. Two forms of lymphocytes in particular, the *T-lymphocytes* and *B-lymphocytes,* are involved in the immune response.

T-lymphocytes circulate throughout the bloodstream and lymphatic system, neutralizing the effects of antigens. The *T-helper* or *T-suppressor* cells either enhance or suppress the immune response of other lymphocytes, aiding in the body's total defense system.

B-lymphocytes produce antibodies that are critical to our whole body defense system. Once stimulated by antigens, B-lymphocytes are converted to plasma cells that secrete *immunoglobulins,* the actual sources of antibody production. There are five major categories of immunoglobulins, the most important of which is immunoglobulin G (IgG).

Although white blood cells and the antigen-antibody response generally work in our favor by neutralizing or destroying harmful antigens, this is not always the case. Sometimes the body makes a mistake and targets its own tissue as the enemy, builds up antibodies against this tissue, and attempts to destroy it. When this occurs, an *autoimmune* (*auto* means "self") disease occurs. Common examples of this type of disease include *rheumatoid arthritis, lupus erythematosus,* and *myasthenia gravis.*

In some cases, the antigen-antibody response completely fails to function. The result is a form of *immune deficiency syndrome.* Perhaps the most dramatic example of this was demonstrated in 1984, with the death of the "bubble boy," a youngster who lived his life inside a protected environment because exposure to the outside world would have proved fatal. An even more frightening example of an immune system disorder is the epidemic of *acquired immune deficiency syndrome* (AIDS), which will be discussed in another section of this chapter.

Hypersensitivity Reactions   More common are those immune responses known as **hypersensitivity reactions,** or allergies. Although hypersensitivity reactions are not communicable by nature, they are disorders that involve the immune system. *Allergic* reactions result from contact with an external, usually harmless *allergen.* Common allergens include pollen, dusts, molds, animal dander, cosmetics, metals, poison oak, poison ivy, and certain foods. Some people may be allergic to a majority of the foods they eat and the chemicals with which they are in constant contact.

The incidence of allergy is estimated to be 10 to 20 percent in the general population. There is often a family tendency toward it, suggesting a hereditary defect in the immune system passed on through generations. Examples of hypersensitivity (allergic) reactions include hay fever, hives, and bronchial asthma (see Chapter 19). However, a more common allergic disorder may include a rash, headache, runny nose, or diarrhea of undetermined cause.

Each of these defense mechanisms may be considered to be part of our natural immune system. To varying degrees, this natural defense mechanism is our strongest ally in the battle against disease, being with us from birth until death. There are periods in our life when the invading organisms are too strong or our own natural immunity is too weak to protect us from "catching" a given disease. It is at that time that we need outside assistance in developing immunity to an invading organism. This assistance generally is given in the form of a **vaccination,** which consists of killed or weakened organisms, given orally or by injection. This form of artificial immunity is termed **acquired immunity,** as distinct from **natural immunity.**

Vaccines: Living versus Nonliving

In response to a deadly polio epidemic of the 1950s, scientists produced two major vaccines. The first of these, developed by Jonas Salk in 1954, contained killed organisms that stimulated antibody production against poliomyelitis (polio). People given this vaccination did not actually develop the disease, but, because they exposed themselves to the organism, their own bodies were able to produce antibodies to protect against later exposure to living polio organisms. Although the Salk vaccine was tremendously effective, the oral vaccine developed a few years later by Albert Sabin, which consisted of weakened (attenuated) polio organisms produced in the laboratory, provided an even more powerful means of stimulating antibody production. Some pathogens, such as tetanus, cause disease, through the toxins they produce. By modifying these toxins, *toxoids* can be formed that also stimulate antibody production and thereby prevent disease.

Today, depending on the virulence of the organism, vaccines containing live, weakened, or dead organisms are given to people for a variety of diseases. In some instances, if a person is already weakened by other diseases, giving a vaccination may provoke an actual case of the disease. This was what happened with the smallpox vaccinations that were given routinely in the 1960s. It was believed that the risk of contracting smallpox from the vaccine was actually greater than was the chance of getting the disease in an environment where it had essentially been eradicated. For this reason, routine smallpox inoculations were eliminated in the late 1960s.

See Table 14.1 for recommended immunization schedules for 7 infectious diseases.

Lymphocytes   White blood cells that aid in the antigen-antibody response.

Hypersensitivity Reactions (Allergies)   Immune reactions caused by usually harmless substances called allergens.

Vaccination   Inoculation with killed or weakened pathogens in order to prevent or lessen the effect of some disease.

Acquired Immunity   Immunity developed in response to disease, vaccination, or exposure.

Natural Immunity   Immunity conferred at birth from the mother.

Table 14.1   Immunization Schedule for Common Infectious Diseases

Age Group	Disease	Type of Immunization	Duration of Protection
6 weeks to 1 year	Diphtheria, tetanus, pertussis (DTP)	4 primary doses given 4 or more weeks apart	10 years
4 to 6 years	DTP	Booster (prior to school)	10 years
14 to 16 years and adults	Tetanus and diphtheria	Booster every 10 years or sooner if exposed	10 years
6 weeks to 2 months	Polio	1st dose (live virus) may be given with DTP	Permanent (once series is complete)
4 months	Polio	2nd dose (live virus)	
6 months	Polio	Optional (killed virus)	
18 months	Polio	3rd dose (killed virus)	
4 to 6 years	Polio	4th dose (killed virus, prior to school)	
15 months	Measles, rubella, mumps	Combined vaccines commonly given	Permanent

Active and Passive Immunity

If you are exposed to an organism, either during your day-to-day life or through vaccination, you will eventually develop an *active acquired immunity* to that organism. Your body will produce its own antibodies, and, in most cases, you will not have to worry about subsequent exposures to the disease.

In some cases, however, the risks of contracting a disease are so severe that you may not be able to wait the days or weeks that are necessary for your own body to produce antibodies. Also, in the situation where a person's resistance is terribly weakened as a result of cancer chemotherapy or for other reasons, the body may be unable to produce its own antibodies. When either of these situations occurs and a victim is in need of immediate aid, antibodies formed in another person or animal are often given. Termed *passive immunity,* this type of immunity is often short-lived but provides the necessary boost for a person to get through a potentially critical period. Antibodies utilized for passive immunity are taken from *gammaglobulins,* proteins synthesized from a donor's blood. A mother also confers passive immunity on her newborn baby through breast-feeding.

SEXUALLY TRANSMITTED DISEASES

Scientists in the last few decades have made great strides in the treatment of communicable diseases. For the most part, we have changed from a country besieged with the communicable diseases of childhood to one of chronic, degenerative diseases typically associated with adulthood or later life.

However, there is still one area of communicable disease that is currently reaching epidemic proportions. The majority of these communicable diseases are sexually transmitted and pose a growing threat among all age groups. The fear of contracting a sexually transmitted disease has had an irrefutable impact on the sexual mores and behaviors of adults over the last decade.

It is estimated that over 10 million people in the United States every year are afflicted with 1 or more of the over 20 different types of **sexually transmitted diseases (STDs)**. Whereas sexually transmitted diseases were once referred to as *venereal diseases,* this newer classification is believed to be broader in scope and more reflective of the number and types of these diseases. STDs are at least 4 times more prevalent than arthritis or respiratory diseases and 10 times more prevalent than heart disease or diabetes. Moreover, at the present rate, the incidence of STDs is expected to double by the year 2000, with more virulent and untreatable strains appearing regularly.

For many victims, symptoms are not serious and range from mild discomfort to annoying itching or discharge. Other less fortunate victims can suffer sterility, blindness, central-nervous-system destruction, disfigurement, and death. Infants born to mothers carrying the organisms for these diseases are at risk for blindness, mental retardation, and death.

Education, responsible action, and prompt treatment when symptoms do occur could do much to reduce the severity of these diseases. Before we can make significant strides in these areas, we must first look at the reasons for the current epidemic of STDs.

Sexually Transmitted Diseases (STD)   Infectious diseases transmitted as a result of some form of intimate, usually sexual, contact.

Possible Causes: Why Me?

Sexually transmitted diseases affect people of both sexes and from all socioeconomic levels, ages, ethnic groups, and regions of the world. Several reasons have been proposed to explain the high rates of STDs. Embarrassment, fear of discovery, or related concerns keep infected people from seeking treatment. Often, these same people fail to accept the seriousness of their problem and continue to remain sexually active, thereby infecting unsuspecting partners.

Another possible reason for this epidemic is our casual attitude toward sex. Bombarded by media hype that glamorizes sexuality, many people become sexually active without considering the consequences. Generally, the more sexual partners a person has, the greater the risk for contracting an STD.

Lack of knowledge, chemical interference, a casual attitude toward responsible sex, and the stresses, strains, and loneliness of everyday life may be significant reasons for the epidemic of STDs in modern society. Another problem is that an infected person may remain asymptomatic and thus be totally unaware that an infection exists. The infected person may unknowingly spread the disease to an unsuspecting partner, who may then ignore or misinterpret the symptoms. By the time either partner seeks medical help, he or she may have infected several others.

Mode of Transmission

Sexually transmitted diseases are generally spread through some form of intimate sexual contact. Sexual intercourse, oral-genital contact, hand-genital contact, and anal intercourse tend to be the most common modes of transmission (means of spreading the disease). In rare instances, pathogens for STDs may also be spread through the mouth or, even more infrequently, through contact with fluids from body sores. STD pathogens prefer the dark, moist body surfaces, especially the mucous membranes lining the reproductive organs. The majority of these organisms are susceptible to light, excess heat, cold, and dryness, and many die quickly on exposure to air. (The toilet seat is *not* a likely breeding ground!)

Characteristics of STDs

To date, there are no vaccinations that effectively prevent STDs. You may get a disease again and again, and you may have several diseases at the same time. As with other communicable diseases, your relative health at the time of contact is an important factor in the likelihood of contracting one of the diseases.

Although all STDs have unique characteristics, they have several things in common with other types of communicable diseases. First, each STD is caused by a specific pathogen. Pathogens for STDs include viruses, bacteria, fungi, and insects, most of which are not visible to the naked eye.

Second, each STD pathogen must have an appropriate environment in which to receive nourishment and grow. From this safe haven, the pathogen must have a means of escaping and being passed on to another person. Like other communicable diseases, STDs have both pathogen-specific incubation periods and periods of time during which transmission is most likely, called *periods of communicability*.

Although there are over 20 different types of sexually transmitted diseases, only those STDs that are most likely to pose a risk for the average adult will be discussed here.

Chlamydia

Often referred to as the "silent epidemic," **chlamydia** is now the most common STD among heterosexual white Americans. The name is derived from the Greek verb *chlamys*, meaning "to cloak," because, unlike most bacteria, chlamydia can only live and grow inside other cells. The Centers for Disease Control in Atlanta, Georgia, estimates that over 3 million Americans have chlamydia, with between 3 million and 10 million new cases occurring every year.

Although many people classify chlamydia as *nonspecific* or *nongonococcal urethritis* (NGU), a person may have NGU without having the organism for chlamydia. In over half of the cases of NGU (infections of the urethra and surrounding tissues that are not caused by gonococcal bacteria), however, *chlamydia trachomatis*, the bacterial organism for chlamydia, is present. For this reason, the two disease terms are often used interchangeably, even though NGU may be caused by other organisms.

The seriousness of the growing epidemic of chlamydia infections cannot be ignored. At present, chlamydia affects 5 times as many people as gonorrhea and 10 times as many people as syphilis. It affects over 10 percent of all college students and is more prevalent than genital herpes and trichomoniasis. What is chlamydia? What are its symptoms? What are the risks?

In males, early symptoms include painful and difficult urination, frequent urination, and a watery puslike discharge from the penis. Symptoms in females include a yellowish discharge, spotting between periods, and occasional spotting after intercourse. Unfortunately, many chlamydia victims display no symptoms and therefore do not seek help until the disease has done secondary damage. Females especially tend to be asymptomatic; over 70 percent do not realize they have the disease until secondary damage has occurred.

Secondary damage resulting from chlamydia is serious for both sexes. Male victims can suffer damage to the

---

Chlamydia Bacterially caused STD of the urogenital tract.

prostate gland, seminal vesicles, and Cowper's glands, as well as arthritislike symptoms and damage to the blood vessels and heart. In females, secondary damage from chlamydia may include inflammation that damages the cervix or fallopian tubes, causing sterility, or damage to the inner pelvic structure, leading to **pelvic inflammatory disease (PID)**, an acute inflammation of the peritoneum (lining) of the abdominopelvic cavity. Severe pain in the lower abdominal cavity, menstrual irregularities, fever, recurring infections, ectopic pregnancy (see Chapter 7), premature need for hysterectomy, and severe depression are just a few of the problems associated with PID. If a woman does become pregnant, her risk for spontaneous abortion and stillbirth increases dramatically. Chlamydia may also be responsible for one type of **conjunctivitis**, an eye infection that affects not only adults but also infants, who can contract the disease from an infected mother during delivery. Untreated conjunctivitis can cause blindness.

Chlamydia can be controlled through responsible sexual behavior and familiarity with the early symptoms of the disease. If detected early enough, the disease itself is readily treatable in 2 to 3 weeks with antibiotics such as tetracycline, doxycycline, or erythromycin. Unfortunately, because so many victims display no symptoms, the disease is often passed on from partner to partner before treatment is effected.

The chlamydia organism is also difficult to diagnose because it can only live and grow inside other cells, a characteristic that, although common in viruses, is not common in bacteria. For this reason, chlamydia is difficult to culture and identify. The cost of testing, coupled with historically inadequate research funding, makes it difficult for doctors and lab technicians to screen patients effectively on a "walk-in" basis. A new diagnostic technique, known as the *microtrak* test, in which the physician swabs the cervix in females or the urethra in males to remove a specimen, has had promising results. Unlike previous tests, the microtrak is able to detect dead organisms. Several new diagnostic techniques are currently being evaluated. These techniques, along with a strong dose of public awareness, may be the necessary steps in the effective control of this disease.

Gonorrhea

Whether you call it "clap," "drip," or anything else, the disease caused by the *Niesseria gonorrhoeae* bacterium is technically referred to as **gonorrhea**. In spite of our vast technology, and in spite of massive education and research efforts, this disease is one of the most prevalent STDs in the United States. In males, the typical symptom is a white milky discharge from the penis, along with painful, burning urination 2 to 9 days after contact. This is enough to send most men to their physician for a heavy dose of antibiotics. Only about 20 percent of all males are asymptomatic for the disease.

In females, the situation is just the opposite. Only about 20 percent of all females experience any form of discharge, and few develop the burning sensation upon urinating until much later in the disease (if ever). The organism can remain in the woman's vagina, cervix, uterus, or fallopian tubes for long periods with no apparent symptoms, except for an occasional slight fever. The woman in this instance is totally unaware that she has been infected and that she may be infecting her sexual partners.

Diagnosis of gonorrhea is done by obtaining a sample of discharge (if present) or through examination of cervical fluids. This sample is cultured, and, after approximately 2 days of incubation, a definitive test is conducted to identify the organism. Antibiotic regimens utilizing penicillin, tetracycline, or other drugs are administered. In some instances, a penicillin-resistant form of gonorrhea may require a particularly strong combination of antibiotic treatments. Treatment is generally completely effective within a short period of time, usually with few problems. This is contingent, however, on early detection of the disease.

Among women, if the disease goes undetected it can spread throughout the genital-urinary tract to the fallopian tubes and ovaries, causing sterility. At the very least, many women end up with severe inflammation and pelvic inflammatory disease symptoms. In the event that an infected woman becomes pregnant, the disease can cause conjunctivitis in her infant. To prevent this, physicians routinely administer silver nitrate or penicillin preparations to the eyes of newborn babies.

Untreated gonorrhea in the male may spread to the prostate, testicles, urinary tract, kidney, and bladder. Blockage of the vas deferens due to scar-tissue formation may cause sterility. In some cases, the penis develops a painful curvature during erection.

Syphilis

Syphilis, the other "well-known" sexually transmitted disease, is also caused by a bacterial organism, the *spirochete* known as *Treponema pallidum*. Because it is extremely delicate and dies readily upon exposure to air, dryness, or cold, this organism is generally transferred through direct sexual contact. Although this typically means contact between sexual organs during intercourse, the organism may, in rare instances, enter the body through a break in the skin, through kissing, or through other transmissions of body fluids.

Pelvic Inflammatory Disease (PID) Infection of the female reproductive tract.
Conjunctivitis Serious inflammation of the eye, caused by any number of pathogens or irritants; can be caused by STDs such as chlamydia.
Gonorrhea Second most common STD in the United States; if untreated, may cause sterility.
Syphilis One of the most widespread STDs; characterized by distinct phases and potentially serious results.

Syphilis is called the "great imitator" because its symptoms resemble those of other diseases. Only an astute physician who has reason to suspect the presence of the disease will order the appropriate tests for a diagnosis. What are the symptoms of this disease? Unlike most of the other STDs, syphilis generally progresses through several distinct stages.

Primary Syphilis The first stage of syphilis, particularly for males, is often characterized by the development of a painless sore known as a **chancre** (pronounced "shank-er"), located most often at the site of the initial infection, such as the penis, vaginal walls, or mouth. This chancre, often about the size of a dime, is oozing with bacteria, ready to be spread to an unsuspecting partner. Usually it appears 3 to 4 weeks after contact. Because the chancre may not be readily apparent, the likelihood of detection is not great. In both males and females, the chancre will completely disappear in 3 to 6 weeks.

Secondary Syphilis From a month to a year after the chancre disappears, secondary symptoms may appear, including a rash or white patches on the skin or on the mucous membranes of the mouth, throat, or genitals. Hair loss may occur, lymph nodes may become enlarged, and the victim may run a slight fever or develop a headache. In rare cases, infectious sores develop around the mouth or genitals. Because symptoms vary so much among individuals, or because any symptoms that do appear are so far removed from previous sexual experience that the victim seldom connects the two, the disease often does its damage over a few weeks or months and then goes into hiding, only to surface at a much later stage.

Latent Syphilis Although the spirochetes appear to be hiding, they actually begin to invade body organs after the secondary stage. There may be occasional periodic recurrences of previous symptoms, including the presence of infectious lesions for between 2 and 4 years after the secondary period. After this period, the disease is rarely transmitted to others, except during pregnancy, when it can be transmitted to the fetus. The child in this situation may be born with *congenital syphilis,* which can cause death or birth defects such as blindness, deafness, or disfigurement. In most cases, the fetus does not become infected until after the first trimester. Thus, treatment of the mother during this period will usually prevent infection of the fetus. In some instances, however, a child born to an infected mother will show no apparent signs of the disease at birth but, within several weeks, will develop body rashes, a runny nose, and symptoms of paralysis.

In some cases, however, the child's immune system will ward off the invading organism, and further symptoms may not surface until the teenage years. Fortunately, most states protect the unborn by requiring pro-spective marriage partners to be tested for syphilis prior to obtaining a marriage license.

In addition to causing congenital syphilis, latent syphilis, if untreated, will continue to progress, infecting more and more organs and leading to the final stage, late syphilis.

Late Syphilis Most horror stories concerning syphilis involve the late stages of the disease. Years after syphilis has entered the body and progressed through the various organs, its net effects become clearly evident. Late-stage syphilis indications may include heart damage, central-nervous-system damage, blindness, deafness, paralysis, premature senility, and ultimately insanity.

Treatment Treatment for syphilis resembles that for gonorrhea. Because the organism is bacterial, it is treated with antibiotics, usually penicillin. Blood tests are used to determine the exact nature of the invading organism, and the doses of antibiotics are much stronger than those given to a typical gonorrhea patient. The major obstacle in treatment is the fact that many physicians initially misdiagnose this "imitator." In 1987, the numbers of reported cases of syphilis in the United States showed an increase.

Venereal Warts

Venereal warts, also known as genital warts or **condylomas,** are caused by a small group of viruses known as *human papilloma viruses (HPV).* A person becomes infected when an HPV penetrates the skin and mucous membranes of the genitals or anus through sexual contact. The virus appears to be relatively easy to catch. Over half of all people with venereal warts catch them from exposure to partners' warts. Typical incubation periods range from 6 to 8 weeks after contact. Many people have no apparent symptoms, particularly if the warts are located inside the reproductive tract. Others may develop a series of small itchy bumps on the genitals, which may range in size from that of a small pinhead to large cauliflowerlike growths that can obstruct normal urinary or reproductive activity. On dry skin (such as on the shaft of the penis), the warts commonly are small, hard, and yellowish gray, resembling warts that appear on other parts of the body.

Typically, these warts are of two different types: (1) *full-blown genital warts* that are noticeable as tiny bumps or growths, and (2) the much more prevalent *flat*

Chancre Sore often found at the site of syphilis infection.
Venereal Warts (Condylomas *or* Genital Warts) STD caused by HPV viruses and characterized by itchy bumps of varying size on the genitals.

Communication

Communicating with Sexual Partners: Reducing Your Risks

The enormous rise in sexually transmitted diseases (STDs) has made it imperative to do everything possible to reduce your risks of infection. Although it is impossible to predict the risk you might take when having intimate relations with another person, there are things that you can do to protect yourself. Use of latex condoms significantly reduces your risk. Knowing what you are getting yourself into *before* you choose to have sexual relations is another key factor in individual risk reduction. Although talking about sex may be more difficult than actually having sex, careful planning and asking the right questions are important first steps. Before beginning a sexual relationship, you should consider the following.

1. *Be direct, honest, and determined in talking about sex before you become involved.* Do not act silly or evasive. Get to the point, ask clear questions, and do not be put off in getting a response. (Remember, a person who does not care enough to talk about sex probably does not care enough to take responsibility for his or her actions.) A good way to start might be by saying, "I'm really concerned about all of the

talk about AIDS and other sexually transmitted diseases. I've been reading about 'safer' sex and how important it is. I'd like to know how you feel. Can we talk about it?" By being direct early in your interaction, you may avoid possible discomfort later. Think about what you are going to say early on, and try to find the best possible way to broach the subject.

2. *Encourage your partner to be honest and share feelings.* This does not happen overnight. If you have never had a serious conversation with your partner before you get into an intimate situation, you cannot expect that you will be comfortable when the lights go off. Setting the stage for a blameless, suspicion-free environment, in which both people feel comfortable, will do a great deal to ease tensions later.

3. *Analyze your own beliefs and values ahead of time.* The worst thing you can do is get yourself into an awkward situation where you have not had time to think about what is important to you and what you believe in. Merely "going with the flow" is inappropriate for a responsible

---

warts that are not usually visible to the naked eye. In females, these flat warts are often first detected by a physician during a routine Pap test. Abnormal Pap re-

Venereal warts have become a growing threat to sexually active people.

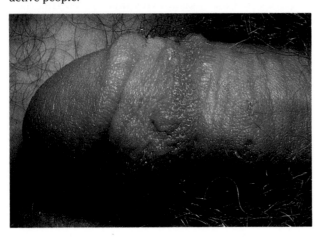

sults may prompt the physician to perform a *colposcopy*. In this procedure, a vinegarlike solution is applied to the insides of the vaginal walls and cervix to bleach potential warts, and the area is then viewed through a special magnifying instrument known as a colposcope. A relatively new photographic procedure known as a *cerviscope* is being used in some clinics to detect venereal warts. During a cerviscope, vinegar is applied to the vaginal and cervical areas, and an image of the area is projected on a screen for a specialist to diagnose. This technique is relatively inexpensive and is believed to be five times more sensitive than standard colposcopy. An even newer method that is being used at medical research centers throughout the United States is the *DNA probe*, a technique that identifies the genetic makeup of possible warts.

Whereas women must see a physician for a diagnosis, males can check for suspicious lesions by wrapping their penis in vinegar-soaked gauze or cloth, waiting for 5 minutes, and checking for white bleached areas indica-

Communication (*Continued*)

adult. Know where you will draw the line on certain actions, and be very clear with your partner about what you expect. If you believe that using a condom is necessary, make sure you communicate this to your partner. Also, decide what you will do if your partner does not agree with you. For example, if you are a female you might say, "I think that safer sex is necessary. If you do not have a condom, I have one with me, and I would like you to use it." If you are a male, you might say, "I have a condom with me, and I believe that it is important to practice safer sex."

4. *Ask questions about past history.* Although it may seem as though you are prying into another person's business, it is essential that you know basic information about your partner's past. An idea of your partner's past sexual involvements and use of intravenous (IV) drugs is very important. Again, it is important to let your partner know why you are concerned and that you are not asking out of jealousy or other ulterior motives. You might ask some of the following types of questions for

starters: "Have you been seriously involved with anyone in the last few months? Do you think that there is any chance that any of your past sexual partners were using IV drugs? Have you ever used IV drugs? Do you think that your past involvements may have exposed you to AIDS or other sexually transmitted diseases?" Although there are no easy ways of asking such intimate questions, the environment that is created early in your relationship will help govern the nature and direction of such questions.

5. *Ask about the importance of monogamy in your partner's relationships.* An important question to ask before becoming involved in a regular sexual relationship relates to the degree of importance that the person places on a committed relationship. People who "sleep around" or use drugs and alcohol heavily may be bad risks in terms of STDs. You will need to decide early about the relationship's importance to you and how much you are willing to work at coming to an acceptable compromise in terms of lifestyle.

---

tive of flat warts. Venereal warts of the rectum must be diagnosed by a physician.

Risks of Venereal Warts   Many venereal warts will eventually disappear on their own. Others will grow and generate unsightly flaps of irregular flesh on the external genitalia. Although these flaps may be a source of embarrassment, they typically do not cause serious problems unless they grow large enough to obstruct urinary flow or become irritated by clothing or sexual intercourse.

The greatest threat from venereal warts may lie in the apparent relationship between these warts and a tendency to *dysplasia,* or changes in cells that may lead to a precancerous condition. Exactly how HPV infection leads to cervical cancer is uncertain. What is known is that within 5 years after infection, 30 percent of all HPV cases will progress to the precancerous stages. Of those that become precancerous and are left untreated, 70 percent will eventually lead to actual malignancy. In addition, venereal warts may pose a threat to a pregnant

woman's unborn fetus if the fetus is exposed to the virus during birth. Cesarean deliveries may be considered in serious cases.

Treatment   Treatment for venereal warts may take several forms.

1. Warts are painted with a medication called *podophyllin* during one or more weekly doctor's visits. This substance is washed off after about 4 hours, and a few days later the warts begin to dry up and fall off. This procedure is relatively painless, but there are potential side effects. Because podophyllin may be absorbed through the skin, pregnant women should not use it. Some patients may experience skin reactions.

2. Warts may be removed by *cryosurgery,* a procedure in which an instrument treated with liquid nitrogen is held to the affected area, "freezing" the tissue. Within a few days, the warts fall off.

3. Depending on size and location, some warts are removed by simple excision.

4. For larger warts, *laser surgery* is often used. This is a major procedure that often requires general anesthesia. The safety of laser use for wart removal is currently being questioned by many health experts. (Precautions must be used to shield medical staff from infection by viral spray during the treatment.)

5. Creams containing *5-Fluoracil* (an anticancer drug) are being used to prevent further precancerous cell development.

6. For warts located externally, injections of *interferon* are sometimes given to keep the virus from spreading to healthy tissue. Although this treatment shows promise, it is expensive and, in large doses, may cause flulike symptoms.

Although treatment methods are available, prevention clearly is a better approach. Fortunately, what is true about protecting yourself from AIDS holds true for protecting yourself from genital warts and other STDs (see the section on AIDS prevention in this chapter).

Candidiasis (Moniliasis)

Unlike many of the other sexually transmitted diseases, the yeastlike fungus caused by the *candida albicans* organism normally inhabits the vaginal tract in most women. Only under certain conditions will these organisms multiply to abnormal quantities and begin to cause problems for the infected person. What are these conditions? What can prevent their occurrence?

The likelihood of **candidiasis** (also known as *moniliasis*) is greatest if a person has diabetes, if the immune system is overtaxed or malfunctioning, if a woman is taking birth-control pills or other hormones, or if the person is taking broad-spectrum antibiotics. Any of the above factors may decrease the acidity of the vagina, making conditions more favorable for a yeastlike infection.

Symptoms of candidiasis include severe vaginal itching, a white cheesy discharge, swelling of the vaginal tissue due to irritation, and a burning sensation. These symptoms are often collectively called **vaginitis.** When this microbe infects the mouth, whitish patches form, and the condition is referred to as *thrush.* This monilial infection also occurs in males and is easily transmitted between sexual partners.

Candidiasis strikes at least 500,000 Americans a year. Antifungal drugs applied on the surface or by suppository usually cure the disease in just a few days. For approximately 1 out of 10 women, nothing seems to work, and the organism returns again and again. In patients with this form of the chronic recurrent infection, symptoms are often aggravated by contact of the vagina

with soaps, douches, perfumed toilet paper, chlorinated water, and spermicides. Tight-fitting jeans and pantyhose can provide the moisture and irritant necessary for continued growth of the organism.

Herpes

Herpes is a general term for a family of diseases characterized by sores or eruptions on the skin. Herpes infections range from mildly uncomfortable to extremely serious. One subcategory, *herpes simplex,* is caused by a virus. Herpes simplex virus type 1 (HSV-1) causes the cold sores and fever blisters that have afflicted so many of us.

Genital herpes, caused by herpes simplex virus type 2, is believed to be one of the most widespread STDs in the world. Thousands of new cases are being discovered every year, and there is little treatment available. What are the symptoms? How does HSV-2 differ from HSV-1? Are there any effective treatments?

Typically, genital herpes is characterized by distinct phases. First, the herpes virus must gain entrance to the body, usually through the mucous membranes of the genital area. Once these organisms invade, the victim will experience the prodromal phase, characterized by a sensation of burning and redness at the site of the infection. This phase is typically followed by the formation of a small blister filled with a clear fluid containing the virus. Picking at this blister or spreading this clear fluid by the hands can autoinoculate other body parts. This is particularly dangerous if the eyes are involved, as blindness may result.

Over a period of days, this blister will crust, dry, and disappear, and the virus will travel to the base of an affected nerve supplying the area and become dormant. Only when the victim becomes overly stressed, when diet is inadequate, when the immune system is overworked, or when there is excessive exposure to sunlight or other stressors will the virus reactivate (at the same site every time) and begin the blistering cycle all over again. This cyclical recurrence can be painful, unsightly, and, most importantly, highly contagious. Fluids from these blisters may readily be transmitted to sexual partners. Through oral sex, herpes simplex type 2 may be transmitted to the mouth. Symptoms are similar to those of herpes simplex type 1.

Genital herpes is especially dangerous for the pregnant female. Because of the danger of infecting the baby as it passes through the vagina during birth, many physicians will recommend cesarean deliveries for infected

---

Candidiasis (Moniliasis) Yeastlike fungal disease often transmitted sexually.

Vaginitis Set of symptoms characterized by vaginal itching, swelling, and burning.

Genital Herpes STD caused by herpes simplex virus type 2.

women. Additionally, women who have a history of genital herpes also appear to have a greater risk of developing cervical cancer.

The many myths and misconceptions surrounding this disease have greatly contributed to the "stigma" associated with it. For many, it is not only embarrassing, painful, and ugly, but it may also be the basis for social ostracism for those who do not understand the disease.

First of all, herpes is not a form of plague. It is a communicable disease for which no cure presently exists, but *it is not transmissible all of the time*. In fact, the only time that sexual partners should refrain from contact is when active lesions are present. At other times, the risk of infection appears to be quite small.

Secondly, it is often just as important to treat the possible psychological problems of the herpes victim as it is to treat the physical symptoms. People with this disease often experience fear, frustration, depression, and a feeling that they have been dealt a "dirty blow" by someone. Counseling and support groups for herpes victims and their intimate partners have proven very effective.

Finally, although no cure for herpes exists at the present time, some degree of success has been indicated using certain drugs such as Acyclovir. However, these drugs have only been effective in reducing symptoms if the disease is confirmed during the first few hours after contact. As might be guessed, this is difficult. Other treatments, such as the use of L-lysine, remain largely unsubstantiated to date. Although lip balms and cold-sore medications may provide temporary anesthetic relief, it is important to remember that rubbing anything on a herpes blister may spread herpes-laden fluids to other tissues, or, via the hands, to other body parts.

Trichomoniasis

Unlike many of the other STDs, **trichomoniasis** is caused by a protozoan. Although as many as half of the women in the United States may have this organism present in the vaginal region, most women remain free of symptoms until their bodily defenses are weakened. Both men and women may transmit the disease, but women are the most likely candidates for infection. In women, the "trich" infection causes a foamy, yellowish discharge with an unpleasant odor that may be accompanied by a burning sensation, itching, and painful urination. These symptoms are most likely to occur during or shortly after menstruation, although they can occur at any time or not at all. Although usually transmitted by sexual contact, this organism may be easily spread by toilet seats, wet towels, or other items that may have discharged fluids on them, or by sitting naked on the bench of the dressing room of your local health spa or locker room. Treatment of "trich" includes oral metronidazole, usually given to both sexual partners to avoid the possible "Ping-Pong" effect that is so typical of the STDs.

General Urinary Tract Infections (UTIs)

Any time invading organisms enter the genital area, there is a risk that they may travel up the urethra and enter the bladder. Similarly, organisms normally living in the rectum, urethra, or bladder may be transmitted to the sexual organs and eventually transmitted to another person.

A common example of a disease being transmitted to yourself by yourself (autoinoculation) often occurs during the simple task of wiping yourself after defecating. Wiping from the anus forward may transmit organisms found in feces to the vaginal opening or to the urethra. Contact between the hands and the urethra or between the urethra and other objects may also transmit bacterial or viral pathogens. Women, with their shorter urethras, are more likely to contract UTIs.

Treatment for these infections is dependent on the nature and type of pathogen. For minor infections, some practitioners have recommended drinking 8 to 10 glasses of fluids per day, particularly those high in acid, such as cranberry juice. Much of this home treatment is controversial. It has been estimated by some authorities that a person would have to drink over 4 quarts of cranberry juice per day over a period of days to even begin to alter vaginal acidity. The cost-benefit ratio of this self-treatment, considering caloric intake, cost of the juice, and minimal effectiveness, may be high when compared to visiting a doctor and obtaining proven medications from a pharmacy.

Pubic Lice

Often called *crabs,* **pubic lice** are more annoying than they are dangerous. Crab lice are small parasites that are most often transmitted during sexual contact. They prefer the dark, moist regions of the body, and during sex they move from partner to partner. They have an affinity for pubic hair, attaching themselves to the base of these hairs and depositing their eggs (nits). Between 1 and 2 weeks after being deposited, these nits develop into adults that lay eggs and migrate, thus perpetuating the cycle. Eventually, lice will infect such body parts as the eyebrows, nose hairs, and the hair on your toes.

Treatment includes washing clothing, furniture, and linens that may harbor the eggs. It usually takes 2 to 3 weeks to kill all larval forms. Although sexual contact is the most common mode of transmission, an innocent roommate may pick up pubic lice from sheets that an infected person has slept on. Hotel and dormitory rooms in which blankets and sheets are not always washed may put you at risk.

Trichomoniasis Protozoan infection characterized by foamy, yellowish discharge and unpleasant odor.
Pubic Lice Parasites that can inhabit body areas, especially the genital areas; also called "crabs."

ACQUIRED IMMUNE DEFICIENCY SYNDROME (AIDS)

In July, 1992, 226,281 cases of **acquired immune deficiency syndrome (AIDS)** were reported in the United States (see Figure 14.3).* Although these numbers are large, it is likely that many more cases go unreported and never show up on the reportable disease listing. In addition, public-health officials estimate that there are currently over 1 million infected people in the United States, the majority of whom have no knowledge that they are infected.

To date, over 124,000 people have died of AIDS in the United States, and despite massive efforts aimed at prevention and treatment, the number of cases continues to escalate. Few regions of the world have been spared, with estimates of over 10 million HIV-infected people globally.** Where did the disease originate? How is it contracted? What is the prognosis once a person is infected? What are the major risk factors? Can it be prevented? What is the prediction for the future?

---

* *HIV/AIDS Surveillance* (Atlanta: Centers for Disease Control, July 1992).

** Ibid.

The Origins of AIDS

Although it is believed that the AIDS virus may actually have been present in the United States since the late 1960s or early 1970s, problems related to the disease were not noted by medical and government officials until the spring of 1981. At that time, federal officials noted increasing requests for an experimental drug used to treat a rare disease called *pneumocystis carinii pneumonia (PCP)*. Caused by a protozoan, PCP appeared to affect significant numbers of previously healthy, young, homosexual males in New York and California.

About the same time, increasing numbers of homosexual men in California were being diagnosed with a rare form of cancer known as Kaposi's sarcoma. People with PCP and Kaposi's sarcoma tended to share many characteristics. They typically were white and homosexual, came from similar geographical regions, used specific types of drugs, and had generalized *lymphadenopathy* (chronic swelling of the lymph nodes) and general malfunctioning of the immune system. Because of this later problem, many of these people developed several diseases at the same time, making diagnosis of one underlying cause extremely difficult.

For many months, epidemiologists investigated possible causes for this apparent "gay plague," including the types of drugs used by individuals, water supplies, and

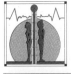

AIDS Alert

AIDS Facts

Did you know that . . .

- In the past year, more than 47,000 people have been diagnosed with AIDS in the U.S., and 40,000 more are believed to have become HIV infected.

- It is estimated that between 1 and 1 1/2 million people in the United States are infected with HIV.

- A total of 19,281 of the AIDS cases reported to the CDC are women with an AIDS diagnosis that meets the current CDC AIDS criteria. Poor women of color are at particularly high risk.

- Worldwide, there have been 371,802 cases of AIDS reported to the World Health Organization (WHO) through June 1991.

- Over 70 percent of prostitutes in New York City are HIV-infected.

- Recent studies of HIV in Africa indicate that there may soon be another differentiation between various forms of the virus. Known as HIV II, this form of the virus has not yet gained widespread acceptance.

- Condom use among 15–24-year-olds has remained steady between 1989–91, at less than 50 percent.

- By the year 2000, experts predict a cumulative total of 40 million to 120 million HIV infections, 90% of them in the developing world.

Source: *HIV/AIDS Surveillance* (Atlanta: Centers for Disease Control, ■■■, 199■).

many other factors. In 1984, two researchers, Robert C. Gallo from the National Cancer Institute in the United States and Luc Montagnier from the Pasteur Institute in Paris, first isolated the retrovirus (a type of slow-acting virus) that causes AIDS. Initially called the human T-cell lymphotropic virus type III (HTLV-III) by most American sources, this virus has been given many names since 1984. Today, most sources prefer to call the virus that causes AIDS the **human immunodeficiency virus (HIV)**. Many health professionals are actually beginning to use the term "HIV Disease" rather than the designation AIDS to describe all the various symptoms that occur once the HIV enters the body.

Although AIDS appeared to infect only homosexuals during the early days of the epidemic, it quickly became apparent that others were not immune to this disease. People with a history of IV drug use, Haitians, hemophiliacs, people who had received whole-blood transfusions, children born to infected mothers, and, more recently, people with no risk factors beyond being sexually active heterosexuals have developed AIDS. In addition, HIV disease is believed to have been present in various regions of the world prior to its diagnosis in the U.S. Equatorial Africa may have been among the first nations whose inhabitants contracted the disease and today experiences one of the world's highest rates of heterosexual transmission. Although theories abound as to the disease's beginning, the actual point of origin may never be known.

Transmission of AIDS

The AIDS virus typically gains entry to the body when an infected person inadvertently deposits body fluids containing HIV at a receptive location on another person. Mucous membranes of the genital organs and the anus appear to be likely spots for such an entry. If there is a break in the mucous membrane (as could occur during sexual intercourse, particularly anal intercourse), the virus begins to multiply.

After initial infection, HIV typically begins to multiply rapidly in the body, invading the bloodstream and cerebrospinal fluid. It progressively destroys helper T-lymphocytes, weakening the body's resistance to disease. The virus also changes the genetic structure of the cell it attacks. In response to this invasion, the body quickly recognizes that a foreign substance is present and begins to process antibodies to destroy it.

Although AIDS poses a growing threat to the world's population, it is not an uncontrollable disease. Several myths have recently been disproved. Countless studies of people living in households with a person with AIDS have shown no documented cases of HIV infection due to casual contact. Investigations also provide overwhelming evidence that insect bites do not transmit the AIDS virus.

The virus itself is actually very selective in the way it is transmitted from person to person. Unless a person en-

gages in certain high-risk activities that are known to spread the virus, the chance of becoming infected is extremely small. These high-risk activities include the following:

Exchange of Body Fluids The exchange of infected body fluids during sexual intercourse appears to provide the greatest risk of HIV infection. Research has provided substantial evidence that blood, semen, and vaginal, cervical, and anal secretions are clearly the major fluids of concern. Saliva and tears are not considered to be high-risk body fluids. However, the virus may be present in saliva and tears; thus caution about engaging in deep, wet kissing seems advisable.

Initially, public-health officials also included breast milk in the list of high-risk fluids due to a small number of infants who apparently contracted AIDS while breast-feeding. Subsequent research has indicated that HIV transmission could have been caused by bleeding nipples rather than actual breast milk.

Feces and urine may be the source of some contact risk. Infection through these routes is believed to be highly unlikely, though technically possible.

Receiving a Blood Transfusion Prior to 1985 Although this group is actually very small, there have been isolated cases of people who became infected with HIV as a result of having received a blood transfusion before 1985, when the Red Cross and other blood-donation programs implemented a stringent testing program for all donated blood. Today, because of these massive screening efforts, the risk of receiving HIV-infected blood is almost nonexistent. In fact, transfusion-related AIDS may be less common than experts have previously thought. CDC researchers looking at 158 people reportedly infected through blood after 1985 found only 15 cases in which people were infected by blood containing undetected HIV.*

Sharing Needles Used for IV Drugs A significant percentage of cases of AIDS in the United States are believed to be the result of sharing HIV-contaminated needles. People who share needles and also engage in sexual activities with members of high-risk groups, such as male homosexuals, increase their risks dramatically.

Mother-to-Infant Transmission (Perinatal) Approximately 80 percent of children who have contracted AIDS received the virus from the infected mother while in the womb or while passing through the vaginal tract during delivery.

Human Immunodeficiency Virus (HIV) The slow-acting virus that causes AIDS.

---

* International Conference on AIDS, Amsterdam. As reported in USA Today, July 27, 1992.

Symptoms of AIDS

A person may go for months or years after infection before any significant symptoms appear. This time period varies greatly from person to person. Children are more severely affected by the virus than adults. Most children with AIDS are newborns and infants. These youngsters are particularly vulnerable because they have not become fully immunocompetent (that is, their immune systems are not fully developed) until they are 6 to 15 months old. New information suggests that some very young children may show the "adult" progression of AIDS.* Current estimates indicate that babies infected with AIDS usually live less than 2 years. The average length of time before older children who become infected develop the actual disease is believed to be about 4 years.

The average period of time for the virus to cause the slow, degenerative changes in the immune system that are characteristic of AIDS is 8 to 10 years. During this time, symptoms of numerous everyday diseases may begin to develop. For example, the person may experience a large number of opportunistic infections (infections that gain a foothold when the immune system is not functioning effectively). Colds, sore throats, fever, tiredness, nausea, night sweats, and other generally non-life-threatening symptoms begin to appear. People who begin to show these combinations of symptoms and display one or more of the opportunistic infections resulting from an HIV-compromised immune system may be diagnosed as having AIDS.

Testing for HIV Antibodies

Once antibodies have begun to form in reaction to the presence of the HIV virus, a blood test known as the ELISA test may detect their presence. If sufficient antibodies are present, the ELISA test will be positive. When a person who previously tested negative (no HIV antibodies having been detected) has a subsequent test that is positive, **seroconversion** is said to have occurred. The majority of persons infected with HIV will seroconvert 3–6 months after infection. In some it may take years for seroconversion to occur.

In such a situation, the person would typically take another ELISA test followed by a more expensive, more precise test known as the Western Blot to confirm the presence of HIV antibodies. Although the ELISA is believed to be quite accurate, the test is designed to have a large number of false positive tests because it was meant to screen for possible problems in the blood supply. Therefore, it was considered wiser to err on the side of protection. There have also been instances of false negative results. Some health professionals feel that there may

be chronic carriers of HIV who continually show false negative results that are not readily detected by either of the above tests. Such speculation raises serious concerns about possible risks for unsuspecting victims.

It is important to note that no test is completely foolproof. It is also important to note that these tests are not AIDS tests per se; they merely detect antibodies for the disease. Whether you actually develop AIDS is dependent to some extent on the strength of your immune system. However, the vast majority of all infected people eventually develop some form of the disease.

Preventing HIV Infection

The number of HIV-infected heterosexuals is steadily increasing, particularly in the 18–24-year-old age group. In fact, AIDS is now a leading cause of death among young adults in America today. Although we used to refer to "high risk **groups**" when discussing who was most susceptible to HIV infection, it is much more appropriate to speak of "high risk **behaviors**." Regardless of your race, gender, sexual orientation, and so on, if you engage in high-risk behaviors, your chances of infection will increase. These people are considered engaging in high-risk behaviors: (1) Anyone who has multiple sex partners where body fluids are exchanged. (2) anyone who has unprotected sex with someone who has contracted or been exposed to the AIDS virus, (3) anyone who shares a needle with an IV drug user, and (4) women who share needles or have multiple sex partners. Although women account for only slightly more than 10 percent of all AIDS cases, these numbers are growing. The vast majority of these women have contracted AIDS through shared needles or sexual relations with bisexual men or men who share needles.

Prevention strategies closely relate to the means by which people contract AIDS. By avoiding high-risk behaviors, individual risk will be greatly reduced.

Where To Go for Help If you are concerned about your possible risk or the risk of a close friend, arrange a confidential meeting with the health educator or other health professional at your college health service. He or she will provide you with the information that you will need to decide whether a test for HIV antibodies is necessary and what you should do to have the test. If the student health service is not an option for you, seek assistance through your local public-health department or community STD clinic. Local physicians, clergy members, counselors, professors, or other responsible people can often provide you with the answers you are looking for.

---

* *HIV/AIDS Surveillance.*

Seroconversion When a previously negative HIV antibody test changes to a positive test.

A Cure for AIDS?

In March 1987, the U.S. government allowed doctors to prescribe the antiviral drug *Zidovudine* (generically referred to as *Azidothymidine*, or *AZT*), a drug that slows down replication of the virus in lymphocytes. Since the introduction of this drug, the lives of many AIDS victims have been extended. Zidovudine is highly toxic and almost prohibitively expensive for many patients, costing over $10,000 per year. Currently, studies are being conducted to determine if the drug can prevent the onset of the disease in people who are HIV-positive but asymp-

Promoting Your Health

Reducing Your Risks for AIDS

AIDS is not an uncontrollable disease. The following list offers ways that you can reduce your risk of contracting the disease.

- Avoid intimate sexual contact involving exchange of body fluids with people who fit the criteria for high risk of infection. Consider that you are effectively exposing yourself to your partner's "history of lovers" whenever you choose to have sexual relations.

- Avoid casual sexual partners. Ideally, only have sex if you are in a long-term committed relationship with someone who is also capable of having a long-term committed relationship.

- All sexually active adults who are not in lifetime, monogamous relationships should practice safer sex by using a condom. Condoms should be purchased based on proven effectiveness, with latex varieties providing the greatest margin of safety.

- Never share hypodermic needles with anyone for any reason.

- Wash your hands before and after sexual encounters. Urinate after sexual relations and if possible, wash your genitals.

- Never share any devices through which blood exchange may occur, including needles, razors, tattoo instruments, ear-piercing instruments, and any other sharp objects.

- Avoid injury to body tissue during sexual activity. The AIDS virus may travel in body fluids through microscopic tears in anal or vaginal tissues.

- Avoid oral sex or any sexual activity where body fluids can penetrate mucous membranes through breaks in the skin.

- Avoid using drugs that may dull your senses and cause you to "forget" to practice reasonable caution with potential sexual partners.

- Do not be afraid to ask intimate sexual questions about your partner's past history. If your partner refuses to answer or is evasive in his or her answers, do not become sexually involved until you are assured that he or she is not infected.

- Although HIV-antibody tests are not routinely recommended for most college students, every situation is different. If you are worried, it is better to be safe and have yourself tested than risk infection with HIV.

- Although total abstinence is the only absolute means of preventing AIDS, this is not a viable alternative for many young adults. It is important to rethink the importance that many people put on the sexual act, however. If you are in doubt about the risks that having sex may pose for you, it may be important to consider other means of intimacy, at least until you are reasonably certain that you will be safe. Massage, social (dry) kissing, hugging, holding and touching, and masturbation (alone or with a partner) can be enjoyable alternatives.

- If you are a woman with a positive HIV-antibody test, you should do everything possible to ensure that you do not become pregnant.

- When going to medical professionals such as dentists or doctors, be assertive. Make sure they take appropriate precautions such as washing their hands, wearing gloves, and sterilizing equipment before coming in contact with you.

- If you suspect that you might become infected or if you test positive, do not donate blood, semen, or body organs.

- Because the status of your immune system is an important factor in whether or not you are susceptible to any of the STDs, it is important that you do everything possible to protect yourself. Adequate nutrition, sleep, stress management, vaccinations, and other preventive maintenance activities can do a great deal to ensure your long-term health.

tomatic and to see if it can prevent seroconversion in people with known exposure, such as infants born to infected mothers.

Although scientists are continually searching for a vaccine to protect people from infection, no such vaccines are available at the present time. Although present methods of treatment have extended life in some patients, these treatments are often tremendously costly, prompting many patients to seek treatments that are questionable and unproven in other countries.

While new treatments such as the drug DDI appear promising, no current treatments have proven significantly effective in reversing the course of HIV infection.

NONINFECTIOUS DISEASES: THE MODERN MALADIES

Typically, when we think of chronic diseases, images of life-threatening situations involving cancer and heart disease immediately come to mind. These graphic pictures often include faces of elderly people, stricken in the waning years of their lives by powerful enemies that they must battle until their death.

Although these "killer" diseases capture much of the media attention, the other forms of chronic diseases often cause us substantial pain, suffering, and disability. Fortunately, the majority of these diseases can be prevented or their onset delayed. Education and reasonable alterations in lifestyle behaviors and improved access to health care can minimize the effects of most chronic diseases.

To prevent the development of noncommunicable and chronic diseases, we must identify common characteristics of these diseases. They are not transmitted by any pathogen or by any form of personal contact. They usually develop over a long period of time, and they cause progressive damage to human tissues. Although these conditions normally do not result in death, they do lead to illness and suffering for many people. Lifestyle, personal health habits, and increased life expectancy appear to be major contributing factors to this general increase in the incidence of chronic diseases in the United States. In this section, we will discuss some of these diseases and the factors that contribute to them.

RESPIRATORY DISORDERS

Allergy-Induced Problems

One of the body's natural defense mechanisms is the antigen–antibody response. When foreign pathogens such as bacteria or viruses invade the body, the body responds by producing antibodies to destroy the invading antigens. Under normal conditions, the production of antibodies is a positive element in the body's defense

system. However, for unknown reasons, in some people the body overreacts by developing an overly elaborate protective mechanism. The resultant hypersensitivity reaction to specific allergens or antigens in the environment is fairly common, as anyone who has awakened with a runny nose or a serious case of itchy eyes will testify. Most commonly, these hypersensitivity, or allergic, responses occur as a reaction to environmental antigens such as molds, animal dander (hair and dead skin), pollen, ragweed, or dust. Once excessive antibodies to these antigens are produced, they trigger the release of **histamines,** chemical substances that dilate blood vessels, increase mucus secretions, cause tissues to swell, and produce other allergylike symptoms. Although many people think of allergies as childhood diseases, allergic responses become chronic in nature, and treatment becomes difficult with age.

Hay Fever

Perhaps the best example of a chronic respiratory disease is **hay fever.** Usually considered to be a seasonally related disease (most prevalent when ragweed and flowers are blooming), hay fever is common throughout the world. Hay-fever attacks, which are characterized by sneezing and itchy, watery eyes and runny nose, cause a great deal of misery and discomfort for countless people. Hay fever appears to run in families, and research indicates that lifestyle is not as great a factor in developing hay fever as it is in other chronic diseases. Instead, a combination of an overzealous immune system and an exposure to environmental allergens such as pet dust, pollen from various plants, or other substances appear to be the critical factors that determine vulnerability.

Asthma

Unfortunately for many hay-fever sufferers, their condition is often complicated by the development of another chronic respiratory disease, **asthma.** Asthma is characterized by short attacks of wheezing, difficulty in breathing, shortness of breath, and coughing spasms. Although most asthma attacks are mild, they can trigger *bronchospasms* (contractions of the bronchial tubes in the lungs) of such a severe nature that, unless treatment is rapid, death may occur.

In the majority of cases, asthma occurs in children under the age of 10, afflicting males nearly twice as often as females. Although many children outgrow the condi-

---

Histamines Chemical substances that dilate blood vessels, increase mucus secretions, and produce other allergylike symptoms.
Hay Fever A chronic respiratory disorder that is most prevalent when ragweed and flowers bloom.
Asthma A chronic respiratory disease characterized by attacks of wheezing, shortness of breath, and coughing spasms.

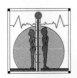

Exercise-Induced Asthma

Friends who bow out of a long run or a tennis game claiming to be allergic to exercise might not be joking. The coughing and wheezing that can strike during or after a workout are, in fact, exercise-induced asthma (EIA), a surprisingly common condition. Unfortunately for your friends' credibility, it is also easily treatable. Track dynamo Jackie Joyner-Kersee, for example, is one of several Olympians who have racked up gold medals despite allergies to exercise.

Doctors do not know what causes EIA or understand its exact connection with allergies. Some athletes without other allergies have EIA, and 35 percent of people with allergies and 90 percent of people with both allergies and asthma suffer from it. Histamines, one of the main symptom-causing chemicals in allergies, also are a known factor in EIA.

Those who suspect they have exercise allergies can find out easily by describing the symptoms to an allergist or sports-medicine doctor, who may perform some simple lung-function tests. Once EIA is diagnosed, breathing easy is no sweat. Cold, dry air is a major cause of EIA, so keeping the air in your lungs moist could stave off an attack. Warming up for at least 10 minutes before working out and breathing through your nose also help. Runners, cross-country skiers, and other outdoor athletes can wear a scarf or light mask. The warm,

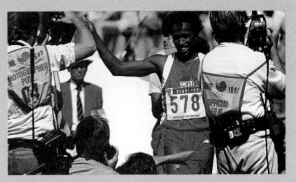

Jackie Joyner-Kersee, an Olympic gold medalist, suffers from exercise-induced asthma.

moist air around swimming pools is one of the best environments for asthmatics.

Drugs may be necessary for serious cases. Doctors warn against using over-the-counter inhalers even though one, Primatene Mist, is promoted by Joyner-Kersee. The medication in inhalers wears off quickly, raises the pulse rate, and stresses the heart. New prescription drugs such as Seldane and inhalers containing albuterol, however, work better without serious side effects. The only obstacle between you and the Olympics will be your athletic ability.

SOURCE: *U.S. News & World Report,* February 20, 1989.

---

tion, a number of them suffer recurrences of the ailment as adults.

Although exposure to allergens such as dust, pollen, and animal dander may trigger many asthmatic episodes, emotional factors and excessive anxiety or stress can also trigger an attack. *Exercise-induced asthma* is a type of asthma that has gained increasing attention. Depending on the underlying causes, asthma may be treated with drugs, such as antihistamines, or through relaxation methods.

Emphysema

If you have ever seen someone hooked up to an oxygen tank and struggling to breathe while climbing a flight of stairs or listened to someone gasping for air during what should be normal breathing, you have probably wit-

nessed an emphysemic episode. **Emphysema** involves the gradual destruction of the *alveoli* (tiny air sacs) of the lungs. As the alveoli are destroyed, the affected person finds it more and more difficult to exhale. The victim typically struggles to take in a fresh supply of air before the air held in the lungs has been expended. The chest cavity gradually begins to expand, producing the barrel-shaped chest characteristic of the chronic emphysema victim.

The exact cause of emphysema is uncertain. There is, however, a strong relationship between the development of emphysema and long-term cigarette smoking and exposure to air pollution. Victims of emphysema often suffer discomfort over a period of many years. What we all take for granted—the easy, rhythmic flow of air in and out of our lungs—becomes a continuous struggle for people with emphysema. Inadequate oxygen supply, combined with the stress of overexertion on the heart, eventually takes its toll on the cardiovascular system and leads to premature death.

Chronic Bronchitis

Although often dismissed as "smoker's cough" or a bad case of the common cold, **chronic bronchitis** may be a serious, if not life-threatening, respiratory disorder. In this ailment, the bronchial tubes become so inflamed and swollen that normal respiratory function is impaired. Excessive use of cigarettes is the major risk factor for this disease, although fumes, dust, and particulate matter in the air are also contributing factors. Victims of chronic bronchitis must often use respiratory devices similar to those used by emphysema patients. They also must avoid those factors, such as cigarettes, that contributed to development of bronchitis. Bronchitis coupled with a severe cold may be serious enough to warrant obtaining immediate medical attention.

Poison-Ivy Allergies

A common case of "poison ivy" may be a response to allergens produced by several different but related plants. If you live in the central or eastern part of the United States, you are likely to have come in contact with true poison ivy. In western states, you are more likely to have come in contact with poison oak. In the South, the culprit may be poison sumac.

In each of these cases, your body comes in contact with the resin (an oily substance) from the leaves of the plant and has an allergic reaction. The more resin you are exposed to, the more likely it is that you will have a reaction. Thus, exposed areas of the skin—ankles and

The method of testing for allergies is to inject small amounts of allergens under the skin.

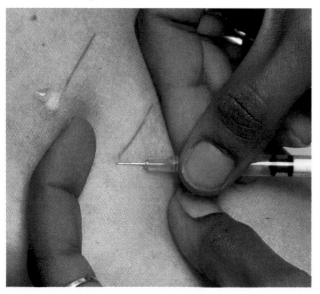

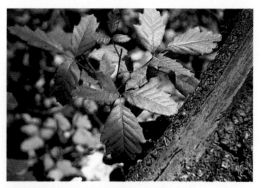

Poison oak.

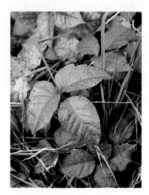

Poison ivy.

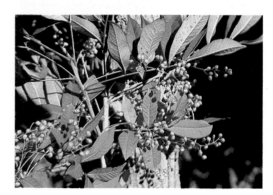

Poison sumac.

wrists, for example—are more vulnerable than covered areas. Also, if you have been exposed before, your next reaction is likely to be more severe.

If you are exposed to any of these plants, wash the affected area with cool water. Avoid spreading the resin to other parts of your body. Using soap is not advised because it may spread the oil to other areas. It is sometimes a good idea to apply rubbing alcohol to the affected area after washing with water to help remove any remaining resin.

If you know that you have been exposed to one of these plants, you can receive oral or injected steroid

Chronic Bronchitis A serious respiratory disorder in which the bronchial tubes become so inflamed and swollen that respiratory function is impaired.

treatments before blisters develop. Once blisters form, the best treatment is calamine lotion, which helps to dry the blisters and prevent any further spread of the resin.

Can you get poison ivy through contact with anything other than the plants themselves? Yes. You can come in contact with the resin if you touch the family dog after it has been exposed to the plant or if you touch clothing that has resin on it. Also, resin can be carried in the air, particularly by smoke from forest fires.

Can you prevent poison-ivy reactions? Prescription pills that contain resinlike substances designed to help immunize you against future outbreaks are available. However, these pills often have side effects or are ineffective. The best method of prevention is to avoid areas known to have poison-ivy plants and to wear appropriate clothing when in these areas to avoid contact with the resin.

▌NEUROLOGICAL DISORDERS

Headaches

Almost all of us have experienced the agony of at least one major headache in our lives. Not all headaches are equal; more important, not all headaches are caused by the same things. Headaches can result from dilated blood vessels within the brain, from underlying organic problems, or from excessive stress and anxiety. The following are the most common forms of headaches and the most effective methods of treatment.

Tension Headache Tension headaches are generally caused by muscle contractions or tension in the neck or head. This tension may be caused by actual strain placed on neck or head muscles because of overuse, static positions held for long periods of time, or tension triggered by stress. The majority of all headaches are caused by excessive tension, be it physical or psychological. Symptoms may vary in intensity and duration, but relaxation is generally the best form of prevention and treatment. Common relaxation methods include sleep, meditation, a hot bath or whirlpool, massage, or certain heat treatments used to relax the affected muscles.

Migraine Headache Experienced by over 20 percent of the American public, **migraine headaches** usually are localized on only one side of the head. Migraines are believed to be caused by unusual alternating dilation and constriction of blood vessels in the brain. Symptoms can range from visual disturbances to excruciating pain that lasts for minutes or hours. The pain often tends to worsen over time and to recur. In some cases, migraines are so severe that the person is unable to work or continue normal activity. Nausea, vomiting, and general weakness often accompany migraines. When true migraines occur, relaxation is only minimally effective as a treatment. Often, strong pain-relieving drugs prescribed by a physician are necessary.

Secondary Headaches Secondary headaches arise as a result of some other underlying condition. A good example is a severe sinus blockage that causes pressure in the sinus cavity. Hypertension, allergies, low blood sugar, diseases of the spine, the common cold, poorly fitted dentures, problems with eyesight, and other types of pain or injury can trigger this condition. Relaxation and pain relievers such as aspirin are of little help in treating secondary headaches. Rather, medications designed to relieve the underlying organic cause of the headache must be included in the treatment regimen.

Psychological Headaches With this type of headache, the "it's all in your head" diagnosis may, in fact, be correct. Rather than having a physical cause, psychological headaches stem from anxiety states, depression, and other emotional factors.

How do these headaches differ from tension headaches? Although it can be difficult to distinguish between the two, psychological headaches result from the stress of severe emotional disturbances, particularly depression. Unlike tension headaches, no muscles or blood vessels appear to be involved, thereby making relaxation and painkillers virtually worthless as treatment.

Victims of depression-related headaches tend to suffer from sleep disturbances and to experience symptoms over a period of years. Only therapy designed to treat the underlying depression or emotional problem appears to be effective in reducing the headache. Depression-related headaches, like all headaches, may indicate a more serious underlying condition. If severe headaches do not improve with aspirin or relaxation techniques, persist for more than 3 days, or are accompanied by visual disturbances, nausea, speech difficulties, numbness or tingling in the face or limbs, you should see your physician.

Seizure Disorders

Epilepsy is derived from the Greek *epilepsia*, meaning "seizure." Reports of epilepsy appeared in Greek medical records as early as 300 B.C. Ancient peoples interpreted seizures as invasions of the body by evil spirits or punishments by the gods. Although much of the mystery surrounding epileptic seizures has been solved in recent years, the stigma and lack of understanding surrounding epilepsy remain for many people. Approximately 1 percent of all Americans suffer from some form of seizure-related disorder.

Migraine Headaches Localized headaches that result from alternation of blood flow, with dilation and constriction of blood vessels.

Epilepsy A neurological disorder caused by abnormal electrical brain activity; can be accompanied by altered consciousness or convulsions.

These disorders are generally caused by abnormal electrical activity in the brain and are characterized by loss of control of muscular activity and unconsciousness. The symptoms vary widely from person to person.

There are several forms of seizure disorders, of which the following two are the most common.

1. *Grand mal,* or *major motor seizure*—often preceded by a shrill cry or a *seizure aura* (body sensations such as ringing in the ears or a specific smell or taste that occurs prior to a seizure). Convulsions and loss of consciousness generally occur.

2. *Petit mal,* or *minor seizure*—no convulsions, minor loss of consciousness that may go unnoticed. Minor twitching of muscles may occur.

Theories concerning the factors that predispose a person to seizure disorders are varied. About half of all cases are of unknown origin. Head injury or trauma is one possible cause; other causes include congenital abnormalities, injury or illness resulting in inflammation of the brain or spinal column, drug or chemical poisoning, tumors, nutritional deficiency, and heredity.

In the majority of cases, people afflicted with seizure disorders can lead normal, seizure-free lives when under medical supervision. Anticonvulsant drugs such as phenobarbital, phenytoin (Dilantin), and primidone (Mysoline) have helped victims to lead normal lives in the absence of a definitive cure. Driving automobiles and similar activities are usually not restricted for people whose seizures are medically controlled. Despite massive educational campaigns in recent years, many people are still afraid to hire people with seizure disorders, and discriminate against them in numerous ways. Public ignorance about these disorders is among the most serious obstacles that confront victims of seizure disorders.

▎COMMON FEMALE DISORDERS

Fibrocystic Breast Condition

Fibrocystic breast condition is a common noncancerous problem among women in the United States. Symptoms range in severity from a small palpable lump to large masses of irregular tissue found in both breasts. The underlying causes of the condition are unknown. Although some experts believe it to be related to hormonal changes that occur during the normal menstrual cycle, many women report that their condition neither worsens nor improves during the cycle. In fact, in most cases the condition appears to run in families and to become progressively worse with age, irrespective of pregnancy or other hormonal disruptions. Although the majority of these cyst formations consist of fibrous tissue, some of them are filled with fluid. Treatment often involves removal of fluids from the affected area or surgical removal of the cyst itself.

The possibility that excessive caffeine consumption might be a contributing factor in fibrocystic breast condition began to be considered in the late 1970s. Subsequent research has indicated that although there may be a relationship between caffeine consumption and specific types of fibrocystic breast conditions, the association is unclear.

Does fibrocystic breast condition predispose a woman to later cancer development? Experts believe that the risks for breast cancer among women with certain types of fibrocystic disease may be slightly higher than among the general populace, but it is likely that a host of other factors, such as a high-fat diet, never having been pregnant, and a family history of breast cancer, present much greater risks.

Premenstrual Syndrome (PMS)

Premenstrual syndrome (PMS), is a condition that has been the basis of a great deal of controversy. Although the monthly problems experienced by many women have been discussed for decades, they have largely been dismissed as insignificant. Psychiatrists and other mental-health professionals who convened for a major conference in 1986 refused, after much debate, to classify PMS as a psychiatric disorder, although they did agree that it was a problem that merited consideration. Currently, PMS still has not been classified as a psychiatric disorder.

Why the sudden interest in PMS? What are the typical signs and symptoms? Why have women in specified situations been acquitted of murder or serious crimes by using PMS as their defense? How legitimate are these claims?

Premenstrual syndrome is characterized by as many as 150 possible physical and emotional symptoms that vary from person to person and from month to month. These symptoms, which usually appear a week to 10 days preceding the menstrual period, affect up to 20 percent of women to some degree. They include depression, tension, irritability, headaches, tender breasts, bloated abdomen, backache, abdominal cramps, acne, diarrhea, and fatigue. It is believed that women who have PMS develop a predictable pattern of symptoms during the menstrual cycle. Severity of symptoms may be influenced by external factors, such as stress.

Women usually experience PMS for the first time after the age of 20. It may remain a regular part of a woman's reproductive life unless she seeks treatment. For many women, the first day of their period brings immediate relief. For others, the depressive symptoms may persist all month and are only heightened prior to the menstrual period.

Most authorities believe that the most plausible cause

Premenstrual Syndrome (PMS) Series of physical and emotional symptoms that may occur in women prior to their menstrual periods.

of PMS is a hormonal imbalance related to the rise in estrogen levels preceding the menstrual period. This theory is substantiated by the fact that women with PMS who are given prescriptions for progesterone (see Chapter 6) often experience relief of symptoms. Critics of this theory argue that controlled research has not yet been conducted on the effects of progesterone on PMS.

Common treatments for PMS include hormonal therapy in addition to drugs and behaviors designed to relieve the symptoms. These include aspirin for pain, diuretics for fluid buildup, decreases in caffeine and salt intake, increases in complex carbohydrate intake, stress-reduction techniques, and exercise.

Endometriosis

Whether the incidence of **endometriosis** is on the rise in the United States or whether the disorder is simply attracting more attention is difficult to determine. Victims of endometriosis tend to be women between the ages of 20 and 40. Symptoms include severe cramping during and between menstrual cycles, unusually heavy or light menstrual flow, abdominal bloating, menstrual pain, infertility, and low back pain. What is this disease? What causes it? What are the common methods of treatment?

Although much remains unknown about the causes of endometriosis, we do know that the disease is characterized by the abnormal growth and development of endometrial tissue in regions of the body other than the uterus. This unusual growth may produce menstrual irregularity, pain, and other symptoms. Among the most widely accepted theories concerning the causes of endometriosis are the transmission of endometrial tissue to other regions of the body during surgery or through the birthing process; the movement of menstrual fluid backward through the fallopian tubes during menstruation; and abnormal cell migration through body-fluid movement.

Treatment of endometriosis ranges from bed rest and reduction in stressful activities to **hysterectomy,** the removal of the uterus, and/or the removal of one or both ovaries and the fallopian tubes. Recently, physicians have been criticized by some segments of the public for being too quick to perform hysterectomies. More conservative treatments that use *dilation and curettage* (surgically scraping endometrial tissue off the fallopian tubes and other reproductive organs) and combinations of hormone therapy have become more acceptable in most regions of the country.

▮ DIGESTION-RELATED DISORDERS

Diabetes

In healthy people, the *pancreas,* a powerful enzyme-producing organ, produces **insulin** in sufficient quantities to allow the body to use or store glucose (blood sugar).

When this organ fails to produce enough insulin to regulate sugar metabolism or the body fails to use insulin effectively, a disease known as **diabetes** occurs. Diabetics exhibit **hyperglycemia,** or elevated blood-sugar levels, and high glucose levels in their urine. Other symptoms include excessive thirst, frequent urination, hunger, tendency to tire easily, wounds that heal slowly, numbness or tingling in the extremities, changes in vision, skin eruptions, and, in women, a tendency toward vaginal yeast infections.

Of the estimated 10 million diabetics in the United States today, nearly 4 million are unaware that they have a problem. Many diabetics remain unaware of their condition until they begin to show overt symptoms. By that time, they may have suffered severe consequences, including impairment in blood circulation, blindness, stroke, kidney damage, loss of limbs due to circulatory problems, and severe infections.

How does a person become diabetic? The more serious form, known as type 1 (insulin-dependent) diabetes, usually begins early in life. Type 1 diabetics typically remain dependent on insulin injections or oral medications for the rest of their lives. Adult-onset (non-insulin-dependent), or type 2, diabetes, tends to develop in later life. Type 2 diabetics often can control the symptoms of their disease, with minimal medical intervention, through a regimen of proper diet, weight control, and exercise, and they may be able to avoid oral medications or insulin indefinitely.

Diabetes tends to run in families, and a tendency toward being overweight, coupled with inactivity, dramatically increases a person's risk. Approximately 80 percent of all patients are overweight at the time of diagnosis. Weight loss and exercise are important factors in lowering blood sugar and improving the efficiency of cellular use of insulin. Both are important aspects of preventing overwork of the pancreas and the development of diabetes. The person who develops diabetes today has a much better prognosis than do those who developed diabetes just 20 years ago. Our understanding of the role that stress, illness, alcohol, smoking, and other lifestyle characteristics may have in the development of diabetes can aid in earlier prevention and earlier diagnosis. Most physicians attempt to control diabetes with a variety of insulin-related drugs. Most of these drugs are taken orally, although self-administered hypodermic injections are prescribed when other treatments are inadequate. Recent breakthroughs in individual monitoring and the implanting of insulin monitors and

---

Endometriosis   Abnormal development of endometrial tissue outside the uterus, resulting in serious side effects.

Hysterectomy   Surgical removal of the uterus and of one or both ovaries and the fallopian tubes.

Insulin   A hormone produced by the pancreas; required by the body for the metabolism of carbohydrates.

Diabetes   A disease in which the pancreas fails to produce enough insulin or the body fails to use insulin effectively.

Hyperglycemia   Elevated blood sugar levels.

insulin infusion pumps that regulate insulin intake "on demand" have provided many diabetics with the opportunity to lead normal lives.

Colitis

Ulcerative **colitis** is a disease of the large intestine in which the mucous membranes of the intestinal walls become inflamed. Victims with severe cases may have as many as 20 bouts of bloody diarrhea a day. Colitis can also produce severe stomach cramps, weight loss, and fever. What causes colitis? Although some experts believe that colitis occurs more frequently in people with high stress levels, this theory is controversial. Hypersensitivity reactions, particularly to milk and certain foods, have also been considered as a possible cause. It is difficult to determine the cause of colitis because the disease goes into unexplained remission and then recurs without apparent reason. This pattern often continues over periods of years and may be related to the later development of colorectal cancer. Because the cause of colitis remains unknown, treatment focuses exclusively on relieving the symptoms and includes dietary monitoring and drugs to reduce intestinal activity and soothe irritated intestinal walls.

Many people develop a condition related to colitis known as *irritable bowel syndrome*, in which diarrhea attacks and cramps occur after eating certain foods or when under unusual stress. Medical advice should be sought whenever such conditions persist.

Diverticulosis

Diverticulosis occurs when the walls of the intestine become weakened for undetermined reasons and small pea-sized bulges develop. These bulges often fill with feces and, over time, become irritated and infected, causing pain and discomfort. If this irritation persists, bleeding and chronic obstruction may occur, either of which can be life-threatening.

Although diverticulosis may appear in any part of the intestinal wall, it most commonly occurs in the small intestine. Often the person affected may be unaware that the problem exists. However, in some cases a person may actually have an attack similar to the pain of appendicitis, except that the pain is on the left side of the body instead of the right, where the appendix is located. Although diverticulosis most frequently occurs during and after middle age, it can appear at any age. If you have a persistent pain in the lower abdominal region, seek medical attention at once.

Peptic Ulcers

An ulcer is a lesion or wound that forms in body tissue as a result of some form of irritant. A **peptic ulcer** is a chronic ulcer that occurs in the lining of the stomach or the section of the small intestine known as the duodenum. It is caused by the erosive effect of digestive juices on these tissues. The lining of these organs becomes irritated, the protective covering of mucus is reduced, and the gastric acid begins to digest the dying tissue, just as it would a piece of food. Typically, this irritation causes pain that disappears when the person eats, only to return about an hour later. Because the exact cause of ulcers is unknown, prevention is difficult. Ulcers do appear to run in families and to be more prevalent in people who are highly stressed over long periods of time and who consume high-fat foods or excessive amounts of alcohol. Treatment of ulcers used to include a diet that consisted of milk and toast or other bland substitutes. This treatment was discarded when it was discovered that stomach acid secretions actually increased when milk was consumed because the lactose and fat in whole milk are difficult to digest. Today, physicians prescribe drugs that reduce stomach secretions, thus allowing patients to eat whatever foods do not irritate their stomachs. People with ulcers should avoid high-fat foods, which cause increased secretion of stomach acids and exacerbate this condition.

Gallbladder Disease

Gallbladder disease, also known as *cholecystitis*, occurs when the gallbladder has been repeatedly irritated by chemicals, infection, or overuse, thus reducing its ability to release *bile* for the digestion of fats. Usually, gallstones, consisting of calcium, cholesterol, and other minerals, form in the gallbladder itself. When the patient eats foods that are high in fats, the gallbladder contracts to release bile, which is necessary for fat digestion; these contractions in turn cause pressure on the stone formations. One of the characteristic symptoms of gallbladder disease is acute pain in the upper right portion of the abdomen after eating fatty foods. This pain may feel like a heart attack or an ulcer attack and is often accompanied by nausea.

Who gets gallbladder disease? The old adage about the "five f's" of risk factors frequently holds true. Anyone who is "female, fat, fair, forty, and flatulent" (prone to passing gas) appears to be at increased risk. However, people who don't fit this picture also get the disease.

Not all gallstones cause acute pain. In fact, small stones that pass through one of the bile ducts and become lodged may be more painful than gallstones that are the size of golf balls. Many people find out that they have gallstones only after undergoing diagnostic X-rays to rule out other conditions. The absence of symptoms is

Colitis An inflammatory disorder that affects the mucous membranes of the large intestine, producing bloody diarrhea.

Diverticulosis A condition in which bulges form in the walls of the intestine; results in irritation and infection of the intestine.

Peptic Ulcer Damage to the stomach or intestinal lining usually caused by digestive juices.

significant because gallstones are considered to be a predisposing factor for gallbladder cancer. In fact, gallstones were present in 75 percent of all gallbladder cancers in 1989.*

Current treatment of gallbladder disease usually involves medication to reduce irritation, restriction of fat consumption, and surgery to remove the gallstones themselves. New medications designed to dissolve small gallstones are currently being used in some patients. In addition, a new technique known as *lithotripsy* is being used, in which small stones are broken up using a series of noninvasive shock waves. Experiments using lasers and other techniques are also being conducted as alternatives to surgery.

DISEASES OF THE BONES AND JOINTS

Arthritis

One of the greatest causes of physical pain and disability in American society, particularly among the elderly, is **arthritis**, an inflammatory disease of the joints. More than 100 different arthritic disorders affect more than 17 million people in the United States alone. These disorders range in severity from slight aches and pains to gnarled and twisted limbs. More than 3 million Americans must restrict their activities because of arthritic problems. The most common forms are *osteoarthritis* and *rheumatoid arthritis*, both of which cause pain and deformed joints.

Osteoarthritis   Osteoarthritis is a progressive deterioration of bones and joints that has been associated with

* Huntington Sheldon, *Boyd's Introduction to the Study of Disease*, 10th ed. (Philadelphia: Lea & Febiger, 1989), p. 486.

the "wear and tear" theory of aging. Weather extremes, excessive strain, and injury often lead to osteoarthritis flare-ups. However, a specific precipitating event does not seem to be necessary. Although age and injury undoubtedly are factors in the development of osteoarthritis, heredity, abnormal use of the joint, diet, abnormalities in joint structure, and impaired blood supply to the joint may also contribute. Extreme disability as a result of osteoarthritis is rare. However, when joints become so distorted that they impair activity, surgical intervention is often necessary. Joint replacement and bone fusion are common surgical repair techniques. For the most part, anti-inflammatory drugs and pain relievers such as aspirin and cortisone-related agents are given to ease discomfort. In some instances, applications of heat, mild exercise, and massage may also relieve discomfort.

Rheumatoid Arthritis   Rheumatoid arthritis is similar to, but far more serious than, osteoarthritis. Rheumatoid arthritis is an inflammatory joint disease that can occur at any age but is most common between the ages of 20 and 45. It is 3 times more common among women than men during early adulthood and equally common among men and women in the over-70 age group. Symptoms may be gradually progressive or sporadic, with occasional unexplained remissions.

Rheumatoid arthritis typically attacks the *synovial membrane* that produces the lubricating fluids for the joints. Advanced rheumatoid arthritis often involves destruction of the bony ends of joints. The remedy for this condition is typically bone fusion, which leaves the joint immobile. In some instances, joint replacement may be a viable alternative. Figure 14.4 illustrates the bone de-

Arthritis   Inflammatory, painful disease of the joints.

Figure 14.4   The stages of rheumatoid arthritis: (a) Normal join; (b) Early stage, cartilage deterioration/synovial inflammation; (c) Bony growth develops; (d) Late stage, bone/joint displacement.

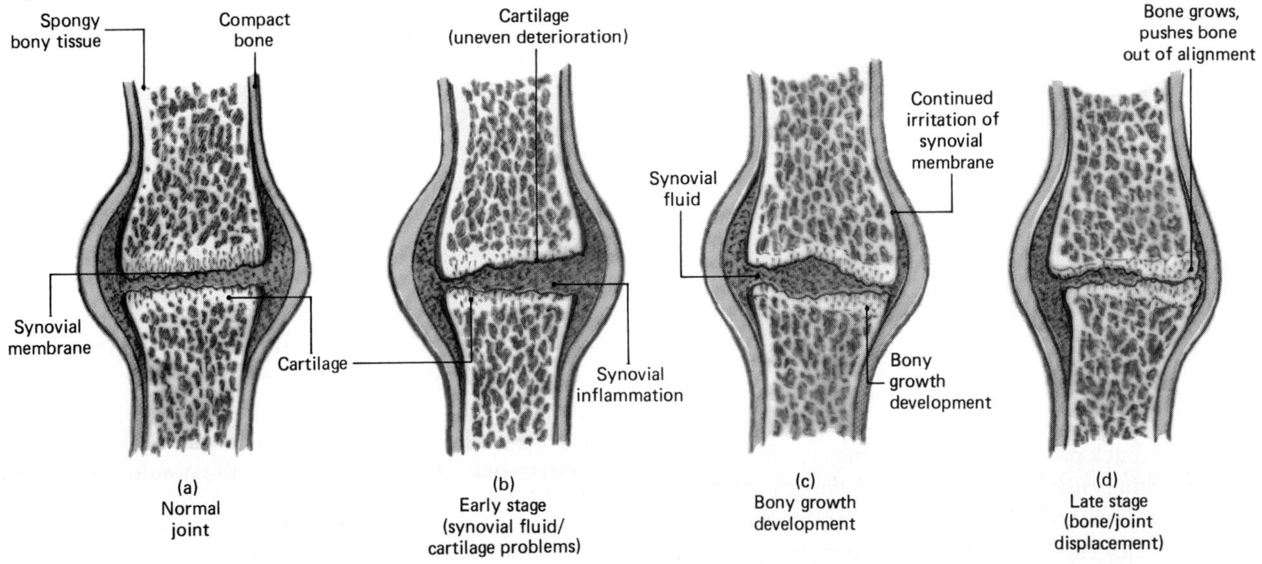

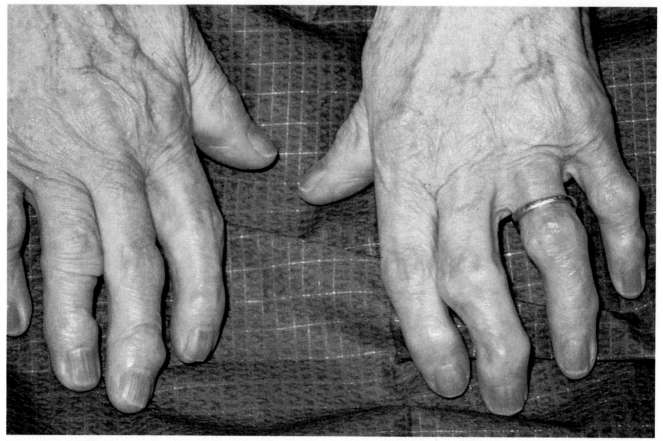

Like many disorders, arthritis occurs at different levels of severity. Serious cases can be extremely painful and disabling.

struction that typically occurs in a joint affected by rheumatoid arthritis.

Although the exact cause of this form of arthritis is unknown, some experts theorize that it is an autoimmune disorder, in which the body responds as if its own cells were the enemy, eventually destroying the affected body parts. Other theorists believe that rheumatoid arthritis is caused by some form of invading microorganism that takes over the joint. Certain toxic chemicals and stress have also been mentioned as possible causes.

Regardless of the cause, treatment of rheumatoid arthritis is similar to that for osteoarthritis. Emphasis is placed on pain relief and attempts to improve the functional mobility of the patient. In some instances, immunosuppressant drugs are given to reduce the inflammatory response.

Low-Back Pain

Approximately 80 percent of all Americans will experience low back pain during their lifetime. Although some of these low-back pain (LBP) episodes may be short-lived and acute, others may be chronic and lifelong. Low-back pain is considered to be epidemic throughout the world and is the major cause of disability for people aged 20 to 45 in the United States.* Young adults suffer more frequently and severely from this problem than do older people.

In 1991, LBP ranked second only to upper respiratory infections as the leading cause of work time lost because of illness in the United States. In fact, costs associated with back injury *exceeded* those associated with all other industrial injuries combined. Back injuries are most frequently mentioned in injury-related lawsuits, with an average cost in medical bills and compensation claims of over $8,000.* Low-back injuries cost business and industry over $15 billion annually. As a result, employers throughout the country have become increasingly interested in preventing these injuries. These figures do not include the costs in human suffering, loss of self-worth, and other emotional problems that occur when a person becomes disabled.

Risk Factors for LBP   Health experts believe that the following factors contribute to LBP:

AGE   People between the ages of 20 and 45 run the greatest risk of LBP. At age 50, the condition becomes

* Bureau of Labor Statistics Bulletin, 1991, and National Council on Compensation Insurance, *Yearly Report,* 1991.

less common. After age 65, the incidence again rises, apparently because of bone and joint deterioration.

GENDER   Men and women are equally susceptible to LBP. However, when women are placed in unusual work situations and must lift heavy objects quickly, their risk appears to increase beyond that of men.

BODY TYPES   Many studies have indicated that people who are very tall, overweight, or have lanky body types run an increased risk of LBP. Much of this research remains controversial.

POSTURE   Poor posture may be one of the greatest risk factors for LBP. People who routinely slouch, particularly during their daily tasks, run an increased risk.

STRENGTH AND FITNESS   People with LBP tend to have lower overall trunk strength than those who do not have LBP. Weak abdominal muscles and weak back muscles also increase your risk. In addition, your total level of fitness and conditioning is a factor. The more fit you are, the lower your risk.

PSYCHOLOGICAL FACTORS   Numerous psychological factors appear to increase risk for LBP. Depression, apathy, inattentiveness, boredom, emotional upsets, drug abuse, and family and financial problems all increase your risk.

OCCUPATIONAL RISKS   Evidence indicates that employees who are new to a particular job run the greatest risk of LBP problems. In addition, the type of work that you do and the conditions under which you work greatly affect your risk. For example, truck drivers, who must endure the bumps and jolts of the road while in a sitting position, and materials handlers, who must routinely lift heavy objects, tend to run the greatest risk. Time of day, exposure to vibration, the size and shape of the object being lifted, and many other factors are also involved. Smokers or people with chronic coughs also run an increased risk.

With so many possible causes, is it possible to prevent LBP? Many industries are attempting to control the environmental conditions that lead to back problems. Some industries are attempting to use diagnostic X-rays and health histories to screen employees who might be susceptible to back problems. Other companies assess such factors as a worker's strength before assigning strenuous jobs. Teaching proper lifting technique is an important part of all industrial prevention efforts.

Personal Prevention   What can you as an individual do to protect yourself from possible back injury? First, you must be knowledgeable about what area of the spinal column is most at risk and attempt to protect that area as much as possible. Almost 90 percent of all back problems occur in the lumbar spine region. Consciously

protecting this region of the body from blows, excessive strain, or sharp twists when muscles are not warmed up is essential. In addition, exercise, particularly exercises that strengthen the abdominal muscles and stretch the back muscles, is important. Consult an exercise physiologist, biomechanist, physical therapist, or physician specializing in bone and joint injuries for recommended exercises.

If you are concerned about your risk, you can also avoid many problems by consciously attempting to maintain good posture. Several guidelines have been proposed to help you protect your spine from undue stress during work, recreation, and sleep:

- *Purchase a firm mattress.* Avoid sleeping on your stomach. Some experts recommend that you sleep in a fetal position on your side, with your knees drawn up slightly to ease spinal pressure. Try to determine what works best for your back.
- *Avoid high-heeled shoes.* These shoes can tilt the pelvis forward, causing excessive curvature of the spine and LBP.
- *Control your weight.* Excessive weight puts an added burden on the back muscles and may lead to LBP.
- *Practice proper lifting techniques.* Bend your knees and keep your back straight, taking the load on your legs rather than your back. Try to hold the object as close to the body as possible.
- *Purchase a car with the right seat.* The structure of the driver's seat and the amount of support that the seat gives to the low back should be a major concern when considering an auto purchase. If possible, buy a car that has adjustable lumbar spine supports, which are common in newer car models.
- *Adjust auto seat for comfort.* If you are driving long distances, move the car seat forward, which elevates your knees slightly, increases circulation, and reduces pressure on the lower back.
- *Warm up before exercising.* This is critical in preventing injury to muscles supporting the back. Stretching back muscles and warming up abdominal and leg muscles may reduce your chances of LBP.

Treating Low Back Pain   If you are plagued with periodic aches and pains in the low back area, the use of heat, massage, or whirlpool baths may help ease your pain by relaxing muscles in the affected area. Rest is a key factor in recovery. In addition, pain relievers such as aspirin may be effective for minor problems. However, if your low-back pain persists, if you have difficulty moving, or if you experience numbness or pain radiating to the extremities, consult a physician. This could be the early indication of a problem with disk alignment, a ruptured disk, or another problem requiring immediate attention.

During the last decade, numerous afflictions have surfaced that seem to be products of our times. Some of these health problems relate to specific groups of people, some are due to technological advances, and some are unexplainable. Still other diseases have been present for many years and continue to cause severe disability (see Table 14.2). Among the conditions that have received the most attention in recent years are chronic fatigue syndrome, disorders related to the use of video display terminals, and sudden-infant-death syndrome.

Chronic Fatigue Syndrome

Fatigue is a subjective condition in which people feel tired before they begin activities, lack energy to accomplish tasks that require sustained effort and attention, and become abnormally exhausted after normal activities. Does this sound familiar? To many Americans, such symptoms are all too common. In the late 1980s, however, a characteristic set of symptoms including chronic fatigue, headaches, fever, sore throat, enlarged lymph nodes, depression, poor memory, general weakness, nausea, and symptoms remarkably similar to mononucleosis were noted in several U.S. clinics. Researchers initially believed that they were really talking about a series of symptoms caused by the same virus as mononucleosis, the Epstein-Barr virus. The disease was initially called chronic Epstein-Barr disease, or the "yuppie flu." This pattern of symptoms appeared to occur most commonly in baby boomers in their early thirties, and in some instances the symptoms were so severe that hospitalization was required. Since those initial studies, researchers have all but ruled out the possibility of a mystery form of the Epstein-Barr virus. Despite extensive testing, a viral cause has never been found.

Today most researchers believe that the illness, now commonly referred to as **chronic fatigue syndrome,** has strong psychosocial roots. According to Harvard psychiatrist Arthur Barsky, our heightened awareness of health makes us scrutinize our bodies so carefully that the slightest deviation becomes amplified. The more we focus on our body and on our perception of health, the worse we feel.* In addition, the growing number of people who suffer from depression seem to be good candidates for chronic fatigue syndrome. Chronic fatigue among college students seems to correlate not with too little sleep or too much work, but with indicators of psychopathology: emotional instability, introversion, anxiety, and depression.**

The diagnosis of chronic fatigue syndrome is associated with 2 major criteria and 8 or more minor criteria. Major criteria include debilitating fatigue that persists or relapses for at least 6 months, and the absence of other diagnoses of illnesses that may cause similar symptoms. Minor criteria include headaches, fever, sore throat, painful lymph nodes, weakness, fatigue after exercise, sleep problems, and rapid onset of the above symptoms. Because an exact cause is not apparent, treatment focuses on improved nutrition, rest, counseling for depression, judicious exercise, and development of a strong support network.

Sudden Infant Death Syndrome (SIDS)

Sudden infant death syndrome (SIDS) is the leading cause of death among infants 1 week to 1 year old. SIDS account for approximately 1 in every 500 infant deaths, or about 15 percent of all deaths in this age group. SIDS is "the sudden death of any infant or young child, which is unexpected by history, and in which a thorough postmortem examination fails to demonstrate an adequate cause of death."* Sudden infant death syndrome does not appear to be hereditary. However, parents who have lost one child to SIDS seem to face a slightly higher risk of having another child die in the same way. It is more common among boys, lower socioeconomic groups, families with several children, and infants born prematurely. Deaths from SIDS appear to occur more frequently during cold weather. There is also some evidence that smoking during pregnancy might contribute to SIDS (see Chapter 11).

Babies whose deaths have been attributed to SIDS almost always die during sleep; they are usually found dead in their cribs. Although no direct causes for these deaths have been established, many possible causes have been suggested, including suffocation in bed linens, sleeping in a face-down position, minor respiratory infections, air pollution, vaccines (such as the diphtheria-pertussis-tetanus vaccine), and allergic reactions to baby formulas. However, none of these causes has been proven.

Current research suggests that several conditions during early pregnancy may increase susceptibility to this syndrome. These conditions are primarily related to disruption of blood and oxygen flow to the fetus. Loss of maternal blood during pregnancy, problems with the placenta that impair fetal circulation, maternal anemia, maternal smoking and drug abuse, and too little time for uterine healing between pregnancies appear to be related to SIDS occurrence.

---

* Arthur J. Barsky, "The Paradox of Health," *New England Journal of Medicine* (1988) 318:414–18.
** G. Holmes, J. Kaplan, N. Gantz et al., "Chronic Fatigue Syndrome: A Working Definition," *Annals of Internal Medicine* (1988) 108(3):387–89.

Chronic Fatigue Syndrome Series of symptoms including debilitating fatigue which affects many adults in their twenties and thirties.

* "Public-Private Partnerships Respond to SIDS," *Public Health Macroview* (July/August 1989) p. 7.

Table 14.2   Other Modern Afflictions

Disease	Victims	Symptoms	Risks	Prevention and Treatment
Parkinson's Disease	Affects 1.5 million Americans; rare before age 40; typically begins after age 55.	Gradual, insidious development of 5 major symptoms: 1. *Tremors*–Typically of hand, leg, foot, chin, thumbs, or fingers when not being used. 2. *Rigidity*—Tightness caused by muscle contractions; cramplike pain. 3. *Slowed movement* (bradykinesia) 4. *Loss of autonomic movements*—Diminished control of blinking, smiling, frowning, and other facial expressions. 5. *Walking difficulties*—Shuffling of feet.	Affects men and women equally. No occupational, ethnic, geographic, or social group is at special risk. Not contagious; no links to a specific dietary or environmental cause; not hereditary.	Emotional upsets cause symptom flare-ups. Because the *cause* is not known, prevention is difficult. Major tranquilizers are useful in controlling nerve responses from affected region of brain.
Multiple Sclerosis	Affects approximately 250,000 Americans per year.	Variable; often sudden onset of unexplained blurred vision or blindness; tingling and numbness in extremitis; sporadic urinary control problems; chronic fatigue; neurological problems characterized by remission and relapse.	Cause unknown, virus suspected; affects more men than women; most common in adults in their thirties.	Stress management may be helpful. Disease is often progressive. Medications can be used to control symptoms.
Cystic Fibrosis	Occurs once in every 1,600 births.	Large amounts of mucus, causing lung complications and infections; digestive disturbances; large greasy stools; excessive sodium excretion.	Inherited disease. If both parents have the gene for cystic fibrosis, there is a 25 percent chance that the child will have disease.	Treatment is geared toward relief of symptoms. Antibiotics are administered for infection.
Cerebral Palsy	Believed to occur in people who suffer from a lack of oxygen at birth; a brain disorder or accident before or after birth; poisoning; or brain infections.	Loss of voluntary control over motor functioning.	(See first column)	Avoidance of risks is best method of prevention.
Graves Disease	Can occur at any age.	Thyroid disorder characterized by swelling of the eyes, staring gaze, retraction of the eyelid; in severe cases, blindness may result.	Cause unknown. Autoimmune dysfunction suspected as cause.	Medication may help to control symptoms. Radioactive iodine supplements can also be administered.
Lupus Erythematosus	Can occur at any age; slightly more prevalent in females.	Progressive systemic disease affecting connective tissue, kidneys, and blood vessels, resulting in pain and chronic fatigue	Autoimmune disease; cause unknown.	Drug treatments, medical supervision.

Because the exact cause of SIDS remains in question, most efforts to reduce the incidence of this problem center on close observation of newborns who are believed to be at risk and the use of electrical warning systems that sound an alarm if breathing stops while the baby sleeps.

▌ SUMMARY

- Communicable disease has always been a part of human existence. We have made remarkable progress in our methods of detection, prevention, and treatment during the last century.

- Heredity, aging, drugs and chemical pollutants, lifestyle, pathogens, and other factors all contribute to the occurrence of diseases.

- Major pathogens include bacteria, viruses, protozoa, rickettsia, parasitic worms, and fungi.

- Defenses against disease or injury include the skin and body linings, body fluids, fever, pain, the immune system, and vaccines.

- It is estimated that over 10 million people in the United States every year are afflicted with one or more of the over 20 different types of sexually transmitted diseases (STDs).

- Most STDs are spread through intimate sexual contact and involve the transmission of body fluids.

- Chlamydia is the most common sexual disease the United States today, followed closely by gonorrhea.

- Condylomas (venereal warts) are on the increase in the United States.

- The herpes simplex type I virus is responsible for the development of cold sores. Genital herpes is caused by the herpes simplex type II virus. There are many other forms of herpes viruses, each of which causes a specific disease.

- Acquired immune deficiency syndrome (AIDS) is a major health problem in the world today. Death rates continue to escalate, and no cure has been found. Scientists believe the disease is caused by the HIV virus.

- Although cancer and heart disease capture most of the media attention, other forms of chronic disease often cause more pain, suffering, and disability.

- Respiratory disorders such as hay fever, asthma, emphysema, and chronic bronchitis cause health problems for millions of people throughout the world.

- Headaches may be caused by a variety of factors, the most common of which are tension, dilation of blood vessels in the brain, and underlying physiological and psychological disorders.

- Seizure disorders may be of several different types, each of which may be controlled with appropriate medication.

- Premenstrual syndrome (PMS) is a condition with a variety of symptoms that appear to be related.

15

Successful Life Transitions

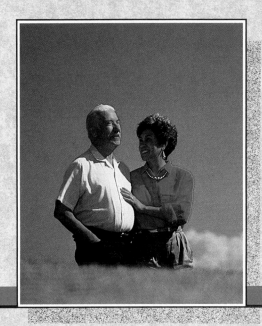

▪ Objectives

- Describe five age-related characteristics, and give a profile of today's elderly. Then describe their impact on society and list the indicators of elder abuse.

- Explain why the traditional use of the term senility reveals an ageist attitude, but why currently the term is still used to describe Alzheimer's disease and other disorders. Then summarize the four biological theories of aging.

- List the physiological and cognitive effects of aging.

- Define death. List its indicators and the definitions that have evolved to facilitate classification of the various phases of biological death.

- Summarize Kubler-Ross's five stages of dying and the three phases common to near-death experiences.

- Distinguish among bereavement, grief, grief work, and mourning.

- List the characteristics of hospice programs and summarize the variety of funeral patterns in the United States. Then discuss some of the decisions that can be made in advance of death to reduce the stress of survivors.

- List the artificial life-support techniques that may be legally refused by competent patients in some states. Then summarize the controversies surrounding each of the following: rational suicide, dyathanasia, and euthanasia.

Each of us has undoubtedly encountered the 80-year-old person who looks and acts like someone who is much younger. Similarly, we have all encountered the 50-year-old who appears to be much older. Determining what we mean when we say that someone is *old* can be difficult. Does aging refer only to chronological years or are there other factors that should be considered? Eventually, everything in the universe—animals, plants, mountain peaks, rivers, planets, and even atoms—undergoes changes over time. This process is commonly referred to as *aging*. The struggle to slow down what are perceived as the negative aspects of the aging process has been a part of human existence since our earliest recorded history. The manner in which we age and the speed with which the inevitable changes of age affect us are largely determined by our history.

From the moment of conception we have genetic predispositions that influence our vulnerabilities to many diseases, our physical characteristics, and many other traits that make us unique as individuals. Maternal nutrition and health habits influence our health while we are in the womb and during the early months after birth. From the time we are born, we begin to take on characteristics that distinguish us from everyone else. We grow, we change, and we pass through many physical and psychological phases. **Aging** has traditionally been described as the patterns of life changes that occur in members of all species as they grow older. Some believe that aging begins at the moment of conception. Others contend that aging begins at birth. Still others believe that true aging does not begin until we reach our forties and

continues until death. Typically, chronological age has been used to assign a person to a particular life-cycle stage. However, it is important to note that people of different chronological ages view age very differently. To a 4-year-old, a freshman in college seems very old. To the 20-year-old, parents in their forties often seem "over the hill." Have you ever raised your eyebrows upon hearing your 65-year-old grandparents talk about those "old people down the street"? Clearly, our traditional definitions of what it means to grow old—to age—need careful reexamination.

AGING REVISITED

Discrimination against people based on age is known as **ageism.** When directed against the elderly, this type of discrimination carries with it social ostracism and negative portrayals of the elderly.

The study of our individual and collective aging processes, known as **gerontology,** explores the reasons for aging and the ways in which people cope with this process. Gerontologists have identified several types of age-related characteristics that should be used in determining where a person is in terms of life-stage devel-

---

Aging   The patterns of life changes that occur in members of all species as they grow older.
Ageism   Discrimination based on age.
Gerontology   The study of our individual and collective aging processes.

Age and Life-Stage Development

Age-Related Characteristics

Biological Age   The relative age or condition of a person's organs and body systems. Arthritis and other chronic conditions often accelerate the aging process. Biological age varies considerably from species to species.

Psychological Age   A person's adaptive capacities, such as coping ability and intelligence, and also a person's awareness of his or her individual capacities, self-efficacy, and general ability to adapt to a given situation.

Social Age   A person's habits and roles relative to society's expectations (e.g., likes and dislikes in music selection, television shows, etc.).

Legal Age   Based on chronological years and the most common definition of age in the United States. Legal age is used to determine voting rights, driving privileges, drinking age, eligibility for Social Security, and a whole host of individual rights.

Functional Age   The ways in which a person compares to others of a similar age. Heart rate, skin thickness, hearing, and other individual characteristics are analyzed and compared.

opment—biological, psychological, social, legal, and functional.*

Normal Aging?

Gerontologists have devised special categories for specific age-related characteristics. For example, people who reach the age of 65 are considered to fit the chronological pattern of "old age" and receive special consideration in the form of government assistance programs such as Social Security and Medicare. People aged 65 to 74 are viewed as the *young-old;* those aged 75 to 84 comprise the *middle-old* group. Those over age 84 are classified as the *old-old.*

Despite these categories, note that chronological age is not the only component to be considered when objectively defining "aging." The question is not how many years a person lives but "how much life" is injected into

———
* Bert Hayslip and Paul Panek, *Adult Development and Aging* (New York: Harper & Row, 1989), p. 14.

those years. This quality-of-life index, combined with the inevitable chronological process, appears to be the best indicator of the "aging gracefully" phenomenon. The eternal question then becomes "How can I age gracefully?" Although there clearly is no fountain of youth, most experts today agree that the best way to experience a productive, full, and satisfying old age is to take appropriate actions to lead a productive, full, and satisfying life prior to old age. Essentially, we are the product of our lifelong experiences, molded over years of happiness, heartbreak, and day-to-day existence.

Profile of Today's Elderly

Whereas the average American could expect to live until age 47 in 1900, the typical American today has an average life expectancy of well over 75 years (see Chapter 1). Where will these elderly people live? Who will pay for their increasing medical costs? How will they support themselves? These questions become more important when other factors we discuss later are considered.

Promoting Your Health

Are You Preparing for Old Age?

Please complete the following self-assessment. Complete statements 1 through 5. Do your responses seem appropriate to you? Why or why not? How do you think others your age might respond? How might your grandfather or grandmother respond?

1. The most important things in life to me right now are _____
   _____ .

2. When I am 70 years old, the most important things to me will probably be _____
   _____ .

3. The things that I look forward to about aging are _____
   _____ .

4. The things that I dread the most about aging are _____
   _____ .

5. The terms that come to mind when I think of "old" people are _____
   _____ .

Answer each of the following questions. How do you think other people might regard your responses? Why?

1. When your parents are too old to care for themselves, what will you be most likely to do? What is the rationale for your decision?

2. How comfortable would you be if you had to bathe your mother or father? Do you think your response is typical of those of others? How do you think your mother or father might feel about your bathing them? What actions might you take now to ease the level of discomfort that you might feel performing such intimate caregiving at a later point in your life?

3. When you are too old to care for yourself, what would you like to have happen? Is your response different from the one you suggested for your parents in the first question? Why or why not?

4. When you reach the age of 70, how would you like to be able to describe yourself? What things might you do now and in the years ahead to ensure that you fulfill the type of life expectations that you have set for yourself?

Promoting Your Health

The Principles of Age

When I Am an Old Woman. . . .

I shall wear purple
With a red hat which doesn't go, and doesn't suit
  me.
And I shall spend my pension on brandy and
  summer gloves
And satin sandals, and say we've no money for
  butter.
I shall sit down on the pavement when I'm tired
And gobble up samples in shops and press alarm
  bells
And run my stick along the public railings
And make up for the sobriety of my youth.
I shall go out in my slippers in the rain
And pick the flowers in other people's gardens
And learn to spit.

You can wear terrible shirts and grow more fat
And eat three pounds of sausages at a go
Or only bread and pickle for a week.
And hoard pens and pencils and beermats and
  things in boxes.

But now we must have clothes that keep us dry
And pay our rent and not swear in the street

And set a good example for the children.
We must have friends to dinner and read the
  papers.

But maybe I ought to practice a little now?
So people who know me are not too shocked and
  surprised
When suddenly I am old and start to wear purple.

From *Warning*
by Jenny Joseph

1. What is this woman saying about the way she has lived her life?

2. In what ways do you think that you are like her? Unlike her?

3. At what times in our lives do you think we suddenly realize that the time and energy spent trying to follow the prescribed path of living might have been put to better use?

4. List five actions you can take in the next month that will help you lead a happier, less stressful life.

How Many Elderly? The older population—people 65 years or older—numbered 30.4 million in 1988. They represented 12.4 percent of the U.S. population, about 1 in every 8 Americans. The number of older Americans had increased by 4.7 million, or 18 percent, since 1980, compared to an increase of 7 percent for the under-65 population.*

In 1988, there were 18 million older women and 12.4 million older men, or a sex ratio of 147 women for every 100 men. The sex ratio increases with age, ranging from 120 women for every 100 men in the 65-to-69-year-old group to a high of 257 women for every 100 men in the 85-and-older age group.

Impact on Society

Retirement Costs When **Social Security** was initiated in 1935, there were approximately 35 people paying into the system for every recipient. At that time, the real

dollars available for recipients were much greater because the costly bureaucratic network had not been established. Fewer people chose to receive benefits from a perceived government "giveaway" program, so payroll deductions to support the system were minimal. Today, approximately three people pay into the Social Security system for every recipient. The system itself is huge and costs billions of dollars to operate. At the same time, people rely on Social Security for their financial security, and the number of recipients continues to grow steadily as the elderly population grows. Consequently, an increasing share of our paychecks is diverted toward supporting the Social Security system. The question arises as to whether the present Social Security system can survive. How much will we be willing to pay to assist the elderly in the future? What impact would abolishment of Social Security have on the elderly? What are the alternatives?

---

* The statistics presented here are from *Profile of Older Americans* (Washington, DC: American Association of Retired Persons, 1989), pp. 1–2.

Social Security A federal system of insurance for elderly persons financed by employees, employers, and the government.

Profile of Older Americans

The Graying of America

The 65+ population has doubled in the past 70 years.
The 85+ population has quadrupled in the past 70 years and will double again by 2010 to reach approximately 21 percent of the population.

INCOME

Households headed by persons 65+ reported a median income in 1989 as follows:
$23,179 (all races)
$23,817 (whites)
$15,766 (blacks)
$19,310 (Hispanics)

About 3.4 million elderly persons were below the poverty level in 1989.

MARITAL STATUS

77 percent of elderly men are married.
42 percent of elderly women are married.

LIVING ARRANGEMENTS

The majority of older persons live in a family setting.
About 30 percent of all noninstitutionalized older persons live alone (6.8 million women, 1.9 million men).
Five percent live in nursing homes.

EDUCATION

Median level of education in 1988 = 12.1 years.
The educational level of the older population has been steadily increasing.

SOURCE: 1990 U.S. Bureau of the Census.

Health Costs Although the elderly represented only 12.7 percent of the U.S. population in 1988, they accounted for over 36 percent of the total national health-care costs. To a large extent, these figures reflect the intense use of expensive medical procedures in treating people with major diseases such as cancer, heart disease, and respiratory ailments. With projected future increases in life expectancy, many analysts fear that health-care costs will skyrocket even more. Will Americans be willing to pay an increased share of the health-care bill for people on fixed incomes who cannot pay for themselves?

Abuse of Older Parents

Although the estimated number of cases varies considerably, it is generally agreed that abuse of elderly parents, grandparents, and other relatives is a hidden aspect of life for many people. This abuse may be overt, such as beatings or physical aggression toward older family members, or it may be of a much more subtle mental or emotional nature. Whereas some elderly parents may show physical bruises, others may actually be driven from the family home and left to fend for themselves with no money or food. Because they are ashamed of what their children are doing to them, or because they fear reprisal, most elderly victims of abuse never report the abuse to the authorities. There are various reasons for such abuse, including revenge for childhood abuse

and a blatant rejection of responsibility on the part of the children. The likelihood of resentment and abuse is greatest for those who have never had a good relationship with their parents, for families in which alcohol and drugs have been a significant factor, and for those who find themselves in serious economic trouble. (See the box entitled, "Detecting Elder Abuse: Causes and Indicators.")

Recognizing the potential risk of abuse, social service organizations have begun to offer counseling and support to adult caregivers, particularly those who must provide care for ailing or disabled parents. In addition, programs designed to help families communicate and work together to solve problems are increasing in many areas of the country.

DISORDERS COMMON TO THE ELDERLY

Senility: An Ageist Attitude

Over the years, the elderly have often been the victims of ageist attitudes. The term **senility** is commonly used to denote a form of mental impairment characterized by memory failure, errors in judgment, and erratic behav-

Senility A term associated with memory loss and judgment and orientation problems occurring in a small percentage of the elderly.

Detecting Elder Abuse

Causes and Indicators

CAUSES

Stress causes caregivers to abuse

Adult child feels powerless

Abusers have individual personality problems

Abusers come from dysfunctional abusive family backgrounds

Abusers exhibit external stress

Elderly isolation

Indicators

HISTORY

Pattern of "physician hopping"

Unexplained delay in seeking treatment

Series of missed medical appointments

Previous unexplained injuries

Explanation of past injuries inconsistent with medical findings

Previous reports of similar injuries

PHYSICAL INDICATORS

Injuries, which may have been inflicted on the patient by others, either maliciously or through neglect
    Fractures, dislocations
    Lacerations, abrasions
    Burns in unusual locations or of unusual shapes
    Injuries to head, scalp, or face
    Bruises

Other
    Poor personal hygiene
    Signs of overmedication, undermedication, misuse of medications
    Sexually transmitted disease
    Pain, itching, or bleeding in genital area

OBSERVATIONAL INDICATORS

Psychological
    Low self-esteem
    Overly anxious or withdrawn
    Extreme changes in mood
    Depression
    Suicidal ideation
    Confusion or disorientation

Interactions between patient and family member/companion
    Patient appears fearful of companion

Conflicting accounts of incident between patient and companion

Absence of assistance, attitudes of indifference, or anger toward patient exhibited by companion

Companion overly concerned with costs of treatment needed by patient

Companion denies patient the chance to interact privately with the physician

SOURCE: J. S. Bloom, P. Ansell, and M. N. Bloom, "Detecting Elder Abuse: A Guide for Physicians," *Geriatrics* (1989) 44(6):40–44, 56.

---

iors. People who were chronologically old were often inadvertently labeled "senile" whenever they displayed any of the symptoms just listed. This term has numerous derogatory connotations. Today, scientists recognize that these same groups of symptoms can occur at any age and for various reasons. For example, a person who is diabetic and suffering from problems with insulin regulation might show temporary signs of disorientation. Other OTC and prescription drugs may cause similar problems, as may a lack of oxygen in people suffering from emphysema. When the underlying problems are corrected, the memory loss and disorientation also improve. Currently, the term *senility* is seldom used except to describe a very small group of organic disorders. It is now considered an imprecise term to describe a problem that may have multiple causes.

Alzheimer's Disease One of the most disabling afflictions threatening older people is **Alzheimer's disease,** a chronic condition involving changes in the nerve fibers that causes mental deterioration, which attacks an estimated 1 in 20 people between the ages of 65 and 75. It may afflict 1 in 5 people over the age of 80, and the disease has been diagnosed in people as early as their late forties and early fifties.

Once Alzheimer's disease strikes, the life expectancy of the victim is cut in half. Tragically, there is little that can be done to treat the disorder. Scientists are experimenting with various drug regimens, but it is unlikely that a drug will be discovered in the foreseeable future

---

Alzheimer's Disease A chronic condition involving changes in nerve fibers of the brain that results in mental deterioration.

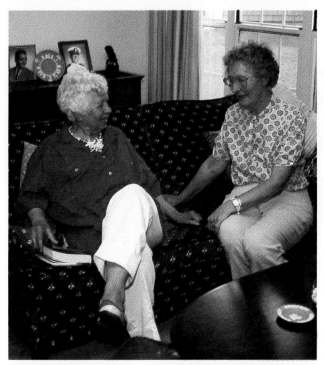

Social interaction is very important among the elderly. These senior citizens have found support by sharing an apartment.

that will undo the damage associated with Alzheimer's disease.

The results of research into the causes of Alzheimer's disease remain inconclusive. Currently, the theories being considered include the following:

- Malfunction of the immune system
- A slow-acting virus

The old woman I shall become will be quite different from the woman I am now. Another I is beginning and so far I have not had to complain of her.

(George Sand)

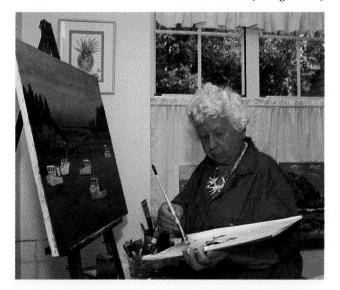

- Exposure to excessive levels of aluminum
- Chromosomal or genetic defects.

Caring for patients with Alzheimer's disease is a challenge for even the most prepared family members. Having to decide between trying to tend to the needs of a loved one at home or seeking the assistance of a long-term-care facility can be difficult. Resources are currently being devoted to helping family members cope with the multiple demands placed on them as caregivers of Alzheimer's patients. Even the best preparation for the final days of our parents and loved ones does not make the process an easy one. Knowing what your options are and recognizing the differences between normal physiological aging and the ravages of certain diseases can help make age-related problems easier to cope with for both the elderly themselves and for family members.

THE AGING PROCESS

"Most people say that as you get old, you have to give up things. I think you get old because you give up things."
(Theodore Francis Green)

The question of what is "typical" or "normal" when applied to aging is highly speculative. In order to assess the typical aging process, we should probably ask ourselves what it is that we can reasonably expect to happen to our bodies as we grow older.

The Aging Body: Physiological Aspects

Although the physiological consequences of aging differ in their severity and timing from person to person, there are standard changes that occur as a result of the aging process.

The Skin As a normal consequence of aging, the skin becomes thinner and loses elasticity, particularly in the outer surfaces. Fat deposits, which add to the soft lines and shape of the skin, begin to diminish. Starting at about the age of 30, lines develop on the forehead as a result of smiling, squinting, and other facial expressions. These lines become more pronounced, with added crow's-feet around the eyes, during the forties. During a person's fifties and sixties, the skin begins to sag and lose color, leading to pallor in the seventies. Body fat in underlying layers of skin continues to be redistributed away from the limbs and extremities and into the trunk region of the body. Age spots become more numerous because of excessive pigment accumulation under the skin. The sun tends to increase pigment production, leading to more age spots.

Bones and Joints Throughout the life span, a person's bones are continually changing because of the addi-

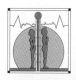

Biological Theories of Aging*

The Wear-and-Tear Theory: The wear-and-tear theory proposes that, like everything else in the universe, the human body wears out. Proponents of this theory agree that activities such as jogging may actually predispose people to premature bone and joint injuries in later years.

The Cellular Theory: According to the cellular theory, we have at birth only a certain number of usable cells which are genetically programmed to divide or reproduce only a limited number of times. Once they reach the end of their reproductive cycle, these cells begin to die, and the organs they comprise begin to show signs of deterioration. The rate of this deterioration depends on the system involved.

The Autoimmune Theory: The autoimmune theory attributes aging to the decline of the body's immunological system. As we age our immune systems become less effective in fighting disease. Eventually, bodies that are subjected to too much stress, coupled with poor nutrition, begin to show signs of disease and infirmity.

The Genetic Mutation Theory: The genetic mutation theory proposes that the number of cells exhibiting unusual or different characteristics increases with age. The greater the mutation, the greater the chance that cells will not function properly, leading to eventual dysfunction of body organs and systems.

* Numerous psychological and sociological factors also have a strong influence on the manner in which people age. Most probably a combination of psychosocial and biological factors, combined with environmental "trigger mechanisms," causes each of us to age in a unique manner.

---

tion and loss of minerals. By the third or fourth decade of life, mineral loss from bones becomes more prevalent than mineral accumulation, resulting in a weakening and porosity (diminishing density) of bony tissue. This loss of minerals (particularly calcium) occurs in both sexes, although it is much more common in females. Loss of calcium can contribute to **osteoporosis** (see box).

The Head   With age, features of the head enlarge and become more noticeable. Increased cartilage and fatty tissue cause the nose to grow a half-inch wider and another half-inch longer. Earlobes get fatter and grow longer, while overall head circumference increases one-quarter of an inch per decade, even though the brain itself shrinks. The skull becomes thicker with age.

The Urinary Tract   At age 70, the kidneys can filter waste from the blood only half as fast as they could at age 30. The need to urinate more frequently occurs because the bladder's capacity declines from 2 cups of urine at age 30 to 1 cup at age 70.

The Heart and Lungs   Resting heart rate stays about the same during a person's life, but the stroke volume (the amount of blood the muscle pushes out per beat) is diminished as heart muscles deteriorate. Vital capacity, or the amount of air that moves when you inhale and exhale at maximum effort, also declines with age. Exer-

cise can do a great deal to reduce potential deterioration in heart and lung function.

Eyesight   By the age of 30, the lens of the eye begins to harden, causing specific problems by the early forties. The lens begins to yellow and loses transparency, while the pupil of the eye begins to shrink, allowing less light to penetrate. Activities such as reading become more difficult, particularly in dim light. By age 60, depth perception declines and farsightedness often develops. A need for glasses usually develops in the forties that evolves into a need for bifocals in the fifties and trifocals in the sixties. **Cataracts** (clouding of the lens) and **glaucoma** (hardening of the eyeball) become more likely. There may eventually be a tendency toward colorblindness, especially for shades of blue and green.

Hearing   The ability to hear high-frequency consonants (for example, *s, t,* and *z*) diminishes with age. Much of the actual hearing loss is in the ability to distinguish not normal conversational tones but extreme ranges of sound.

Osteoporosis   A degenerative bone disorder characterized by increasingly porous bones.
Cataracts   Clouding of the lens that interrupts the focusing of light on the retina, resulting in blurred vision or eventual blindness.
Glaucoma   Elevation of pressure within the eyeball, leading to hardening of the eyeball, impaired vision, and possible blindness.

Taste The sense of taste begins to decline as a person gets older. At age 30, each tiny elevation on the tongue (called *papilla*) has 245 taste buds. By the age of 70, each has only 88 left. The mouth gets drier as salivary glands secrete less fluid. The ability to distinguish sweet, sour, bitter, and salty tastes diminishes. Elderly people often compensate for their diminished sense of taste by adding excessive amounts of salt, sugar, and other flavor enhancers to their food.

Smell and Touch The sense of smell also diminishes with age. As a result of this loss, coupled with the loss of the sense of taste, food is often less appealing to older people. Pain receptors also become less effective. The tactile senses decline.

Sexual Changes with Age As men age, they experience notable changes in sexual functioning. Whereas the degree and rate of change vary greatly from person to person, the following changes generally occur.

1. The ability to obtain an erection is slowed.
2. The ability to maintain an erection is diminished.
3. The amount of time required for the refractory period between orgasms increases.
4. The angle of the erection declines with age.
5. The orgasm itself grows shorter in duration.

The female body also undergoes several changes.

1. Menopause occurs between the ages of 45 and 55. Women may experience such symptoms as hot flashes, mood swings, weight gain, development of facial hair, and other hormone-related problems.
2. The walls of the vagina become less elastic, and the epithelium thins, making painful intercourse more likely.
3. Vaginal secretions during sexual activity diminish.
4. The breasts decrease in firmness. Loss of fat in various areas leads to fewer curves, with a decrease in the soft lines of the body contours.

Body Comfort Because of the loss of body fat, thinning of the epithelium, and diminished glandular activity, elderly people experience greater difficulty in regulating body temperature. This change means that their ability to withstand extreme cold or heat may be very limited, thus increasing the risks of hypothermia, heatstroke, and heat exhaustion.

The Aging Body: Cognitive Perspectives

Intelligence Stereotypes concerning inevitable intellectual decline among the elderly have been largely refuted. Recent research has demonstrated that much of our previous knowledge about elderly intelligence was based on inappropriate testing procedures. Given an appropriate length of time, elderly people may learn and develop skills in a similar manner to younger people. It has also been determined that what many elderly people may lack in speed of learning they make up for in practical knowledge—that is, the "wisdom of age."

Memory Have you ever wondered about your grandfather's inability to remember what he did last weekend while he can graphically depict the details of a social event that occurred 40 years earlier? This phenomenon is not unusual among the elderly. Research indicates that although short-term memory may fluctuate on a daily basis, the ability to remember events from past decades seems to remain largely unchanged in many elderly people.

Flexibility versus Rigidity Although it is widely believed that people become more homogeneous as they age, nothing could be further from the truth. Having lived through a multitude of experiences and having faced diverse joys, sorrows, and obstacles, the typical elderly person has developed unique methods of coping with life. These unique adaptive variations make for interesting differences in how the elderly confront the many changes brought on by the aging process. As a group, the elderly are extremely *heterogeneous*. The idea that they become religious, white-haired conservatives with similar political ideologies and moral doctrines is erroneous.

Environment versus Biology

Although each of the changes outlined in the preceding sections occurs to some extent, we do not know the degree to which each is inevitable or preventable. Distinguishing between those conditions that occur as a natural part of the aging process and those that occur as a result of environmental factors and lifestyle is difficult. For example, the changes that occur in the elasticity and texture of the skin are certainly related to age. However, the relative impact that smoking, exposure to ultraviolet light, and skin deterioration have on the rate and severity of this process remains difficult to determine.

DEATH DEFINED

Dying and death are complex topics that raise questions without simple answers. Throughout history, humans have attempted to determine the nature and meaning of death. The questions continue today. Moral and philosophical questions about death must be addressed and will be touched on, but we do not explore these issues in depth. Instead, we present dying and death as normal components of life and discuss how we can cope with these events.

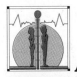
Osteoporosis: An Epidemic Among Older Women

A question often asked, especially by women is, "How much milk should I drink every day to get enough calcium?" The answer, which often elicits a gasp, is that you should consume the amount of calcium contained in five glasses of milk. Few adult Americans consume anywhere near that level of calcium. Current statistics indicate that we pay a high price for our neglect of this vital nutrient.

Osteoporosis, a weakened condition of the bones in which small fractures occur, results from a slow, insidious loss of calcium and has become an epidemic among American women. Depending on how long they live, up to 40 percent of American women develop osteoporosis, the first sign of which is usually a broken bone or collapsed vertebra. Although men are not immune to this problem, the disease is far more common among females, probably due in part to the hormonal changes that accompany menopause. After menopause, the average American woman loses an inch and a half in height each decade as a result of vertebral collapse. Far more serious are the millions of fractures and tens of thousands of deaths that occur as weakened bones break in response to the strains of normal living.

Women at highest risk are those who are white, thin, petite, sedentary, postmenopausal, and cigarette smokers, and who have a family history of osteoporosis.

The disease, however, can occur whenever anyone fails to take advantage of known protective factors. The following are the main preventive considerations.

Dietary Calcium

The average middle-aged American female consumes only one-third of the calcium she needs to maintain normal bone strength. Even teenaged girls are commonly deficient in calcium. The recommended daily dietary allowance (RDA) for calcium for adult women who are neither pregnant nor nursing is 800 milligrams per day. Recent studies have indicated that in order to ensure absorption, this RDA should be closer to 1,000 mg/day before menopause and 1,200 to 1,500 mg/day after menopause. Typical consumption among American women over 45 is only 450 mg/day.

The best sources of calcium are milk, yogurt, hard cheese, sardines, canned salmon (with lots of bones), and certain dark green leafy vegetables (collards, kale, turnip greens, mustard greens, and broccoli). For those who cannot eat enough calcium-rich foods, calcium supplements such as calcium carbonate supply the most calcium per tablet at the least cost. Calcium is best absorbed if consumed throughout the day, rather than all at once, with one dose taken before bedtime.

The student who is looking for "the right way" to approach death will not find the answer in this text, because there *is* no right way. Confrontations with death elicit different feelings depending on many factors, including age, religious beliefs, family orientation, health, personal experience with death, and the circumstances of the death itself. To cope effectively with dying, we must address the individual needs of those involved. We identify some of those needs and offer information and suggestions that have been helpful to many people as they face the final transition of life.

Dying is the process of decline in body functions resulting in the death of an organism. **Death** can be defined as the "final cessation of the vital functions" and also refers to a state in which these functions are "incapable of being restored."* This definition has become more significant as medical and scientific advances have made it increasingly possible to postpone death.

Traditional indicators of biological death include the following:

> Cessation of vital functions such as heartbeat and respiration
>
> Unresponsiveness of the senses to stimuli (for example, of the eyes to light)
>
> Cyanosis (bluing) of the lips and extremities.

These indicators of biological death were universally accepted until high-technology societies developed sophisticated death-prevention techniques, resulting in the

---

* *Oxford English Dictionary,* 1969, pp. 72, 334, 735.

Dying   The act or state of losing one's physical life; to face death.
Death   A permanent cessation of all vital functions; the state of being dead.

A Medical Problem of the Elderly (*Continued*)

Salt, coffee, alcohol, lack of vitamin D, frequent low-calorie diets, excessive consumption of phosphorus (such as in soft drinks), undue stress, and smoking more than one pack of cigarettes per day all interfere with calcium absorption.

Prevention and Intervention

Other than direct consumption of calcium, perhaps the best way to strengthen bones and increase bone mass is through exercise. Like muscles, bones weaken. Activities that stress the long bones of the body—for example, walking, jogging, bicycling, jumping rope, tennis, basketball, and dancing—are most effective in preventing osteoporosis.

Although moderate amounts of exercise are good, excessive exercise can be counterproductive. Women who exercise to a point of ultrathinness and who lose their menstrual periods as a result actually suffer a loss of calcium, probably because of hormonal deficiency. Moderate exercise, combined with sensible attention to calcium ingestion, is perhaps the most effective means of avoiding excessive bone deterioration.

To date, the best method for preventing or slowing the progress of osteoporosis is estrogen replacement therapy. In the absence of exercise, estrogen therapy is remarkably effective. Women who have a history of breast or cervical cancer are typically unable to have estrogen replacement therapy, due to increased risk for recurrence of cancer. Recently, researchers have noted a possible breakthrough compound called *Etidronate* (a biophosphonate) that appears to slow the process of bone loss and may, in fact, improve bone mass in women with osteoporosis.

New Controversies

Recent research has forced scientists to reconsider some accepted ideas concerning osteoporosis. For example, in certain other countries where dairy products and calcium-rich products are virtually nonexistent, osteoporosis occurs much less frequently than in the United States. This research opens the door for a more careful assessment of the roles of heredity, environment, and exercise in the development of osteoporosis. It also raises the question of whether too much calcium, like too much of any of our overused vitamin supplements, is really the answer to a serious problem.

Sources: Nelson Watts et al., "Intermittent Cyclical Etidronate Treatment of Postmenopausal Osteoporosis," *New England Journal of Medicine* (1990) 323(2):73–80; L. J. Melton et al., "Epidemiology of Vertebral Fractures in Women," *American Journal of Epidemiology* (1989) 129:1000–11.

---

introduction of the *absence of brain function* as an additional indicator of death.

In response to legal and ethical questions related to death and dying, a presidential commission developed the Uniform Determination of Death Act in 1981, with endorsement by the American Medical Association, the American Bar Association, and the National Conference for Commissioners on Uniform State Laws. This act, which has been adopted by several states, reads as follows: "An individual who has sustained either (1) irreversible cessation of circulatory and respiratory functions, or (2) irreversible cessation of all functions of the entire brain, including the brainstem, is dead. A determination of death must be made in accordance with accepted medical standards."* The following definitions have subsequently evolved to facilitate classification of various phases of biological death.

CELL DEATH   Death of a cell after all metabolic activity has ceased. The rate of cellular death varies according to the type of tissue involved. For example, higher brain cells die 5 to 8 minutes after respiration stops; striated muscle cells die after 2 to 4 hours; kidney cells die after

---

* Uniform Determination of Death Act (1981) in *Deciding to Forgo Life-Sustaining Treatment,* by the President's Commission for the Study of Ethical Problems in Medicine and Biomedical and Behavioral Research. (New York: Concern for Dying—An Educational Council, 1983), p. 9.

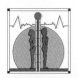

Health Strategies

Activities for Health Enhancement

Keep physically fit: If we are in good physical shape, exercise regularly, and have good muscle strength and agility, the likelihood we will be able to perform optimally is greatly enhanced. Although we may never prove that exercise by itself extends life, the positive benefits to be derived from lifelong regular exercise cannot be denied.

Eat an appropriate diet: Eating a proper diet throughout the life span ensures that we maintain strong bones, healthy organs, and optimal weight. Controlling the consumption of alcohol and fats are examples of behaviors that people can adopt to maximize their potential for good health.

Keep mentally active: For some people, keeping mentally active means they are also socially active. Some people are happy to let others be their source of mental stimulation. Others find pleasure in reading, going to plays, and engaging in other activities by themselves.

Maintain a variety of support networks: Relationships with friends, family, church, and other social contacts is important. We all need a friend or someone we can call on when we need help, or when we just want to talk.

Take care of known afflictions early: Regardless of whether you are 20 or 45, if you notice a small lump in your breast, you should have it checked immediately. If your arm aches excessively after playing tennis, make sure it is not the first warning sign of arthritis.

Have regular checkups: Everyone, regardless of age, should know his or her risk factors and have periodic medical examinations.

Learn to accept help when help is needed: Seek advice or assistance when needed and don't feel foolish or intimidated. If you acquire these skills early in life, they will help carry you through the later years.

Take positive steps now to plan for your secure retirement: Although living for the moment may be enjoyable, financial problems that result may cause undue strain and may seriously limit mobility and socialization later in life.

Do not allow yourself to stagnate: Stagnation can occur at any age. Change is always stressful, but if planned for can add to the spice of life.

---

about 7 hours; and epithelial cells (hair and nails) die after several days. **Rigor mortis,** the temporary stiffening of muscles, is associated with cell death.

LOCAL DEATH   Death of a body part or portion of an organ without the death of the entire organism. For example, a kidney might fail, part of the heart muscle might die, or a limb or section of intestine might die as a result of loss of circulation.

SOMATIC DEATH   The death of the entire organism, as opposed to death of a part of an organ or an extremity.

APPARENT DEATH   Cessation of vital physiologic functions, particularly spontaneous cardiac and respiratory activities, which produces a state simulating actual death, but from which *recovery is possible* through the use of resuscitative efforts.

FUNCTIONAL DEATH   Extensive and *irreversible* damage to the central nervous system, with respiration and circulatory function maintained only by artificial means.

BRAIN DEATH   The termination of brain function, as evidenced by loss of all reflexes and electric activity of the brain or irreversible coma. Brain death is confirmed by an **electroencephalogram** (EEG) reading of electrical activity of brain cells. As determined in 1968 by the Ad Hoc Committee of the Harvard Medical School, brain death must meet the following criteria:

1. Unreceptivity and unresponsiveness; that is, no response even to painful stimuli
2. No movements for a continuous hour after observation by a physician and no breathing after 3 minutes off a respirator
3. No reflexes, including brainstem reflexes; pupils are fixed and dilated.
4. A "flat" EEG for at least 10 minutes

Rigor Mortis   The temporary stiffening of muscles that occurs after death.

Electroencephalogram   The tracing of brain waves made by an electronic sensing apparatus designed to detect electrical activity of the cells near the surface of the brain (the cerebral cortex).

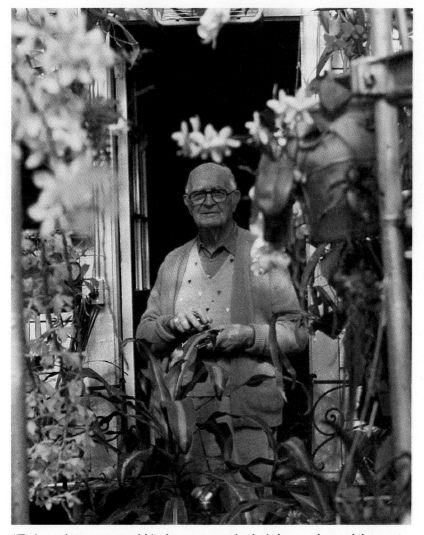

"To know how to grow old is the masterwork of wisdom, and one of the most difficult chapters in the great art of living."

(*Amiel*)

5. All of these tests repeated at least 24 hours later with no change
6. Certainty that hypothermia (extreme loss of body heat) and depression of the central nervous system through use of drugs such as barbiturates are not responsible for the conditions.*

Most of these criteria are relatively easy to understand, but the term *flat* (isographic) *EEG* is often incorrectly interpreted by the general public. Part of our misconception may stem from exposure to dramatic medical crises on television, in which frantic attempts to save a victim are suddenly discontinued when the EEG tracing drags across the graph paper in an unerring straight line. The patient is declared "dead" at this point, and we logically conclude that a "flat EEG" can be equated with total brain death—that is, a complete absence of electrical activity anywhere in the brain.

This conclusion is inaccurate. In actuality, an EEG records electrical activity only in the outermost layers of the brain. These layers, the cortex and neocortex, are composed of highly differentiated cells that integrate sensory input in an individually characteristic manner, thereby producing a unique personality. It is accepted by most experts that the loss of function of these outer layers of the brain results in death of the *person*, but not necessarily in death of the physical body. Lower brain centers may still retain some degree of electrical activity, thus preserving some vital functions such as breathing, cardiac function, digestion, elimination of wastes, and reflex action. Although a flat EEG is valuable when used in conjunction with other criteria for brain death, it cannot be considered an adequate indicator of death when used alone.

Despite the development of these specific death indicators, the issue of death determination remains prob-

* Ad Hoc Committee of the Harvard Medical School to Examine the Definition of Brain Death, "A Definition of Irreversible Coma," *Journal of the American Medical Association*, vol. 205, 1968, p. 377.

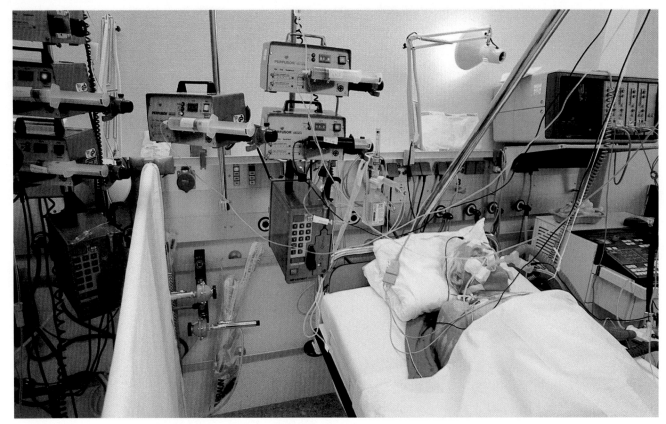

A patient in an intensive care unit.

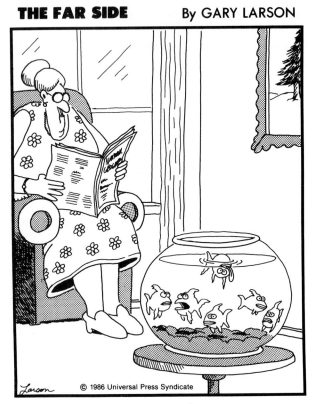

THE FAR SIDE   By GARY LARSON

© 1986 Universal Press Syndicate

"Dang, that gives me the creeps.
... I wish she'd hurry up and scoop that guy out."

lematic and surrounded by ethical dilemmas. In the 1980s, experts modified the standards for death determination in response to ethical questions resulting from organ-transplant technology. The new rules stated that the signs of death for an organ donor must be affirmed by two physicians, neither of whom is on the transplant team. We can expect continued controversy and further modification of policy as medical technology progresses.

▌ THE PROCESS OF DYING

Dying is a complex process that includes physical, intellectual, social, spiritual, and emotional dimensions. Accordingly, the process of dying must be considered from several perspectives. Although the preceding section primarily examined the physical indicators of death, consideration of the emotional aspects of dying and "social death" is essential in establishing an appreciation for the multifaceted nature of life and health.

Stages in an Emotional Experience

Science and medicine have enabled us to understand changes associated with growth, development, aging, and social roles throughout the life span, but they have not revealed the nature of death. This may partially explain why the transition from life to death evokes so much mystery and emotion. Although emotional reactions to dying do vary, there seem to be many similarities in this process.

Much of our knowledge about reactions to dying stems from the work of Elisabeth Kübler-Ross, a major figure in modern **thanatology,** the study of death and dying. In 1969, Kübler-Ross published *On Death and Dying,* a sensitive analysis of the reactions of terminally ill patients. This pioneering work encouraged the development of death education as a discipline and prompted efforts to improve the care of dying patients. In her book, Kübler-Ross identified five psychological stages that terminally ill patients often experience as they approach death: denial, anger, bargaining, depression, and acceptance (see Figure 15.1). The health-care profession immediately embraced this "stage theory" and hastily applied it in clinical settings. Although inappropriate applications of the untested theory resulted in numerous problems, Kübler-Ross's observations are still useful. A summation of the five stages follows.

Denial This is usually the first stage, experienced as a sensation of shock and disbelief. A person intellectually accepts the impending death but cannot accept it on an emotional level. The patient is too confused and stunned to comprehend "not being" and thus rejects the idea. Within a relatively short time, the anxiety level diminishes, enabling the patient to sort through the powerful web of emotions.

Anger Anger is another common reaction to the realization of imminent death. The patient becomes angry at having to face death while others, including loved ones, are healthy and not threatened. The dying person perceives the situation as "unfair" or "senseless" and may be hostile to friends, family, or the world in general.

Bargaining This stage occurs toward the middle of the progression toward acceptance of death. During this stage, the patient may resolve to be a better person in return for an extension of life or may secretly pray for a short reprieve from death in order to see a loved one or experience a special event.

Depression Depression eventually sets in as vitality diminishes and the patient begins to experience distressing symptoms with increasing frequency. The patient's deteriorating condition becomes impossible to deny, and feelings of doom and tremendous loss may become unbearably pervasive. Feelings of worthlessness and guilt are also common in this depressed state, because the dying person may feel responsible for the emotional suffering of loved ones and the arduous but seemingly futile efforts of caregivers.

Acceptance This is the final stage in the progression. At this point, the patient stops battling with emotions and becomes very tired and weak. The need to sleep increases, and wakeful periods become shorter and less frequent. With acceptance, the patient does not "give up" and become sullen or resentfully resigned to death, but rather becomes passive. According to one dying patient, the acceptance stage is "almost void of feelings . . . as if the pain had gone, the struggle is over, and there comes a time for the final rest before the long journey."*

Thanatology The study of death and dying.

---

* Elisabeth Kübler-Ross, *On Death and Dying* (New York: Macmillan, 1969), p. 113.

Figure 15.1 Kübler-Ross's stages of dying.

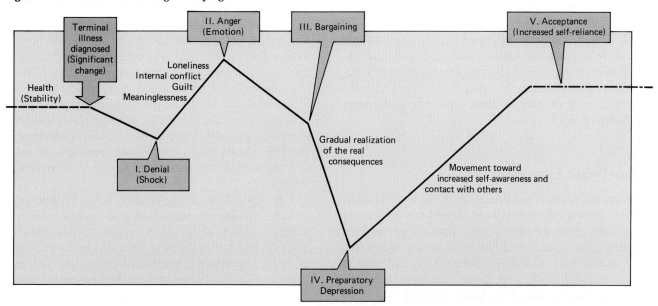

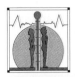

Protecting the Dying

The Dying Person's Bill of Rights

As we face death, what are our rights as human beings? This bill of rights was created at a workshop on "The Terminally Ill Patient and the Helping Person," sponsored by the Southwestern Michigan Insurance Education Council and conducted by Amelia J. Barbus.

• I have the right to be treated as a living human being until I die.

• I have the right to maintain a sense of hopefulness, however changing its focus may be.

• I have the right to be cared for by those who can maintain a sense of hopefulness, however changing this might be.

• I have the right to express my feelings and emotions about my approaching death in my own way.

• I have the right to participate in decisions concerning my care.

• I have the right to expect continuing medical and nursing attention even though "cure" goals must be changed to "comfort" goals.

• I have the right not to die alone.

• I have the right to be free from pain.

• I have a right to have my questions answered honestly.

• I have the right not to be deceived.

• I have the right to have help from and for my family in accepting my death.

• I have the right to die in peace and dignity.

• I have the right to retain my individuality and not be judged for my decisions which may be contrary to beliefs of others.

• I have the right to discuss and enlarge my religious and/or spiritual experiences, whatever these may mean to others.

• I have the right to expect that the sanctity of the human body will be respected after death.

• I have the right to be cared for by caring, sensitive, knowledgeable people who will attempt to understand my needs and will be able to gain some satisfaction in helping me face my death.

SOURCE: Copyright © 1975 by American Journal of Nursing Company; reproduced with permission from *American Journal of Nursing,* January 1975, vol. 75, no. 1.

The dying person may no longer welcome visitors and may not wish to engage in conversation. Death usually occurs quietly and painlessly while the victim is unconscious.

Some of Kübler-Ross's contemporaries considered her stage theory to be too neat and orderly. Subsequent research indicated that the experiences of dying people do not fit so easily into specific categories and that patterns vary from person to person. Even if it is not accurate in all its particulars, however, Kübler-Ross's theory offers valuable insights for those seeking to understand or deal with death.

Near-Death Experiences

One cannot speak of the process of dying without mention of *near-death experiences.* Thousands of reports have been given by people who almost died or were actually pronounced dead but subsequently recovered. The descriptions of feelings, perceptions, and visions associated with being near death have many common features. Three phases have been identified in a large number of reports of near-death accounts: resistance, life review, and transcendence. During the initial phase, *resistance,* the dying person is aware of extreme danger and struggles desperately to escape from the unseen threat. A sensation of expanding fear is commonly reported. The second phase, *life review,* has been described as a feeling of being outside of one's body and beyond danger. During this period the dying person feels a sensation of security while observing his or her physical body from an emotionally detached perspective. The dying person's lifetime of experiences may also seem to pass by in rapid review. The last phase, *transcendence,* is characterized by a reported feeling of euphoria, contentment, and even ecstasy. Some people have recalled a sensation of being unified with nature and having an awareness of infinity.

Life After Life, a provocative book by Raymond Moody, recounts the near-death and "out-of-body" experiences of over 150 people who were resuscitated after being declared clinically dead. Moody's book, published in 1975, stimulated a great deal of interest and controversy about this phenomenon. Subsequent investigations indicate that many people experience sensations

Health in the Community

Communicating with the Dying and Their Families

Helping people cope with death includes being able to communicate with the dying and their families. A few guidelines for supportive communication are presented here:

1. Be sincere. Follow your feelings rather than rules that commonly dictate behavior.
2. Remember that dying people are still alive and need to be treated like living people.
3. Don't avoid the reality of imminent death, but let the dying person set the pace in communications about dying and related matters.

4. Be aware that crying is a natural reaction to loss and is understood as an expression of caring.
5. Offer support and assistance when needed, but don't try to assume control. The dying person needs to have as much control of the situation as possible in order to maintain self-esteem.
6. Don't confuse the dying person's needs and values with your own. As previously stated, there is no single "right way" to die. Each person must deal with death individually, according to his or her own needs and desires.

similar to those previously described, suggesting that these perceptions are not uncommon. Various theories have been proposed to explain the occurrence of these hallucinations, including the release of beta-endorphin, a morphinelike chemical produced in the brain that is known to block or reduce the sensation of pain.

COPING WITH LOSS

The losses resulting from the death of a loved one may be extremely difficult to cope with. The dying person, as well as close family and friends, frequently suffers emotionally and physically from the impending loss of critical relationships and roles. Words used to describe feelings and behavior related to losses as a result of death include *bereavement, grief, grief work,* and *mourning.* These terms are related but differ in meaning. An understanding of them may be helpful in comprehending the emotional processes associated with loss and the cultural constraints that often inhibit normal coping behavior.

Bereavement, Grief, Grief Work, and Mourning—What Is Normal?

Bereavement is generally defined as the loss or deprivation that is experienced by a survivor when a loved one dies. Because relationships vary in type and intensity, reactions to losses also vary. The death of a parent, a spouse, a sibling, a child, a friend, or a pet will result in different kinds of feelings. In the lives of the bereaved or of close survivors, "holes" will be left by the loss of loved

ones. We can think of bereavement as the empty space that is left from these holes. Time and courage are necessary to fill in these spaces.

A special case of bereavement occurs in old age. Loss is an intrinsic part of growing old. The longer we live, the more losses we are likely to experience. These losses include physical, social, and emotional losses as our bodies deteriorate and more and more of our loved ones die. The theory of *bereavement overload* has been proposed to explain the effects of multiple losses and the accumulation of sorrow in the lives of some elderly people. This theory suggests that the gloomy outlook, disturbing behavior patterns, and apparent apathy that is characteristic of these people may be related more to bereavement overload than to intrinsic physiological degeneration in old age.*

Grief is a mental state of distress that occurs in *reaction* to significant loss, including one's own impending death, the death of a loved one, or a quasi-death experience. Grief reactions include any adjustments that are necessary in order to "make it through the day" and may include changes in patterns of eating, sleeping, working, and even thinking.

What is "normal" grief? This is a difficult question to answer. Grief responses vary widely from person to person (see Figure 15.2). Despite these differences, a classic

Bereavement Deprivation or loss caused by the death of a significant other.

Grief A mental state of distress that occurs in reaction to the loss of a loved one, therefore a reaction to bereavement.

* Robert J. Kastenbaum, *Death, Society, and Human Experience,* 3rd ed. (Columbus, OH: Chas. E. Merrill, 1986), p. 153.

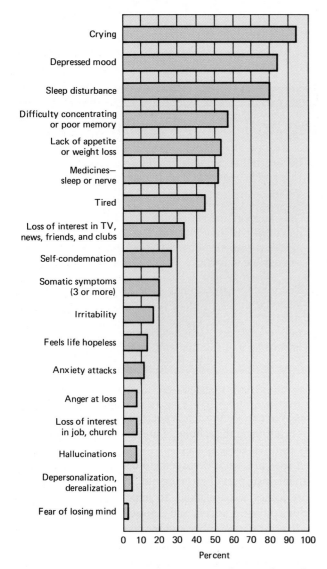

Figure 15.2 Common grief responses of bereaved people. These responses are normal and can be expected to occur as people cope with the death of a loved one. The percentages of specific responses shown in this graph represent expressions of recently widowed people. Do you think the reaction percentages might vary individually? For children? For very old people?

acute grief syndrome often occurs when a person acknowledges a loss. This common grief reaction can include the following symptoms:

Periodic waves of physical distress, lasting from 20 minutes to an hour

A feeling of tightness in the throat

Choking and shortness of breath

A frequent need to sigh

A feeling of emptiness in the abdomen

A feeling of muscular weakness

An intense feeling of anxiety that is described as actually painful.

Other common symptoms of grief include insomnia, memory lapse, loss of appetite, difficulty in concentrating, a tendency to engage in repetitive or purposeless behavior, an "observer" sensation or feeling of unreality, difficulty in making decisions, lack of organization, excessive speech, social withdrawal or hostility, guilt feelings, and preoccupation with the image of the deceased. susceptibility to disease increases with grief and may even be life threatening in severe and enduring cases.

A person may suffer emotional pain and may exhibit a variety of grief responses for many months after the death of a loved one. The rate of the healing process depends on the amount and quality of **grief work** that a person does. Grief work is the process of integrating the reality of the loss with everyday life and learning to feel better. The bereaved person must deliberately and systematically work at reducing denial and coping with the pain that results from memories of the deceased. This process takes time and requires emotional effort.

The term **mourning** is often incorrectly equated with the term *grief*. As we have noted, *grief* refers to a wide variety of feelings and actions in response to bereavement. *Mourning,* in contrast, refers to culturally prescribed and accepted time periods and behavior patterns for expression of grief. In Judaism, for example, a designated period of mourning is initially seven days of "sitting shiva." However, various other rituals may continue for up to a year, depending on a person's relationship with the deceased.

Social and Emotional Support for Readjustment

Symptoms of grief vary in severity and duration, depending on the situation and the individual. However, the bereaved person can benefit from emotional and social support from family, friends, clergy, employers, and the traditional support organizations, including the medical community and the funeral industry. The larger and stronger the support system, the easier readjustment is likely to be (see Figure 15.3).

Religion provides comfort to many dying and grieving people. Although some people question the existence of an afterlife, others gain support from religious beliefs that provide a purpose and meaning to life. By accepting dying as a part of the continuum of life, many people are able to make necessary readjustments after the death of a loved one. This holistic concept, which accepts dying as a part of the total life experience, is shared by both believers and nonbelievers.

Grief Work The process of accepting the reality of a person's death and coping with memories of the deceased.

Mourning The culturally sanctioned display of grief for a person's death.

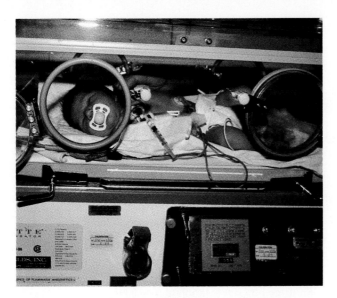

Our modern technology requires us to make decisions regarding how far we should go to preserve human life.

Living with Death and Loss

The reality of death and loss touches everyone. Although the accompanying grief causes painful emotions, it can also bring strength. C. M. Parkes, a British researcher in the psychiatric aspects of bereavement, observed that "the experience of grieving can strengthen and bring maturity to those who have previously been protected from misfortune. The pain of grief is just as much a part of life as the joy of love; it is, perhaps, the price we pay for love, the cost of commitment. To ignore this fact, or to pretend that it is not so [would] leave us unprepared for the losses that will inevitably occur in our lives and unprepared to help others cope with the losses in theirs."*

* C. M. Parkes, *Bereavement* (New York: International Universities Press, 1972), p. 6.

Figure 15.3 Stages of grief. People react differently to losses, but most eventually adjust. The common stages of grief and relief are depicted in this diagram. Generally, the stronger the social support system, the smoother the progression through the stages of grief.

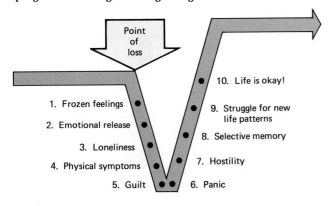

Point of loss

1. Frozen feelings
2. Emotional release
3. Loneliness
4. Physical symptoms
5. Guilt
6. Panic
7. Hostility
8. Selective memory
9. Struggle for new life patterns
10. Life is okay!

TAKING CARE OF BUSINESS

Caring for dying people and dealing with the practical and legal questions surrounding death can be difficult and painful. The problems of the dying person and the bereaved loved ones include a wide variety of psychological, legal, social, spiritual, economic, and interpersonal issues. This section examines some practical problems associated with death and presents a humanitarian alternative that has been offered as a possible solution.

Alternative Care for the Dying

An increasing number of people are considering the **hospice** philosophy as an acceptable alternative to modern "high-tech" death. The objective of hospice programs is to maximize the quality of life when it has already been determined that death is inevitable. The Dying Person's Bill of Rights (see box) reflects the sort of humanitarian idealism upon which the hospice philosophy was founded. The primary goals of the hospice program are to relieve the dying person's pain, to offer emotional support to the dying person and loved ones, and to restore a sense of control to the dying person, the family, and friends. Although home care with maximum involvement by loved ones is emphasized, hospice programs are under the direction of cooperating physicians, coordinated by specially trained nurses, and fortified with the services of counselors, clergy, and trained volunteers. Hospital inpatient beds are available if necessary. Hospice programs usually include the following characteristics:

1. The patient and family constitute the unit of care, because the physical, psychological, social, and spiritual problems of dying confront the family as well as the patient.

2. Emphasis is placed on symptom control, primarily the alleviation of pain. Curative treatments are curtailed as requested by the patient, but sound judgment must be applied to avoid a feeling of "abandonment."

3. There is overall medical direction of the program, with all health care being provided under the direction of a qualified physician.

4. Services are provided by an interdisciplinary team, because no one person can provide all the needed care.

5. Coverage is provided 24 hours per day, 7 days per week, with emphasis on the availability of medical and nursing skills.

6. Carefully selected and extensively trained volunteers are an integral part of the health-care team, augmenting staff service but not replacing it.

Hospice A concept of care for terminally ill patients designed to maximize the quality of life.

Communication

Death Denial as a Barrier to Effective Communication

In the United States, there is a high level of discomfort associated with death and dying. As a result, we may avoid speaking about death in an effort to limit our own discomfort. This form of death denial can take many forms in our communications, including the following:

- Avoiding people who are grieving after the death of a loved one, so we won't have to talk about it.
- Failing to validate a dying person's frightening situation by talking to the person as if nothing were wrong.

- Substituting euphemisms for the term *death*. A few examples include "passing away," "kicking the bucket," "no longer with us," "going to heaven," or "going to a better place."
- Giving false reassurances to people who are dying by saying things like "everything is going to be okay."
- Shutting off conversation about death by silencing people who are trying to talk about it.
- Not touching people who are dying.

7. Care of the family extends through the bereavement period.

8. Patients are accepted on the basis of health needs, not their ability to pay.

Although a growing number of people are considering the hospice option, many people prefer to go to a hospital to die. Others choose to die at home, without the intervention of medical staff or life-prolonging equipment. Each dying person and his or her family should decide as early as possible what type of terminal care is most desirable and feasible. This will allow time for necessary emotional, physical, and financial preparations.

Funeral Arrangements

Anthropological evidence indicates that all cultures throughout history have developed some sort of funeral ritual. For this reason, social scientists agree that funerals must somehow assist survivors of the deceased in coping with their loss. Arranging the funeral, however, is not often perceived as beneficial and may even compound an already difficult situation. The stress involved in making funeral arrangements for a loved one is multiplied if the deceased did not previously indicate specific preferences concerning body disposal and memorial services.

In the United States, with its diversity of religious, regional, and ethnic customs, funeral patterns are quite

WIZARD OF ID   **BY BRANT PARKER & JOHNNY HART**

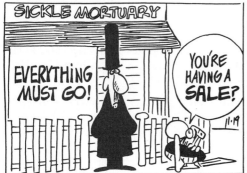
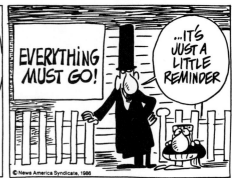

varied. Prior to body disposal, the deceased may be displayed to formalize last respects and increase social support to the bereaved. This part of the funeral ritual is referred to as a *wake* or *viewing*. The body of the deceased is usually embalmed prior to viewing to retard decomposition and minimize offensive odors.

The funeral service may be held in a church, in a funeral chapel, or at the burial site. Some people choose to replace the funeral service with a simple memorial service held within a few days of the burial. Social interaction associated with funeral and memorial services is valuable in helping survivors cope with their losses.

Common methods of body disposal include burial in the ground, entombment above ground in a mausoleum, cremation, and anatomical donation. Expenses involved in body disposal vary according to the method chosen and the available options that may be selected. Examples of options and their costs are listed in Table 15.1. It should be noted that if burial is selected, an additional charge may be assessed for a burial vault. Burial vaults—concrete or metal containers that hold the casket—are required by most cemeteries to limit settling of the gravesite as the casket disintegrates and collapses.

The Burden of Planning

Stress related to funeral ritual varies culturally as well as individually. In traditional societies, funeral rites and preparation of the body are quite specific. These practices limit the stress on survivors because few decisions have to be made. Bereaved people fully understand their individual roles in funeral customs and may even anticipate carrying out expected duties. In contrast, funeral practices in the United States today are extremely varied. A great number of decisions have to be made, usually within 24 hours. These decisions relate to method and details of body disposal, type of memorial service, display of the body, site of burial or body disposition, cost of funeral options, organ donation decisions, ordering of floral displays, contacting friends and relatives, planning for arrival of guests, choosing markers, gathering and submitting obituary information to newspapers, printing of memorial folders, as well as numerous other details. Even though funeral directors are available to facilitate decision making, the bereaved may incur undue stress, especially in the event of a sudden death. In our society, people who make their own funeral arrangements can save their loved ones from having to deal with unnecessary problems. Even making the decision regarding method of body disposal can greatly reduce the stress on survivors.

The Living Will

Another decision that can be made in advance concerns the use of artificial life-support treatment to prolong life. The common use of highly developed death-prevention

---

Table 15.1 Body Disposal Costs

Services of Funeral Director and Staff	Price
1. Removal from place of death	$205
2. Basic care and minimum services Includes filing death certificate, obtaining permits, arrangement conference, claims-notifications-benefits assistance, temporary care of remains (first 24 hours)	$540
3. Embalming	$290
4. Other preparation	
Autopsy repair	$220
Modified preparation for limited viewing	$230
Dressing and handling	$205
5. Funeral director and staff for memorial service	$180–205
6. Funeral coach	$140
7. Limo service	$145–200
Facilities Charges	$150–215
Immediate Burial	$1095–1492

An "immediate burial" is a disposition of human remains by burial, without formal viewing, visitation, or ceremony with the body present, except for a graveside service. Immediate burial includes removal of the remains to the mortuary.

Direct Cremation	$865–1262

A "direct cremation" is a disposition of human remains by cremation, without formal viewing, visitation, or ceremony with the body present. Direct cremation includes removal of the remains to the mortuary and transportation to the crematory.

This represents a partial list of costs associated with body disposal from a 1992 price list of a large West Coast corporation. Other costs include caskets and burial vaults (a major expense), vehicle expenses for transportation of body, memorial marker, engraving, and many other items.

SOURCE: DeMoss-Duran Garden Chapel; Member: Uniservice Corp.; 815 N.W. Buchanan Avenue; Corvallis, OR 97330.

Accidental deaths may require survivors to make quick decisions on funeral arrangements at a time when they are under great stress.

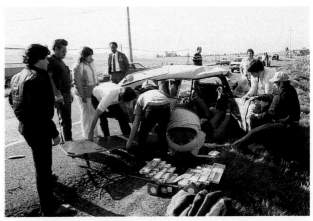

technology, including artificial respirators, nasogastric tube feeding, and intravenous fluid replacement, raises serious questions concerning the artificial extension of a terminal patient's life. Because patients can be kept technically alive almost indefinitely, many people are beginning to weigh quality of life against quantity of life. The *living will,* which has been recognized in many states, assists physicians and family members in making life-and-death decisions about artificial life support in cases in which the patient has lost the power to communicate. Figure 15.4 offers a sample copy of a living will. Special considerations and practical issues regarding living wills are presented in the section on "The Right to Die."

Organ Donation

Organ-transplant techniques have become so refined, and the demand for transplant tissues and organs has become so great, that many people are being encouraged to donate these "gifts of life" upon their death. Uniform donor cards are available through the National Kidney Foundation, donor information is printed on the backs of drivers' licenses, and many hospitals have included the opportunity for organ-donor registration as a part of their admission procedures. Although some people are opposed to organ transplants and tissue donation, others experience a feeling of personal fulfillment knowing that their organs might extend and improve someone else's life after their own death (see Figure 15.5).

▌ SPECIAL ETHICAL CONCERNS

Life-and-death questions are serious, complex, and often expensive. As stated in the introduction to this chapter, we do not attempt to present the "answers" to death-related moral and philosophical questions. Instead, we offer topics for your consideration. It is hoped that the preceding discussion of the needs of the dying person and the bereaved will help you make difficult decisions in the future. A few topics that are problematic or controversial are the right to die, the concept of rational suicide, and euthanasia.

The Right to Die: A Right to Refuse Treatment

Few people would object to a proposal for the right to a dignified death. Going beyond that concept, however, many people today believe they should be *allowed to die* if their condition is inevitably terminal and their existence is dependent on mechanical life-support devices or artificial feeding or hydration systems. Artificial life-support techniques that may be legally refused by competent patients in some states include the following:

Electrical or mechanical resuscitation of the heart

Mechanical respiration by machine

Nasogastric tube feedings

Intravenous nutrition

Gastrostomy (tube feeding directly into the stomach)

Medications to treat life-threatening infections.

As long as a person is conscious and competent, he or she has the legal right to refuse treatment, even if this decision will hasten death. However, when a person is in a coma or is otherwise incapable of speaking on his or her own behalf, treatment will be dictated by medical personnel and administrative policy.

This issue has evolved into a battle involving personal freedom, legal rulings, health-care administration policy, and physician responsibility. The living will, described in the previous section, was developed to assist in solving conflicts among these people and agencies. For the American Medical Association (AMA) position on physician responsibility in these cases, see the box entitled "The Physician and the Right to Die: The AMA Position."

Cases have been reported in which the wishes of people who have signed a living will indicating their desire not to receive artificial life support were not honored by the physician or medical institution. This problem can be avoided by choosing both a physician and a hospital that will carry out the directives of the living will. Taking this precaution and discussing your personal philosophy and wishes with your family should eliminate anxiety about how you will be treated at the end of your life.

Rational Suicide

Suicide has been discussed in earlier chapters. The concept of *rational suicide* as an option to an extended dying process, however, deserves mention here. Although exact numbers are not known, medical ethicists, experts in rational suicide, and specialists in forensic medicine (the study of legal issues in medicine) estimate that every year thousands of terminally ill people decide to kill themselves rather than endure constant pain and slow decay. To these people the prospect of an undignified death is unacceptable. But does anyone have the right to end his or her life? This issue has been complicated by advances in death-prevention techniques that allow terminally ill patients to exist in an irreversible disease state for extended periods of time. Medical personnel, clergy, lawyers, and patients all must struggle with this ethical dilemma.

Intestate The situation in which a person dies without having made a will.

GUIDE TO THE LIVING WILL

To get a copy of your state's living will you have to ask; request one from your hospital, nursing home, physician, lawyer, or state government or write to the Society for the Right to Die, 250 West 57th Street, New York, New York 10107. Filling out a living will should not in any way affect the provisions of your life insurance policy.

Thirty-eight states and D.C. have living wills. All the remaining states (KY, MA, MI, MN, ND, NE, NJ, NY, OH, PA, RI, SD) are considering living will law statutes. Living wills are binding only within state boundaries, but some states honor those from elsewhere. If your state does not have a living will or if you are traveling, you can get a generic form from the Society for the Right to Die that you can use to express your wishes, though it may not be binding. Keep a copy of your living will on file with your next of kin, lawyer, or physician.

Except in CA, where they must be renewed every five years, living wills are effective until they are revoked. Still, it's considered a good idea to initial and date your living will every few years to show that it still expresses your wishes.

"Life-sustaining procedures" are those that only prolong the process of dying. Most states include feeding and hydration tubes in this definition. But CO, CT, GA, ID, ME, MO, and WI specifically rule them out, though courts in CO have affirmed a patient's right to have feeding tubes disconnected.

"Imminent" is used on many living wills to express the inevitability and timing of death, but it is open to varying interpretations. A recent VA court decision found that it does not necessarily mean "immediately, at once, within a few days," and that a comatose person who is within a few months of death falls within the definition.

Except in CA, ID, and OR, living wills have a space to specify treatment you do or don't want. Ask your physician what to include here. You can:
- ask for or prohibit use of artificial feeding tubes, cardiopulmonary resuscitation, antibiotics, dialysis, and respirators;
- ask for pain medication to keep you comfortable;
- state whether you would prefer to die in the hospital or at home;
- designate a proxy—someone to make decisions about your treatment when you are unable;
- donate organs or other body parts.
If your directions are contrary to state law they will be ignored, but the rest of the document will stand.

You can revoke or amend your living will at any time simply by making a statement to a physician or nurse or other health care worker.

In some states a physician who will not carry out a patient's wishes must make a "good faith effort" to locate a doctor who will; other states require the physician to actually *find* someone and specify penalties—in some cases jail terms—for failure to do so.

In AZ, CO, ME, TN, VA, DC, LA, NM, NC, OR, VT, WV the living will is valid for pregnant women. Others exclude women during all or part of their pregnancy, although that has been challenged on the grounds that a woman's right to privacy doesn't end when she becomes pregnant.

Eight states (AR, DE, FL, LA, TX, UT, VA, WY) provide for the appointment of a proxy. In CA, RI, IL, ME, and NV, decisions may be delegated through a document called a Durable Power of Attorney. These forms are commonly used instead of living wills in RI, which has no living will law, and CA, whose law is extremely restrictive.

In HI, ID, NH, NC, OK, SC, TN, WV your signature must be notarized. Elsewhere, the signature of the witnesses is adequate, although if you are in a hospital or nursing home in some states you may need as an additional witness the chief of staff or medical director.

TEXAS

DIRECTIVE TO PHYSICIANS

Directive made this _____ day of _____ (month, year). I, _____, being of sound mind, wilfully and voluntarily make known my desire that my life shall not be artificially prolonged under the circumstances set forth below, and do hereby declare:

If at any time I should have an incurable condition caused by injury, disease, or illness certified to be a terminal condition by two physicians, and where the application of life-sustaining procedures would serve only to artificially prolong the moment of my death and where my attending physician determines that my death is imminent whether or not life-sustaining procedures are utilized, I direct that such procedures be withheld or withdrawn, and that I be permitted to die naturally.

In the absence of my ability to give directions regarding the use of such life-sustaining procedures, it is my intention that this directive shall be honored by my family and physicians as the final expression of my legal right to refuse medical or surgical treatment and accept the consequences from such refusal.

If I have been diagnosed as pregnant and that diagnosis is known to my physician, this directive shall have no force or effect during the course of my pregnancy.

Other directions: [See reverse side for suggested Proxy Designation form.]

This directive shall be in effect until it is revoked.

I understand the full import of this directive and I am emotionally and mentally competent to make this directive.

I understand that I may revoke this directive at any time.

Signed _____

City, County, and State of Residence _____

The declarant has been personally known to me and I believe him/her to be of sound mind. I am not related to the declarant by blood or marriage, nor would I be entitled to any portion of the declarant's estate on his/her decease, nor am I the attending physician of the declarant or an employee of the attending physician or a health facility in which the declarant is a patient, or a patient in the health care facility in which the declarant is a patient, or any person who has a claim against any portion of the estate of the declarant upon his/her decease.

Witness _____ Witness _____

RESEARCH BY FRANCESCA BANNERMAN

Figure 15.4 This is an example of a "living will," so named because the directives of the will are to be carried out while the testator is still living. Because living wills are not legally binding in many states, you should check its status in your state before filing the document with your physician and lawyer.

Figure 15.5 Organ-donor card provided by the National Kidney Foundation.

Still, questions remain. If terminally ill patients wish to die, should they be allowed to commit suicide? Is a person in this situation *capable* of making a rational decision about suicide? If terminally ill patients are allowed to commit suicide legally, what other groups will demand this option? Should the courts be involved in private decisions? Should any organization be allowed to distribute information that may encourage suicide?

Dyathanasia and Euthanasia

Should loved ones or medical caregivers be allowed to assist the person who wants to die by providing the means? This question refers to **dyathanasia,** a form of so-called mercy killing in which someone plays a passive role in the death of a terminally ill person. This passive role may include providing necessary lethal drugs, hypodermic paraphernalia, or weapons. Dyathanasia may also include withdrawal of life-sustaining medical support, thereby allowing the person to die. Recent court rulings have allowed dyathanasia in certain cases.

Euthanasia is the active form of mercy killing. An example of euthanasia is direct administration of a lethal

---

Dyathanasia The passive form of "mercy killing" in which life-prolonging treatments or interventions are not offered or are withheld, thereby allowing a terminally ill person to die naturally.

Euthanasia The active form of "mercy killing" in which a person or organization knowingly acts to hasten the death of a terminally ill person.

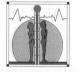

The Dying Patient's Best Interests

The Physician and the Right to Die: The AMA Position

The social commitment of the physician is to sustain life and relieve suffering. Where the performance of one duty conflicts with the other, the preferences of the patient should prevail. If the patient is incompetent to act in his own behalf and did not previously indicate his preferences, the family or other surrogate decisionmaker, in concert with the physician, must act in the best interest of the patient.

For humane reasons, with informed consent, a physician may do what is medically necessary to alleviate severe pain, or cease or omit treatment to permit a terminally ill patient to die when death is imminent. However, the physician should not intentionally cause death. In deciding whether the administration of potentially life-prolonging medical treatment is in the best interest of the patient who is incompetent to act in his own behalf, the surrogate decisionmaker and physician should consider several factors, including: the possibility for extending life under humane and comfortable conditions; the patient's values about life and the way it should be lived; and the patient's attitudes toward sickness, suffering, medical procedures, and death.

Even if death is not imminent but a patient is beyond doubt permanently unconscious, and there are adequate safeguards to confirm the accuracy of the diagnosis, it is not unethical to discontinue all means of life-prolonging medical treatment.

Life-prolonging medical treatment includes medication and artificially or technologically supplied respiration, nutrition or hydration. In treating a terminally ill or permanently unconscious patient, the dignity of the patient should be maintained at all times.

SOURCE: *Current Opinions of the Council on Ethical and Judicial Affairs of the American Medical Association,* 1989: "Withholding or Withdrawing Life-Prolonging Medical Treatment," p. 13. Reprinted with permission.

Promoting Your Health

How Do You Feel about Death and Dying?

The statements below are indicative of how some people feel about dying and death. Read each statement and check the blank that indicates how you feel about the item.

	Very Acceptable	Acceptable	Unsure	Unacceptable	Very Unacceptable
1. Attending a funeral	___	___	___	___	___
2. Living forever	___	___	___	___	___
3. Seeing a dead person	___	___	___	___	___
4. Writing a living will	___	___	___	___	___
5. Telling someone that he or she is dying	___	___	___	___	___
6. Visiting a hospital for the terminally ill	___	___	___	___	___
7. Dying quickly	___	___	___	___	___
8. Living with a disability	___	___	___	___	___
9. Visiting a cemetery	___	___	___	___	___
10. Being able to choose when you will die	___	___	___	___	___
11. Dying before your spouse	___	___	___	___	___
12. Talking with a dying person	___	___	___	___	___
13. Dying after your spouse	___	___	___	___	___
14. Planning for your own funeral	___	___	___	___	___
15. Being unhooked from a life-support system	___	___	___	___	___
16. Dying in your sleep	___	___	___	___	___
17. Being told that you have a terminal illness	___	___	___	___	___
18. Dying with the hope that there's an afterlife	___	___	___	___	___
19. Refusing to try a "miracle" drug that might work	___	___	___	___	___

Of course, there are no right or wrong answers to these questions. Reactions to issues of death and dying vary considerably. Compare *your* responses to the following "most frequently selected responses" from other college students.

Most frequent responses:
(1) very acceptable; (2) unsure; (3) acceptable; (4) very acceptable; (5) unsure; (6) acceptable; (7) very acceptable; (8) unacceptable; (9) acceptable; (10) unsure; (11) unsure; (12) acceptable; (13) unsure; (14) acceptable; (15) very acceptable; (16) very acceptable; (17) acceptable; (18) very acceptable; (19) unsure.

SOURCE: D. A. Read, *Looking In: Exploring One's Personal Health Values* (Englewood Cliffs, NJ: Prentice-Hall, 1977).

drug overdose with the objective of hastening the death of a suffering person. Euthanasia is illegal and is viewed as murder. Despite this restriction, euthanasia continues to occur. In fact, some experts believe that certain doctors induce euthanasia upon the request of the patient.

This type of euthanasia is accomplished by administering large doses of painkillers that depress the central nervous system to the extent that basic life-sustaining regulatory centers cease to function. The heart stops beating, breathing ceases, and total brain death follows shortly.

- Aging has traditionally been described as the characteristic pattern of life changes that occur normally in all species as they grow older.

- Modern-day gerontologists have begun to recognize that the process of aging involves much more than an analysis of the number of chronological years a person has lived.

- Biological, psychological, social, legal, and functional age are all types of aging that must be considered when we look at human development.

- Adults typically go through several developmental phases during a lifetime.

- Although many of the negative aspects of aging are inevitable, there is a great deal that can be done to enhance the quality of the later years.

- Ageist attitudes prevalent in American society promote many negative beliefs concerning the aging process.

- Continued problems in mastering developmental tasks often lead to problems with self-efficacy and internal locus of control and a general lack of confidence throughout life.

- Although people age 65 and older made up 12.7 percent of the U.S. population in 1990, by 2030 they are projected to make up 20.7 percent of the population.

- Mental health at any age involves interpersonal relationships and the ability to share your life with others.

- Those who have developed self-confidence, self-reliance, and mentally healthy attitudes about themselves and others, as well as effective coping mechanisms, typically lead active, mentally healthy lives.

- Numerous theories purport to explain the physiological changes that occur with aging. These theories attempt to explain the biological, psychosocial, cognitive, and environmental factors that contribute to the aging process.

- Death and dying are normal components of life.

- Confrontations with death elicit different feelings depending on many factors, including age, religious beliefs, family orientation, health, previous experience with death, and the circumstances of the death itself.

- Changes in family structure and advances in science and medicine during this century have produced an attitude of "death denial" in many industrialized nations.

- Our present system of death prevention is so effective that, under ideal conditions, it may be possible to keep a body artificially "alive" for an indefinite period.

- Death determination can be a complicated task in cases involving brain death or irreversible coma. The Harvard criteria for brain death were developed in 1968 in an attempt to facilitate such decisions.

- Reactions to death are variable, reflecting each person's unique personality and beliefs.

- Bereavement and grief vary among individuals, whereas mourning is a culturally prescribed reaction to death.

- Emotional stages of dying may include denial, anger, bargaining, depression, and acceptance.

- Preplanning of funerary details reduces the stress on survivors and is becoming more acceptable in our culture.

- More Americans are rejecting "high-tech" death in favor of a more "dignified" and natural death. One alternative is the hospice concept, which emphasizes comfort, symptom relief, and support rather than curative measures.

- Living wills are becoming increasingly accepted but are not legally binding in many states. It is important to be certain that your doctor and your family agree with the terms of the living will.

- The "right to die," euthanasia, dyathanasia, and rational suicide are all controversial concepts that we cannot escape.

16

Environmental Health

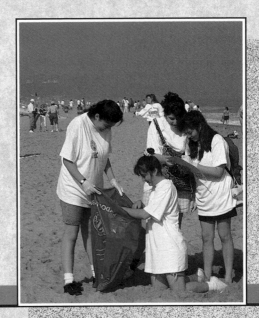

Objectives

- Explain why the earth's most challenging environmental problem is its population, and describe the factors contributing to population growth in developing nations.

- List each of the main air pollutants and describe its harmful health effects.

- Discuss why there is concern over the ozone layer and global warming.

- List each of the main water pollutants and describe its harmful health effects.

- Describe the harmful effects of short- and long-term noise pollution.

- Describe the methods for disposal of hazardous and solid wastes. Identify what parts of our trash are recyclable.

- Discuss why stockpiles of nuclear weapons and radioactive waste dumps are endangering the health of the planet.

- Discuss what steps can be taken to improve the environment.

M anagement of our environment and stewardship of the earth's resources are recognized as two of the most important problems facing humanity as the century draws to a close. In the wake of toxic spills, nuclear accidents, and rapidly expanding landfills and trash heaps, many people feel powerless to exert any control over the environment. Environmentalists are encouraging us as individuals to "think globally and act locally" and to "live as if the earth mattered." In order to behave this way we must first understand how our environmental problems have developed and then resolve to do our part to contribute to planet management.

▌POPULATION

The earth's most challenging environmental problem is its population. The late anthropologist Margaret Mead once wrote. "Every human society is faced with not one population problem but two: how to beget and rear enough children and how not to beget and rear too many."*

Globally, our population is out of control. In early 1990, the world population was nearly 5.3 billion and is increasing by three people every second, about a quarter of a million every day or 145 million people every year.** This rate leaves the planet with an annual net population gain of 93 million people. Population experts believe that unless current birth and death rates change radically, 10.4 billion people will be competing for the world's diminishing resources by the year 2029.*** Table 16.1 shows the world population growth rate by decade, with projections through the year 2029.

The population explosion is not occurring equally around the world. The United States and Western Europe have the lowest birthrates. At the same time, these two regions have more grain and other foodstuffs than their populations consume. Countries that can least afford an increased birthrate in economic, social, health, and nutritional terms are the ones with the most rapidly expanding populations.

As the population expands, so does the competition for the earth's resources. Our world economy is based on three biological systems: croplands, forests, and grasslands. With the exception of fossil fuels and minerals, these three systems supply all the raw materials for industry. They provide all of our food except for seafood. Environmental degradation through loss of topsoil, pesticides, toxic residues, deforestation, global warming, air pollution, and acid deposition (acid rain) seriously threatens the food supply and undermines world health.

Nowhere are these threats more visible than in Third World countries in Africa, Asia, and Latin America. The combination of falling economic levels and rising grain prices due to grain scarcity has led to starvation and famine in these areas. An estimated 40,000 children under the age of 5 die *each day* in these countries from severe nutritional deprivation and related infectious diseases.†

Controlling the Population Explosion

At first examination, it might seem that there is little we can do as individuals to control the population explosion in Third World countries. We can begin to do our part, however, by recognizing that the United States consumes far more energy and raw materials than does any other nation on earth. Many of these resources come from other parts of the world, and our consumption depletes

---

† Lester R. Brown, "The Illusion of Progress," *State of the World, 1990,* Lester R. Brown, ed. (New York: Norton, 1990), p. 11.

Starvation is a major threat in Third World countries with large populations.

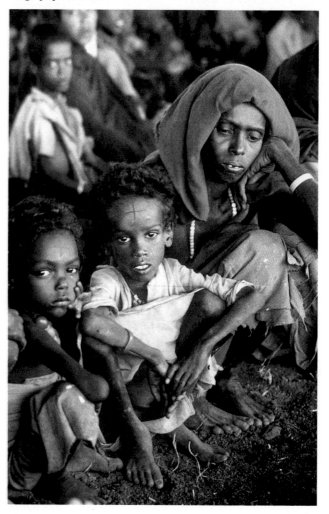

---

* Ruth Caplan, *Our Earth, Ourselves* (New York: Bantam, 1990), p. 247.

** Nafis Sadik, "World Population Continues to Rise," *The Futurist,* March/April 1991, pp. 9–14.

*** Caplan, pp. 247–50.

Table 16.1 World Population Growth by Decade, 1950–1990, with Projections to 2029

Year	Population (billion)	Increase by Decade (million)	Average Annual Increase (million)
1950	2.5		
1960	3.0	504	50
1970	3.7	679	68
1980	4.5	752	75
1990	5.3	842	84
2000	6.3	959	96
2029	10.4	(not available)	

SOURCES: Lester Brown, "The Illusion of Progress," *State of the World, 1990,* Lester R. Brown, ed. (New York: Norton, 1990), p. 5; Ruth Caplan, *Our Earth, Ourselves* (New York: Bantam, 1990), p. 248.

the resource balances of other countries. We must start by living environmentally conscious lives.

Perhaps the simplest course of action we can take is to control our own reproductivity. The concept of *zero population growth* (ZPG) was born in the 1960s. Proponents of this idea believed that each couple should produce only two offspring. When the parents die, the two offspring are their replacements, and the population stabilizes. In recent years, federal officials have cut population control funding dramatically for developing countries.

Supporting policies that are aimed at educating people in other countries about the dangers of rapid population growth and starvation is also important.

Several factors contribute to population growth in developing nations. Many of these countries believe that their wealth lies in their children. Although they often cannot clothe and feed their young, they continue to reproduce because they believe a large population gives them national unity and strength. Women in developing countries frequently bear large numbers of children because they know that many of their offspring will not survive infancy and childhood. (The same was true in preindustrial America.) Religious beliefs control reproductive behaviors as well. Asking people to avoid having children may violate their religious tenets. In addition, representatives of some developing nations feel that overpopulation does not present as great a problem as does inequitable distribution of wealth and resources both within their countries and worldwide.

AIR POLLUTION

In late 1970, Congress passed the Clean Air Act to help reduce the air pollution caused by urbanization, industrial development, and increasing use of motor vehicles.

Your Environmental IQ

Do You Know

One in 6 people drink water with excessive amounts of lead, a heavy metal that impairs children's IQ and attention span.

In a recent study conducted on fish, 43 percent of salmon samples contained PCBs, 90 percent swordfish contained mercury, and 50 percent of lake whitefish were contaminated with PCBs.

Since 1950, U.S. energy consumption has increased 60 percent.

Every day Americans buy about 62 million newspapers and throw away 44 million of them. That's the equivalent of dumping 500,000 trees into landfills each week.

According to *Home Energy Magazine* we could save over 250 million gallons of water every day if Americans installed faucet aerators.

Americans throw out 28 million tons of grass, dead leaves, and branches every year. All of it could be composted.

Fourteen thousand tons of garbage are dumped into the world's oceans every year—most of it in the Northern Hemisphere.

Dishwashers use about 6 fewer gallons of water than handwashing, but they should be used only when full and on economic settings.

Showers use one-third the water that baths do, but only if you are sensible about how much time you spend in the shower. Water-saving shower heads help conserve water.

Front-loading washing machines use up to 40 percent less water than top-loading machines.

Widespread Air Pollutants

The Clean Air Act was amended in 1977. The act and its amendments were designed to develop standards for six of the most common and widespread air pollutants: sulfur dioxide, particulates, carbon monoxide, nitrogen dioxides, ozone, and lead. Each of these pollutants has serious health effects.

Sulfur Dioxide Sulfur dioxide is a yellowish-brown gas that is a by-product of coal-powered electrical generating stations, smelters, refineries, and industrial boilers. In humans, sulfur dioxide aggravates symptoms of heart and lung disease, obstructs breathing passages, and increases incidences of respiratory diseases such as colds, asthma, bronchitis, and emphysema. It is toxic to plants, destroys some paint pigments, corrodes metals, impairs visibility, and is a precursor to acid deposition, which is discussed later in this chapter.

Particulates As we discussed in Chapter 11, cigarette smoke releases particulate matter, or **particulates**, into the air. These particulates are tiny solid particles or liquid droplets that are suspended in the air. They are the products of some industrial processes and the internal combustion engine. Approximately 7 percent of particulates exist in the form of windblown dust and ash from forest fires or volcanoes. Particulates carry heavy metals and carcinogenic agents deep into the lungs. When combined with sulfur dioxide, they exacerbate respiratory diseases. Particulates can also corrode metals and obscure visibility.

Carbon Monoxide Carbon monoxide is an odorless, colorless gas that originates primarily from motor vehicle emissions. Carbon monoxide interferes with the blood's ability to absorb and carry oxygen and can impair thinking, slow reflexes, and cause drowsiness, unconsciousness, and death. If the air contains 80 ppm (parts per million) of carbon monoxide, the body's supply of oxygen is reduced by 15 percent. In heavily congested traffic, the levels of carbon monoxide may reach as high as 400 ppm, causing headaches for many commuters stuck in traffic. When inhaled by pregnant women, it may threaten the growth and mental development of the fetus. Long-term exposure can increase the severity of circulatory diseases.

Vehicle emissions may be cut down by car pooling, riding a bicycle, walking, or using public transportation. Regular maintenance and tune-ups increase vehicle efficiency. In addition, the catalytic converter has been found to decrease harmful emissions significantly.

Nitrogen Dioxide Nitrogen dioxide is an amber-colored gas emitted by electrical utility boilers (coal-powered)and motor vehicles. High concentrations of nitrogen dioxide can be fatal. Lower concentrations increase susceptibility to colds and flu, bronchitis, and pneumonia. Nitrogen dioxide is also toxic to plant life and causes a brown discoloration in the atmosphere. It is a precursor to the formation of ozone, and, along with sulfur dioxide, to acid deposition.

Ozone Ozone is a form of oxygen that is formed when nitrogen dioxide reacts with hydrogen chloride. These gases release oxygen, which is altered by sunlight to produce ozone. In the lower atmosphere, ozone irritates the mucous membranes of the respiratory system, causing coughing and choking. It can impair lung functioning, reduce resistance to colds and pneumonia, and aggravate heart disease, asthma, bronchitis, and pneumonia. Ozone corrodes rubber and paint and can injure or kill vegetation, including crops, trees, and shrubs. It is also one of the irritants found in smog. The ozone found in the upper atmosphere, however, serves as a protective membrane against heat and radiation. This atmospheric layer is called the ozone layer and is discussed later in this chapter.

Lead Lead is a metal found in motor vehicle exhaust and in the emissions from lead smelters and processing plants. Today, the major source of lead pollution is lead-contaminated air, 98 percent of which comes from lead gasoline. The lead in this gasoline also settles on produce grown close to highways, which must then be thoroughly washed to remove it. There is evidence that lead-free gasoline has reduced the levels of lead in the U.S. population. But other sources of lead exist such as lead-based paint. In addition, the drinking systems in older homes, where plumbing was installed before 1930, are often contaminated by lead. Lead affects the circulatory, reproductive, and nervous systems. It can affect the blood and kidneys and can accumulate in bone and other tissues. The presence of lead is particularly harmful to children and fetuses. It can cause birth defects, behavioral abnormalities and decreased learning abilities.

Hydrocarbons Although not listed as one of the six major air pollutants in the Clean Air Act, hydrocarbons encompass a wide variety of chemical pollutants in the air. Sometimes known as *volatile organic compounds* (VOCs), **hydrocarbons** are chemical compounds containing different combinations of carbon and hydrogen. The principal source of hydrocarbons is the internal

---

Sulfur Dioxide A yellowish-brown gaseous by-product of the burning of solid wastes.

Particulates Nongaseous air pollutants.

Carbon Monoxide An odorless, colorless gas that originates primarily from motor vehicle emissions.

Nitrogen Dioxide An amber-colored gas found in smog; can cause eye and respiratory irritations.

Ozone A gas formed when nitrogen dioxide interacts with hydrogen.

Lead A metal found in exhausts and emissions.

Hydrocarbons Chemical compounds that contain carbon and hydrogen.

combustion engine. Most automobile engines emit hundreds of different types of hydrocarbon compounds. By themselves, hydrocarbons seem to cause few problems. When combined with sunlight and other pollutants, however, they form such poisons as formaldehyde, various ketones, and peroxyacetylnitrate (PAN), all of which are respiratory irritants. Hydrocarbon combinations such as benzene and benzopyrene are carcinogenic. In addition, hydrocarbons play a major part in the formation of smog.

Photochemical Smog Photochemical smog is a brown, hazy mix of particulates and gases that forms when oxygen-containing compounds of nitrogen and hydrocarbons react in the presence of sunlight. Photochemical smog is sometimes called "ozone pollution" because ozone is created when vehicle exhaust reacts with sunlight. Smog is most likely to develop on days when there is little wind and high traffic congestion. In most cases, smog forms in areas that experience a **temperature inversion,** in which a cool layer of air is trapped under a layer of warmer air, preventing the air from circulating. When gases such as the hydrocarbons and nitrogen oxides are released into the cool air layer, they cannot escape, and thus they remain suspended until wind conditions move away the warmer air layer. Sunlight filtering through the air causes chemical changes in the hydrocarbons and nitrogen oxides, which results in smog. Smog is more likely to be produced in valley regions blocked by hills or mountains—for example, the Los Angeles basin, Denver, and Tokyo.

Photochemical Smog   The brownish-yellow haze resulting from the combination of hydrocarbons and nitrogen oxides.

Temperature Inversion   A weather condition occurring when a layer of cool air is trapped under a layer of warmer air.

Promoting Your Health

Watch Out for These Polluters

You can help cut air pollution by avoiding, whenever possible, use of the following household, personal care, and automotive products. They contain solvents and alcohol, both of which emit air-polluting hydrocarbons. The list is based on 27 products now regulated by the state of California. The products are ranked according to their average daily contributions of hydrocarbon emissions in the state. Some suggested alternatives are given in parentheses.

1. Hair sprays
2. Windshield washer fluids
3. Insecticides (Sweeping, vacuuming, and beating carpets, and storing food in containers will keep most pests at bay.)
4. Air fresheners
5. Perfumes and colognes
6. Antiperspirants and deodorants
7. General-purpose cleaners (For surfaces, a mixture of vinegar and salt. For a deodorizing solution, 4 tablespoons of baking soda in 1 quart water.)
8. Engine degreasers
9. Charcoal lighter fluid (Electric coil charcoal starter)
10. Floor polishes
11. Glass cleaners (1 teaspoon of lemon juice or vinegar in 1 quart of water.)
12. Laundry prewashers
13. Laundry starches
14. Carburetor choke cleaners
15. Household adhesives
16. Nail polish removers
17. Oven cleaners
18. Brake cleaners
19. Aerosol cooking sprays (Use nonstick cooking surfaces or oil, butter, or margarine.)
20. Hair mousses
21. Dusting aids
22. Bathroom and tile cleaners (To disinfect: baking soda and water; lemon juice or vinegar and water; 1/2 cup of borax in 1 gallon water.)
23. Aerosol insect repellents
24. Hair styling gels
25. Shaving creams
26. Fabric protectants

SOURCES: *Blueprint for a Green Planet* by John Seymour and Herbert Girardet and *Design for a Livable Planet* by John Naar.

The most noticeable adverse effects of exposure to smog are difficulty in breathing, burning eyes, headaches, and nausea. Long-term exposure to smog poses the most serious health risks, particularly for children, the elderly, pregnant women, and people with chronic respiratory disorders, such as asthma or emphysema. According to the American Lung Association, continued exposure to smog accelerates aging of the lungs and increases susceptibility to infections by hindering the functions of the immune system.*

Despite local efforts to reduce the problem, smog pollution in the United States repeatedly surges above the federal standards for safety. In the early 1970s, the Environmental Protection Agency (EPA) established 0.12 parts of smog per million parts of air as the "safe" standard. Table 16.2 shows 15 cities in the United States that failed the federal ozone standard from 1986 to 1988. These cities are representative of the estimated 382 cities (home to more than half of all Americans) that exceed federal standards every year.

The EPA has also developed a numerical scale for measuring air pollution called the Pollutant Standards Index (PSI). The PSI measures hourly concentrations of carbon monoxide, hydrocarbons, sulfur oxides, particulates, nitrogen oxides, and photochemical smog, with the total amounts ranging from zero to 500 serving as indicators of air quality. Values below 100 are regarded as safe; values above 100 are increasingly unhealthy. Values above 300 indicate the air is hazardous to the health of people breathing it.

Acid Deposition (Acid Rain)

The poet Alfred, Lord Tennyson once referred to rain as a "useful trouble." Most people have thought of rain this way, feeling that it was sometimes a wet, bothersome nuisance, but that it was also life-giving, cleansing, and nurturing. Since the 1950s, however, people have begun to reexamine their feelings, as a menace called acid deposition, or acid rain, has been threatening human health, damaging crops, destroying forests, decimating wildlife, and straining international relationships.

Acid deposition (acid rain) is precipitation that has fallen through acidic air pollutants, particularly those containing sulfur dioxides and nitrogen dioxides. This precipitation in the form of rain or snow has a more acidic composition than unpolluted rain or snow. When introduced into lakes and ponds, acid deposition gradually acidifies the water. When the acid content of the water reaches a certain level, plant and animal life cannot survive. Ironically, lakes and ponds that are acidified become a crystal-clear deep blue, giving the illusion of beauty and health.

Table 16.2   U.S. Cities that Failed Federal Ozone Standards of 0.12 Parts per Million from 1986 to 1988

City or Area	Highest Ozone Level (Parts per Million)	Average Number of Days above Standard Each Year
Los Angeles, CA	.340	145.4
New York, NY	.217	18.0
Chicago, IL	.193	21.2
Houston, TX	.190	12.6
Milwaukee, WI	.183	9.1
Baltimore, MD	.181	13.3
San Diego, CA	.180	11.1
Muskegon, MI	.180	9.0
Philadelphia, PA	.180	8.9
Portsmouth/ Dover/Rochester, NH-ME	.179	7.8
Hartford, CT	.179	6.9
Louisville, KY	.171	5.6
Fresno, CA	.170	11.6
El Paso, TX	.170	8.1
Parkersburg/ Marietta, WV-OH	.169	7.2

SOURCE: Environmental Protection Agency.

Acidity is measured in terms of pH, the number of hydrogen ions concentrated in a given substance. The pH scale ranges from values of 0 to 14.0. for life to be sustainable, the pH of water must be near neutral, or near pH 7.0. Values below 7.0 indicate acidity, whereas values above 7.0 indicate alkalinity.

Sources of Acid Deposition   More than 95 percent of acid deposition comes from human sources, mostly originating in the burning of fossil fuels. The single greatest source of acid deposition in the United States is coal-fired power plants, followed by ore smelters, steel mills, and other industries. Figure 16.1 shows those areas in North America which are most vulnerable to acid deposition because of their geology and proximity to industries that produce sulfur and nitrogen dioxide.

Effects of Acid Deposition   The damage caused to lake and pond habitats is not the worst of the problems created by acid deposition. Each year, acid deposition is responsible for the destruction of millions of trees in forests in Europe and North America. For example, in 1982, an estimated 8 percent of trees in West German forests were in poor health. By 1985, this figure had

---

* *Breath in Danger* (New York: American Lung Association, 1989), p. 2.

Acid Deposition   Precipitation contaminated with both nitric acid and sulfuric acid.

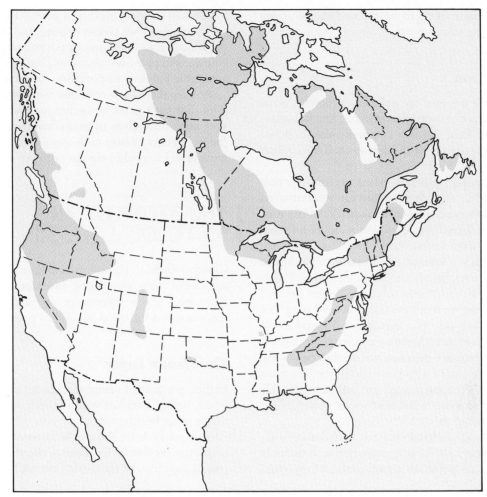

Figure 16.1 Areas of North America most vulnerable to acid deposition. Lakes and streams in the shaded areas on this map are most vulnerable to acid deposition because the bedrock of these areas has low acid neutralizing capacity.

increased to 52 percent.* Damage in North American forests is not yet as widespread, but it does appear to be a growing concern.

Although at the present time, precise data regarding adverse effects of acid deposition on human health are not available, medical doctors believe that acid deposition aggravates and may cause bronchitis, asthma, and other respiratory problems. People with emphysema and those with a history of heart disease may also suffer from exposure to acid deposition. Acid deposition may also be hazardous to a pregnant woman's unborn child.

A final consequence of acid deposition is the destruction of public monuments and structures. Damage to buildings in the United States alone is estimated to be more than $5 billion annually.**

Air pollution is obviously a many-faceted problem. Because we breathe approximately 15,000 to 20,000 liters of air per day (compared to drinking 2 liters of

Acid rain has destroyed thousands of acres of forests and continues to pose a significant threat to the environment.

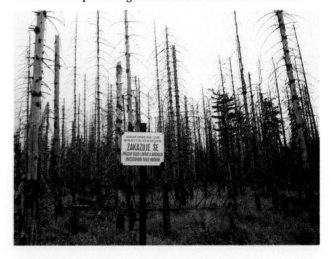

* Lawrence Pringle, *Rain of Trouble* (New York: Macmillan, 1988), pp. 60–61.
** Pringle, *Rain of Trouble*, p. 78.

water), we are more likely to be exposed to pollutants through breathing than any other way.

National Action

The roots of our national air pollution problems lie in our use of energy, transportation systems, and industrial technology. We must develop comprehensive national strategies to clear the air for the nineties and the coming century.

Modern technology provides means to reduce air pollution levels. Sulfur dioxide emissions can be controlled by *scrubbers,* devices installed in smokestacks of coalfired facilities. *Selective catalytic reduction* removes nitrogen oxide emissions from smoke. And, particular matter can be removed from smokestack emissions through the use of electrostatic precipitators and baghouse filters. These, however, are only short-term solutions at best because they can create environmental hazards of their own. For example, scrubber ash is a hazardous byproduct of scrubber use. Moreover, these three technologies do not reduce carbon dioxide emissions; nor do they help solve the problems associated with global warming. We must support policies that encourage the use of renewable resources such as solar, wind, and water power as the providers of most of the world's energy.

Most experts agree that shifting away from automobiles as the primary source of transportation is the only way to reduce air pollution significantly. Many cities have taken steps in this direction by setting high parking fees, imposing bans on city driving, and establishing high road-usage tolls. Community governments should be encouraged to provide convenient, inexpensive, and easily accessible public transportation for their citizens.

Auto makers must continue to manufacture automobiles that have good fuel economy and low toxic emission rates. Incentives to manufacturers, and tax breaks for purchasers, along with gas-guzzler taxes on inefficient vehicles, could help spur growth in this direction.

THE OZONE LAYER AND GLOBAL WARMING

Closely related to air pollution are the growing problems associated with the ozone layer and gradual global warming. These problems are interrelated and pose serious questions for the earth and its population.

The Ozone Layer

Earlier, we defined ozone as a chemical that is produced when oxygen interacts with sunlight. Close to the earth, ozone poses health problems such as respiratory distress. Farther away from the earth, however, ozone forms a protective membranelike layer in the earth's stratosphere (the highest level of the earth's atmosphere). This layer is

Conservation

Tips for Conserving Electrical Energy

- Keep your thermostat set between 65 and 68 degrees during daytime hours and between 50 and 60 degrees at night. Be sure your heating system is frequently serviced and maintained.

- Minimize your use of air conditioning. Set your thermostat at no lower than 78 degrees. Keep the system clean and free from leaves and debris that may clog vents.

- Consider alternatives to air conditioning including shades, ceiling fans, and shutting the doors to unoccupied rooms.

- Maintain an airtight home. Caulk, weatherstrip, and maintain windows and doors.

- Keep draft guards at the base of all outside doors.

- Insulate your attic according to levels recommended for your geographical area.

- Plant trees around your house to keep it cooler in the summer.

- Conserve water as much as possible, especially hot water. Install a water-saver showerhead to cut water flow from 40 to 60 percent. Repair leaky faucets. Invest in water-saving toilets.

- When you purchase new appliances, buy the most energy-efficient ones you can afford. This is especially important for refrigerators, because this appliance runs 24 hours a day, 365 days a year.

- Use energy-efficient light bulbs.

- Turn off lights in unused rooms.

located from 12 to 30 miles above the earth's surface and protects the earth and its inhabitants from ultraviolet B (UV-B) radiation, a primary cause of skin cancer.

Recently, the United Nations Environment Program predicted a 26 percent rise in the incidence of non-melanoma skin cancers worldwide if overall ozone levels drop 10 percent. UV rays can cause the lens of the eye to cloud up with cataracts, which leads to blindness if un-treated. Excess UV radiation may also damage DNA and be linked to weakened immune systems in humans and animals.* Ultraviolet B radiation may also damage DNA and it, too, may be linked to weakened immune systems in humans and animals.

In addition to visible health effects, the ozone layer affects how well the atmosphere absorbs heat. Without the ozone layer, the atmosphere absorbs less heat, mak-ing the surface of the earth hotter, thereby contributing to global warming. Global warming is discussed in more detail in the next section.

Chlorofluorocarbons In the early 1970s, scientists began to warn of a depletion in the earth's ozone layer. Special instruments developed to test atmospheric con-tents indicated that specific chemicals used on earth were contributing to the rapid depletion of the vital protective layer. These chemicals are called **chlorofluorocarbons (CFCs)**.

Chlorofluorocarbons were first believed to be miracle chemicals. They were used as refrigerants (Freon), aerosol propellants in products such as hair sprays and deodorants, cleaning solvents, medical sterilizers, rigid foam insulation, and Styrofoam. Along with halons

(used in many fire extinguishers), methyl chloroform, and carbon tetrachloride (organic cleaning solvents), CFCs were found to be the major cause of depletion of the ozone layer.

When released into the air through spraying our out-gassing, CFCs migrate upward toward the ozone layer, where they decompose and release chlorine atoms. These atoms cause ozone molecules to break apart.

In 1979, a satellite photograph showing a large hole in the ozone layer over Antarctica shocked and worried scientists. Since then, satellites have taken regular photo-graphs of the ozone layer, which show an increase in the size of the hole (Figure 16.2). The latest findings imply that the ozone layer over some regions including the northernmost parts of the United States, Canada, and Europe, could be temporarily depleted soon by as much as 40 percent.**

In the early 1970s, the U.S. government banned the use of aerosol sprays containing CFCs in an effort to reduce ozone depletion. CFCs are still used in various foam products, refrigerators, and air conditioners. The United States still has the highest per capita use of CFCs in the world, generating approximately 30 percent of emissions of ozone-depleting chemicals, with Japan close behind.

In 1987, after much international negotiation, a group of 24 nations agreed to freeze all production of CFCs immediately and to reduce CFC outputs by 50 percent by the year 1998. This agreement was called the Montreal Protocol. The Protocol was further strength-

---

Chlorofluorocarbons Chemicals that contribute to the depletion of the ozone layer.

---

* "The Ozone Vanishes," *Time*, February 17, 1992, pp. 60–63.

** Ibid.

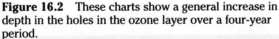

Figure 16.2 These charts show a general increase in depth in the holes in the ozone layer over a four-year period.

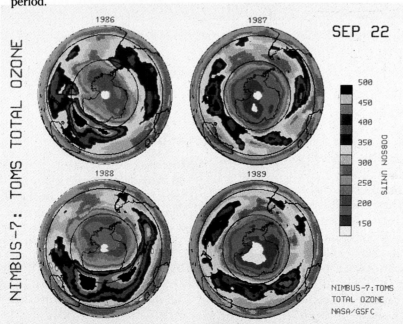

Environmental Watch Inside Your Home

Indoor Air Pollution

Combating the problems associated with air pollution begins at home. Indoor air can be 10 to 40 times more hazardous than outdoor air, and there are between 20 and 100 potentially dangerous chemical compounds present in the average home.

Woodstove Smoke Woodstove smoke is a serious air pollution problem in some metropolitan areas. Woodstoves emit significant levels of particulates and carbon monoxide in addition to other pollutants, such as sulfur dioxide. People who rely on wood for heating should make sure that their

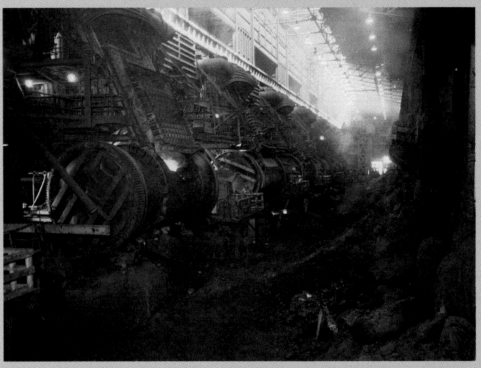

A copper smelting plant. Many industrial processes, such as copper smelting, release gases that contribute to the greenhouse effect.

ened in May 1989, when 81 nations signed the Helsinki Declaration, a document that pledged to completely phase out CFCs by the year 2000.

In 1990 a law was passed that called for an accelerated phaseout of CFCs if new scientific evidence revealed a greater threat to the ozone layer than expected. Based on such evidence the United States may seek to end CFC production by 1996. Although it will take several years before alternative chemicals can be substituted for CFCs, some of the alternatives, as Table 16.3 shows, are not without environmental hazards of their own.

Global Warming

More than 100 years ago, scientists theorized that carbon dioxide emissions from fossil-fuel burning would create a buildup of greenhouse gases in the earth's atmosphere. This accumulation, in turn, would have a warming effect on the earth's surface.

The Greenhouse Effect The century-old predictions have now begun to come true, with alarming effects. Average global temperatures are higher today than at

Environmental Watch Inside Your Home (*Continued*)

stove is properly installed, vented, and maintained. Proper adjustments and emission controls to recombust potential pollutants can also help to reduce pollution levels from woodstoves. In addition, burning properly seasoned wood reduces particulates released into the air.

Asbestos Asbestos is another indoor air pollutant that poses serious threats to human health. It is a mineral that was commonly used in insulating materials in homes built before 1970. If the tiny asbestos fibers become airborne, they can embed themselves in the lungs and cannot be expelled. Their presence leads to cancer of the lungs, stomach, and chest lining. To eliminate asbestos hazards in your home, have an asbestos testing lab (usually listed in the yellow pages) come to inspect. If there is asbestos present, it should be removed by a qualified contractor.

Passive Smoke Exposure to cigarette smoke can significantly increase the risks of developing cancer. (For more information on passive smoke, see Chapter 11.) People who are exposed to other indoor pollutants, such as radon and asbestos, are particularly at risk. If you smoke, quit. Ask guests who smoke to do so outside.

Formaldehyde Formaldehyde is a colorless, strong-smelling gas. It is present in carpets, draperies, furniture, particleboard, plywood, wood

paneling, countertops, and many adhesives. Exposure to formaldehyde can cause respiratory problems, dizziness, fatigue, nausea, and rashes. Long-term exposure can lead to central nervous system disorders and cancer.

To reduce exposure to formaldehyde, avoid the purchase of products containing this gas. Ask about formaldehyde content in the products you purchase. If your home has urea-formaldehyde, remove it and replace it with a safer substance. If you experience symptoms of formaldehyde exposure, have your home tested by a city, county, or state health agency.

Radon Radon has been recognized as one of the most serious forms of indoor air pollution. This odorless, colorless gas is the natural by-product of the decay of uranium and radium in the soil. Radon penetrates homes through cracks, pipes, sump pits, and others openings in the foundation. Between 5,000 and 20,000 cancer deaths per year have been attributed to radon. A home testing kit from a hardware store will enable you to test your home yourself. If your home tests high in radon levels, you should have a professional seal cracks in the floor of the basement or foundation and cover and seal other openings, such as floor drains or sump pumps. Exposed soil should be covered with concrete.

---

any time since 1862, and a radical change in atmospheric temperature is taking a toll on human beings and crops. Climate researchers have predicted since 1975 that the buildup of greenhouse gases would produce life-threatening natural phenomena, including drought in the midwestern United States, more frequent and severe forest fires, flooding in India and Bangladesh, extended heat waves over large areas, and superhurricanes. In 1988 and 1989, the planet experienced all five of these phenomena.

Greenhouse gases include carbon dioxide, CFCs, ground-level ozone, nitrous oxide, and methane. They become part of a gaseous layer that encircles the earth, allowing solar heat to pass through and then trapping the heat close to the earth's surface.

The most predominant of the gases is carbon dioxide, which accounts for 50 percent of the greenhouse gases. Eastern Europe and North America are responsible for approximately half of all carbon dioxide emissions. Since the late nineteenth century, carbon dioxide concen-

Greenhouse Gases Gases in the upper atmosphere that contribute to global warming by trapping heat near the earth's surface.

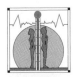
Guidelines for Protecting Yourself Against the Sun

Ozone depletion is cause for caution, but it's no reason to stay barricaded indoors or put on a body shield before venturing outside. Excessive exposure to the sun's ultraviolet (UV) rays is dangerous, depletion of the ozone just adds to the risk.

Even if there were no damage to the ozone layer, an estimated one-sixth of all Americans would still develop skin cancer during their lifetime. Most of these cases are curable if detected early. The 4 to 8 percent loss of ozone over the past decade could raise the risk at least 15 percent. A significant increase in cataracts, which now afflict 1 of every 10 Americans, is also possible.

As the ozone depletion worsens, health risks will rise. Experts suggest the following guidelines for protecting yourself:

1. When out in the sun for prolonged periods of time, put on protective clothing. Choose clothes made of tightly woven fabric and wear a wide-brimmed hat. Baseball caps and visors are inadequate, as they can leave the scalp and rims of the ears exposed.

2. Use a broad spectrum sunscreen with sun protection factor of at least 15, especially from 10 A.M. to 3 P.M. Remember to reapply the sunscreen after swimming or sweating.

3. Wear sunglasses when outdoors in the bright sunlight. Use glasses treated to absorb UV radiation or that meet the American National Standards Institute Guidelines for eye wear. Glasses that are not treated to block UV rays can do more harm than good, as the dark lens can cause the eyes to dilate, allowing the damaging UV rays to harm the retina.

SOURCE: "The Ozone Vanishes," *Time,* February 17, 1992, p. 62.

Table 16.3 CFC Alternatives

HCFCs (hydrochlorofluorocarbons)
PRO Because they break down more quickly in the atmosphere, they pose less danger in the ozone layer.
CON If overused, they can damage ozone. Repaired appliances may use more energy than original appliances.

HFCs (hydrofluorocarbons)
PRO Because they do not contain chlorine, they are "ozone safe."
CON Safety questions such as flammability and toxicity remain unsolved.

Hydrocarbons (such as butane and propane)
PRO They are cheap and readily available.
CON They can be flammable and poisonous. Some add to ground-level pollution.

Ammonia
PRO It is an easy alternative to refrigerators.
CON It has to be handled carefully.

Water and steam
They are effective for some cleaning applications.

---

trations in the atmosphere have increased 25 percent, with half of this increase occurring since the 1950s. Not surprisingly, these greater concentrations coincide with world industrial growth.

Rapid deforestation in the tropical rain forests of Central and South America, Africa, and Southeast Asia is contributing to the rapid rise in the production of greenhouse gases. Without those forests, there is no way to dissipate carbon dioxide. Trees take in carbon dioxide, transform it, store the carbon for food, and then release oxygen into the air.

The consequences of global warming are dire. Scientists predict an increase in natural disasters, such as superhurricanes like Hurricane Hugo, which struck the eastern United States and the Caribbean in 1989. Increased energy use in response to warming (air conditioners) will exacerbate levels of greenhouse gases in the atmosphere. Forest fires will increase. Rapid global warming will affect large mammals, especially in the middle latitudes, stifling their reproductive capabilities. Melting polar ice caps will cause the sea levels to rise, inundating many low-lying areas, which are primary food-producing regions in some countries.

WATER POLLUTION

Seventy-five percent of the earth is covered with water in the form of oceans, seas, lakes, rivers, streams, and wetlands. Beneath the landmass are reservoirs of groundwater. We draw our drinking water from either underground or surface freshwater sources. The status of our water supply is ultimately a reflection of the pollution level of our earth and communities.

In 1986, the National Wildlife Federation concluded a study revealing that the major environmental concern of Americans was the quality of their drinking water. The Federation followed up on their study with an additional 18-month probe into the quality of drinking water in the United States. This study found more than 100,000 violations of federal public health standards for drinking water. Over 40 million people were affected by these violations.*

---

* *Danger on Tap* (Washington, DC: National Wildlife Federation, 1988).

Human and industrial waste have had a significant negative impact on waterways such as Lake Michigan.

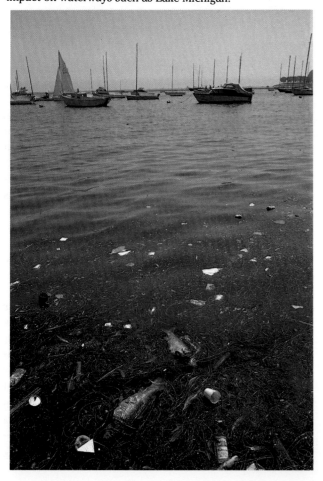

How Contamination Occurs

Any substance that gets into the soil has the potential to get into the water supply. Contaminants that settle from industrial air pollution and acid deposition eventually work their way into the soil and then to the ground water. Pesticides sprayed on crops wash through the soil into the ground water. Spills of oil and other hazardous wastes flow into local rivers and streams. Underground storage tanks for gasoline may develop leaks. The list continues. The major water pollutants include chemical pollutants, such as organic solvents and chemicals and pesticides, and gasoline and petroleum products, but water supplies are contaminated by other pollutants as well (see Figure 16.3).

Dumps and Landfills   Landfills and dumps generate a liquid called **leachate,** a mixture of soluble chemicals that come from household garbage, office waste, biological waste, and industrial waste. Leachate trickles through the layers of garbage in a landfill and into the water supply.

Lead   Significant lead levels in drinking water are much more common than once assumed. Levels once thought to be safe are now known to threaten health, especially in infants and children. The EPA estimates that drinking water now accounts for 15 to 25 percent of a child's total lead intake, much more if the water is highly contaminated.* Soft or acidic water is very effective at corroding pipes thereby allowing lead to invade the drinking water. Copper pipes connected by lead solder or brass faucets leaches lead into water. A solution to this problem is to let tap water run each morning for about a minute, or until it is as cold as possible, to clear out the lead that has accumulated overnight. Use only cold water for cooking and drinking.**

Nitrates   Nitrate contamination occurs mainly in groundwater. In a recent survey conducted by the EPA, nitrate showed up in more than half of the drinking water wells tested across the country.*** Fertilizers are designed to add nitrogen to the soil, thereby increasing plant yield. Wastes leaking from septic tanks also add nitrogen to groundwater. Nitrogen leaches into the soil and combines with oxygen to form nitrates and, later, nitrosamines, chemicals associated with cancer. Nitrate levels are also a threat to newborn infants and developing fetuses. Distillation and digging a deeper well to

---

Leachate   A liquid consisting of soluble chemicals from garbage and industrial waste that seeps into the water supply from landfills.

---

* "The Pollutants That Matter Most: Lead, Radon, Nitrate," *Consumer Reports* (1990) 55 (1):30–34.
** "Is Your Water Safe?" *U.S. News and World Report* (1991) 3(5):44–55.
*** Ibid.

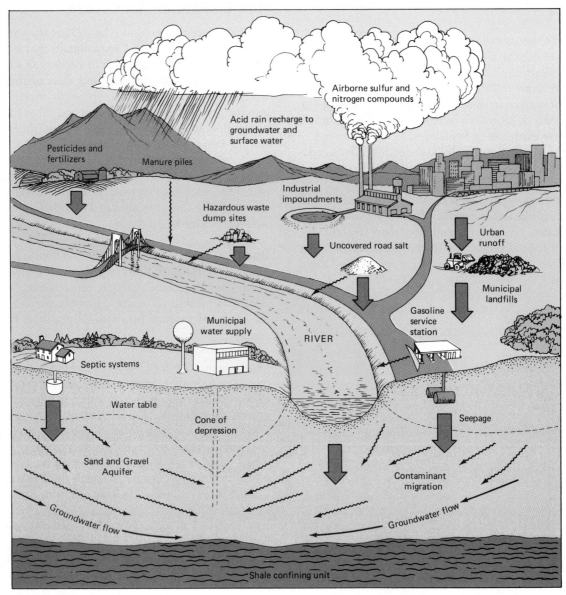

Figure 16.3 Sources of groundwater contamination.

an uncontaminated water source are alternatives for avoiding nitrate-contaminated water.

Radon Radon poses a greater health risk than any other environmental pollutant. Not only does radon pollute the air, but this radioactive gas also permeates groundwater. The EPA estimates that as many as 17 million people may have excessive levels of radon in their water. It is most likely to be present in water from private wells or from community water systems serving fewer than 500 people. Between 100 and 1,800 deaths a year are attributed to radon from household water. Showering, dishwashing, and laundering agitate water and release radon into the air. Simple measures may reduce exposure to waterborne radiation. Ventilating your bathroom, laundry, or kitchen may be all that is needed. Water treatment may be necessary. All water entering a

house needs to be treated, with either home aerators or granular-activated carbon units.

Gasoline and Petroleum Products In the United States, there are more than 2 million underground storage tanks for gasoline and petroleum products, most of which are located at gasoline filling stations. One quarter of these underground tanks are thought to be leaking.*

Most of these tanks were installed between 25 and 30 years ago. They were made of fabricated steel that was unprotected from corrosion. Pinpoint holes may develop, and the petroleum products can leak into the groundwater. The most common way to detect the presence of petroleum products in the water supply is to

* John Naar, *Design for a Livable Planet* (New York: Harper & Row, 1990), p. 68.

test for benzene, a component of oil and gasoline. Benzene is highly toxic and is associated with the development of cancer.

As long as the world's oceans are used as transportation lanes for crude oil tankers, the danger of oil spills exists. In March 1989, the *Exxon Valdez,* an oil supertanker, ran aground on Bligh Reef in Prince William Sound, near the town of Valdez, Alaska. The ruptured tanker spilled 11 million gallons of crude oil into the sound. Cleanup operations were slow, and thousands of miles of wilderness coastline were fouled with oil. Hundreds of seals, otters, and seabirds were killed. Commercial fishing operations in the area were completely shut down for the 1989 season. The 1990 herring season took place on schedule, but each fish was tested for contamination before being released for marketing.

Chemical Pollutants

Chemicals designed to dissolve grease and oil are called organic solvents. These extremely toxic substances, such as carbon tetrachloride, tetrachloroethylene, and trichlorethylene (TCE), are used to clean clothing, paint equipment, plastics, and metal parts. Many household products, such as stain and spot removers, degreasers, drain cleaners, septic system cleaners, and paint removers, contain these toxic chemicals.

Organic solvents work their way into the water supply in different ways. Consumers often dump leftover

In March 1989, the oil tanker *Exxon Valdez* ran aground and spilled 11 million gallons of crude oil into Alaska's Prince William Sound.

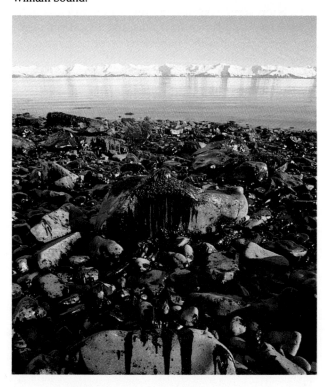

products into the toilet. Industries pour leftovers into large barrels, which are then buried. After a while, the chemicals eat their way out of the barrels and leach into the groundwater system.

Organic chemicals are a related group of toxic substances that contain chlorinated hydrocarbons. The most notorious of these substances are the **polychlorinated biphenyls** (PCBs), their cousins the *polybromated biphenyls* (PBBs), and the **dioxins.**

PCBs PCBs are fire-resistant and stable at high temperatures and are used as insulating materials in high-voltage electrical equipment such as transformers. PCBs bioaccumulate, meaning that the body does not excrete them, but rather stores them in fatty tissues and the liver. PCBs are associated with birth defects, and exposure to them is known to cause cancer. The manufacture of PCBs was discontinued in the United States in 1977, but associated problems have not disappeared. Between 300 million and 540 million kilograms of PCBs are still in use, and still have the potential to enter the environment.*

Dioxins Dioxins are chlorinated hydrocarbons that are used in herbicides (chemicals employed to kill vegetation), paper processors, and garbage incinerators. Today these chlorine by-products are lodged in the body of every American who eats fish, meat, or dairy products.* Dioxins are associated with birth defects and cancer. Dioxins now appear more dangerous to human health than ever. Not only are they potential carcinogens, the newest research indicates they have substantial immunological, developmental, and neurological effects that may actually pose the greater public health threat.** Like PCBs, dioxins have the ability to bioaccumulate. But dioxins are much more toxic than PCBs, as a smaller concentration of dioxin is required to reach toxicity levels. Dioxins have been called some of the most toxic chemicals known to humans.

The long-term effects of bioaccumulation of these toxic substances are extremely serious. However, exposure to high concentrations of PCBs or dioxins for a short period of time can also have severe consequences, including nausea, vomiting, diarrhea, painful rashes and sores, and chloracne, an ailment in which the skin develops hard, black, painful pimples that may be permanent. In 1979, the EPA banned the use of two herbicides

Polychlorinated Biphenyls (PCBs) Industrial chemicals used in electrical transformers, lubricants, and plastics; can cause cancer.
Dioxin A toxic chemical used in some herbicides; can cause cancer.

* Joseph M. Moran, Michael Morgan, and James H. Wiersma, *Introduction to Environmental Science* 2nd ed. (New York: W.H. Freeman, 1986), p. 227.
* Karen Schmidt, "Puzzling over a Poison," *U. S. News and World Report* (1992) 112(13): 60–61.
** Ibid.

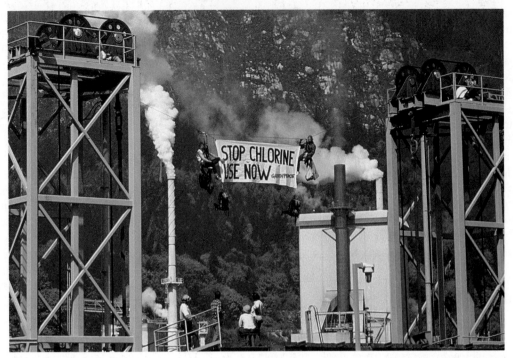

Dioxin is a byproduct of chlorine bleaching, used by pulp and paper plants to manufacture white goods for consumers.

that contain dioxin, 2,4,5-T and 2,4-D, after citizen action groups spoke out on their hazards to vegetation, animals, and humans.

Pesticides Pesticides are chemicals that are designed to kill insects, rodents, plants, and fungi. More than 1.2 billion pounds of pesticides are used each year, but only 10 percent actually reach the targeted organisms. The remaining 1.1 billion pounds of pesticides settle on the land and in the water supplies. Pesticide residues also cling to many fresh fruits and vegetables and are ingested when people eat these items.

Most pesticides accumulate in the body. Potential hazards associated with long-term exposure to pesticides include birth defects, cancer, liver and kidney damage, and nervous system disorders. Children are more at risk because of their small body sizes. Children consume large amounts of fresh fruits and vegetables, and many receive four times more exposure in pesticide residues in food than adults.

▍ NOISE POLLUTION

Noise has become commonplace in our lives. We are often painfully aware of construction crews in the streets, jets departing, blaring stereos, and the drone of trucks on nearby freeways. Our bodies have definite physiological responses to noise, and noise can become a source of physical or mental distress.

Prolonged exposure to some noises results in hearing loss. Short-term exposure reduces productivity, concentration levels, and attention spans, and may affect mental and emotional health. Symptoms of noise-related distress include disturbed sleep patterns, headaches, and tension. Physically, our bodies respond to noises in a variety of ways. Blood pressure increases, blood vessels in the brain dilate, and vessels in other parts of the body constrict. The pupils of the eye dilate. Cholesterol levels in the blood rise, and some endocrine glands secrete additional stimulating hormones, such as adrenaline, into the bloodstream.

At this point, it is necessary to distinguish between *sound* and *noise*. Sound is anything that can be heard. Noise is sound that can damage the hearing or cause mental or emotional distress. When sounds become distracting or annoying, they become noise.

Sounds are measured in decibels. Table 16.4 shows the decibel levels for various sounds. Hearing can be damaged by varying lengths of exposure to sound. If the duration of allowable daily exposure to different decibel levels is exceeded, hearing loss will result.

Pesticides Chemicals that kill insect pests.

Table 16.4 Noise Levels of Various Activities (in Decibels)

Decibels (db) measure the volume of sounds. Decibel levels of some common sounds are presented here.

Type of Sound	Noise Level (db)
Carrier deck jet operation	150
Jet takeoff from 200 feet	140
	120 painful
Rock music	110
Auto horn (3 feet)	110 extremely loud
Motorcycle	100
Garbage truck	100
Pneumatic drill	90
Lawnmower	90
Heavy traffic	80
Alarm clock	80
Shouting, arguing	80 very loud
Vacuum cleaner	75 loud
Freight train from 50 feet	70
Freeway traffic	65
Normal conversation	60
Light auto traffic	50 moderate
Library	40
Soft whisper	30 faint

HAZARDOUS AND SOLID WASTES

Hazardous waste dump sites are merely an indication of the severity of the toxic chemical problem in the United States. There are approximately 12,000 chemical manufacturing facilities in this country. These facilities produce 70,000 kinds of chemicals, including nearly 40,000 pesticides. American manufacturers generate more than 1 ton of chemical waste per person per year (approximately 260 million tons).†

Hazardous Waste Disposal

There are three principal methods for disposal of hazardous wastes: secure landfills, incineration, and deep-well injection. **Secure landfill** sites are controlled by strict regulations and regularly inspected. They must be located above the 100-year floodplain for the region and away from fault zones. Solid hazardous wastes such as solvents, pesticides, and petroleum-refinery waste, as well as combustible liquid wastes, are disposed of through burning, or **incineration.** Incineration reduces the volume of toxic wastes and destroys organic chemicals by converting them to carbon dioxide, water, and gases, which are then removed by scrubbers. The third method of hazardous waste disposal is **deep-well**

injection. This method forces hazardous wastes into wells that are at least 1,000 meters (3,000 feet) deep. Deep wells can be located only in certain areas, and they must be drilled into rock that is deep, porous enough to hold the injected chemicals, and sandwiched between layers of impermeable rock.

Solid Waste

Solid waste is the trash that accumulates in landfills throughout the country. It includes plastics, wrappers, aluminum foil, glass, cans, disposable diapers, paper, tires, batteries, used appliances, and many more items that take up space in dumps.

Each day, the United States creates approximately 450,000 tons of residential and commercial solid waste. Experts believe this figure may reach 530,000 tons per day by the year 2000.* Eighty percent of this trash is buried in landfills. Cities and smaller communities throughout the country are in danger of exhausting their landfill space. Some cities have already run out of landfill space. Philadelphia, for example, must ship its garbage to landfills in Ohio, Maryland, and Virginia at an annual cost of more than $44 million.

Garbage is heaped on barges and sent to landfills in other parts of the country. When this method fails, the garbage is hauled to sea and dumped, or taken to landfills in developing countries for dumping.

Figure 16.4 shows the composition of our trash and what happens to our garbage after disposal. Recycling now accounts for only 10 percent of garbage treatment. Experts believe that as much as 90 percent of our trash is ultimately recyclable. Recycling is not a new word or concept in the American vocabulary. Americans have been recycling for years. During World War I, the Great Depression, and World War II, scrap materials, bottles, clothing, and other goods were recycled regularly because of scarcity of products. In today's throwaway society, we need to become aware of the amount of waste generated by each of us every day and look for ways to recycle, reuse, and most desirable of all, reduce the need for the products we use.

Aluminum Aluminum, especially that found in cans, is very valuable. Approximately 95 percent less energy is needed to make a new aluminum can from recycled aluminum than to make a can from ore. The aluminum industry is geared to purchase and process all the alumi-

Secure Landfills Landfill sites designated for hazardous waste disposal.

Incineration Burning or solid hazardous wastes.

Deep-well Injection A method of hazardous waste disposal that forces wastes into deep wells.

Solid Waste The trash that accumulates in landfills and dumps.

---

† Naar, *Design for a Livable Planet*, p. 38.

* Patricia H. Hynes, *Earthright* (Rocklin, CA: Prima Publishing and Communications, 1990), p. 47.

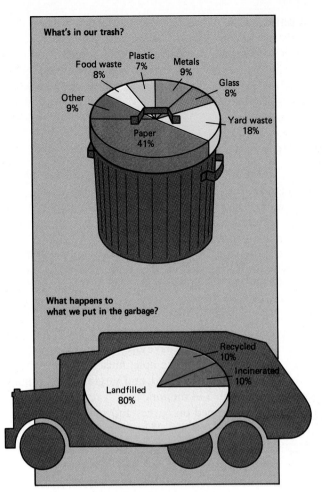

What's in our trash?

Food waste 8%
Plastic 7%
Metals 9%
Glass 8%
Other 9%
Paper 41%
Yard waste 18%

What happens to what we put in the garbage?

Recycled 10%
Incinerated 10%
Landfilled 80%

Figure 16.4 The composition and disposition of our trash.

num in the country, including recyclable aluminum. Recycling aluminum cans is an easy way consumers can help conserve energy and stop solid waste pollution. Other products made from aluminum are also recyclable, including aluminum siding, gutters, downspouts, storm doors, window frames, and lawn furniture frames. Most communities have dealers who will pay for such products.

Iron and Steel Scrap metal dealers are the most visible recyclers today. The metals we use in pipes, automobiles, and tin food cans is all recyclable. New tin can be manufactured from old tin, and new steel can be reprocessed from old steel.

Paper Paper is the largest component of the American trash heap. There are five broad grades of wastepaper that can be recycled: newspaper; corrugated cardboard; office paper; mixed paper from cereal boxes, telephone books, junk mail, and grocery bags; and high grade wastepaper from commercial printers. Many communities have paper recycling programs, and there is a strong export market for recyclable papers, especially in Japan, Taiwan, and South Korea.

Glass Approximately 10 percent of our national trash heap is composed of glass from bottles, jars, and other containers. Glass is made from sand, soda ash, and limestone and is easy to recycle. Old crushed glass melts at a lower temperature than do the individual components of glass. Therefore less energy is required to recycle glass products.

Plastics Plastics make up approximately 7 percent of our total waste, but they are the most troublesome of wastes because they endure for long periods of time without breaking down. Plastics in the environment pose hazards to animals, birds, and fish. Creatures can become tangled in plastic six-pack holders or plastic fishing line and can suffocate.

Recycling of plastics has not been pursued as diligently as has recycling of other materials, but the public is pushing for more recycling projects, and the industry is complying slowly. Three types of plastics can be recycled. The polyethylene terephthalate (PET) in soft-drink bottles can be recycled into carpet backing and fiberfill (a lightweight filling made of synthetic fibers) for such items as sleeping bags and jackets. It can also be recycled into refrigerator insulation, fiberglass, paintbrushes, and kitchen scouring pads.

High-density polyethylene (HDPE) is another type of plastic that can be recycled. HDPE can be made into trash cans, flowerpots, pipes, traffic cones, plastic lumber, pier decking, and fencing.

The polystyrene foam found in cups, plates, fast-food containers, and various packaging is also recyclable. This material can be cleaned and converted into little pellets that can be combined into plastic lumber, building insulation, and packing material.

Plastic recycling does have its drawbacks, however. Some plastic resins cannot be combined with one another. Also, recycling of plastic generally does not reduce the amount of plastics manufactured, nor the volume of plastic waste. Consumer pressure must influence manufacturers to slow the manufacture of plastics.

Motor Oil Motor oils can be recycled through a process called **rerefining** and can be used again as motor oil, or as an acceptable fuel for some incinerators.

Scrap Tires More than 1 billion scrap tires have accumulated throughout the United States. Abandoned tires have a tendency to collect water and become breeding grounds for mosquitoes and other insects. Burning tires is not a solution, because tires can burn for months, fouling the air with noxious fumes. Old tires can be recycled by grinding, shredding, and pulverizing. They are then turned into sheet rubber and used to make new tires or as an ingredient in asphalt or concrete. The federal Intermodal Surface Transportation Efficiency Act, signed into law in December 1991, requires that 5 percent of asphalt laid using federal aid in 1994 must contain scrap rubber from tires. This translated into more than 3,000 miles of rubberized roadway for that year, with the law requiring the percentage to increase over time.* Some cities pay about 10 cents per pound to dispose of old tires. This cost amounts to approximately $700,000 per year for a medium-sized city. A rubber recycling plant could add up to $3 million to the local economy, thus providing recycling services and jobs for the community.

NUCLEAR HAZARDS

The discoveries of the X ray in 1895 by Wilhelm Roentgen and of radium in 1898 by Madame Marie Curie marked the beginning of the atomic age. Later, in the 1940s, physicists at Los Alamos, New Mexico, succeeded in turning theory into the reality of nuclear weapons. Those physicists had hoped that once they created a bomb to end the war, nuclear energy would be put to peaceful uses, such as the generation of electricity. Instead, stockpiles of nuclear weapons and radioactive waste dumps are endangering the health of the planet.

Radiation

Radiation is not a new phenomenon. The earth has been subjected to various types of radiation throughout its history, including cosmic rays and background radiation from elements in the soil. **Radiation** is caused by the release of particles and electromagnetic rays from atomic nuclei during the normal process of disintegration. Some naturally occurring elements, such as uranium, emit radiation. Other radiation-producing elements, such as deuterium, develop as part of the decay process of uranium or are created by humans in laboratories. Radiation, whether naturally occurring or made by humans, can damage the genetic material in the reproductive cells of living organisms. Radiation can also cause mutations, miscarriages, physical and mental deformities, cancer, eye cataracts, gastrointestinal illnesses, and shortened life expectancies.

These sources of radiation are not as worrisome to us as the radiation associated with nuclear energy production or the use of nuclear weapons. A substance is said to be *radioactive* when it emits high-energy particles from the nuclei of its atoms. Three types of radiation exist: alpha particles, beta particles, and gamma rays. Alpha particles are the slowest moving and are not capable of penetrating human skin. They pose health hazards only when inhaled or ingested. Beta particles are capable of slight penetration of the body and are harmful if ingested or inhaled. Gamma rays are the most dangerous radioactive particles because they can pass straight through the human body, causing serious damage to organs and other vital structures.

Scientists cannot agree on a "safe" level of radiation. Reactions to radiation differ from person to person. Exposure is measured in **radiation absorbed doses,** or *rads* (also called roentgens). Recommended maximum "safe" dosages range from 0.5 rads to 5 rads per year. Approximately 50 percent of the radiation to which we are exposed comes from natural sources, such as building materials. Another 45 percent comes from medical and dental X rays. The remaining 5 percent comes from computer display screens, microwave ovens, television sets, luminous watch dials, and radar screens and waves (see Table 16.5). For most of us, exposure to radiation is far below the recommended maximum per year.

Radiation can cause damage at dosages as low as 100 to 200 rads. At this level, signs of radiation sickness include nausea, diarrhea, fatigue, anemia, sore throat, and occasional hair loss. Death is unlikely at this dosage. At 350 to 500 rads, these symptoms become more severe, and death may result. Death and disease frequently result when radiation affects the bone marrow's ability to produce the white blood cells necessary to protect us from disease. Dosages above 600 to 700 rads are invariably fatal. The effects of long-term exposure to relatively low levels of radiation are unknown. Some scientists believe that such exposure can cause lung cancer, leukemia, skin cancer, bone cancer, and skeletal deformities.

Table 16.5 Everyday Doses of Radiation

Most of us believe that radioactivity is only associated with nuclear weapons or power plants. In fact, we receive doses of radioactivity from various other sources. Below are listed common sources of radiation in our environment. All values are expressed in rads (radiation absorbed doses). Recommended "safe" dosages are between 0.5 and 5 rads per year.

Source	Rads
Cosmic rays	0.45
Soil	0.15
Water, food, air	0.25
Air travel (round trip New York to London)	0.04
Medical X rays	0.10
Nuclear power plant in vicinity	0.01
Brick structures	0.50–1.0
Concrete structures	0.70–1.0
Wooden structures	0.30–0.50

SOURCE: *Radiation—A Fact of Life* (The American Nuclear Society, 1981).

Radiation Rays emitted from the release of fast-moving particles from atomic nuclei during decay.

Radiation Absorbed Doses (Rads) Units that measure radioactivity.

---

* Elizabeth Pennisi, "Rubber to the Road," *Science* (1992) p. 155.

Nuclear Power Plants

One source of radioactive emissions is nuclear power plants. At present, these plants account for less than 1 percent of the total radiation to which we are exposed. Disposal of radioactive wastes created by nuclear power plants and the possibility of reactor core meltdown are the two most serious threats these plants pose to the environment.

Electricity can be generated in many ways. Dams and other hydroelectric methods use the force of falling water to turn the turbines that generate electricity. Coal, natural gas, and oil-fired power plants use steam heat to turn similar turbines. Nuclear power plants also use heat to generate electricity, but the heat generated in such plants comes from atomic chain reactions in uranium fuel rods. When enough uranium or other radioactive material is combined, the escaping radioactive particles move to atomic nuclei, causing splitting or **fission** of other atoms. Once fission has occurred, the released atomic particles travel to other nuclei, producing self-sustaining chain reactions. This process liberates tremendous amounts of energy, which is then used to generate steam and turn generating turbines.

Proponents of nuclear energy believe that it is a safe and efficient way to generate electricity. Once the initial expense for building a power plant is out of the way, actual power generation is relatively inexpensive. One 1-inch pellet of uranium fuel produces as much electricity as 3 barrels of oil, 1 ton of coal, 2.5 tons of wood, or 17,000 cubic feet of natural gas. A 1,000-megawatt reactor produces enough energy for 650,000 homes and saves 420 million gallons of fossil fuels each year. In some areas where nuclear power plants have been decommissioned, electricity bills tripled when power companies were forced to turn to hydroelectric or fossil fuel sources to generate electricity.

Nuclear reactors also discharge fewer carbon monoxide emissions into the air than fossil fuel generators. Advocates believe that conversion to nuclear power could help slow the global warming trend. During the past 15 years during which nuclear power was popular, carbon emissions were reduced by 298 million tons, or 5 percent.*

The advantages of nuclear energy must be weighed against the disadvantages. First, disposal of nuclear wastes is extremely problematic for the entire world. Additionally, the chances of a reactor core meltdown pose serious threats to a plant's immediate environment and to the world in general.

Accidents at nuclear power plants are not rare occurrences. In 1985, United States plants experienced nearly 3,000 mishaps and 765 emergency shutdowns. At least 18 of the shutdowns were reported to be the result of serious accidents that could have led to reactor core damage.

▌ TAKING INDIVIDUAL ACTION

Environmental health begins at home. One celebrant of the 1990 Earth Day stated that in order to save the planet, we will all have to overcome our inertia and make sacrifices that contribute to the good of the planet. Examine your behaviors that contribute to pollution, change those behaviors, and take community action to improve your local environment. Showing your concern for the earth by living an environmentally conscious life will have a positive impact on the rest of the world.

Politically, we need to understand how various policies affect the environment. We can exert pressure on leaders to change policies that affect the environment. For example, environmentalist pressure forced the World Bank to stop issuing development loans that were leading to the destruction of rain forests. Some of our national policies should be reexamined. Exporting American agricultural techniques, for example, has led to disaster in some areas because of fertilizer and pesticide pollution. Discussing issues with lawmakers and making decisions at the polls are two ways we can help influence national policy.

Saving the Ozone Layer

On an individual level, you can reduce the release of ozone-depleting chemicals into the atmosphere by reading labels and refusing to purchase products containing such chemicals. Also, the use of halon fire extinguishers should be limited to commercial or public use where water or chemical damage to paper and other products needs to be minimized, such as in libraries.

Nationally, we should urge our senators and representatives to work for a ban on production and use of ozone-depleting chemicals by 1996. We must also demand that such products not be imported into the United States from other countries. Even these measures do not guarantee the safety of the ozone layer, as CFCs and halons used in the early 1990s will remain in the upper atmosphere well into the twenty-first century.

Reducing Water and Air Pollution

Groundwater contamination is another extremely complex problem. Levels of contamination depend on the type of soil, the amount of water in the area, the concentrations of pollutants, and the rate of flow of the groundwater in question. Preventing contamination is better

---

* Christopher Flavin, "Slowing Global Warming," in *State of the World, 1990,* Lester R. Brown, ed., pp. 23–24.

Fission   The splitting of atoms; results in release of atomic energy.

Questions for Consumers

Shopping Checklist for Environmentally Conscious Consumers

1. Do I really need this product?
2. Is the package recyclable or returnable?
3. Is there a similar product with less packaging?
4. Can I reuse this disposable product?
5. Is there a nondisposable alternative?
6. How many times can I use this product before throwing it away?
7. How long will this product last?
8. Can this product be repaired rather than discarded?
9. If the product is something I seldom use, can I borrow or rent it?
10. Will the disposal of this product be a hazard to the environment? If so, is there a safer alternative?

SOURCE: Patricia H. Hynes, *Earthright* (Rocklin, CA: Prima Publishing and Communications, 1990), p. 59.

than trying to correct the problem at a later date. For example, a town in Massachusetts had to close down its public well in 1980 when benzenes from a leaking service station tank were found in the water supply. Ten years and $5 million later, the problem had not been solved.

Individually, you must first start by understanding where your drinking water originates. Then, identify possible sources of pollution, and eliminate or minimize your personal use and disposal of toxic substances.

Work in your community to help create and enforce laws that protect drinking water and prohibit the manufacture, use, storage, transport, or disposal of hazardous substances related to industries such as metal plating shops, machine shops, printing operations, biological laboratories, pesticides, and dry cleaning in your water supply area. Your water supply area should also be free from sanitation landfills, wastewater treatment facilities, junk and salvage yards, service stations, and underground storage tanks for hazardous materials.

Encourage action in your community to sponsor household hazardous waste collection sites. Each year, U.S. households generate more than 2 million tons of hazardous waste chemicals from such products as old car batteries, car wax, household cleansers, paint, weed killers, fertilizers, and pesticides. Many communities sponsor annual or semiannual household hazardous waste pickup days during which citizens can bring their waste products to a central location for proper disposal.

Instead of using fertilizer on your lawn and garden, consider alternatives such as composting (using vegetable garbage as fertilizer). For gardening, there are alternatives to pesticides, including homemade foliage sprays using peppers, onions, and garlic. Natural pesticides, such as diatomaceous earth, pyrethrins (extracts from

chrysanthemums), and insect-eating predators, such as ladybugs and praying mantises, can be used in your garden. Minimize your use of toxic nonbiodegradable products. If you must use any toxic products in your home, use the smallest amount necessary to get the job done. Consider donating surplus products to community groups.

America's thirst for soft drinks provides a major source of solid waste. Recycling is one method of dealing with the problem in many states.

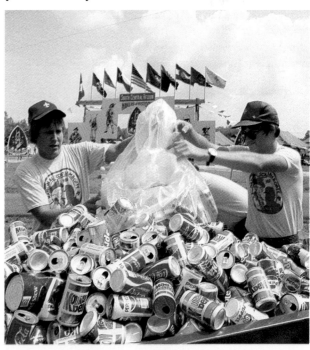

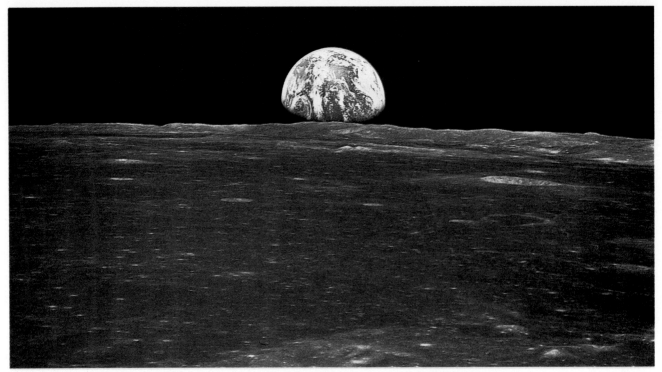

Preserving the delicate balances present in our environment is the challenge of the future. Without responsible actions today, tomorrow's world may be unfit for all forms of life.

Recycling

Be sure that your community has recycling opportunities. Use your political right to know to discover what kinds of hazardous waste dump sites exist in your community. Find out what is being done about them. If nothing is being done, take action by starting or joining a community activist group whose purpose is to eliminate hazardous waste in your community.

Recycling advocates promote the three Rs of recycling: reduce, reuse, and recycle. We are all capable of making an impact on the solid-waste problems in our communities if we follow these rules.

We need to learn to shop selectively. The box entitled "Shopping Checklist for Environmentally Conscious Consumers" includes questions each consumer should ask before making a purchase. When you shop, take your own cloth shopping bag to the store, or take old grocery bags. Buy sensibly packaged products with less plastic in the packaging material and reuse plastics products, such as produce bags, as often as possible.

Recycling and reuse are the other cornerstones of individual solid-waste management. Whenever possible, buy used and rebuilt products, and resell your unused items at yard or garage sales. Your trash may be someone else's treasure. Things that are not sold can be donated to charities. You should also urge your community to set up mandatory recycling programs, with garbage fees for people who do not recycle.

Reducing Energy Consumption

You can improve the environment by reducing your energy consumption. Start by using energy-efficient transportation. Purchase automobiles that get 30 to 35 miles per gallon of gasoline, and keep your car well tuned and maintained. Consider starting a car pool, taking public transportation, walking, or riding your bicycle. You can also maintain a fuel-efficient home, replacing inefficient light bulbs and purchasing energy-efficient appliances. Finally, support policies that encourage renewable energy such as solar, wind, and water power.

Appendix:
First Aid and Emergency Care

In certain situations, it may be necessary to administer first aid. Ideally, first-aid procedures should be performed by someone who has received formal training from the American Red Cross or some other reputable institution. If you do not have such training, you should contact a physician or call your local emergency medical service (EMS) by dialing 911 or your local emergency number. In life-threatening situations, however, you may not have time to call for outside assistance.

In cases of serious injury or sudden illness, you may need to initiate first aid immediately and continue at least until help arrives. This appendix contains basic information and general steps to follow for various emergency situations. It is important to remember that simply reading these directions may not prepare you fully to handle these situations. For this reason, you should consider enrolling in a first-aid course.

Calling for Emergency Assistance

When calling for emergency assistance, you should be prepared to give exact details. Be clear and thorough, and do not panic. Never hang up until the dispatcher has all the information needed. You should be ready to answer the following questions:

1. Where are you and the victim located? This is the most important information the EMS will need.
2. What has apparently happened? Was there an accident or illness?
3. What is the victim's apparent condition?
4. What has already been done to help the victim?
5. Are there any life-threatening situations that the EMS should know about (for example, fires, explosions, or fallen electrical lines)?
6. Do you know the victim's name?
7. Does the victim wear a medic-alert tage (a tag indicating a specific medical problem such as diabetes)?

Are You Liable?

According to the laws in most states, you are not required to administer first aid unless you have a special obligation. For example, parents must provide first aid for their children, and a lifeguard must provide aid to a swimmer.

Before administering first aid, you should obtain the victim's consent. If the victim refuses aid, you must respect that person's rights. However, you should make every reasonable effort to persuade the victim to accept your help. In emergency situations, consent is *implied* if the victim is unconscious.

Once you begin to administer first aid, you are required by law to continue. You must remain with the victim until someone of equal or greater competence takes over.

Can you be held liable if you fail to provide adequate care or if the victim is further injured? To help protect people who render first aid, most states have "good Samaritan" laws. These laws grant immunity (protection from civil liability) if you act in good faith to provide care to the best of your ability, according to your level of training. Because these laws vary from state to state, you should become familiar with the good Samaritan laws in your state.

When Someone Stops Breathing

If someone has stopped breathing, you should perform mouth-to-mouth resuscitation. This involves the following steps:

1. Check for a response by gently tapping or shaking the victim. Ask loudly, "Are you OK?"
2. Ask someone to call for help.
3. Roll victim onto back and pull slowly toward you.
4. Open an airway by tilting the victim's head back and lifting the chin.

5. Check for breathing: look, listen, and feel for breathing for 3 to 5 seconds.

6. Give 2 full breaths.
   • Keep victim's head tilted back.
   • Pinch victim's nose shut.
   • Seal your lips tightly around victim's mouth.
   • Give 2 full breaths for 1 to 1 1/2 seconds each.

7. Check for pulse at side of neck; feel for pulse for 5 to 10 seconds.

8. Phone EMS for help.

9. Begin rescue breathing.
   • Keep victim's head tilted back.
   • Lift victim's chin.
   • Pinch victim's nose shut.
   • Give 1 full breath every 5 seconds.
   • Look, listen, and feel for breathing between breaths.

10. Recheck pulse every minute.
    • Keep victim's head tilted back.
    • Feel for pulse for 5 to 10 seconds.
    • If victim has pulse but is not breathing, continue rescue breathing. If there is no pulse, begin CPR.

There are some variations when performing this procedure on infants and children. For children ages 1 to 8, at step 9, you should give one slow breath every 4 seconds. For infants, you should not pinch the nose. Instead, seal your lips tightly around the infant's nose and mouth. Also, at step 9, you should give one small breath every 3 seconds.

In cases in which the victim has no pulse, cardiopulmonary resuscitation (CPR) should be performed. This technique involves a combination of artificial respiration and chest compressions. You should not perform CPR unless you have received training. You cannot learn CPR simply by reading directions, and without training, you could cause further injury to the victim. The American

Red Cross offers courses in mouth-to-mouth resuscitation and CPR as well as general first aid. If you have taken a CPR course in the past, you should be aware that certain changes have been made in the procedure. You should consider taking a refresher course.

When Someone Is Choking

Choking occurs when an object obstructs the trachea (windpipe), thus preventing normal breathing. Failure to expel the object and restore breathing can lead to death within 6 minutes. The universal signal of distress related to choking is the clasping of the throat with one or both hands. Other signs of choking include not being able to talk and/or noisy and difficult breathing. If a victim can cough or speak, do not interfere. The most effective method for assisting choking victims is the Heimlich maneuver, which involves the application of pressure to the victim's abdominal area to expel the foreign object (see Figure A.1).

The Heimlich maneuver involves the following steps:

If the victim is standing or seated:

1. Wrap your arms around the victim's waist, making a fist with one hand.

2. Place the thumb side of the fist on the middle of the victim's abdomen, just above the navel.

3. Cover your fist with your other hand.

4. Press upward with a quick, thrusting motion, Repeat these abdominal thrusts until the obstruction is removed.

5. If the victim becomes unconscious, gently lower him or her to the ground.

6. Try to clear the airway by using your finger to sweep the object from the victim's mouth or throat.

Figure A.1 The Heimlich maneuver.

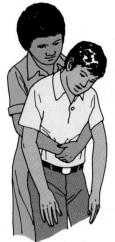
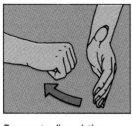

First aid for the choking victim
The Heimlich maneuver

Rescuer standing- victim standing or sitting

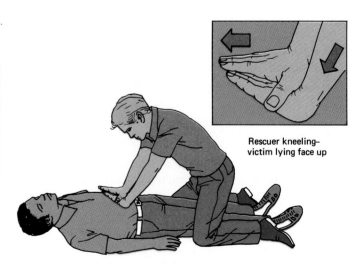

Rescuer kneeling-
victim lying face up

7. Then, try to inflate the lungs. If the passage is still blocked and air will not go in, proceed with the Heimlich maneuver as follows:

If the victim is lying down:

8. Facing the person, kneel with your legs astride the victim's hips. Place the heel of one hand against the abdomen, covering it with the other hand.

9. Press inward with quick upward thrusts. Do not push to either side. Repeat 6 to 10 times.

10. Repeat the following steps in this sequence until the airway becomes clear:
    a. attempt to clear airway using a finger sweep
    b. try to inflate the lungs
    c. perform 6 to 10 abdominal thrusts
    d. repeat

Controlling Bleeding

External Bleeding   Control of external bleeding is an important part of emergency care. Survival is threatened by the loss of 1 quart of blood or more. There are three major procedures for the control of external bleeding: direct pressure, elevation, and use of pressure points.

DIRECT PRESSURE   The best method is to apply firm pressure by covering the wound with a sterile dressing, bandage, or clean cloth. Apply pressure for 5 to 10 minutes to stop bleeding.

ELEVATION   Elevating the wounded section of the body can slow bleeding. For example, a wounded arm or leg should be raised above the level of the victim's heart. This technique can be used in combination with direct pressure.

PRESSURE POINTS   Pressure points are places over a bone where arteries are close to the skin. Pressing the artery against the bone can limit the flow of blood to the injury. This technique should be used only as a last resort when direct pressure and elevation have failed to stop bleeding.

Knowing where to apply pressure to stop bleeding is critical (see Figure A.2). For serious wounds, seek medical attention immediately.

Internal Bleeding   Although internal bleeding may not be immediately obvious, you should be aware of the following signs and symptoms:

- Symptoms of shock (discussed later in this appendix)
- Coughing up or vomiting blood
- Blood in urine
- Black, tarlike stools
- Abdominal discomfort or pain (rigidity or spasms).

In some cases, a person who has suffered an injury (such as a blow to the head, chest, or abdomen) that does not cause external bleeding may experience internal bleeding.

If you suspect that someone is suffering from internal bleeding, follow these steps:

1. Have the person lie on a flat surface with knees bent.
2. Keep the victim warm. Cover the person with a blanket, if possible.
3. Do *not* give the victim any medications or fluids.
4. Send someone to call for emergency medical help immediately.

Nosebleeds   To control a nosebleed, follow these steps:

1. Have the victim sit down and lean slightly forward to prevent blood from running into the throat. The person's nose should be pinched firmly closed using the thumb and forefinger. Keep the nose pinched for at least 5 minutes.
2. While the nose is held closed, apply a cold compress to the surrounding area.
3. If pinching does not work, gently pack the nostril with gauze or a clean strip of cloth. Do not use absorbent cotton, which will stick. Be sure that the ends of the gauze or cloth hang out so that it can be easily removed later. Once the nose is packed with gauze, pinch it closed again for another 5 minutes.
4. If the bleeding persists, seek medical attention.

Treatment for Burns

Minor Burns   For minor burns caused by fire or scalding water, apply running cold water or cold compresses for 20 to 30 minutes. Never put butter, grease, salt water, aloe vera, or topical burn ointments or sprays on burned skin. If the burned area is dirty, gently wash it with soap and water and blot it dry with a sterile dressing.

Major Burns   For major burn injuries, call for help immediately. Wrap the victim in a dry sheet. Do not clean the burns or try to remove any clothing attached to burned skin. Remove jewelry near the burned skin immediately, if possible. Keep the victim lying down and calm.

Chemical Burns   Remove clothing surrounding the burn. Wash skin that thas been burned by chemicals by flushing with water for at least 20 minutes. Seek medical assistance as soon as possible.

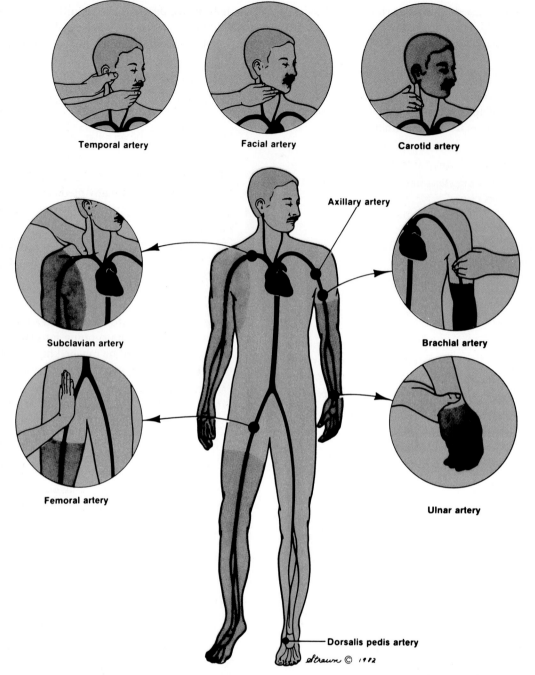

Figure A.2 Pressure points. This figure shows the points at which pressure can be applied to stop bleeding. Unless absolutely necessary, you should avoid applying pressure to the carotid arteries, which supply blood to the brain. Also, *never* apply pressure to both carotid arteries at the same time.

Shock

Shock is a condition in which the cardiovascular system fails to provide sufficient blood circulation to all parts of the body. Victims of shock display the following symptoms:

- Dilated pupils
- Cool, moist skin
- Weak, rapid pulse

- Vomiting
- Delayed or unrelated responses to questions.

All injuries result in some degree of shock. Therefore, treatment for shock should be given after every major injury. The following are basic steps for treating shock:

1. Have the victim lie flat with his or her feet elevated approximately 6 to 10 inches. (In the case of chest

injuries, difficulty breathing, or severe pain, the victim's head should be slightly elevated.)

2. Keep the victim warm. If possible, wrap him or her in blankets or other material. Also, keep the victim calm and reassured.

3. Seek medical help.

Electrical Shock

Do not touch a victim of electrical shock until the power source has been turned off. Approach the scene carefully, avoiding any live wires or electrical power lines. Pay attention to the following steps:

1. If the victim is holding on to the live electrical wire, do not remove it unless the power has been shut off at the plug, circuit breaker, or fuse box.

2. Check the victim's breathing and pulse. Electrical current can paralyze the nerves and muscles that control breathing and heartbeat. If necessary, give mouth-to-mouth resuscitation. If there is no pulse, CPR might be necessary. (Remember that only trained people should perform CPR.)

3. Keep the victim warm and treat for shock. Once the person is breathing and stable, seek medical help or send someone else for help.

Poisoning

Of the 1 million cases of poisoning reported in the United States each year, about 75 percent occur in children under age 5, and most are caused by household products. Most cases of poisoning involving adults are attempted suicides or attempted murders.

You should have emergency telephone numbers for the poison control center and the local EMS ready. Many people keep these numbers on labels on their telephones. The National Safety Council recommends that you be prepared to give the following information when calling for help:

- What was ingested? Have the container of the product and the remaining contents ready so you can describe it. You should also bring the container to the emergency room with you.
- When was the substance taken?
- How much was taken?
- Has vomiting occurred? If the person has vomited, save a sample to take to the hospital.
- Are there any other symptoms?
- How long will it take to get to the nearest emergency room?

When caring for a person who has ingested a poison, keep these basic principles in mind:

1. Maintain an open airway. Make sure the person is breathing.

2. Call the local poison control center. Follow their advice for neutralizing the agent.

3. If the poison control center or another medical authority advises inducing vomiting, then do so. In general, if the victim has ingested poison within the previous 3 to 4 hours, you should induce vomiting to empty the stomach. However, never induce vomiting if the person is unresponsive, unconscious, or has swallowed acids or alkalies (such as drain and toilet cleaners, ammonia, lye, or oven cleaners) or petroleum products (such as floor polish, gasoline, lighter fluid, or paint thinner).

4. For most other ingested poisons (cosmetics, ink, rat poison, medicines, or illicit drugs), use syrup of Ipecac to induce vomiting. The recommended dose for an adult is 2 tablespoons with two or three glasses of water. For a child over the age of 1 year, the dose is 1 tablespoon with one or two glasses of water. If vomiting does not occur within 20 minutes, the dose should be repeated. Do not give more than two doses. If you do not have syrup of Ipecac, do not use other techniques or home remedies to induce vomiting. Transport the victim to the nearest health facility.

Injuries of Joints, Muscles, and Bones

Sprains   Sprains result when ligaments and other tissues around a joint are stretched or torn. The following steps should be taken to treat sprains:

1. Elevate the injured joint to a comfortable position.

2. Apply an ice pack or cold compress to reduce pain and swelling.

3. Wrap the joint firmly with a (roller) bandage.

4. Check the fingers or toes periodically to ensure that blood circulation has not been obstructed. If the bandage is too tight, loosen it.

5. Keep the injured area elevated, and continue ice treatment for 24 hours.

6. Apply heat to the injury after 48 hours if there is no further swelling.

7. If pain and swelling continue or if a fracture is suspected, seek medical attention.

Fractures   Any deformity of an injured body part usually signals a fracture. A fracture is any break in a bone, including chips, cracks, splinters, and complete breaks. Minor fractures (such as hairline cracks) might be difficult to detect and might be confused with sprains. Whenever there is any doubt, treat the injury as a fracture until X rays have been taken.

Do not move the victim if a fracture of the neck or

back is suspected because this could result in a spinal cord injury. If the victim must be moved, splints should be applied to immobilize the fracture, to prevent further damage, and to decrease pain. Following are some basic steps for treating fractures and applying splints to broken limbs:

1. If the person is bleeding, apply direct pressure above the site of the wound.

2. If a broken bone is exposed, do not try to push it back into the wound. This can cause contamination and further injury.

3. Do not try to straighten out a broken limb. Splint the limb as it lies.

4. The following materials are needed for splinting:
   • Splint: wooden board, pillow, magazine, or newspaper
   • Padding: towels, blankets, socks, or cloth
   • Ties: cloth, rope, or tape.

5. Place splints and padding above and below the joint. Never put padding directly over the break. Padding should protect bony areas and the soft tissue of the limb.

6. Tie splints and padding into place.

7. Check the tightness of the splints periodically. Pay attention to the skin color, temperature, and pulse below the fracture to make sure the blood flow is adequate.

8. Elevate the fracture, and apply ice packs to prevent swelling and reduce pain.

Head Injuries

A head injury can result from an auto accident, a fall, an assault, or a blow from a blunt object. All head injuries can potentially lead to brain damage, which may result in a cessation of breathing and pulse.

For minor head injuries:

1. For a minor bump on the head resulting in a bruise without bleeding, apply ice to decrease the swelling.

2. If there is bleeding, apply even, moderate pressure. Because there is always the danger that the skull may be fractured, excessive pressure should not be exerted.

3. Observe the victim for a change in consciousness. Observe the size of pupils and note signs of inability to think clearly. Assess for any signs of numbness or paralysis. Allow the victim to sleep, but wake him or her periodically to check for awareness.

For severe head injuries:

1. If the victim is unconscious, check the airway for breathing. If necessary, perform mouth-to-mouth resuscitation.

2. If the victim is breathing, check the pulse. If it is less than 55 or more than 125 beats per minute, the victim may be in danger.

3. Check for bleeding. If fluid is flowing from the ears or nose, do not stop it.

4. Do not remove any objects imbedded in the person's skull.

5. Cover the victim with blankets to maintain body temperature, but guard against overheating.

6. Seek medical help as soon as possible.

Temperature-Related Emergencies

Frostbite Frostbite is damage to body tissues caused by intense cold. Frostbite generally occurs at temperatures below 32°F. The body parts most likely to suffer frostbite are the toes, ears, fingers, nose, and cheeks. When skin is exposed to the cold, ice crystals form beneath the skin. Avoid rubbing frostbitten tissue, because the ice crystals can scrape and break blood vessels.

To treat frostbite, follow these steps:

1. Bring the victim to a place of treatment as soon as possible.

2. Cover and protect the frostbitten area. If possible, apply a steady source of external warmth, such as a warm compress. The victim should avoid walking if the feet are frostbitten.

3. If the victim cannot be transported, you must rewarm the body part by immersing it in warm water (100°F to 105°F). Continue to rewarm until the part is warm to the touch when removed from the bath. Do not allow the body part to touch the sides or bottom of the container. After rewarming, dry gently and wrap in bandages to protect from refreezing.

Hypothermia Hypothermia is a temperature-related emergency that can be prevented with proper precautions. Hypothermia is a condition of generalized cooling of the body resulting from exposure to cold temperatures or immersion in cold water. It can occur at any temperature below 65°F and can be made more severe by wind chill and moisture. The following are key symptoms of hypothermia:

• Shivering
• Vague, slow, slurred speech
• Poor judgment
• Lethargy, or extreme exhaustion
• Slowed breathing and heartbeat
• Numbness and loss of feeling in extremities.

You should take the following steps to provide first aid to a victim of hypothermia:

1. Replace any wet clothing. Make sure the person is warmed evenly, using whatever sources of heat are available (blankets, heating pads, or hot water bottles). If possible, give the victim a warm bath. The temperature of the fluids or the heating sources should not exceed 110°F (43°C).

2. Give the victim hot drinks. Do not give the victim alcohol or caffeinated beverages, and do not allow the victim to smoke.

3. Do not allow the victim to exercise.

Heat-Related Emergencies

Temperature-related problems common in the summer months include heatstroke, heat exhaustion, and heat cramps. These conditions result from prolonged exertion or exposure to high temperatures and humidity.

Heatstroke   Heatstroke, the most serious heat-related disorder, results from the failure of the brain's heat-regulating mechanism (the hypothalamus) to cool the body. The signs and symptoms of heatstroke are as follows:

- Rapid pulse
- Hot, dry, flushed skin (absence of sweating)
- Disorientation leading to unconsciousness
- High body temperature

As soon as these symptoms are noticed, the body temperature should be reduced as quickly as possible. The victim should be immersed in a cool bath, lake, or stream. If there is no water nearby, a fan should be used to help lower the victim's body temperature.

Heat Exhaustion   Heat exhaustion results from excessive loss of salt and water. The onset is gradual, with the following symptoms:

- Gradual fatigue and weakness
- Anxiety
- Nausea
- Profuse sweating
- Clammy skin
- Normal body temperature.

To treat heat exhaustion, get the victim out of the sun. Have the victim lie down flat or with feet elevated. Replace lost fluids slowly and steadily.

Heat Cramps   Heat cramps result from excessive sweating, resulting in an excessive loss of salt and water.

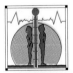

Promoting Your Health

Plan of Action for Positive Health Change

An important part of any behavior change strategy is to make a realistic assessment of what your risks are and begin to plan a step-by-step approach to improve. Answering the following questions and carefully considering your responses may provide the basis for a solid beginning for your own personal behavior change.

1. Based on the information presented in this chapter, what would you say are your most important health risks?
   a.
   b.
   c.
   d.

2. Of these risks, which ones would it be possible for you to change?
   a.
   b.
   c.
   d.

3. Which ONE risk do you think is the one that you need to act on NOW?
   _____
   _____

4. What things are you currently doing, or what resources are available to help you change?

5. What factors will make it difficult for you to change?

6. List the names of people who can help you change. What will you ask them to do?

7. What is your goal for next month at this time? Next year?

8. Outline the steps that you will need to take . . . . starting now.

Although heat cramps are the least serious heat-related emergency, they are the most painful. The symptoms include muscle cramps, usually starting in the arms and legs. To relieve symptoms, the victim should drink electrolyte-rich beverages or a light saltwater solution or eat salty foods.

First-Aid Supplies

Every home, car, or boat should be supplied with a basic first-aid kit. In order to respond effectively to emergencies, you must have the basic equipment. This kit should be stored in a convenient place, but it should be kept out of the reach of children. Following is a list of supplies that should be included:

- Bandages, including triangular bandages (36 inches by 36 inches), butterfly bandages, a roller bandage, rolled white gauze bandages (2- and 3-inch widths), adhesive bandages
- Sterile gauze pads and absorbent pads

- Adhesive tape (2- and 3-inch widths)
- Cotton-tip applicators
- Scissors
- Thermometer
- Antibiotic ointments
- Syrup of Ipecac (to induce vomiting)
- Aspirin
- Calamine lotion
- Antiseptic cream or petroleum jelly
- Safety pins
- Tweezers
- Flashlight
- Paper cups
- Blanket.

You cannot be prepared for every medical emergency. However, these essential tools and a knowledge of basic first aid will help you cope with many emergency situations.

Index

The **boldface** pages refer to tables; the *italicized* pages refer to figures.

starvation, 142
Dietary calcium, 318
Dietary chaos syndrome (bulimia), 142, 143
Dietary Goals for the United States, 115
Dieter's Dilemma, The, 153
Diethylstilbesterol (DES), 104
Diet pills, *231*
Digestion-related disorders, 301–3
Digestive system, 117–18, *119*
Dilation and curettage (D & C), 107, 301
Dilation and evacuation (D & E), 107
Dioxin, 349–50
Disaccharides, 121
Discrimination, 44
Disease(s), 271–308. *See also* Acquired immune deficiency syndrome (AIDS); Heart disease
  autoimmune, 283
  body defense mechanisms against, 273, 281–84
  chronic, 5–6
  course of, 282
  factors contributing to, 272–74
  iatrogenic, 274
  immunization schedules for common, **284**
  noninfectious, 296–308, **307**
    bone and joint diseases, 303–5
    chronic fatigue syndrome, 306
    common female disorders, 300–301
    digestion-related disorders, 301–3
    neurological disorders, 299–300
    respiratory disorders, 296–99
    sudden infant death syndrome (SIDS), 217, 306–8
  pathogens, 274–81
    bacteria, 275–76
    fungi, 281
    parasitic worms, 281
    protozoa, 281
    rickettsia, 281
    viruses, 276–80
  sexually transmitted (STDs), 284–91
    candidiasis (moniliasis), 281, 290
    characteristics of, 285
    chlamydia, 285–86
    condom use and, 96–98
    general urinary tract infections (UTIs), 291
    gonorrhea, 286
    herpes, 290–91
    mode of transmission of, 285
    possible causes of, 285
    pubic lice (crabs), 291
    spermicides and, 99
    syphilis, 286–87
    trichomoniasis, 281, 291
    venereal warts, 287–90
Disease model of addiction, 194
Distillation, 202
Distress, 38. *See also* Stress
  assessing, 51
  managing reactions to, 49–59
  recognition and assessment of, 49

Distressors, 44–45
Disulfiram (Antabuse), 212, 226
Diuretics, 232
Diverticulosis, 124, 302
Divorce, 68–69
  parenthood and, 86
  by sex and age, **67**
Divorce litigation, 66
DNA probe, 288
Down's syndrome, 89, 90
Drug profile, 225
Drugs, 222–46. *See also* Addiction; Alcohol; Tobacco
  actions of, 223
  alternatives to, 227
  antidepressant, 31
  caffeine and caffeinism, *231*, 232–33
  categories of, 224
  defined, 223
  disease and, 274
  fertility, 110
  gateway, 191, 194, 220
  generic, 230
  hypersensitivity to, 225
  illicit, 224, 233–46
    deliriants, 242–43
    depressants, 238–41
    designer drugs, 243
    inhalants and solvents, 243, 259
    lure of, 233–34
    marijuana, 191, 194, 237–38, 239, 244
    psychedelics, 241–42
    stimulants, 235–37
    use in the U.S., 243–46
  interactions of, 226
    with alcohol, **202**
  intravenous, HIV transmission and, 293
  labeling of, 228, 231
  over-the-counter, 224, 230–32, *231*
  pregnancy and, 88
  prescription, 224, 228–30
  psychoactive, 225–26
  recreational, 224
  routes of administration of, 226–28
  sexuality and, 79
  stress and, 57
  teratogenic effects of, 88, **88**
  use and abuse of, 25–27, 224–26
Drug therapy for alcoholism, 1, 212
Dumps, 347
Duodenum, 118
Dyathanasia, 332
Dyes, 259
Dynamic muscular contractions, 176
Dysfunction, sexual, 79–80
Dysfunctional family, 196–97
  intimacy and, 62
Dyspareunia, 80
Dysphoria, 242
Dysplasia, 289

Eating. *See also* Diet(s); Nutrition; Weight management
  changing eating behavior, 156–59
  compulsive, 191–92
  "Eating right pyramid," 126–27, 137

Eccentric muscular contractions, 176, 178
Economic status, Type A behavior and, 43
Ecstasy (drug), 243
Ectopic pregnancy, 95
Education about drugs, 244–45
Egg sacs, 72
Ego, 18
Ejaculation, 74
  premature, 80
Ejaculatory duct, 74
Elderly, 311–15. *See also* Aging
  abuse of, 313, 314
  disorders common to, 313–15
  impact on society, 312–13
  osteoporosis among, 318
  profile of today's, 311–12
  suicide among, 27, *28*
  vegetarianism and, 131
Electrical shock, first aid for, 361
Electricity, conserving, 342
Electrocardiogram (ECG), 256
Electroconvulsive therapy (ECT), 31–32
Electrodesiccation, 264
Electroencephalogram (EEG), 320–21
Eliot, Robert S., 253
ELISA test, 294
Embolism, *255*
Embolus, 255
Embryo, 91
Embryo freezing, 110
Embryo transfer, 110
Emergency care. *See* First aid and emergency care
Emotional attachment, 60
Emotional availability, 61
Emotional development, 62
Emotionality, 20
Emotional responses to stress, 51–52
Emotional stress, cardiovascular disease and, 252
Emotional well-being, 16–36
  achieving, 21–24
    communication and, 24
    problem solving and decision making, 23–24
    self-esteem development and maintenance, 21–22
    understanding and expressing emotions, 22–23
  adaptations to problems, unsound, 24–28
    defense mechanisms, 25, **27**
    drug abuse, 25–27
    suicide, 27–28
  foundations of, 17–18
  mental illness, 28–33
    anxiety disorders, 29–30, 31
    depression, 6, 30–33, 93, 259
    manic-depressive mood disorder, 32
    obsessive-compulsive disorders, 29
    schizophrenia, 33
    seasonal affective disorder (SAD), 32–33

CREDITS

Figure 1.4 From *Changing Health Behavior* by D. Girdano and D. Dusek. Copyright © 1988 by Gorsuch Scarisbrick Publishers, Scottsdale, AZ. Reprinted with permission.

Table 2.1 From *The Life Cycle Completed, A Review,* by Erik H. Erikson, by permission of W. W. Norton & Company, Inc. Copyright © 1982 by Rikan Enterprises Ltd.

Figure 2.2 National Center for Health Statistics.

Chapter 4 Box "Learning to Relax" and Figures 3.2, 3.3, and 3.7 adapted from Girdano/Everly/Dusek, *Controlling Stress and Tension: A Holistic Approach,* 3rd ed. Copyright © 1990, pp. 12, 35, 214, 220–21. Reprinted by permission of Prentice-Hall, Inc., Englewood Cliffs, NJ.

Figures 4.1, 4.2, 4.4, 4.5 From J. Geer, J. Heiman, and H. Leitenberg, *Human Sexuality* (Englewood Cliffs, NJ: Prentice Hall, 1984), pp. 30, 31, 35, 41, 45, 46. Reprinted by permission of Prentice-Hall, Inc.

Figures 5.2, 5.4, 5.5, 5.6, 5.7, 5.8, 5.9 From J. Geer, J. Heiman, and H. Leitenberg, *Human Sexuality* (Englewood Cliffs, NJ: Prentice Hall, 1984), pp. 111, 130, 132, 136, 138, 142. Reprinted by permission of Prentice-Hall, Inc.

Chapter 5 Box "Choosing a Method of Birth Control" from *Contraceptive Technology 1988–1989* by R. A. Hatcher, G. Guest, F. Stewart, G. K. Stewart, J. Trussell, S. C. Bowen, W. Cates. Reprinted with permission of the authors.

Figure 10.1 From *The Addictive Personality* by Craig Nakken, C.C.D.P., M.S.W. Copyright © 1988 by Hazelden Foundation, Center City, MN. Reprinted by permission.

Figure 10.2 Adapted from *Concepts of Chemical Dependency* by H. E. Doweiko. Copyright © 1990 by Wadsworth, Inc. Adapted by permission of Brooks/Cole Publishing Company, Pacific Grove, CA 93950.

Figure 10.4 The Graham model of addiction is used by permission of Cheryl A. Graham, M.S.C.H.E.S.

Chapter 12 Bayer ad courtesy Drug Enforcement Administration.

Chapter 12 Comtrex label courtesy Bristol-Myers.

Figure 11.4 From *The American Medical Association Encyclopedia of Medicine,* edited by Charles B. Blayman. Reprinted by permission of Random House, Inc.

Table 11.5 Copyright © 1988 by Mike Samuels, M.D. and Nancy Samuels. Reprinted by permission of Summit Books, a division of Simon & Schuster, Inc.

Chapter 11 Box "Do You Have a Problem with Alcohol?" adapted by Cheryl Graham of Oregon State University from an instrument developed at Arizona State University, with permission.

Table 11.2 Reprinted with permission of Macmillan Publishing Company from *Drugs and the Human Body,* 2nd ed. by Ken Liska. Copyright © 1986 by Ken Liska.

Figure 11.1 Copyright © 1989, Center for Science in the Public Interest.

Table 11.3 Oakley Ray and Charles Ksir, *Drugs, Society & Human Behavior,* 5th ed. St. Louis, 1990, Times Mirror/Mosby College Publishing.

Chapter 6 Box "The Cholesterol/Saturated Fat Index." Copyright © 1986 by Sonja L. Connor, M.S., R.D., and William E. Connor, M.D. Reprinted by permission of Simon & Schuster, Inc.

Figure 6.2 From Barrett/Abramoff/Kumaran/Millington, *Biology,* © 1986, p. 266. Prentice Hall, Englewood Cliffs, NJ.

Figure 6.3 From *The Barbara Kraus Sodium Guide to Brand Names and Basic Foods* by Margaret Markham. Copyright © 1983 by Margaret Markham and Margaret Ternes. Reprinted by arrangement with NAL Penguin, Inc., New York, NY.

Figure 6.5 Copyright © 1988, CSPI. Reprinted from *Nutrition Action Healthletter,* 1875 Connecticut Ave. N.W., Suite 300, Washington, DC 20009-5728.

Tables 6.4 and 6.6 Adapted from *Jane Brody's Nutrition Book* by Jane Brody, by permission of W. W. Norton & Company, Inc. Copyright © 1982 by Jane E. Brody. Reprinted by permission of the Wendy Weil Agency, Inc.

Figure 7.2 Courtesy Year Book Medical Publishers.

Chapter 7 Garfield cartoon by Jim Davis reprinted by permission of UFS, Inc.

Figure 13.1 Reproduced with permission from "1990 Heart and Stroke Facts." Copyright © 1989 American Heart Association.

Figure 13.3 Adapted from American Heart Association, *1987 Heart Facts,* p. 19. Reproduced with permission.

Table 16.1 Reprinted by permission of *The Wall Street Journal.* © 1990 Dow Jones & Company, Inc. All rights reserved worldwide.

Chapter 13 Box "What to Do in the Event of a Heart Attack" reproduced with permission from "1991 Heart and Stroke Facts." Copyright © 1990 American Heart Association.

Figure 13.4 Courtesy of the American Cancer Society, Inc.

Figure 13.5 Copyright © 1982. Wyeth Laboratories. All rights reserved.

Figure 13.7 Courtesy of the American Cancer Society, Inc.

Figure 14.3 Reprinted with permission of Macmillan Publishing Company, a Division of Macmillan, Inc. from *Epidemiology: Man and Disease* by John P. Fox, Carrie Hall & Lila R. Elveback. Copyright © 1970 by Macmillan Publishing Company.

Chapter 14 Box "Exercise-Induced Asthma." Copyright © Feb. 20, 1989, *U.S. News & World Report.*

Chapter 15 Poem "Warning" by Jenny Joseph in *Rose in the Afternoon,* published by J. M. Dent & Sons. Copyright © 1974 by Jenny Joseph.

Chapter 15 Cartoon "The Far Side" by Gary Larson. © 1986 Universal Press Syndicate.

Figure 15.1 Adapted from Elisabeth Kübler-Ross, *Death: The Final Stage of Growth* (Englewood Cliffs, NJ: Prentice Hall, 1975). Reprinted by permission of Simon & Schuster, Inc.

Figure 15.2 Adapted from Clayton/Halikes/Maurice, "The Bereavement of the Widowed," *Diseases of the Nervous System* (1971), 32(9):597–604.

Figure 15.3 Cremation Association of North America.

Chapter 15 Box "The Dying Person's Bill of Rights." Copyright © 1975 by American Journal of Nursing Company, reproduced with permission from *American Journal of Nursing,* January 1975, Vol. 75, No. 1. Used with permission. All rights reserved.

Chapter 15 Cartoon "The Wizard of Id" by Brant Parker and Johnny Hart by permission of Johnny Hart and NAS, Inc.

Figure 15.4 Research by Francesca Bannerman. Reprinted from *In Health* Magazine. Copyright © 1988.

Chapter 15 Box "The Physician and the Right to Die" from *Current Opinions of the Council on Ethical and Judicial Affairs of the American Medical Association.* Copyright © 1986 by the American Medical Association.

Figure 16.1 Reprinted with permission of Macmillan Publishing Company from *Rain of Troubles: The Science and Politics of Acid Rain* by Laurence Pringle. Copyright © 1988 by Laurence Pringle.

Figure 16.3 From Patricia H. Hynes, *Earth Right,* 1990, p. 103. By permission of Prima Publishing and Communications.

Figure 16.4 Environmental Protection Agency.

Chapter 16 Box "Shopping Checklist for Environmentally Conscious Consumers" From Patricia H. Hynes, *Earth Right,* 1990, p. 59. By permission of Prima Publishing and Communications.

Figure A.2 From *First Responder: A Skills Approach,* 3rd ed. by Keith J. Karren and Brent Q. Hafen. Copyright © 1990 by Morton Publishing Company. Reprinted with permission.

Photographs

Chapter 1: *1* Ken Cooper/The Image Bank; *11* Bob Daemmrich/Stock, Boston

Chapter 2: *16* Laima Druskis; *18* Tom Hollyman/Photo Researcher; *22* Bob Daemmrich/Stock, Boston; *31* John Griffin/Image Works; *32* Ellis Herwig/Stock, Boston; *34* Rick Browne/Stock, Boston

Chapter 3: *37* Bob Daemmrich/Uniphoto; *40* Janeart/The Image Bank; *43* Jack Liu; *46* Gail Grieg/Monkmeyer Press; *47* United Nations; *52* Mike Greenlar/The Image Works; *53* Jack Liu; *58* Grant Leduc/Monkmeyer Press